Handbook of
Neonatal Clinical Practices

Handbook of Neonatal Clinical Practices

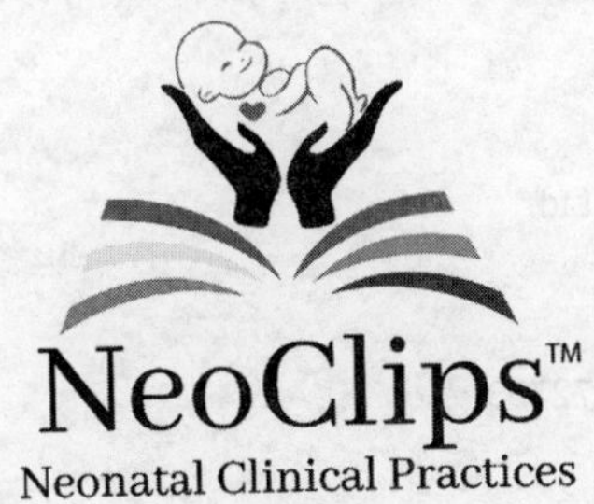

Editor

Ravi Sachan MD MBA FNNF
Fellowship in Clinical Neonatology
Associate Professor
Neonatal Division
Department of Pediatrics
University College of Medical Sciences and
Guru Teg Bahadur Hospital
New Delhi, India

Co-Editor

Kumar Ankur MD DNB (Neonatology)
Associate Director and Head
Department of Neonatology
BLK-Max Super Specialty Hospital
New Delhi, India

Foreword

Piyush Gupta

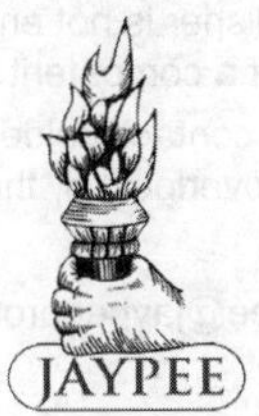

JAYPEE BROTHERS MEDICAL PUBLISHERS
The Health Sciences Publisher

New Delhi | London

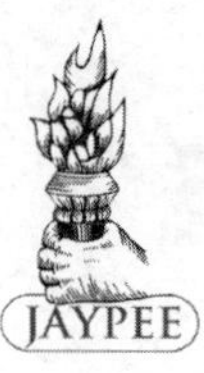 **Jaypee Brothers Medical Publishers (P) Ltd**

Headquarters

Jaypee Brothers Medical Publishers (P) Ltd
EMCA House, 23/23-B
Ansari Road, Daryaganj
New Delhi 110 002, India
Landline: +91-11-23272143, +91-11-23272703
+91-11-23282021, +91-11-23245672
Email: jaypee@jaypeebrothers.com

Corporate Office

Jaypee Brothers Medical Publishers (P) Ltd
4838/24, Ansari Road, Daryaganj
New Delhi 110 002, India
Phone: +91-11-43574357
Fax: +91-11-43574314
Email: jaypee@jaypeebrothers.com

Overseas Office

JP Medical Ltd
83 Victoria Street, London
SW1H 0HW (UK)
Phone: +44 20 3170 8910
Fax: +44 (0)20 3008 6180
Email: info@jpmedpub.com

Website: www.jaypeebrothers.com
Website: www.jaypeedigital.com

Inquiries for bulk sales may be solicited at: jaypee@jaypeebrothers.com

Handbook of Neonatal Clinical Practices

First Edition: **2023**

ISBN: 978-93-5465-911-9

Printed at: Rajkamal Electric Press, Kundli, Haryana.

Reviewers

Alok Bhandari FIAP FNNF
Secretary NNF, 2017-2018
National Joint Secretary IAP 2022-2023

Amit Upadhyay MD DNB DM (Neonatology)
Director
Neutema Hospital
Meerut, Utter Pradesh, India

Arti Maria DM (Neonatology)
Professor and Head
Department of Neonatology
Atal Bihari Vajpayee Institute of Medical Sciences
and Ram Manohar Lohia Hospital
New Delhi, India

Ashish Jain DM (Neonatology)
Associate Professor
Department of Neonatology
Maulana Azad Medical College
New Delhi, India

Avneet Kaur MD
Consultant Neonatologist and In-Charge NICU
Apollo Cradlle
New Delhi, India

Dinesh Tomar MD (Pediatrics)
Consultant
Department of Pediatrics
Aastha Hospital
Rohtak, Haryana, India

Girish Gupta (Retd) NM VSM DM
Head, Department of Neonatology
Himalayan Institute of Medical Sciences
Dehradun, Uttarakhand, India

Jagjit Singh Dalal MD DM (Neonatology)
Senior Professor and Head
Department of Neonatology
Pandit Bhagwat Dayal Sharma
Post Graduate Institute of Medical Sciences
Rohtak, Haryana, India

Lalan Bharti MD FIAP FNNF
Head
Department of Pediatrics
Jag Pravesh Chandra Hospital
Government of Delhi
New Delhi, India

Manoj Modi MBBS MD DNB
Senior Consultant
Department of Neonatology
Sir Ganga Ram Hospital
New Delhi, India

Pankaj Paul DCH
Owner
Dr Ravi Paul Children Hospital
Jalandhar, Punjab, India

Poonam Sidana
MD (Pediatrics) Neonatology Fellowship (Australia)
Director Neonatology and Pediatrics
CK Birla Hospital
New Delhi, India

Pradeep Debata MD DM
Professor
Vardhman Mahavir Medical College and
Safdarjung Hospital
New Delhi, India

Pradeep Suryawanshi
MD DCH FNNF FRCPCH Fellowship in Neonatology (Australia)
Professor and Head
Department of Neonatology
BVU Medical College, Pune
Head
Department of Pediatrics and Neonatology
Sahyadri Hospital
Department of Pediatrics
BLDE University, Vijapur

Ravindra Kumar MD (Pediatrics)
In-Charge
Neonatal Division
Hindu Rao Hospital
New Delhi, India

Sanjay Wazir MD DM
Medical Director
Neonatology and Pediatrics
Mother Hood Hospital
Gurugram, Haryana, India

Sourabh Dutta MD DM
Professor
Department of Neonatology
Postgraduate Institute of Medical
Education and Research
Chandigarh, India

Somashekhar Nimbalkar MD
Head
Department of Neonatology
Bhaikaka University
Anand, Gujarat, India

Sunil Duta Sharma MD DCH
Professor
Department of Pediatrics
Government Medical College
Jammu, Jammu and Kashmir, India

Surender Singh Bisht MD DNB
Senior Consultant and In-Charge NICU
Department of Pediatrics
Swami Dayanand Hospital
New Delhi, India

Sushil Srivastava MD
Professor
Department of Pediatrics
University College of Medical Sciences and
Guru Teg Bahadur Hospital
New Delhi, India

Sushma Nangia MD DM
Director Professor and Head
Department of Neonatology
Lady Harding Medical Collage
New Delhi, India

Utkarsh Sharma MD (Pediatrics)
Professor and Head
Department of Pediatrics and Neonatology
Shri Guru Ram Rai Institute of Medical and
Health Sciences
Dehradun, Uttarakhand, India

VC Manoj MD DM
Professor and Head
Department of Neonatology
Jubilee Mission Medical College
Thrissur, Kerala, India

Vikram Datta MD
Director Professor
Department of Neonatology
Lady Hardinge Medical College
New Delhi, India

Vinay Kumar Rai
MBBS MD (Pediatric) DNB (Neonatology)
Consultant
Department of Neonatology
Manipal Hospital
New Delhi, India

Aaradhana Singh MD (Pediatrics)
Associate Professor
Department of Pediatrics
University College of Medical Sciences
and Guru Teg Bahadur Hospital
New Delhi, India

Aashish Sethi
MD (Pediatrics) Fellowship in Pediatric Endocrinology
Assistant Professor
Department of Pediatrics
SGRR Institute of Medical and Health Sciences
Dehradun, Uttarakhand, India

Aheed Khan DNB (Pediatrics)
Senior Registrar
Department of Pediatrics
Apollo Cradle Royale Children's Hospital
New Delhi, India

Amanpreet Sethi DM (Neonatology)
Assistant Professor
Department of Neonatology
Guru Gobind Singh Medical College
Faridkot, Punjab, India

Amarnath Saran MD Fellowship in Neonatology
Associate Consultant
Department of Neonatology
Motherland Hospital
Noida, Utter Pradesh, India

Amit Yadav MBBS MD Fellowship in Neonatology
Consultant
East Delhi Advance NICU
New Delhi, India

Anantika Garg MD
Senior Resident
Department of Pediatrics
University College of Medical Sciences and Guru
Teg Bahadur Hospital
New Delhi, India

Anil Batra DNB (Neonatology)
Senior Consultant
Department of Neonatology
Madhukar Rainbow Children Hospital
New Delhi, India

Anita Singh MD DNB (Neonatology)
Additional Professor
Department of Neonatology
Sanjay Gandhi Postgraduate Institute
of Medical Sciences
Lucknow, Uttar Pradesh, India

Anita Yadav MD (Pediatrics)
Associate Professor
Department of Pediatrics
Vardhman Mahavir Medical College and
Safdarjung Hospital
New Delhi, India

Ankit Gupta MD (Pediatrics)
MTI Neonatal Clinical Fellow
John Radcliffe Hospital
Oxford University Hospitals NHS Trust
Headley Way, Oxford, UK

Anu Sachdeva DM (Neonatology)
Associate Professor
Department of Pediatrics
All India Institute of Medical Sciences
New Delhi, India

Anunaya Katiyar Fellow Pediatrics Nephrology
Consultant
Department of Pediatric Nephrologist
Indraprastha Apollo Hospitals
New Delhi, India

Anup Thakur MD (Pediatrics) DNB (Neonatology)
Senior Consultant and Associate Professor
(GRIPMER)
Department of Neonatology
Institute of Child Health
Sir Ganga Ram Hospital
New Delhi, India

Anuradha Bansal MD MRCPCH
Associate Professor
Department of Pediatrics
Punjab Institute of Medical Sciences
Jalandhar, Punjab, India

Aparna Prasad MD
Senior Consultant
BLK-Max Super Specialty Hospital
New Delhi, India

Arti Uniyal Postgraduate MD (Pediatrics)
Department of Pediatrics
University College of Medical Sciences and Guru
Teg Bahadur Hospital
New Delhi, India

Arun Gautam MD (Pediatrics)/PDCC (Neonatology)
Associated Consultant
Department of Neonatology
Medanta Hospital
Lucknow, Uttar Pradesh, India

Arvind Kant Manipal
DCH Fellowship in NICU (NNF)
Associate Consultant
Department of Pediatrics and Neonatology
CK Birla Hospital
New Delhi, India

Ashish Jain DM (Neonatology)
Associate Professor
Department of Neonatology
Maulana Azad Medical College
New Delhi, India

Ashok C DNB (Neonatology)
Associate Professor
Department of Neonatology
SRM Medical College Hospital
and Research Centre
Chengalpattu, Tamil Nadu, India

Athira Thilakan BSc Nursing
Staff Nurse
Neonatal Intensive Care Unit
Fortis La-Femme Hospital
New Delhi, India

Atif Majit
Starship Children Hospital
Auckland, New Zealand

Avadhesh Ahuja Fellowship in Neonatology
Consultant Neonatology
Fortis La-Femme Hospital
New Delhi, India

Bhavya Kukreja Fellow NNF
Associate Consultant
Department of Neonatology
Max Superspecialty Hospital
New Delhi, India

Bikrant Bihari Lal MD PDCC DM
Associate Professor
Department of Pediatric Hepatology
and Liver Transplantation
Institute of Liver and Biliary Sciences
New Delhi, India

Boby Varghese GNM
Nursing Officer
Department of Pediatrics
Guru Teg Bahadur Hospital
New Delhi, India

Chanchal MD MRCOG FICOG
Lead Consultant, Fetal Medicine
Madhukar Rainbow Children's Hospital and
Birth Right by Rainbow Hospitals
New Delhi, India

Chinmay Chetan DM (Neonatology)
Assistant Professor
Department of Neonatology
Himalayan Institute of Medical Sciences
Dehradun, Uttarakhand, India

Deepika Kainth MD DM (Neonatology)
Research Consultant
All India Institute of Medical Sciences
New Delhi, India

Deepika Rustogi
MD Fellowship in Neonatal-Perinatal Medicine
Senior Consultant
Department of Neonatology
Yashoda Superspeciality Hospital
Ghaziabad, Uttar Pradesh, India

Enboklang Suting MD (Pediatrics)
Pediatrician
Department of Pediatrics
Ganesh Das Government Maternal and
Child Health Hospital
Shillong, Meghalaya, India

Garima Saxena MD
NNF Senior Fellow
Fortis Hospitals
Noida, Uttar Pradesh, India

Gaurav Jawa MD
Senior Consultant
Department of Neonatology
Apollo Cradle Royale
New Delhi, India

Gunjan Srivastava DCH DNB
Senior Resident
Department of Pediatrics
Guru Teg Bahadur Hospital
New Delhi, India

Gurleen Sikka RCPCH Fellowship in Neonatology
Consultant
Department of Pediatrics and Neonatology
CK Birla Hospital
New Delhi, India

Jay Kishore DNB (Neonatology)
Senior Consultant
Department of Neonatology and Pediatrics
Cloudnine Hospital
New Delhi, India

Jubilant James
NNF Nursing Fellowship-2021 (Gold Medalist)
Nursing Officer
Neonatal Intensive Care Unit
All India Institute of Medical Sciences
New Delhi, India

Kalathingal Thaslima Aboobacker MD
Assistant Professor
Department of Neonatology
Lokmanya Tilak Municipal Medical College and
General Hospital
Mumbai, Maharashtra, India

Kamal Arora MD DM (Neonatology)
Professor
Division of Neonatology
Department of Pediatrics
Dayanand Medical Collage
Ludhiana, Punjab, India

Kaushaki Shankar DM (Neonatology)
Consultant and In-charge
Department of Neonatology
Max Super Specialty Hospital
New Delhi, India

Kiran More MD FRACP AFRACMA
Neonatal Senior Consultant and Head
Department of Neonatology
BJ Wadia and NJ Wadia Hospital
Mumbai, Maharashtra, India

Kritika Famra MD (Pediatrics)
Neonatology Fellow (NNF)
Neonatal Intensive Care Unit
Cloudnine Hospital
Bengaluru, Karnataka, India

Kumar Ankur MD DNB (Neonatology)
Associate Director and Head
Department of Neonatology
BLK-Max Super Specialty Hospital
New Delhi, India

Kunal P Ahya MD (Pediatrics) Fellow in Neonatology
Director and Consultant Neonatologist
MAAHI Newborn Care Centre
Rajkot, Gujarat, India

Kunal S Chawla MBBS DCH DNB (Pediatrics)
Consultant Pediatrician
Kiddy Care Clinic
Ulhasnagar, Maharashtra, India

Lovish Gupta MD (Pediatrics)
Senior Fellow
Department of Neonatology
Fortis Hospital
Noida, Uttar Pradesh, India

Mahendra Jain DM (Neonatology)
Associate Professor
Department of Neonatology
All India Institute of Medical Sciences
Bhopal, Madhya Pradesh, India

Malvika Haldwani MD (Pediatrics)
Senior Resident
Department of Pediatrics
University College of Medical Sciences and Guru
Teg Bahadur Hospital
New Delhi, India

Mamta Jajoo DNB FNNF
Professor and NICU In-charge
Department of Pediatrics
Chacha Nehru Bal Chikitsalaya
New Delhi, India

Manan Parikh Fellowship in Neonatology
Director Neonatologist
Neonatal Intensive Care Unit
Lotus Hospital for Newborn and Children
Vadodara, Gujarat, India

Manish Diwedi
Consultant Neonatologist
Medanta Hospital
Lucknow, Uttar Pradesh, India

Manisha Garg MD DM (Neonatology)
Consultant
Jaswant Rai Specialty Hospital
Meerut, Uttar Pradesh, India

Mayank Priyadarshi DM (Neonatology)
Assistant Professor
Department of Neonatology
All India Institute of Medical Sciences
Rishikesh, Uttarakhand, India

Meena Joshi BSc (Nursing)
Department of Neonatology
All India Institute of Medical Sciences
New Delhi, India

Mrinal Sinha MD
Senior Resident
Department of Pediatrics
University College of Medical Sciences and Guru
Teg Bahadur Hospital
New Delhi, India

Mudita Arora
DrNB (Neonatology) Fellow Neonatology
Sir Ganga Ram Hospital
New Delhi, India

Murugesan A DM
Assistant Professor
Department of Neonatology
Jawaharlal Institute of Postgraduate Medical
Education and Research
Puducherry, India

Naveen Parkash Gupta DNB (Neonatology)
Senior Consultant
Department of Neonatology
Madhukar Rainbow Children Hospital
New Delhi, India

Neha Jain
Senior Resident
Department of Pediatrics
University College of Medical Sciences
and Guru Teg Bahadur Hospital
New Delhi, India

Nidhi Jain DM (Neonatology)
Consultant
Department of Neonatology
Sitaram Bhartia Institute of Science and
Research
New Delhi, India

Pinky Meena
PDCC Pediatric and Adolescent Endocrinology
Assistant Professor
Department of Pediatrics
All India Institute of Medical Sciences
Rajkot, Gujarat, India

Pratima Anand DM (Neonatology)
Consultant Neonatology
Department of Pediatrics
Vardhman Mahavir Medical College and
Safdarjung Hospital
New Delhi, India

Preetha Joshi Fellowship in Pediatric Cardiac and
Neonatal Critical Care, Australia and Canada
Lead Consultant
Kokilaben Dhirubhai Ambani Hospital
Mumbai, Maharashtra, India

Prince Pareek DM (Neonatology)
Consultant Neonatologist
Department of Pediatrics
ESIC Medical College and Hospital
Faridabad, Haryana, India

Purvi Patel MD (Pediatrics)
Associate Professor
Department of Pediatrics
Pramukhswami Medical College
Karamsad, Gujarat, India

Rachit Mehta DCH FICCM
Neonatal Intensive Care
Kokilaben Dhirubhai Ambani Hospital
Mumbai, Maharashtra, India

Raktima Chakrabarti
MD (Pediatrics) Fellowship Neonatology (Germany)
Senior Consultant
Department of Pediatrics and Neonatology
Miracle Apollo Cradle Spectra Hospital
Gurugram, Haryana, India

Ramesh Choudhary MD (Pediatric Medicine)
Associate Professor
Department of Pediatric Medicine
Sawai Man Singh Medical College
Jaipur, Rajasthan, India

Ramji Bhardwaj MBBS DCH Fellow Neonatology
Consultant
Department of Pediatrics and Neonatology
East Delhi Advance NICU
New Delhi, India

Rashi Gupta DM (Neonatology Resident)
3rd Year DM Resident
Department of Neonatology
Atal Bihari Vajpayee Institute of Medical Sciences
and Ram Manohar Lohia Hospital
New Delhi, India

Ravi Sachan
MD MBA FNNF Fellowship in Clinical Neonatology
Associate Professor
Neonatal Division
Department of Pediatrics
University College of Medical Sciences and Guru
Teg Bahadur Hospital
New Delhi, India

Ravinder Yadav MD (Pediatrics) FNNF FACEE
Pediatrics Consultant
Aastha Hospital and IVF Centre
New Delhi, India

Rema S Nagpal
MD (Pediatrics) IAP Fellowship Neonatology
Associate Professor
Department of Pediatrics
BJ Medical College and Sassoon General
Hospital
Pune, Maharashtra, India

Richa Malik Fellow NNF
Consultant
Department of Neonatology and Pediatrics
Neonest Hospital
New Delhi, India

Ronak Patel Fellowship in Neonatal Medicine
Chief Neonatologist
NeoKids Children Hospital
Palanpur, Gujarat, India

Sachin Garg
MD (Pediatrics) Fellowship in Clinical Neonatology
Consultant
Shashikant Super Specialty Hospital
New Delhi, India

Sana Ibad Khan MD (Pediatric) FNNF
Senior Resident
Department of Pediatrics
Guru Teg Bahadur Hospital
New Delhi, India

Sanjeev Chetry DNB (Neonatology)
Senior Consultant and In-Charge
Neonatal Intensive Care Unit
Fortis Hospital
Noida, Uttar Pradesh, India

Sankalp Dudeja DM (Neonatology)
Consultant
Department of Neonatology
Amrita Hospital
Faridabad, Haryana, India

Saraswati Kini MD
Senior Resident
Chacha Nehru Bal Chikitsalaya
New Delhi, India

Sarvani Sattiraju
PG Resident
Department of Pediatrics
University College of Medical Sciences and Guru
Teg Bahadur Hospital
New Delhi, India

Seema Rai MBBS MD (Pediatrics)
Associate Professor
Department of Pediatrics
Guru Gobind Singh Medical College
Faridkot, Punjab, India

Shikha Handa
MD (Pediatrics) Fellow Neonatology (NNF)
Associate Consultant
Department of Pediatrics
Cloudnine Hospital
Faridabad, Haryana, India

Shilpa Kalane DrNB (Neonatology)
Chief Consultant Neonatology
Division of Neonatology
Department of Pediatrics
Deenanath Mangeshkar Hospital
Pune, Maharashtra, India

Shriyan Ashvij
MD (Pediatrics) Fellowship in Neonatology
Consultant Neonatologist
AJ Hospital and Research Center
Mangaluru, Karnataka, India

Sidharth Nayyar DrNB (Neonatology)
Chief Neonatologist
Cloudnine Hospital
Faridabad, Haryana, India

Smita Ramachandran
MD (Pediatrics) Fellowship in Pediatric and Adolescent
Endocrinology (FIPAE)
Consultant Pediatric and Adolescent
Endocrinologist
Department of Pediatrics
Venkateshwar Hospitals
New Delhi, India

Smriti Saryan MD
PG Resident
Department of Pediatrics
Guru Teg Bahadur Hospital
New Delhi, India

Somalika Pal DM (Neonatology)
Consultant
Department of Neonatology and Pediatrics
Cloudnine Hospital
New Delhi, India

Somosri Ray DM (Neonatology)
Assistant Professor
Department of Neonatology
Medical College
Kolkata, West Bengal, India

Sonali Verma
Fellowship Pediatric and Adolescent Endocrinology
Senior Resident
Department of Pediatric Endocrinology
Sanjay Gandhi Postgraduate Institute
of Medical Sciences
Lucknow, Uttar Pradesh, India

Sonia Thomas MSc Nursing (Pediatrics)
Nursing Officer
Neonatal Intensive Care Unit
Department of Pediatrics
Guru Teg Bahadur Hospital
New Delhi, India

Souradip Banik
MD Fellowship in Neonatology
BLK-Max Super Specialty Hospital
New Delhi, India

Sreedhara MS DM (Neonatology)
Consultant Neonatologist
Rainbow Children's Hospital
Bengaluru, Karnataka, India

Srishti Goel
DM (Neonatology) Gold Medalist
Consultant
Department of Neonatologist
Lifeline and Kidney Hospital
Jalandhar, Punjab, India

Sujoy Neogi DNB Pediatric Surgery
Associate Professor
Department of Pediatric Surgery
Maulana Azad Medical College
New Delhi, India

Sukena Susnerwala DM Neonatology
Assistant Professor
Lokmanya Tilak Medical College and
General Hospital
New Delhi, India

Suprabha Patnaik
Fellowship (Neonatology)
Associate Professor (Neonatology)
Bharati Vidyapeeth (Deemed to be University)
Medical College
Pune, Maharashtra, India

Susanta Kumar Badatya DNB (Neonatology)
Consultant Neonatologist
Department of Neonatology
Apollo Cradle
New Delhi, India

Swati Bhayana
MBBS MD FNB (Pediatric Hematology and Oncology)
Senior Resident
Department of PHO and BMT Unit I
Sir Ganga Ram Hospital
New Delhi, India

Swati Jangra PG
Resident
Department of Pediatrics
University College of Medical Sciences
and Guru Teg Bahadur Hospital
New Delhi, India

Swati Manerkar MD
Professor and Head
Department of Neonatology
Lokmanya Tilak Municipal Medical College
and General Hospital
Mumbai, Maharashtra, India

Swati Upadhyay
MD (Pediatrics) DNB (Neonatology)
Consultant and Head
Department of Neonatology
Max Super Specialty Hospital
New Delhi, India

Sweta Kumari MD (Pediatrics)
Assistant Professor
Department of Pediatrics
University College of Medical Sciences and
Guru Teg Bahadur Hospital
New Delhi, India

Tanushree Joshi Bahuguna MD (Pediatrics)
Senior DMO and Head
Department of Pediatrics
Northern Railway Central Hospital
New Delhi, India

Tapas Bandyopadhyay DM (Neonatology)
Associate Professor
Department of Neonatology
Atal Bihari Vajpayee Institute of Medical Sciences
and Ram Manohar Lohia Hospital
New Delhi, India

Tejo Pratap DM (Neonatology)
Head
Department of Neonatology
Fernandez Hospital
Hyderabad, Telangana, India

Utkarsh Sharma
MD (Pediatrics and Neonatology)
Professor and Head
Department of Pediatrics and Neonatology
SGRR Institute of Medical and Health Sciences
Dehradun, Uttarakhand, India

Varun Vij
MD (Pediatrics) Fellowship in Neonatology
Senior Consultant Neonatologist
Department of Pediatrics
Max Smart Super Specialty Hospital
New Delhi, India

Vikram Bedi MD Fellowship Neonatology
Head Level III
Neonatal Intensive Care Unit
Bedi Hospital
Chandigarh, India

Vikrant Sood DM (Pediatric Hepatology)
Associate Professor
Department of Pediatric Hepatology and Liver
Transplantation
Institute of Liver and Biliary Sciences
New Delhi, India

Vinay Joshi
DM (Neonatology) Fellowship PICU and Cardiac ICU Canada
Consultant
Department of NICU, PICU and Cardiac ICU
Cloudnine Hospital
Wadia Hospital
Mumbai, Maharashtra, India

Vishal Gupta DrNB (Neonatology)
Consultant
Department of Neonatology
Delhi Newborn Centre
New Delhi, India

Vishal Kaushik MD (Pediatrics)
Assistant Professor
Department of Pediatrics
Government Doon Medical College and
Doon Hospital
Dehradun, Uttarakhand, India

Vivek Choudhury DNB (Neonatology)
Senior Consultant
Department of Neonatology and Pediatrics
Apollo Cradle
New Delhi, India

Neonatology has evolved tremendously over the last decades. There is great need for the residents and neonatal healthcare providers to understand the basic approach to the diagnosis and management of common neonatal problems. Apart from understanding clinical approach, students need guidance on presenting neonatal case and understanding the necessary investigation and outline preliminary management.

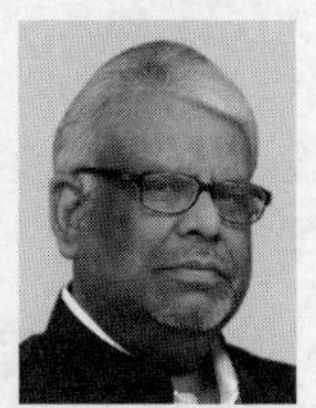

I am very happy to know that the first edition of the *Handbook of Neonatal Clinical Practices* is being released, and this will add to the overall knowledge and practice of every neonatal healthcare provider. This book is an attempt to gather the most practical aspect of the neonatology in a comprehensive and simplified manner.

I congratulate the Editor, Dr Ravi Sachan, and the Co-Editor, Dr Kumar Ankur as well as all the esteemed authors who have contributed to this handbook.

I am sure this handbook will serve as an import source of knowledge to clinicians and academicians alike as well as residents and students and will stimulate a holistic interest in the subject.

Piyush Gupta MD FIAP FNNF FAMS
Principal
University College of Medical Sciences
Delhi University, New Delhi, India
President
Indian Academy of Pediatrics, 2021

It gives us great pleasure to bring to you the first edition of *Handbook of Neonatal Clinical Practices*. This is an earnest, humble and hard-working attempt to bring the latest knowledge in the field of neonatal care. Neonatal Clinical Practices (Neo-Clips), which is based on treatment flow with the aim of guiding decision in the diagnosis and management of common neonatal diseases. This algorithmic approach will of immense benefit of all the neonatal healthcare providers at all levels of healthcare facility. The book has many sections and each section focuses on the clinical approach on a specific neonatal condition highlighting the points to be covered in history and clinical examination.

We thank Professor Anju Aggrawal, Head, Department of Pediatrics, University College of Medical Sciences and Guru Teg Bahadur Hospital, New Delhi, India, for her support and encouragement. We thankful to all the authors and reviewers, who have done a marvelous job in the time available. Our sincere thanks to them Ms Chetna Malhotra (Senior Director—Professional Publishing, Marketing and Business Development), and Ms Saima Rashid (Development Editor), have allowed us remarkable latitude in our writing and submission schedules.

We thank Dr Aradhana (W/O Dr Ravi Sachan) and Dr Sweta Rani (W/O Dr Kumar Ankur) and children have been supportive with us during the preparation of the book. The readers are the ultimate judges of the contents of all they read, will hopefully like this latest offering from us and hopefully some of the content will benefit their patients. This is the first edition, and we will be happy to rectify any unintentional and unknown errors in the book. Please let us know your thoughts, critical comments, and suggestions to drravisachangtbh@gmail.com

Ravi Sachan
Kumar Ankur

Contents

Neurological and Renal Disease

Hepatic and Hematological Disease

Section 3 Supportive Management

Neonatal Infection

Neonatal Nutrition

Section 4 Diagnostic Management

Section 8　National Health Program

Section 9　Annexures

17-OHP:	17-hydroxyprogesterone
A/REDF:	Absent or reversed end diastolic flow
AA:	Arachidonic acid
AaDO$_2$:	Alveolar-arterial oxygen difference
AAP:	American Academy of Pediatrics
ABG:	Arterial blood gas
AC:	Abdominal circumference
ACD:	Alveolar capillary dysplasia
ACE:	Angiotensin-converting enzyme
ACT:	Activated clotting time
ADHD:	Attention deficit hyperactivity disorder
AED:	Antiepileptic drug
AFB:	Acid-fast bacilli
AFV:	Amniotic fluid volume
AL:	Argininosuccinate lyase
AP:	Anteroposterior
APH:	Antepartum hemorrhage
ART:	Antiretroviral therapy
AS:	Argininosuccinate synthetase
ASA:	Argininosuccinic acid
ATT:	Antitubercular treatment
AXR:	Abdominal X-ray
BASD:	Bile acid synthesis defect
BCG:	Bacillus Calmette-Guérin
BF:	Breastfeeding
BMV:	Bag-mask ventilation
BPD:	Bronchopulmonary dysplasia
BPM:	Beats per minute
CAC:	Comprehensive abortion care

CAH:	Congenital adrenal hyperplasia
CBC:	Complete blood count
CBNAAT:	Cartridge-based nucleic acid amplification test
CCHD:	Cyanotic congenital heart disease
CCTV:	Closed circuit television
CDC:	Choledochal cyst
CDH:	Congenital diaphragmatic hernia
CHC:	Community health center
CHD:	Congenital heart disease
CMV:	Cytomegalovirus
CNS:	Central nervous system
CO:	Cardiac output
CPAP:	Continuous positive airway pressure
CPK-MB:	Creatine phosphokinase-MB
CPS:	Carbamoyl phosphate synthetase
CRP:	C-reactive protein
CRT:	Capillary refill time
CSF:	Cerebrospinal fluid
CT:	Computed tomography
CTVS:	Cardiothoracic vascular surgery
CVS:	Cardiovascular system
CXR:	Chest X-ray
DBF:	Direct breastfeeding
DBS:	Dried blood spot
DCC:	Delayed cord clamping
DDH:	Developmental dysplasia of the hip
DH:	District hospital
DHA:	Docosahexaenoic acid
DHEAS:	Dehydroepiandrosterone sulfate
DHT:	Dihydrotestosterone
DIC:	Disseminated intravascular coagulation
DORV:	Double outlet right ventricle
DOTS:	Directly observed treatment-short course
DR:	Delivery rooms
DRCPAP:	Derived nasal continuous positive airway pressure
DSD:	Differences of sex development

EBM:	Expressed breast milk
ECMO:	Extracorporeal membrane oxygenation
EEG:	Electroencephalogram
EISF:	Early initiation of breastfeeding
ELISA:	Enzyme-linked immunosorbent assay
ETT:	Endotracheal tube
FAO:	Fatty acid oxidation defects
FBM:	Fetal breathing movements
FFP:	Fresh frozen plasma
FGR:	Fetal growth restriction
FiO$_2$:	Fraction of inspired oxygen
FISH:	Fluorescence in situ hybridization
FM:	Fetal movements
FRC:	Functional residual capacity
FRU:	First referral unit
FSH:	Follicle stimulating hormone
FT:	Fetal tone
G6PD:	Glucose-6-phosphate dehydrogenase
GA:	Gestational age
GDM:	Gestational diabetes mellitus
H:	Hydrocephalus
HFI:	Hereditary fructose intolerance
HHHFNC:	Heated Humidified high flow nasal cannula therapy
HIV:	Human immunodeficiency virus
HR:	Heart rate
HRZ:	Isoniazid, rifampicin and pyrazinamide
HRZE:	Isoniazid, rifampicin, pyrazinamide, and ethambutol
HSD:	Hydroxysteroid dehydrogenase
HSV:	Herpes simplex virus
HWC:	Health and wellness center
IAP:	Indian academy of pediatrics
ICP:	Intracranial pressure
Ig:	Immunoglobulin
IgA:	Immunoglobulin A
IgG:	Immunoglobulin G
IGRA:	Interferon-gamma release assay

IHPS:	Idiopathic hypertrophic pyloric stenosis
IMV:	Invasive mechanical ventilation
INH:	Isoniazid
INO:	Inhaled nitric oxide
INSURE:	INtubation, SURfactant, Extubation
ITP:	Immune thrombocytopenia
IU:	International unit
IUGR:	Intrauterine growth restriction
IV:	Intravenous
IVF:	In vitro fertilization
IVH:	Intraventricular hemorrhage
IVRT:	Isovolumic relaxation time
KMC:	Kangaroo mother care
LA:Ao:	Left atrial to aortic root ratio
LBW:	Low birth weight
LFT:	Liver function test
LGA:	Large for gestational age
LH:	Luteinizing hormone
LISA:	Less invasive surfactant administration
LR:	Labor room
LSCS:	Lower segment cesarean section
LV:	Left ventricular
LVF:	Left ventricular failure
LVO:	Left ventricular output
MAP:	Mean airway pressure
MAS:	Meconium aspiration syndrome
MBP:	Mean blood pressure
MCT:	Medium-chain triacylglycerols
MDR:	Multidrug resistant
MDR TB:	Multidrug resistant tuberculosis
MIST:	Minimal invasive surfactant therapy
MLD:	Metabolic liver disease
MODS:	Multiple organ dysfunction syndrome
MOM:	Mother's own milk
MRI:	Magnetic resonance imaging
MSL:	Meconium-stained liquor

MTx:	Mantoux test
n-CPAP:	nasal continuous positive airway pressure
NAGS:	N-acetylglutamate synthetase
NAIT:	Neonatal alloimmune thrombocytopenia
NEC:	Necrotizing enterocolitis
NICCD:	Neonatal intrahepatic cholestasis caused by citrin deficiency
NICE:	National Institute for Health and Clinical Excellence
NICU:	Neonatal intensive care unit
NIMV:	Nasal Intermittent mandatory ventilation
NIPPV:	Noninvasive positive pressure ventilation
NNF:	National neonatology forum
NNPD:	National neonatal perinatal database
NRP:	Neonatal resuscitation program
NS:	Normal saline
NSAID:	Nonsteroidal anti-inflammatory drug
NST:	Nonstress test
OG/NG:	Orogastric/nasogastric
OR:	Operating room
OTC:	Ornithine transcarbamylase
PA:	Alveolar pressure
Pa:	Pulmonary arterial pressure
PAH:	Pulmonary arterial hypertension
PaO_2:	Partial pressure of oxygen in arterial blood
PCO_2:	Partial pressure of carbon dioxide
PCR:	Polymerase chain reaction
PCV:	Packed cell volume
PDA:	Patent ductus arteriosus
PDC:	Predelivery counseling
PDSA:	Plan-do-study-act
PEEP:	Positive end-expiratory pressure
PFA:	Platelet function analysis
PFIC:	Progressive familial intrahepatic cholestasis
PFO:	Patent foramen ovale
PF ratio:	PaO_2/FiO_2 ratio
PGE3:	Prostaglandin E3
PHC:	Primary health center

PICC:	Peripherally inserted central catheter
PIH:	Pregnancy-induced hypertension
PIP:	Peak inspiratory pressure
PMA:	Postmenstrual age
PNC:	Postnatal care
PPE:	Personal protective equipment
PPH:	Postpartum hemorrhage
PPHN:	Persistent pulmonary hypertension of the newborn
PPROM:	Premature rupture of membrane
PPV:	Positive pressure ventilation
PROM:	Prolonged rupture of membrane
PS:	Pressure support
PSARP:	Posterior sagittal anorectoplasty
PT:	Prothrombin time
PTT:	Partial thromboplastin time
PV:	Pulmonary venous pressure
PVR:	Pulmonary vascular resistance
Qp:Qs ratio:	Difference between systemic and pulmonary pressures
RAT:	Rapid antigen test
RDS:	Respiratory distress syndrome
RHD:	Rheumatic heart disease
RNTCP:	Revised national tuberculosis program
ROP:	Retinopathy of prematurity
RPM:	Rotation per minute
RR:	Respiratory rate
RT-PCR:	Reverse transcription-polymerase chain reaction
RV:	Right ventricular
RVF:	Right ventricular failure
SAM:	Severe acute malnutrition
SAS:	Silverman-Anderson score
SDH:	Subdistrict hospital
SIMV:	Synchronized intermittent mandatory ventilation
SLE:	Systemic lupus erythematosus
SNCU:	Special newborn care unit
SOP:	Standard operating protocol
SPAP:	Systolic pulmonary artery pressure

SpO_2:	Oxygen saturation
SSC:	Skin-to-skin contact
SSRI:	Selective serotonin reuptake inhibitor
TABC:	Temperature, airway, breathing, and circulation
TAPSE:	Tricuspid annular plane systolic excursion
TAPVC:	Total anomalous pulmonary venous connection
TB:	Tuberculosis
TEF:	Tracheoesophageal fistula
TFI:	Total fluid intake
TGA:	Transposition of the great arteries
Ti:	Inspiratory time
TMP:	Transmembrane pressure
TPN:	Total parenteral nutrition
TSH:	Thyroid stimulating hormone
TST:	Tuberculin sensitivity test
TTM:	Target temperature management
TTNB:	Transient tachypnea of the newborn
TV:	Tidal volume
UAC:	Umbilical arterial catheter
UAC:	Umbilical artery catheterization
UCHC:	Urban community health center
USG:	Ultrasonography
UTI:	Urinary tract infection
UVC:	Umbilical venous catheter
VACTERL:	Vertebral, anorectal, cardiac, tracheoesophageal, renal, and limb abnormalities
VBG:	Venous blood gas
VDRL:	Venereal disease research laboratory test
VILI:	Ventilator-induced lung injury
VKDB:	Vitamin K deficiency bleeding
VLBW:	Very low birth weight
VT:	Ventilator rate
VT:	Volume targeted
vWD:	von Willebrand disease
VZIG:	Varicella zoster immunoglobulin
WHO:	World health organization

Management of Neonatal Emergencies

Chapter 1

Neonatal Assessment and Triaging

Ravi Sachan

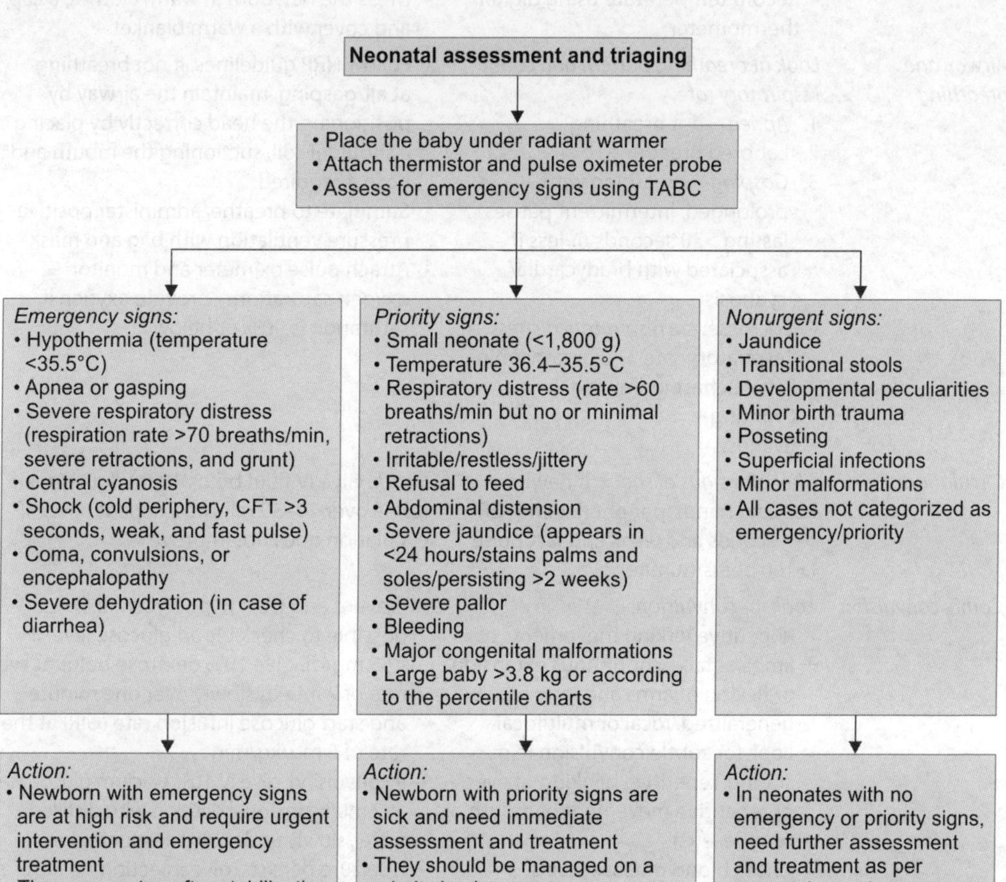

ASSESSMENT AND MANAGEMENT OF NEWBORN WITH EMERGENCY SIGNS

Emergency signs	Assessment	Management
Temperature	*Check for hypo/hyperthermia:* • Place under radiant warmer in servo control mode • Perform hand hygiene • Attach the thermistor probe to the skin over upper right side of the abdomen Or • Record temperature using digital thermometer	• Maintain temperature under radiant (if warmer not available, provide skin to skin contact) • Monitor axillary temperature every hour till it reaches 36.5°C—if hypothermic • *Prevent hypothermia:* Remove cold or wet clothing • Dress the newborn in warm clothes, a cap, and cover with a warm blanket
Airway and breathing	*Look at breathing pattern and count respiratory rate:* 1. *Apnea*—not breathing 2. Labored breathing 3. *Gasping*—breathing with prolonged, intermittent pauses lasting >20 seconds or less if associated with bradycardia/cyanosis *Check for severe respiratory distress:* • Respiratory rate >70 breaths/min • Severe chest indrawing • Grunting • Cyanosis	• Follow NRP guidelines. If not breathing at all/gasping, maintain the airway by positioning the head correctly by placing a shoulder roll, suctioning the mouth and nose if required • Stimulate to breathe, administer positive pressure ventilation with bag and mask • Attach pulse oximeter and monitor oxygen saturation—provide oxygen if saturation is 90% or below
Circulation	*Check for signs of shock:* If newborn has cold hands/peripheries with CRT >3 seconds and weak and fast pulse (>160 beats/minute)	*Shock:* Give IV fluid bolus 10 mL/kg normal saline over 20–30 minutes. Repeat bolus, if circulation does not improve
Coma, convulsion	*Look for convulsion:* • Repetitive jerking movements of limbs or face, continuous extension or flexion of arms and legs; may be generalized, focal or multifocal • Look for subtle convulsion (e.g., staring, repetitive blinking of eyes, or repetitive movement of mouth or tongue, etc.) • Check blood glucose levels • *Check for consciousness level:* Assess whether the baby is sleeping, lethargic or unconscious	• Prevent and treat hypoglycemia. If not possible to check blood glucose level if <45 mg/dL give 10% dextrose bolus at the rate of 2 mL/kg slowly over one minute and start glucose infusion rate (GIR) at the rate of 6 mg/kg/min • If convulsing, give IV 10% calcium gluconate at 2 mL/kg in equal dilution with distilled water, slowly under cardiac monitoring • If seizure persists, give injection phenobarbitone at a dose of 20 mg/kg (diluted with normal saline) slowly over 15–20 minutes
Dehydration/ diarrhea	• Assess signs of dehydration: weight loss, frequency of urine output, etc. • Look for lethargy, sunken eyes, and skin pinch (If history of diarrhea)	• Consider frequent breast feeding • Consider calculated expressed mother's own milk (MOM), If baby is lethargic • Consider IV fluid if newborn is unable to accept orally

ASSESSMENT AND MANAGEMENT OF NEWBORN WITH NONEMERGENCY SIGNS

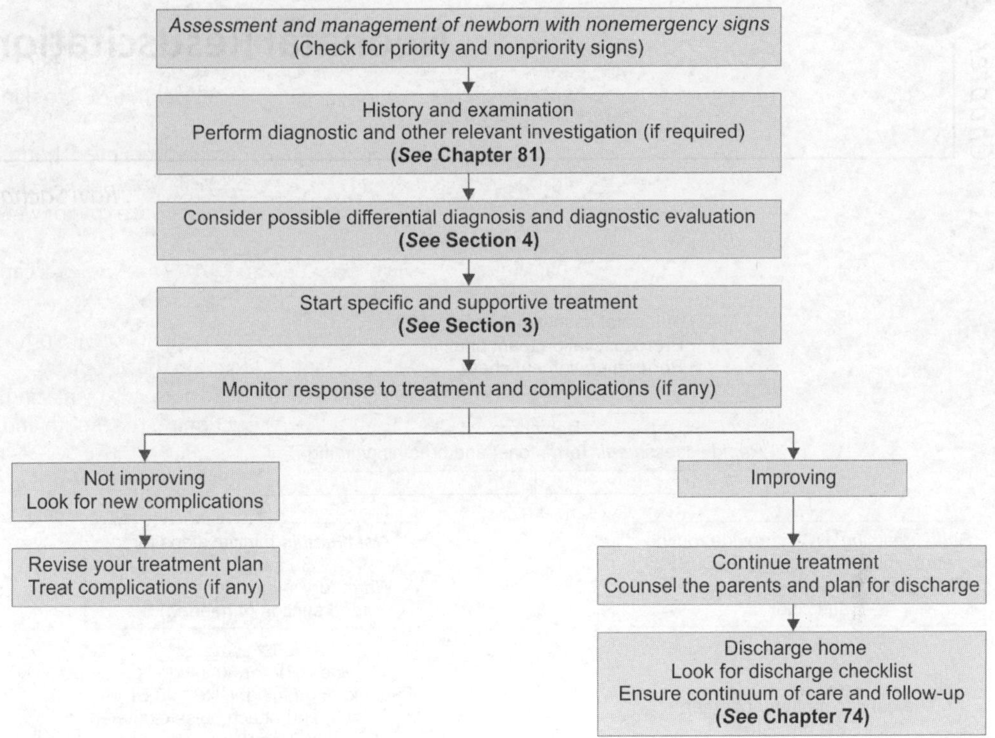

Key Points to Remember

- A sick newborn can present with one or more emergency signs.
- Always give priority to small and sick newborn during triage.
- Attend the neonate immediately as it brought to the facility.
- Maintain TABC, in addition to specific management.
- Maintain SpO_2 between 91 and 95%.
- Prevent and treat hypothermia and hypoglycemia.
- Consider referral after initial stabilization if adequate facility is not available. Administer prereferral dose of antibiotics and provide IV fluids or oxygen support as required during transport.
- Give injection vitamin K1 if not given earlier, around birth.
- If a newborn has surgical emergency (*See* Chapter 5), discuss with pediatric surgeon and follow surgical guidelines.

FURTHER READING

1. Facility based newborn care, training module for doctors & nurses. MOHFW, GOI. 2014.

Neonatal Resuscitation

Ravi Sachan

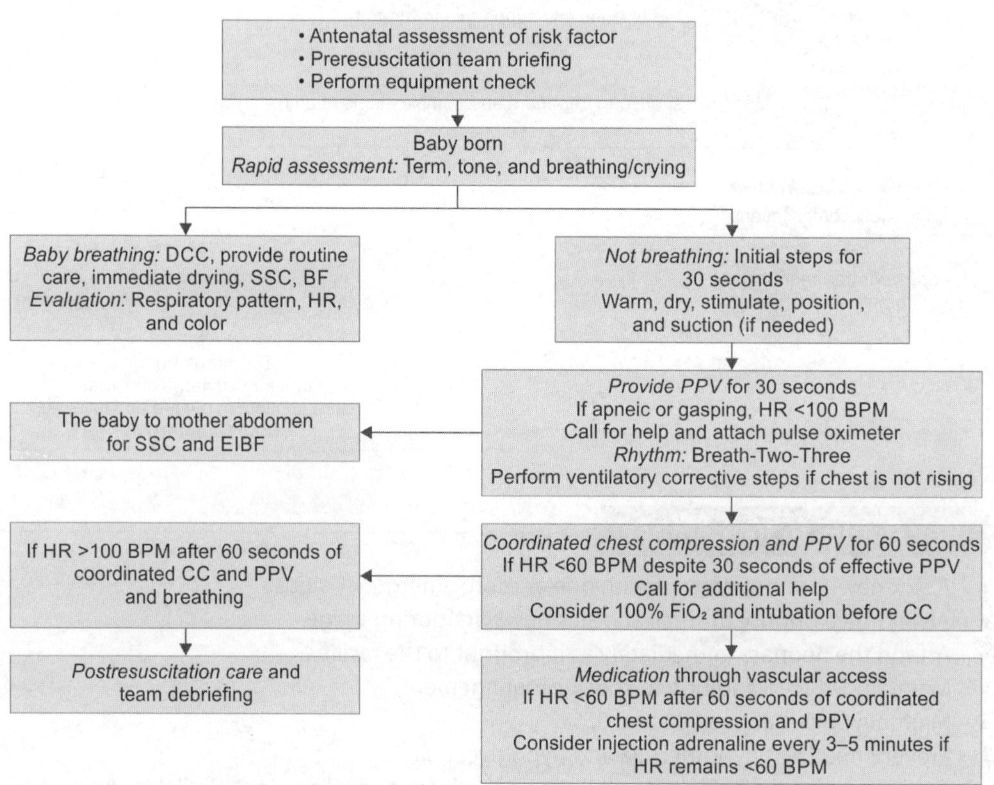

Simplified approach to neonatal resuscitation in the delivery room.

■ SPECIAL CONSIDERATION—RESUSCITATION OF PRETERM NEONATES

Issue with preterm neonate in the delivery room.

Problem	Contributing factors
Hypothermia	Less subcutaneous brown fat, thin skin, large surface area relative to body mass, and limited thermal response
Asphyxia	Poor respiratory drive, poor tone, and immature brain control
Breathing difficulty	Immature and surfactant deficient lungs, weak breathing muscles, and immature respiratory drive
Hypovolemia	Smaller blood volume loss, increases risk of hypovolemia
Hypoglycemia	Limited reserve and immature compensatory mechanism
Sepsis	Immature immune system

Preterm-specific resuscitation interventions.

Performance step	Intervention
Temperature	• Ensure room is draft free and warm (26–28°C) • Use plastic wrap and a thermal mattress (<32 weeks) • Use heated and humidified resuscitation gases (If available) • Record temperature at the end of resuscitation and on admission • Avoid hyperthermia (>38°C)
DCC	DCC for at least 30–60 seconds of birth
Initial steps	• No drying the baby (<32 weeks), all resuscitation is done with the plastic bag in situ • Place infant under preheated warmer. Cover the head with a cap • Place the baby in plastic bag/wrap, food grade immediately at birth
Respiratory support	• Consider using CPAP (PEEP of 5–7 cmH$_2$O) in spontaneously breathing baby with labored breathing or low oxygen saturation and has at least HR 100 BPM, by using T-piece/ short bi-nasal prong • If fails to initiate spontaneous breathing consider PPV via appropriate size face mask • Use of air oxygen blender (if available) and pulse oximeter for SpO$_2$ monitoring • Use 21–30% for <35 weeks with PPV
Drugs	• Avoid rapid infusions of fluid (slowly over 5–10 minutes) • If baby requires intubation for stabilization, consider giving surfactant in the DR
Handling	Handle gently to prevent neurological injury. Maintain head in neutral position
Transport	Rewarmed transport incubator with blended oxygen and a pulse oximeter after initial stabilization

Key Points to Remember

- At least one person who can initiate resuscitation should attend the delivery.
- If risk factors are present, at least two qualified person should be present. The number will be determined by the risk factors.
- Ask four key questions to obstetrician before birth:
  1. What is the expected gestational age?
  2. Is the amniotic fluid clear?
  3. Are there any additional risk factors?
  4. What is our umbilical cord management plan?
- Ventilation of the newborn's lungs is the single most important and most effective step in neonatal resuscitation.
- The most important indicator of successful PPV is a rising heart rate.
- Rhythm for PPV: *"Breathe-two-Three……"*
- Rhythm for CC and PPV: *"One*-and-*Two*-and-*Three*-and-*Breathe*-and……."
- Intubation is strongly recommended before chest compression.

OSCE/Checklist 1: Anticipation and preparation for birth.		
Name of the participant: _______________________________		
S. No.	*Performance steps*	*Yes*	*No*
1.	Assessment of perinatal risk factors		
2.	Assemble team based on risk factors		
3.	Preresuscitation team briefing		
4.	Hand washing		
5.	Check functionality of all equipment and supplies: Ensure that an equipment check has been done prior to every birth		
	Temperature:		
	Preheated warmer, prewarm towels or blankets, and cap		
	Thermal mattress, plastic bag, or plastic wrap (<32 weeks' gestation)		
	Airway:		
	Suction catheter/mucus aspirator		
	10 F or 12 F suction catheter attached to wall suction, set at 80–100 mm Hg		
	Auscultation:		
	Stethoscope		
	Ventilation:		
	Self-inflating bag (PPV device) with appropriate size mask (term and preterm)		
	5 F/6 F and 8F feeding tube and 20-mL syringe		
	Oxygen blender (21–30% if <35 weeks' gestation)		

Contd...

Contd...

S. No.	Performance steps	Yes	No
	T-piece resuscitator, flowmeter set to 10 L/min		
	Oxygenation:		
	Equipment to give free-flow oxygen		
	Pulse oximeter with sensor and target oxygen saturation table		
	Intubation:		
	Laryngoscope with size 0 and size 1 straight blades (size 00, optional)		
	Endotracheal tubes (sizes 2.5, 3.0, and 3.5)		
	Measuring tape and/or endotracheal tube insertion depth table		
	Scissors and tape for securing ET tube		
	Medication:		
	Injection adrenaline [1:10,000 (0.1 mg/mL)], normal saline		
	Supplies for emergency insertion of UVC and administering medications		
	Total score		

OSCE/Checklist 2: Birth and routine care.

Name of the participant: _______________________________

S. No.	Performance steps	Yes	No
1.	Call out the time of birth		
2.	Receive the baby in prewarm linen		
3.	Place the baby prone on mother's abdomen		
4.	Turn the head to one side		
5.	Clear the secretion- if present		
6.	Rapid Assessment of neonates, *if baby is breathing/crying—Yes*		
7.	Cover the baby with fresh prewarm linen and continue SSC		
8.	Ensure airway is open by positioning head and neck		
9.	Clamp and cut the cord after 1–3 minutes		
10.	Facilitates early initiation of breastfeeding		
11.	Check for breathing pattern (spontaneous and sustained), HR and color		
	Total score		

OSCE/Checklist 3: Birth and initial steps of resuscitation.

Name of the participant: _______________________________

S. No.	Performance steps	Yes	No
1.	Call out the time of birth		
2.	Receive the baby in prewarm linen		

Contd...

Contd...

S. No.	Performance steps		Yes	No
3.	Place the baby prone on mother's abdomen			
4.	Turn the head to one side			
5.	Clear the secretion, if present			
6.	Rapid assessment of neonates, *if baby is breathing/crying—No*			
7.	Immediately cut the cord and place the baby under radiant warmer			
8.	Dry the baby and remove the wet linen			
9.	Stimulate the baby by gently rubbing the back			
10.	Position the head and neck to open the airway			
11.	Clear airway by suctioning mouth and then nose—if needed			
12.	Assess the newborn's response to the initial steps—respiration and HR			
13.	Assess breathing pattern	Spontaneous and sustained: Yes		
		Apneic or gasping : Start PPV		
		Labored: Consider CPAP		
14.	Auscultates HR-	Above 100 BPM: Yes		
		Below 100 BPM: Start PPV		
15.	Check central cyanosis, if persisting, attach a pulse oximeter probe on right hand to confirm and provide free flow oxygen as per targeted oxygen saturation			
16.	If yes—Replace the baby over the mother's abdomen for observational care			
	Total score			

OSCE/Checklist 4: Positive pressure ventilation (PPV).				
Name of the participant: ______________________________________				

S. No.	Performance steps		Yes	No
1.	Indicate the need for PPV by assessing breathing and HR (apneic/gasping or HR below 100 BPM)			
2.	Call for additional help			
3.	Select the appropriate size mask and applies correctly			
4.	Start PPV with room air (GA ≥ 35 week) with proper rhythm			
5.	Request assistant to place pulse oximeter probe on right hand/wrist and adjust FiO_2 as per target saturation (if GA<35 weeks 21–30%)			
6.	Check HR -within 15 seconds of PPV	If HR increasing—continue PPV for 15 seconds		
		If HR is not increasing—look for the chest rise		
7.	Takes ventilation corrective steps, if chest is not rising			
8.	Mask adjustment			
9.	Reposition the head and neck			

Contd...

Contd...

S. No.	Performance steps		Yes	No
10.	Give 5 breath and look for chest rise, if chest is rising now continue PPV for 30 seconds. If not takes other corrective steps			
11.	Suction the mouth and nose			
12.	Open the mouth			
13.	Give 5 breath and look for chest rise, if chest is rising now continue PPV for 30 seconds. If not takes other corrective steps			
14.	Increase *Pressure* to squeeze the bag			
15.	Takes *Alternative* airway (perform intubation), if chest is not rising			
16.	Give 5 breath and look for chest rise, if chest is rising now continue PPV (with B & T Ventilation) for 30 seconds			
17.	Assess the HR after 30 seconds of effective PPV	Breathing: Spontaneous effort—Yes		
		HR: >100 BPM—Yes		
		HR: <60 BPM—start chest compression		
		Oxygenation: As per target saturation		
18.	If yes, gradually discontinue PPV			
19.	Plan postresuscitation care			
20.	Debrief the resuscitation team and communicate with parents			
		Total score		

OSCE/Checklist 5: Intubation, chest compression, and medication.

Name of the participant: ____

S. No.	Performance steps	Yes	No
1.	Indicate the need for chest compression by assessing breathing (no spontaneous respiratory effort) and HR (HR below 60 BPM), after 30 seconds of effective positive pressure ventilation		
2.	Call for additional help (may be needed for vascular access and medication)		
3.	Preferably intubate for better coordination with ventilation		
4.	Ask assistant to increase FiO_2 to 100%		
5.	Ask the assistant to place temperature sensor probe on body		
6.	Compressor moves to head end of the baby		
7.	Locate the area of compression and administer chest compression by two thumb technique		
8.	Compress sternum one third of the AP diameter of the chest		
9.	Ask one of the team member to prepare for umbilical venous catheterization		
10.	Continues coordinated chest compression with effective ventilation (3:1) for 60 seconds		
11.	Pause compression, continue PPV (higher rate 40–60), and check HR after 60 seconds		

Contd...

Contd...

S. No.	Performance steps		Yes	No
12.	Check breathing HR and oxygenation	If spontaneous breathing movement—Yes		
		If HR increasing >60 BPM—discontinue CC and continue PPV Plan postresuscitation care		
		If HR is not increasing <60 BPM, give medication		
13.	Administer injection adrenaline (0.2 mg/kg) followed by flushes (3 mL/kg) via UVC and announce the medication given			
14.	Continues coordinated chest compression with effective ventilation (3:1) for 60 seconds			
15.	Pause compression, continue PPV (higher rate 40–60), and check HR			
16.	If HR not increasing, administer injection adrenaline (0.2 mg/kg) every 3–5 minutes followed by flushes (3 mL/kg) via UVC and announce the medication given			
17.	Continues coordinated chest compression with effective ventilation (3:1) for 60 seconds			
18.	Administer volume expander NS (10 mL/kg) via UVC over 5–10 minutes			
19.	Check HR after every 60 seconds	Breathing : No spontaneous effort		
		HR: >60 BPM—stop chest compression and continue PPV		
20.	Plan postresuscitation care			
21.	Debrief the resuscitation team and communicate with parents			
		Total score		

Golden Hour Management

Ravi Sachan

- The "concept of golden hour" includes practicing all the evidence-based intervention for term and preterm neonates, in the first 60 minutes after birth for better long-term outcome
- Initial first hour of postnatal life includes neonatal resuscitation, postresuscitation care, transportation to neonatal intensive care unit, stabilization of cardiopulmonary system, and initial course in nursery

Term delivery with no significant antenatal risk factors

- Newborn cried immediately after birth
- Perform routine care as per NRP guideline

- In addition to the routine care, the following action need to performed in the labor room
- Care in the postnatal ward (please see in subsequent section)

- Significant antenatal history
- High-risk pregnancy
- Preterm delivery

- Inform the NICU team
- Discuss management plan with obstetrician and parents
- Preresuscitation team briefing

Resuscitation as per latest NRP guideline

Postresuscitation team debriefing
Parents counseling about newborn condition and plan of management

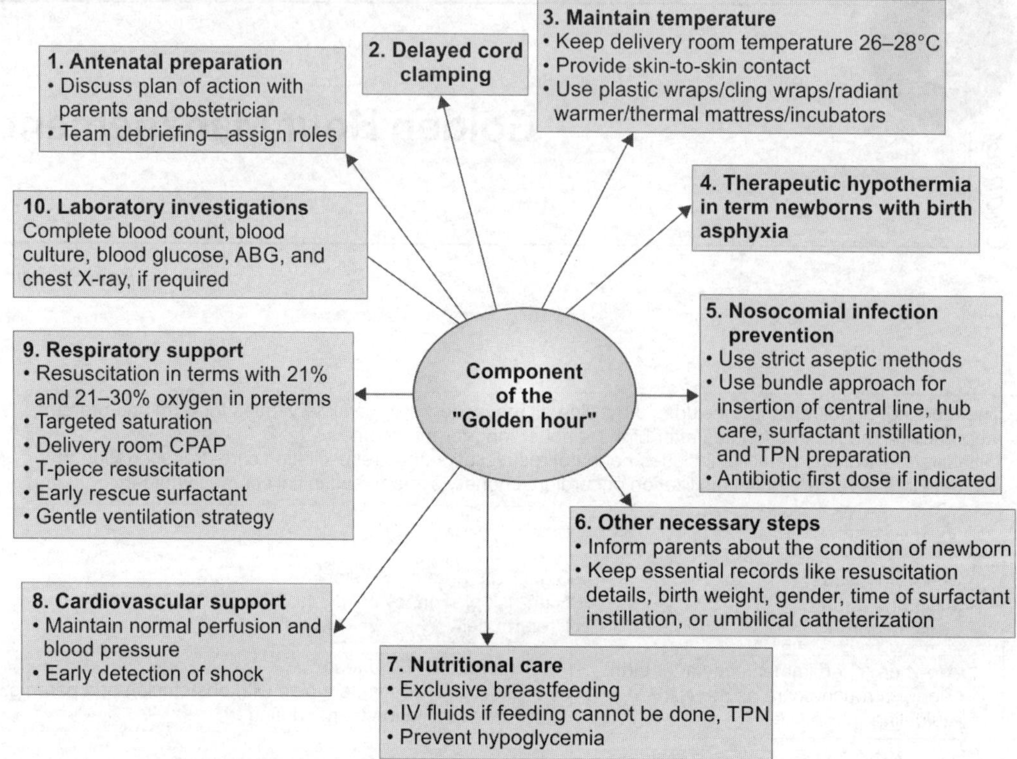

Golden hour interventions to be done at the time of birth.

Transitional Care from Delivery Room and Early Stabilization in NICU

Ravi Sachan

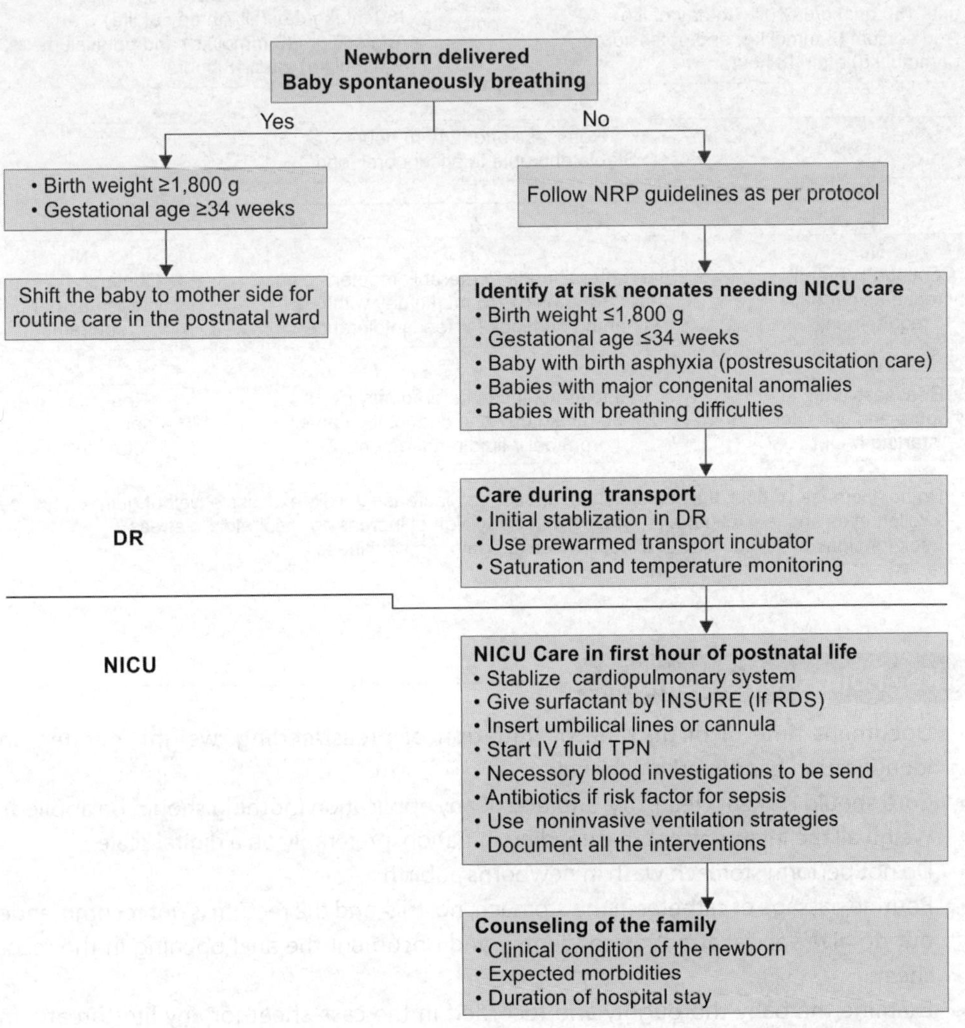

IV fluid therapy in newborn after initial stabilization.

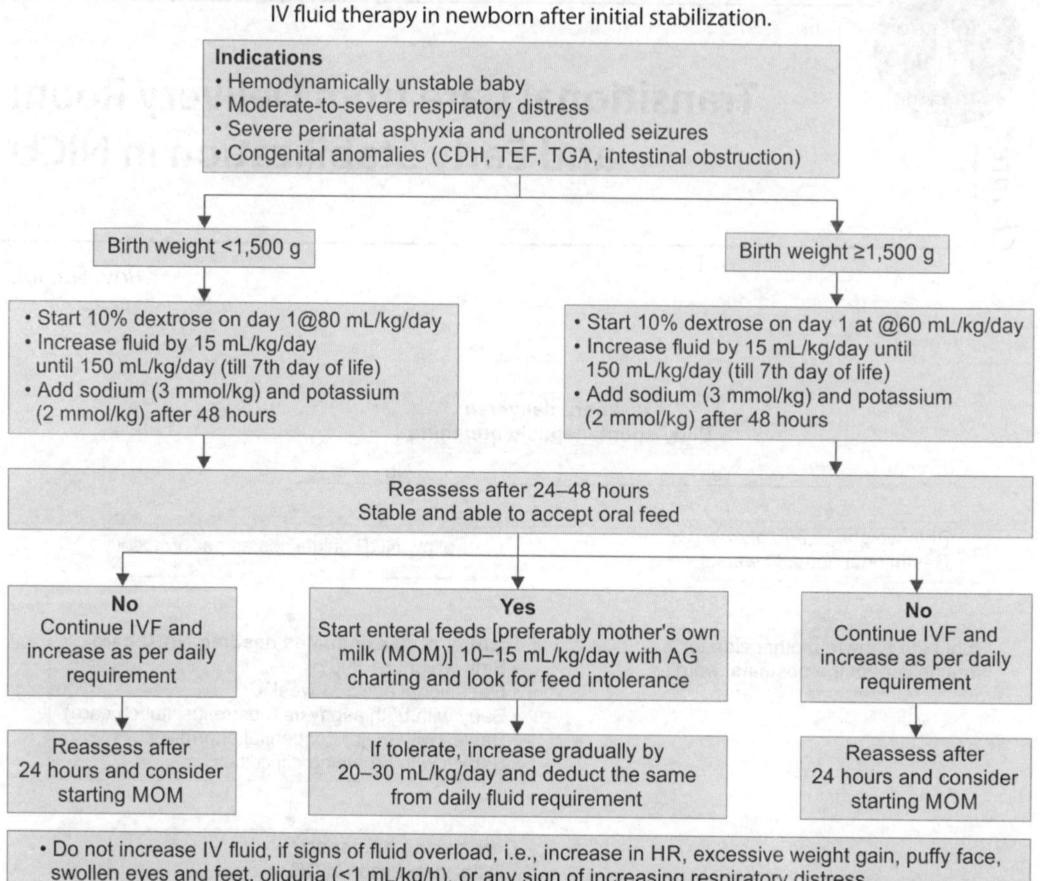

Key Points to Remember

- Document time of birth, time of initiation of breastfeeding, weight, gender, and identification band/marking for baby.
- Cord should be kept clean, dry, and free of any application (nothing should be applied).
- Weigh all the infants after breastfeeding initiation, preferably on a digital scale.
- Do not perform stomach wash in newborns at birth.
- Routine passage of catheter in the stomach, nostrils, and the rectum is not recommended but do give special attention to identify and document the anal opening in the record sheet.
- Examine the baby thoroughly and recorded in the case sheet for any life-threatening congenital anomalies, and birth injuries (cephalohematoma, brachial plexus injury, facial paralysis, fracture, and dislocation of hip).

- Injection vitamin K1 should be administered intramuscularly (0.5 mg for babies weighing <1,000 g 1.0 mg for those weighing above 1,000 g at birth) on the anterolateral aspect of the thigh using a 26-gauge needle and 1-mL syringe.
- Health provider must show the newborn to the mother and other family members, with particular attention to the identity tag on the newborn and must communicate to them the time, birth weight, gender, and condition of the newborn.

Admission checklist for a sick neonate at the time of admission	Yes	No
• *Before arrival*		
– NICU team informed about anticipated admission		
– Warmer on manual mode		
– Crib made ready		
– Standby ventilator/CPAP with new circuit and humidifier		
• *On Admission*		
– Check baby identification/name tagged		
– Suction if required		
– Oxygen by nasal prongs, if indicated		
– Temperature and pulse oximeter probe attached		
– Warmer mode shifted to servo		
– IV/UVC cannula inserted and dated		
– RBS on arrival checked		
– Necessary investigations collected		
– NIBP recorded		
– IV fluids started, if Indicated		
– Feeding tube inserted, if indicated		
– Consider CPAP and surfactant, if indicated		
– Injection vitamin k given, if not given earlier		
– Time of first dose of antibiotic after arrival noted		
– Weight, length, HC checked, and documented		
– Any injuries, previous cannula extravasations noted, and documented		
– X-ray chest and abdomen according to clinical scenario		
• *Admission formalities and counseling*		
– Counsel the parents for the need of admission		
– Plan of management and expected complications		
– Expected duration of NICU stay		
– Expected cost of care		

Contd...

Contd...

Admission checklist for a sick neonate at the time of admission	Yes	No
– Explained about daily visiting hours, time of daily counseling		
– Explained regarding feeding plan and expression of milk and storage of milk		
– Written informed consent taken regarding initial support, invasive procedures		
– Baby shown to attendants after initial stabilization		
– Admission slip, medication slip given to attendants, if any		
– Signature of the attending doctor/nurses:		

■ FURTHER READING

1. Facility-based newborn care, training module for doctors & nurses. MoHFW, GoI; 2022.

Surgical Emergencies

Sujoy Neogi

Many surgical neonates are referred to the tertiary care center due to lack of medical facility. Following are the common surgical conditions, where newborn needs surgical management:

- *Gastrointestinal tract (GIT)*
  - Tracheoesophageal fistula (TEF)
  - Idiopathic hypertrophic pyloric stenosis (IHPS)
  - Bowel atresia
  - Anorectal malformation
  - Peritonitis
  - Abdominal wall defects (Exomphalos, Gastroschisis)
- *Respiratory system*
  - Congenital diaphragmatic hernia (CDH)
  - Congenital lung disease
- *Urological system*
- Posterior urethral valves (PUV)

■ TRACHEOESOPHAGEAL FISTULA

- Antenatal diagnosis:
  - Polyhydramnios
  - Absence of gastric bubble
- Postnatal diagnosis:
  - Failure to negotiate nasogastric tube in (preferably size 9/10 or red rubber catheter) to the stomach during newborn resuscitation
  - Any newborn with excessive frothing from the mouth, failure to feed

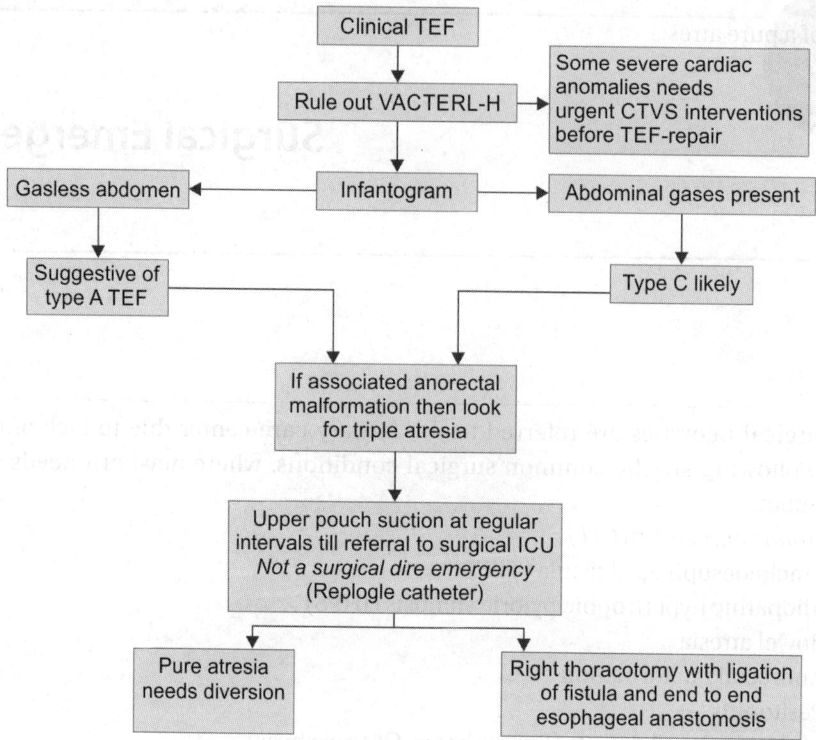

Classification of TEF

- Gross classification

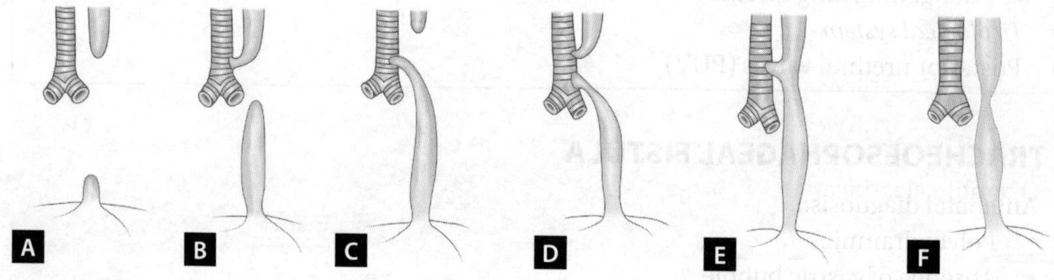

VACTERL-H

Incidence of associated anomalies	
Cardiovascular	≈24%
Genitourinary	≈21%
Gastrointestinal	≈21%
Musculoskeletal	≈14%
Central nervous system	≈7%
VACTERL association	≈20%
Overall incidence	50–70%
Source: From textbook Coran	

X-ray of a pure atresia showing no gas shadow in the abdomen.

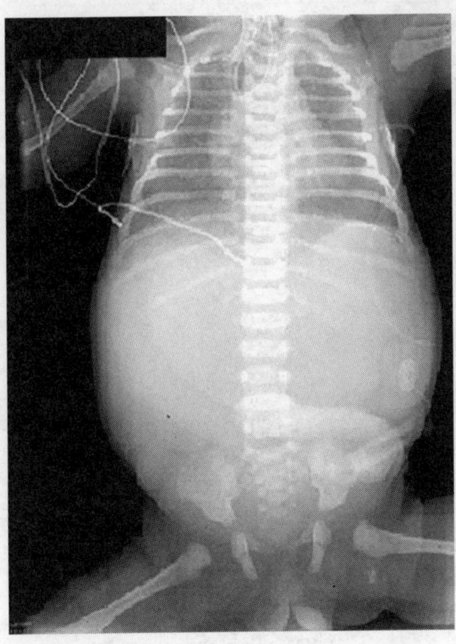

Prognostic Classification

- Spitz classification

Spitz classification system		
Group	**Features**	**Survival**
I	Birth weight >1,500 g, no major cardiac disease	97%
II	Birth weight <1,500 g, or major cardiac disease	59%
III	Birth weight <1,500 g, and major cardiac disease	22%

- Okamoto classification

Okamoto modification of the Spitz classification: Predictors of survival in cases of esophageal atresia			
Class	**Description**	**Risk**	**Survival**
Class I	No major cardiac anomaly, BW ≥ 2000 g	Low	100%
Class II	No major cardiac anomaly, BW < 2000 g	Moderate	81%
Class III	Major cardiac anomaly, BW ≥ 2000 g	Relatively high	72%
Class IV	Major cardiac anomaly, BW < 2000 g	High	27%

- Replogle tube

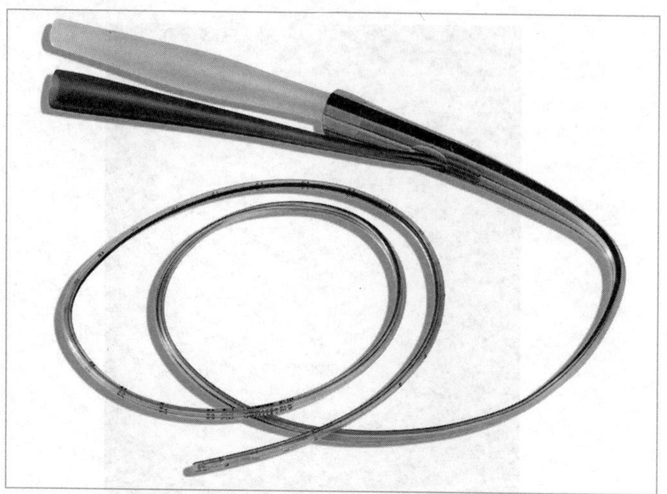

IDIOPATHIC HYPERTROPHIC PYLORIC STENOSIS

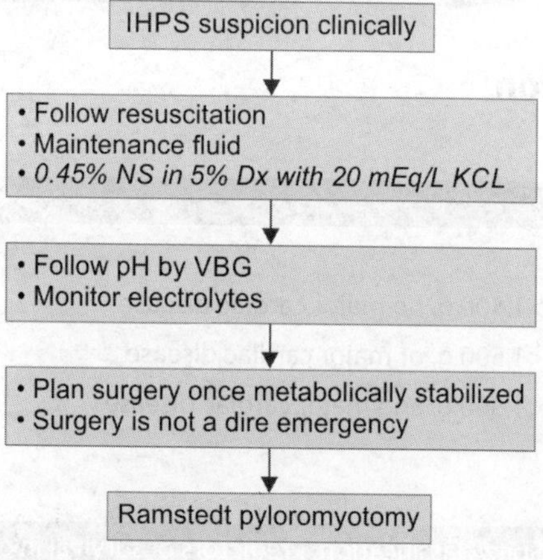

■ BOWEL ATRESIAS

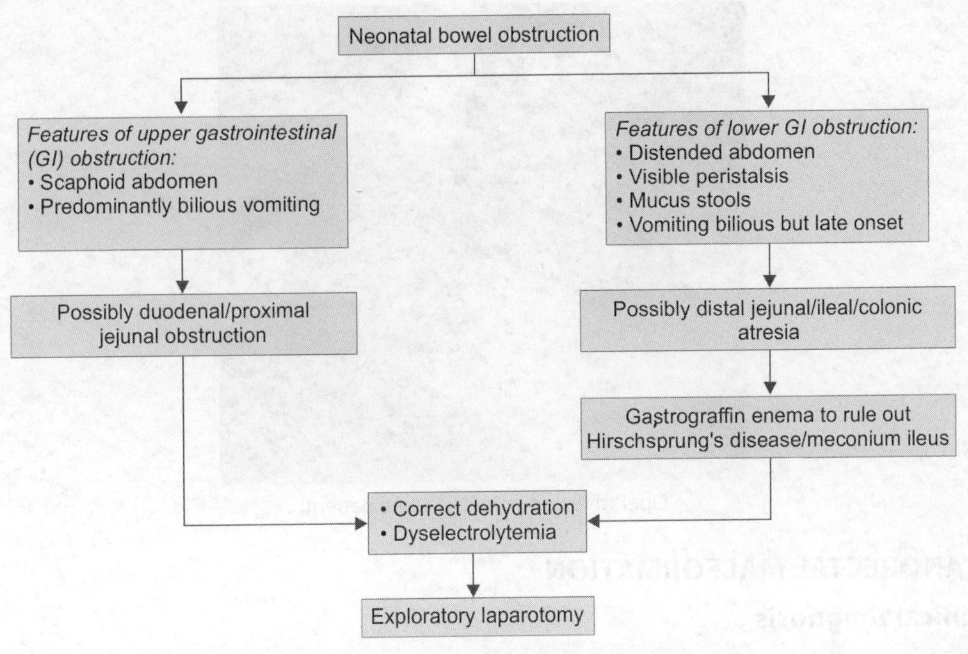

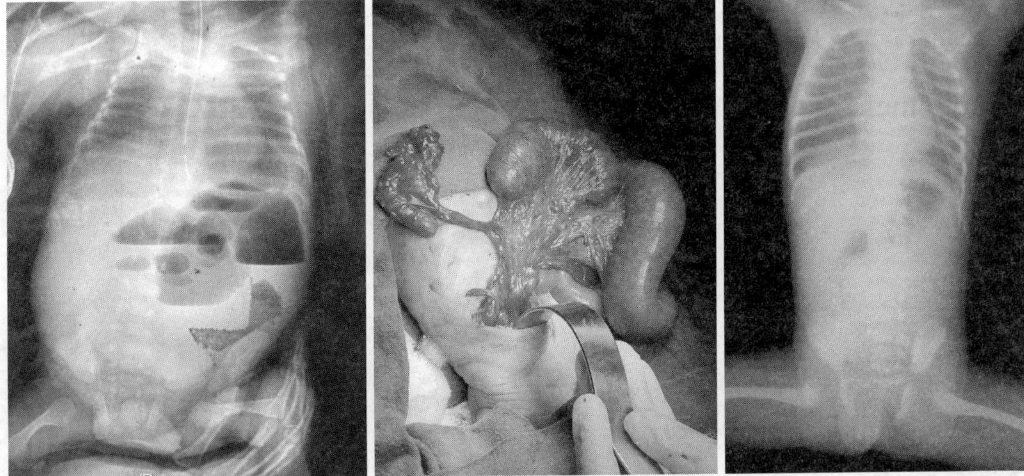

Duodenal atresia (Double bubble sign).

Differential diagnosis: Duodenal atresia, annular pancreas, and malrotation of gut.

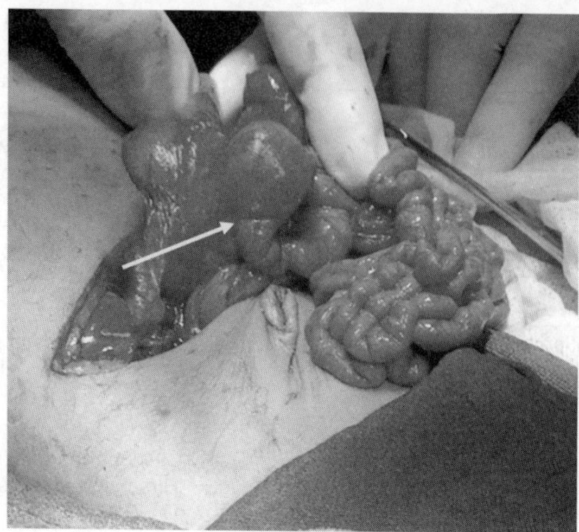

Operative finding of the same patient.

ANORECTAL MALFORMATION

Clinical Diagnosis

- Feeding tube should be put into the anal opening to confirm anal opening and meconium.
- Perineal examination of all neonates with lower GI obstruction
- Ruling out VACTER-H is mandatory.

Management of Male Anorectal Malformation

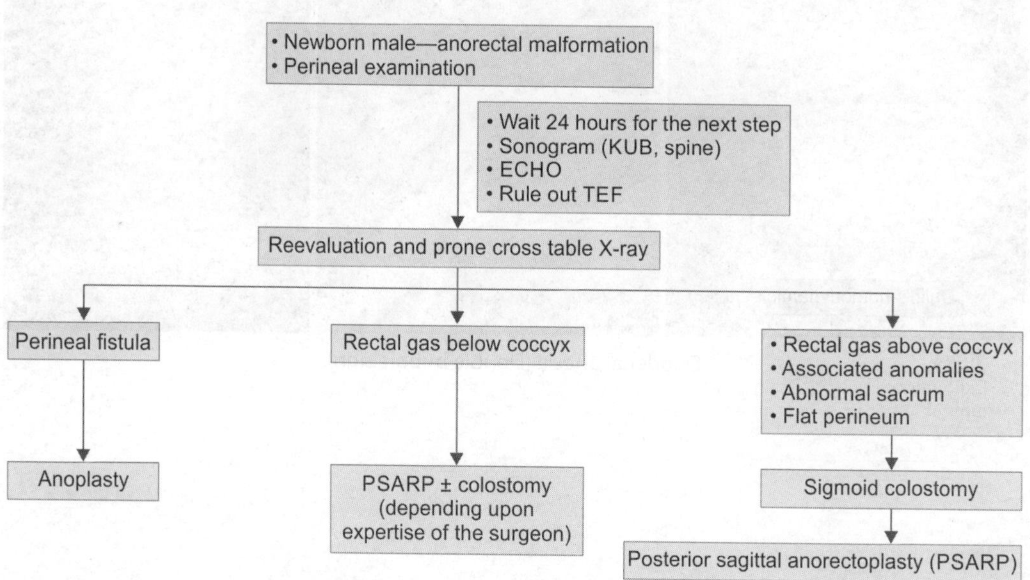

Management of Female Anorectal Malformation

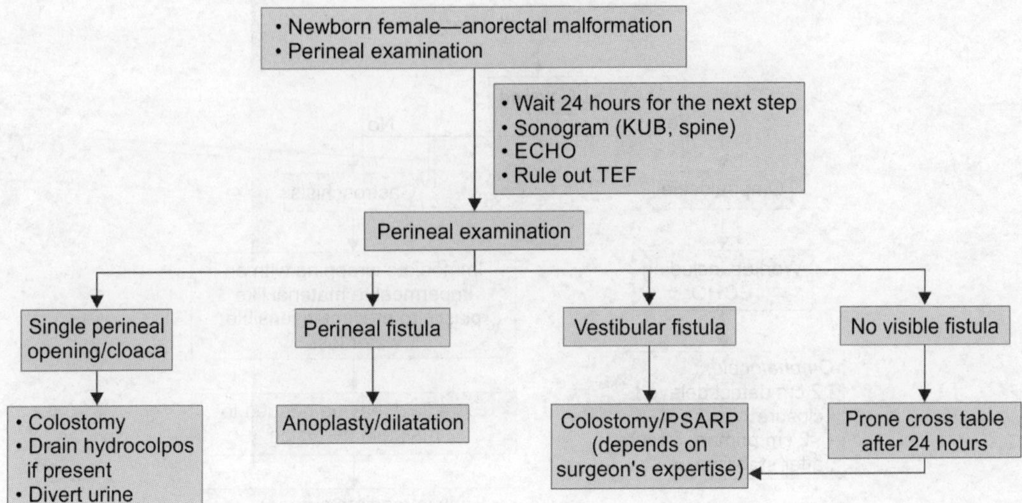

■ NEONATAL PERITONITIS

Clinical Features

- Neonatal peritonitis unlike adults are mostly indistinguishable from neonatal obstruction
- Grossly distended abdomen without visible loops of intestines
- Shiny abdomen
- Signs of septicemia

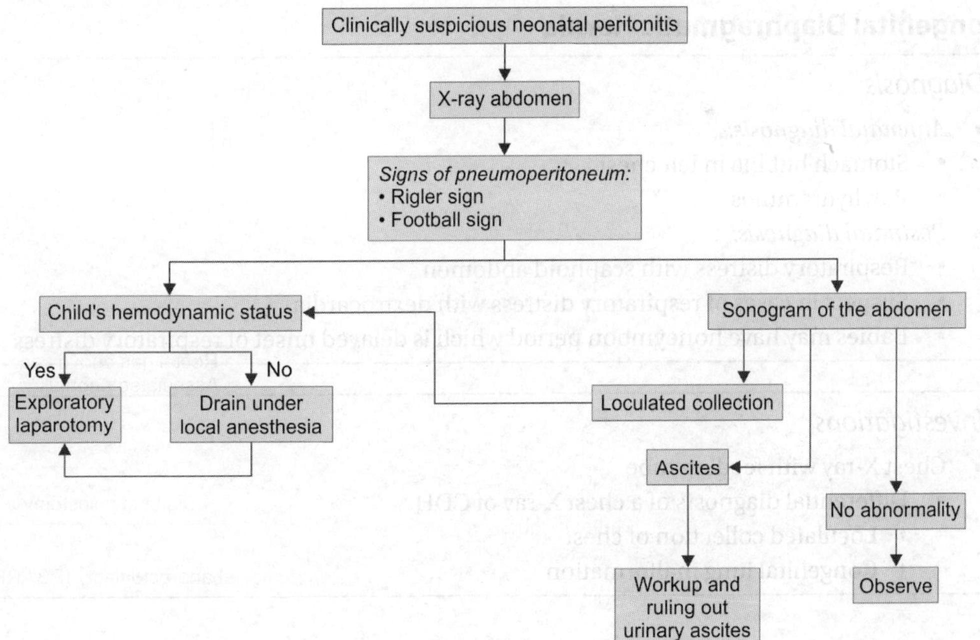

■ ABDOMINAL WALL DEFECTS

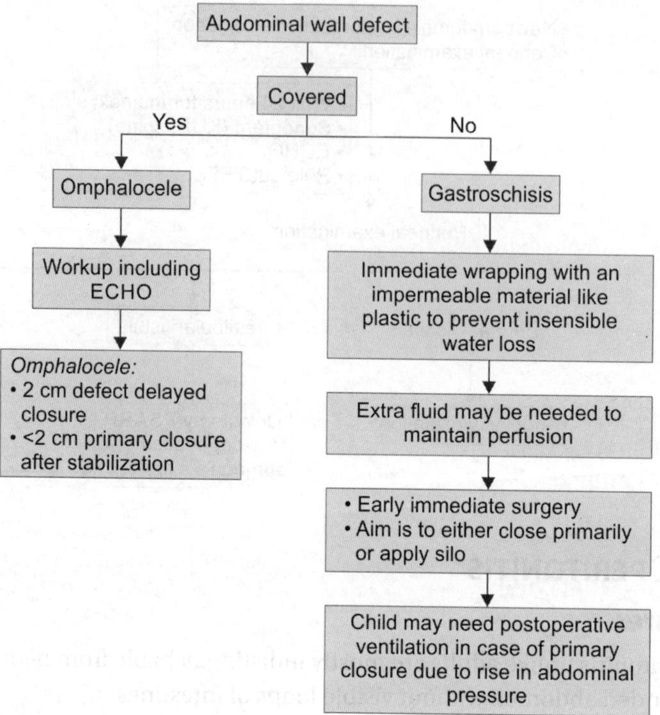

■ RESPIRATORY SYSTEM

Congenital Diaphragmatic Hernia

Diagnosis

- *Antenatal diagnosis:*
  - Stomach bubble in left chest
  - Polyhydramnios
- *Postnatal diagnosis:*
  - Respiratory distress with scaphoid abdomen
  - Suspect in cases of respiratory distress with dextrocardia
  - Babies may have honeymoon period which is delayed onset of respiratory distress

Investigations

- Chest X-ray with feeding tube
  - Differential diagnosis of a chest X-ray of CDH
    - Loculated collection of chest
    - Congenital lung malformation

- Contrast-enhanced computed tomography (CT) scan
  - Right-sided CDH
  - Older babies with eventration

Important Quotes Pertaining to Management of CDH

- "For the patient in whom the hernia makes its appearance at birth, little or nothing can be done from a surgical standpoint."
  - Greenwald and Steiner
- CDH is a physiological emergency and not a surgical emergency.

Prognostic Factors

- *Anatomical factors:*
  - LHR (lung–head ratio):
    - >1 good prognosis
    - <1 bad prognosis
  - Cardioventricular index
  - McGoon index
  - Pulmonary artery index
- *Physiological factors:*
  - Alveolar-arterial oxygen gradient
  - Ventilatory index
  - Modified ventilatory index (MVI) (most commonly used)
    - $MVI = (\text{respiratory rate} \times PIP \times PaCO_2)/1{,}000$
      - $MVI < 40 \rightarrow 96\%$ survival
      - $MVI > 80 \rightarrow 100\%$ mortality

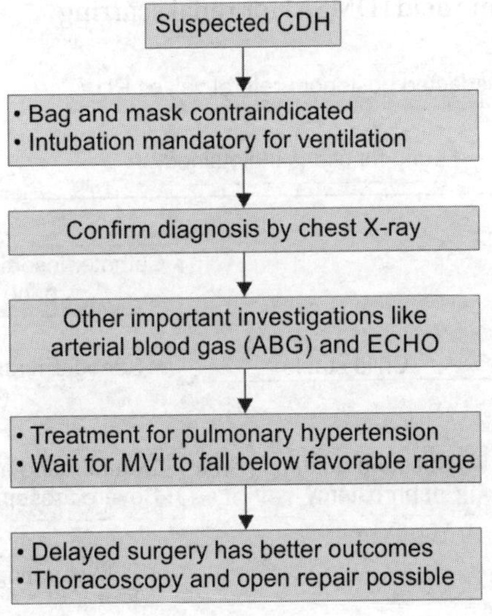

Congenital Lung Malformations

Congenital lung malformations are three types, which include:

1. Congenital lobar emphysema:
   - True surgical emergency
   - Child needs urgent thoracotomy and lobectomy
2. Congenital pulmonary adenoid malformation
3. Sequestrated lung

■ UROLOGICAL SYSTEM

Posterior Urethral Valves

Diagnosis

- *Antenatal:*
  - Fetal hydronephrosis (usually bilateral)
  - Echogenic kidney
  - Thick-walled bladder without inability to empty urine
  - Keyhole sign (posterior urethra dilated)
  - Urinary ascites
- *Postnatal:*
  - Sonogram
  - Micturating cystourethrogram
  - Urine routine and cultures
  - Other ancillary investigations for associated renal compromise:
    - Serum creatinine
    - Venous blood gases
    - Blood pressure charting
    - Complete blood count and serum electrolytes
    - Dimercaptosuccinic acid (DMSA) for renal scarring

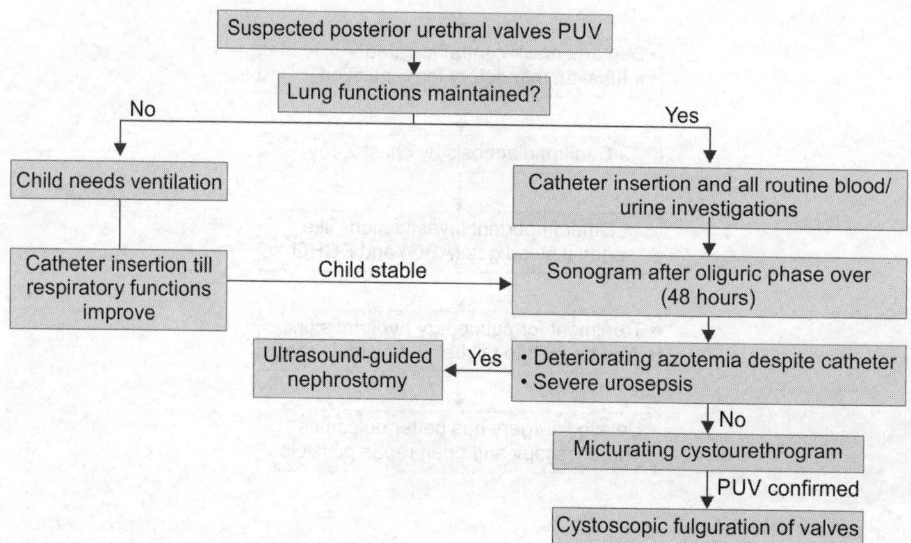

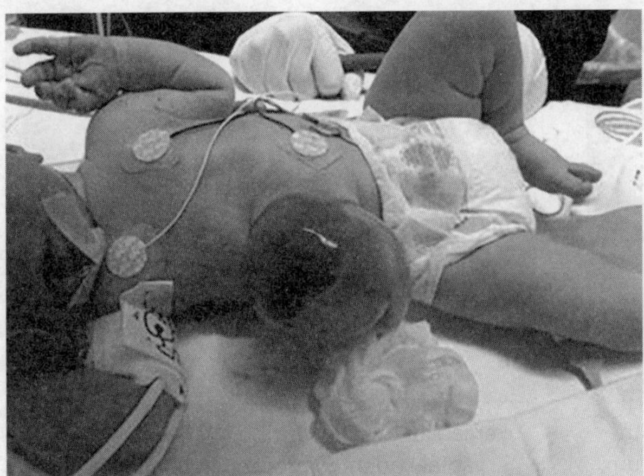

Omphalocele major.

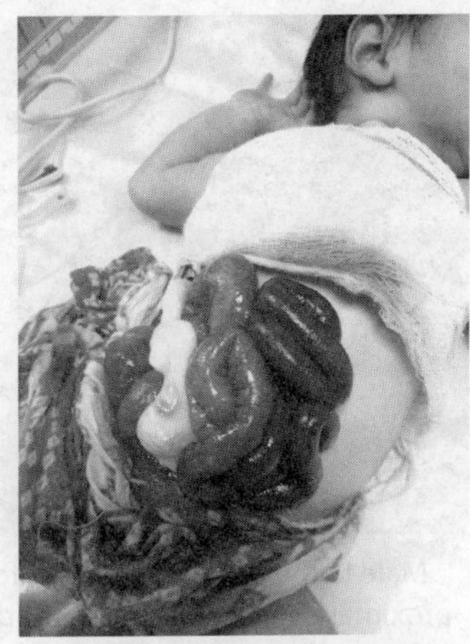

Gastroschisis referred from outskirts with bowel edema.

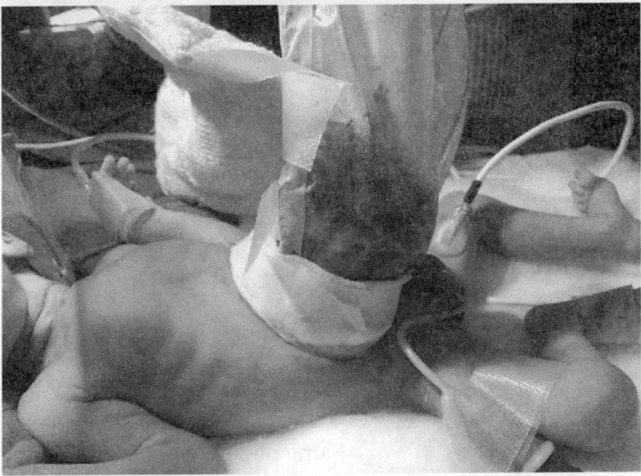

Makeshift silo application (urobag) to prevent insensible water loss.

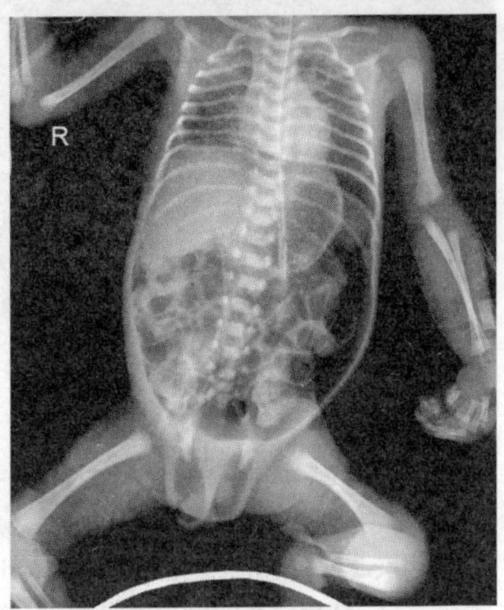

Infantogram showing football sign suggestive of perforation of bowel.

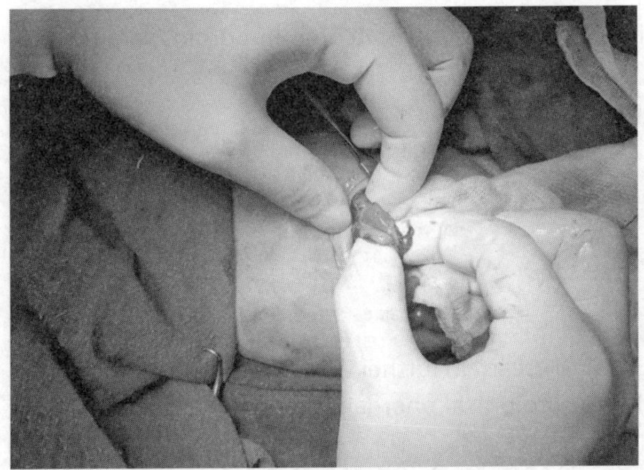

Same patient's perforation in the transverse colon.

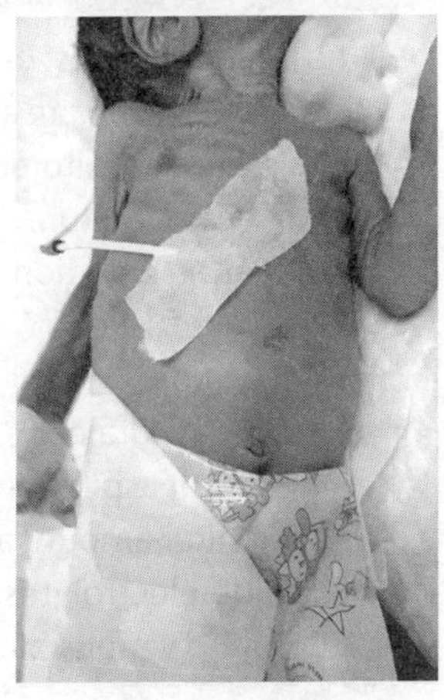

Suspected peritonitis (shining tense abdomen).

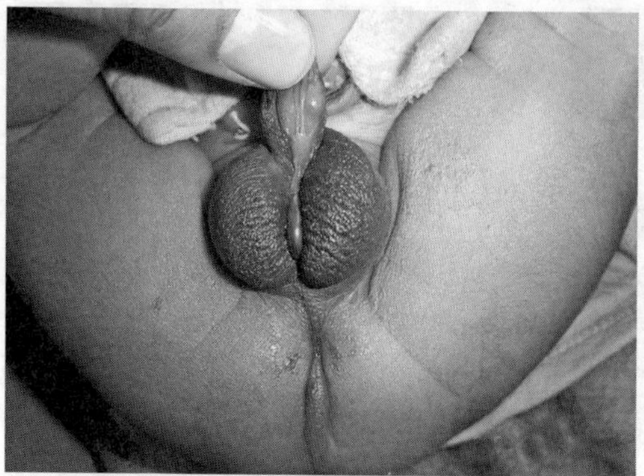

Male baby with anorectal malformation with proximal penile hypospadias with bifid scrotum.

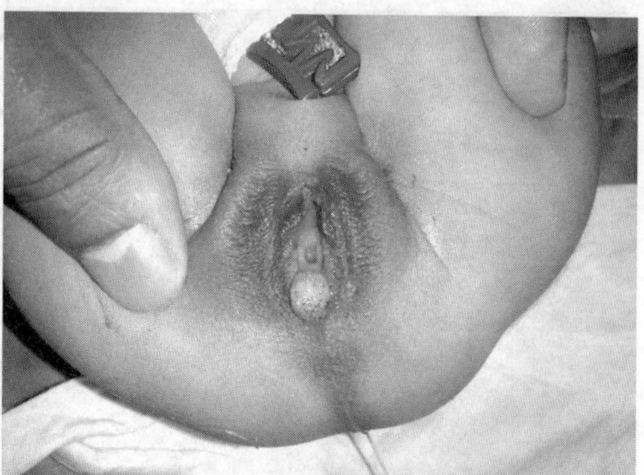

Female baby with vestibular anus (just below vaginal opening meconium coming out).

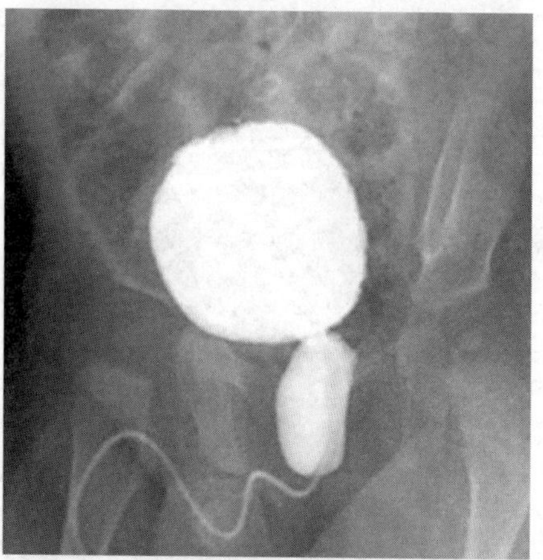

Keyhole sign suggestive of posterior urethral valves (PUV).

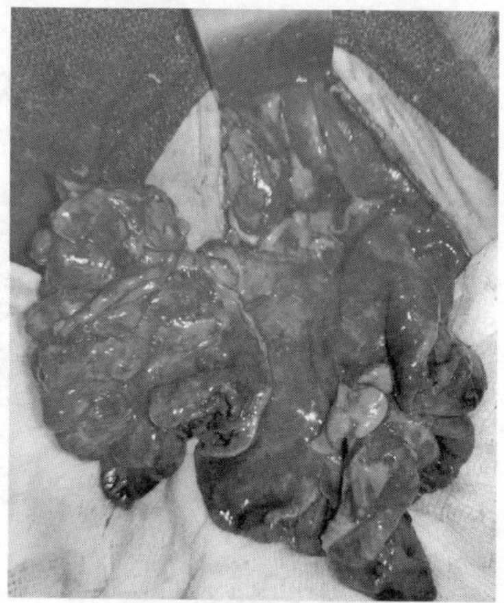

Same patient with extensive necrotizing enterocolitis.

Key Points to Remember

All the newborns must be stabilized before referral for better outcome. Important parameters to be stressed upon are as follows:

- Vitals to be monitored during transport: TOPS
  - T—Temperature
  - O—Oxygenation
  - P—Perfusion
  - S—Sugar
- Nasogastric drainage to:
  - Prevent aspiration
  - Monitor amount and color of output to ascertain further course of action
- Baseline electrolytes, kidney profile (for urological anomalies), arterial blood gas (for CDH), and venous blood gas (if facility available)

Neonatal Transport

Ronak Patel

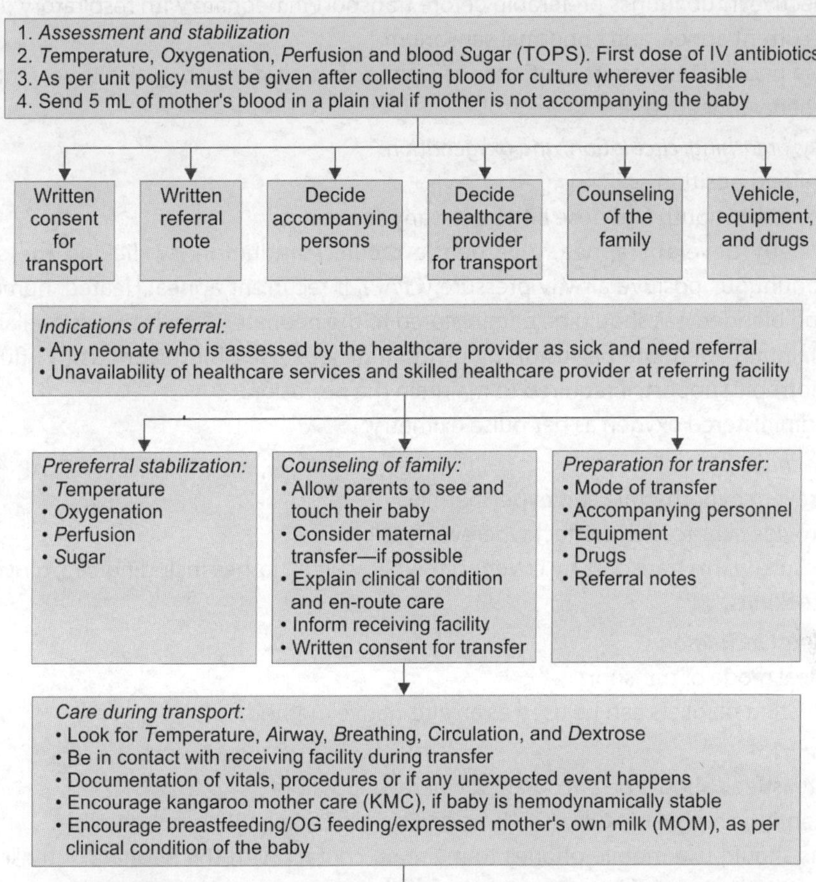

Key Points to Remember

Types of transfers
- Interfacility transfer—from community to hospital/hospital to other hospital
- Intrafacility transfer—transport within hospital
- Transport for specialized care
- Reverse transport after treatment
- In utero transfer—expected high-risk baby delivery is always better to transfer in utero

Care during transport
- *Stabilization during transport:*
  - Elective intubation is preferable before transport in neonate with respiratory distress, recurrent apnea, and abnormal sensorium.
  - Use neonatal transport ventilator or T-piece resuscitator or bag and tube ventilation wherever needed.
- *Airway, breathing, circulation, and oxygenation:*
  - Sniffing position
  - Clear the mouth and nose if there are any secretions.
  - If baby develops apnea, give gentle tactile stimulation by flicking the sole or continuous positive airway pressure (CPAP), if recurrent apnea. Heated, humidified, and blended gas should be administered to the neonate, if the facility is available.
  - Maintain adequate perfusion by giving judicious use of intravenous (IV) fluid and inotropic support, if required to maintain the perfusion.
  - Administered oxygen as per pulse oximetry.
- *Warm chain:*
  - Prevent hypothermia and hyperthermia.
  - Provide skin-to-skin contact wherever feasible.
  - Ensure warm transport by covering the baby with clothes including cap, gloves, and stockings.
- *Transport incubator:*
  - Ideal mode of transport
  - Heating blankets can be used as an alternative method.
- *Feeds:*
  - Breastfeed should be encouraged wherever possible.
  - Continue orogastric tube (OGT) feeds if breastfeeding (BF) is not possible.
- Teams should use mobile phones to maintain contact with the neonatal intensive care unit (NICU) and seek advice for unexpected events.
- Document all events and procedures done along with monitoring charting.

OSCE/checklist for neonatal transport.			
S. No.	*Performance steps*	*Yes*	*No*
1.	Transport incubator/embrace		
2.	Thermometer and/or temperature monitor and probes		
3.	Plastic wraps, insulating blankets, and heat shield		
4.	Oxygen cylinders with indicators of line pressure and gas contents		
5.	Flow meters, oxygen tubing, and adapters		
6.	Oxygen hood, all size neonatal size masks, and cannula and appropriate nasal prongs		
7.	Oxygen analyzer and pulse oximeter		
8.	Ambu bags (250 mL and 500 mL)		
9.	Transport mechanical ventilator with back up circuit		
10.	CPAP/T-piece machine		
11.	Laryngoscope with size 00, 0, and 1 blades and extra batteries		
12.	*Endotracheal tubes*: 2.5, 3.0, 3.5, and 4.0 mm with fixation tape		
13.	Mucus suction trap and suction catheters (5, 6, 8, 10, and 12 F)		
14.	Regulated suction with pressure regulator		
15.	Feeding tube (8 Fr) for orogastric decompression		
16.	Sterile gloves and sterile water		
17.	Stethoscope and cardiac monitor		
18.	Glucometer and its strips		
19.	Intracaths (No. 24 and 26 guaze)		
20.	Disposable syringes (2, 5, 10, 20, and 50 mL)		
21.	Splint, transparent dressings, or micropore		
22.	Three-way stopcocks, extension tubings		
23.	IV chamber sets and microdrip sets		
24.	Intravenous administration tubings compatible with infusion pump		
25.	Injection calcium gluconate 10%		
26.	Epinephrine (1:10,000) prefilled syringes, sodium bicarbonate		
27.	Dopamine, dobutamine, morphine, and midazolam		
28.	Normal saline, phenobarbitone, and levetiracetam surfactant		

■ FURTHER READING

1. National Neonatology Forum of India. Transport of sick neonates. Clinical practice guidelines 2020.

Chapter 7

Management of Cyanosis

Anita Yadav

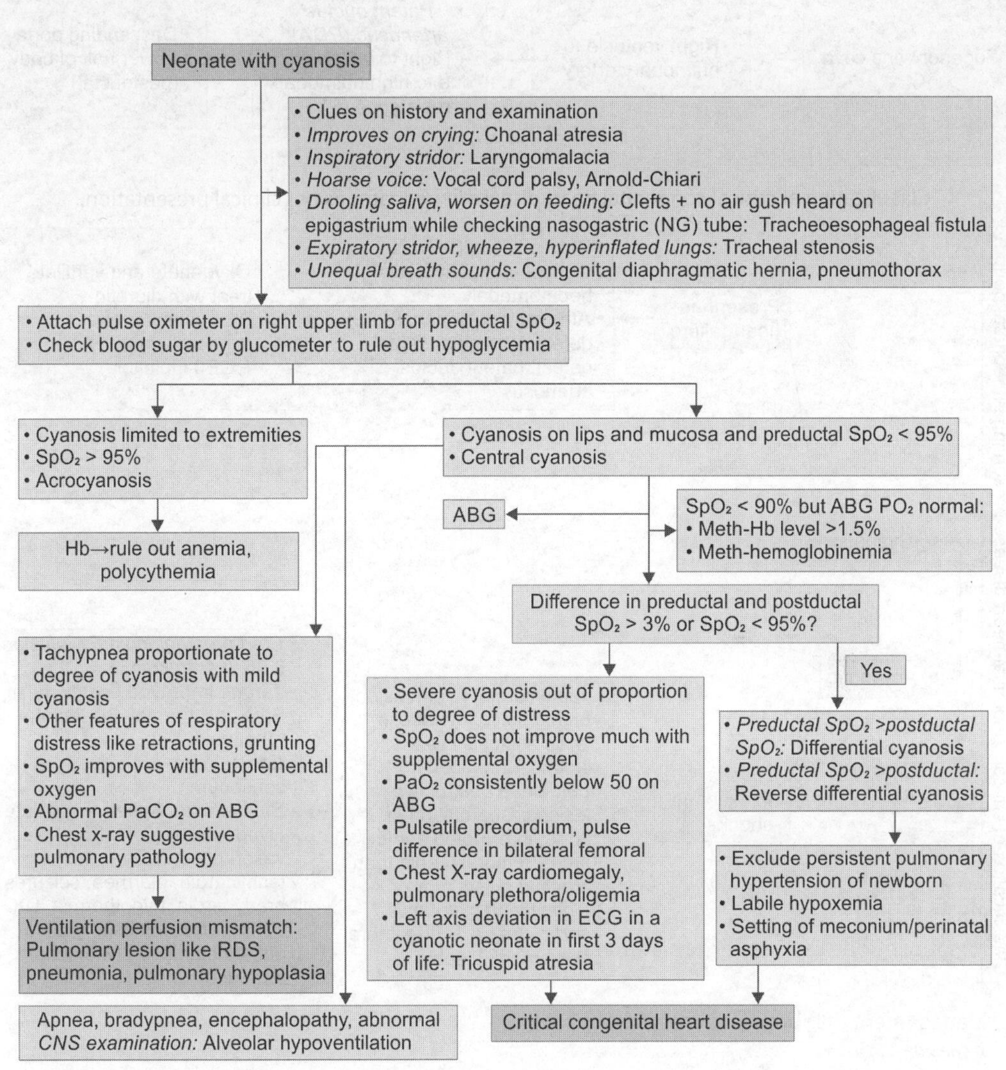

Fetal circulation.

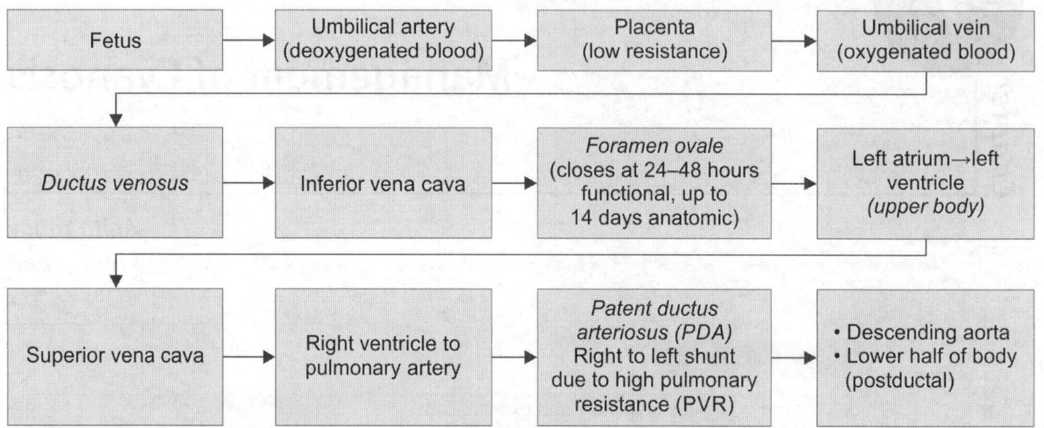

Fetus
Umbilical artery (deoxygenated blood)
Placenta (low resistance)
Umbilical vein (oxygenated blood)
Ductus venosus
Inferior vena cava
Foramen ovale (closes at 24–48 hours functional, up to 14 days anatomic)
Left atrium→left ventricle *(upper body)*
Superior vena cava
Right ventricle to pulmonary artery
Patent ductus arteriosus (PDA) Right to left shunt due to high pulmonary resistance (PVR)
• Descending aorta
• Lower half of body (postductal)

Classification of critical congenital heart disease in neonates as per clinical presentation.

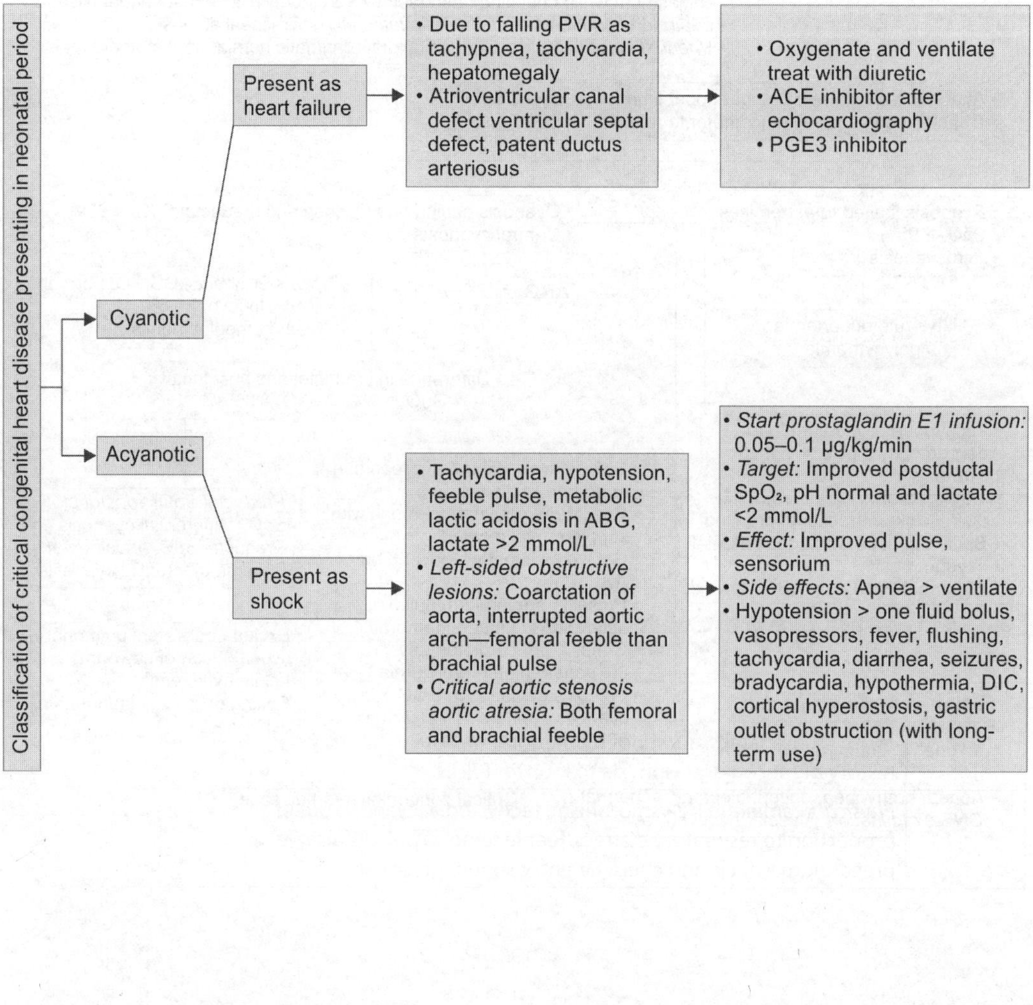
Classification of critical congenital heart disease presenting in neonatal period
Cyanotic
Acyanotic
Present as heart failure
• Due to falling PVR as tachypnea, tachycardia, hepatomegaly
• Atrioventricular canal defect ventricular septal defect, patent ductus arteriosus
• Oxygenate and ventilate treat with diuretic
• ACE inhibitor after echocardiography
• PGE3 inhibitor
Present as shock
• Tachycardia, hypotension, feeble pulse, metabolic lactic acidosis in ABG, lactate >2 mmol/L
• *Left-sided obstructive lesions:* Coarctation of aorta, interrupted aortic arch—femoral feeble than brachial pulse
• *Critical aortic stenosis aortic atresia:* Both femoral and brachial feeble
• *Start prostaglandin E1 infusion:* 0.05–0.1 μg/kg/min
• *Target:* Improved postductal SpO_2, pH normal and lactate <2 mmol/L
• *Effect:* Improved pulse, sensorium
• *Side effects:* Apnea > ventilate
• Hypotension > one fluid bolus, vasopressors, fever, flushing, tachycardia, diarrhea, seizures, bradycardia, hypothermia, DIC, cortical hyperostosis, gastric outlet obstruction (with long-term use)

Approach to cyanosis and pathophysiology with management.

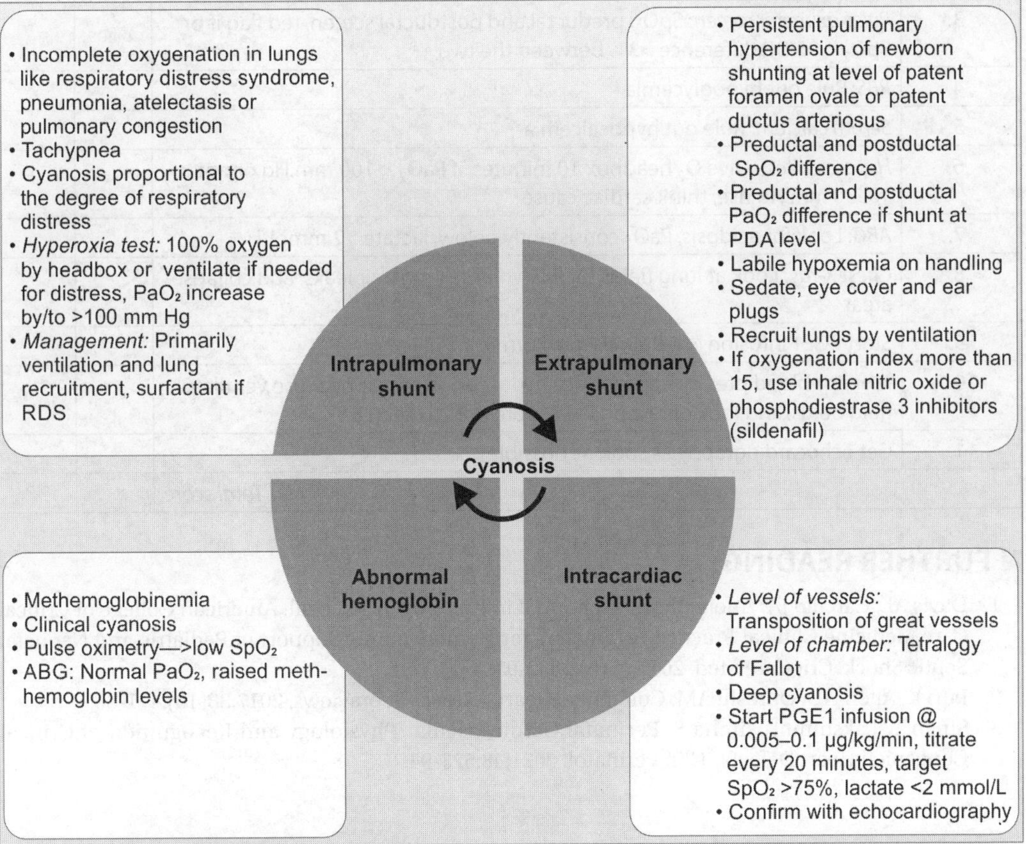

Key Points to Remember

- Keep a high index of suspicion for critical congenital heart disease in neonates presenting with shock and persistent cyanosis.
- Start prostaglandin infusion without waiting for echocardiography, if not available immediately.

OSCE/Checklist: Approach to Cyanotic Newborn

*Name of the participants:*____

S. No.	Performance steps	Yes	No
1.	*History:* Antenatal scan, sudden deterioration with cyanosis or shock, history of meconium/asphyxia to look for PPHN		
2.	*Physical examination:* Dysmorphism, tachycardia, cyanosis out of proportion to respiratory distress, feeble femoral pulse, pulsatile precordium, shock, and check air entry should be equal		

Contd...

Contd...

3.	*Pulse oximeter screen:* SpO$_2$: preductal and postductal screen, red flag if or SpO$_2$ < 95 OR difference >3% between the two		
4.	*RBS:* Rule out hypoglycemia		
5.	*Serum calcium:* Rule out hypocalcemia		
6.	*Hyperoxia test:* Give O$_2$ headbox 10 minutes, if PaO$_2$ < 100 mm Hg or not 10–30 mm Hg rise, think cardiac cause		
7.	*ABG:* Look for acidosis, PaO$_2$ consistently below, lactate >2 mmol/L		
8.	*Chest X-ray:* Look at lung fields for low volume lungs, air leaks, and collapse areas		
9.	Start PGE1 infusion @ 0.005–0.1 µg/kg/min		
10.	Monitor blood pressure actively for hypotension and apnea (use ventilator, fluid bolus, and look of response/vasopressors to keep BP)		
11.	Get echocardiography as soon as possible		
	Total score		

■ FURTHER READING

1. Davis AL, Carcillo JA, Aneja RK, DEyman AJ, Lin JC, Nyugen TC, et al. American College of Critical Care Medicine Clinical Practice Parameters for Hemodynamic Support of Pediatric and Neonatal Septic Shock. Crit Care Med. 2017;45(6):1062-93.
2. Puri K, Allen HD, Qureshi AM. Congenital heart disease. Neoreviews. 2017;38(10):471-86.
3. Singh Y, Lakshminrusimha S. Perinatal Cardiovascular Physiology and Recognition of Critical Congenital Heart Defects. Clin Perinatol. 2021;48:573-94.

Management of Shock

Naveen Prakash Gupta

Definition

It is an unstable pathophysiologic state characterized by cellular or tissue hypoxia due to reduced oxygen delivery and/or increased oxygen consumption or inadequate oxygen utilization

↓

History and clinical pointers

Preterm Neonates
- *Baby well (BP low but other parameters within normal limits):* Transient circulatory compromise in first 24 hours is common in extremely low birth weight (ELBW) and very low birth weight (VLBW) infants
- *Sick preterm:* Sepsis, intraventricular hemorrhage (IVH), large patent ductus arteriosus (PDA), and adrenal insufficiency
- *Extremely low birth weight infant with excessive weight loss:* Hypovolemic shock

Term Neonates <24 hours
- History of hypoxic ischemic encephalopathy (HIE), Meconium aspiration syndrome (MAS), persistent pulmonary hypertension of the newborn (PPHN)
- >24 hours, initially normal but gradual onset—sepsis; sudden onset—suspected duct-dependent cardiac disease
- Look for etiology and type of shock (*see* **Table 1**)

Interventions in the Immediate Past
- Surfactant administration/mechanical ventilation—excessive peak inspiratory pressure/positive end-expiratory pressure (PIP/PEEP) and obstructive shock, and pneumothorax
- Postcentral line insertion—pneumothorax in subclavian line insertion, cardiac tamponade in PICC line/umbilical line insertion
- Postdouble volume exchange transfusion (DVET) —air embolism

↓

Clinical assessment

Clinical parameters	• Tachypnea, tachycardia, and variable heart rate (HR) • Prolonged capillary refill time (CRT) • Poor peripheral pulses • Cold peripheries • Mottling of skin • Lethargy • Hypotension • Decrease in urine output
Laboratory parameters	• Blood gas (lactic acidosis)
Newer parameters now being used in clinical practice	• Functional echocardiography (*see* **Table 2**) • Near infrared spectroscopy (rSO_2)

Contd...

Contd...

Initial stabilization and management (see Table 3):
• Establish vascular access
• Restore perfusion by administering 10–20 mL/kg of normal saline over 30–60 minutes (depending upon your assessment about etiology of shock)
• Correct hypothermia/hyperthermia
• Evaluate airway and breathing—provide appropriate support if needed (supplemental oxygen or intubation and positive pressure ventilation)

Clinical monitoring (see Table 4):
• Temperature, heart rate (HR), respiratory rate (RR), noninvasive blood pressure (NIBP), oxygen saturation (SpO2), CRT, and peripheral pulses
• Urine output (in last 6 hours)

• Start thinking about etiology of shock
• In case of suspected cyanotic congenital heart disease and duct dependent circulation, plan for prostin (PGE1) infusion

Focused evaluation, laboratory testing, and imaging:
• Blood gas (one including lactate is preferable)
• Complete blood count (CBC), SE, kidney function test (KFT), liver function test (LFT), and sepsis screen
• Chest X-ray
• Functional echocardiography (if available)
• Start Empiric antibiotics (as per your unit policy)

Correct any abnormality detected on initial evaluation:
• Hypo/Hyperthermia
• Hypo/Hyperglycemia
• Electrolyte abnormality
• Pneumothorax
• Significant anemia

Assess response to initial interventions

Adequate response (improvement in the clinical parameter)

Inadequate response (worsening in the clinical parameter)

• Continue supportive care
• Continue monitoring (see Table 4)

Are there signs of fluid overload (crepts, hepatomegaly) and/or clinical deterioration with administration of fluid bolus

Yes

No

Start vasoactive therapy Chose inotrope based on suspected etiology (see Table 3)

• Consider the second bolus
• After the second bolus if inappropriate response, consider fluid refractory shock and chose inotrope/vasopressor based on suspected etiology (see Table 3)

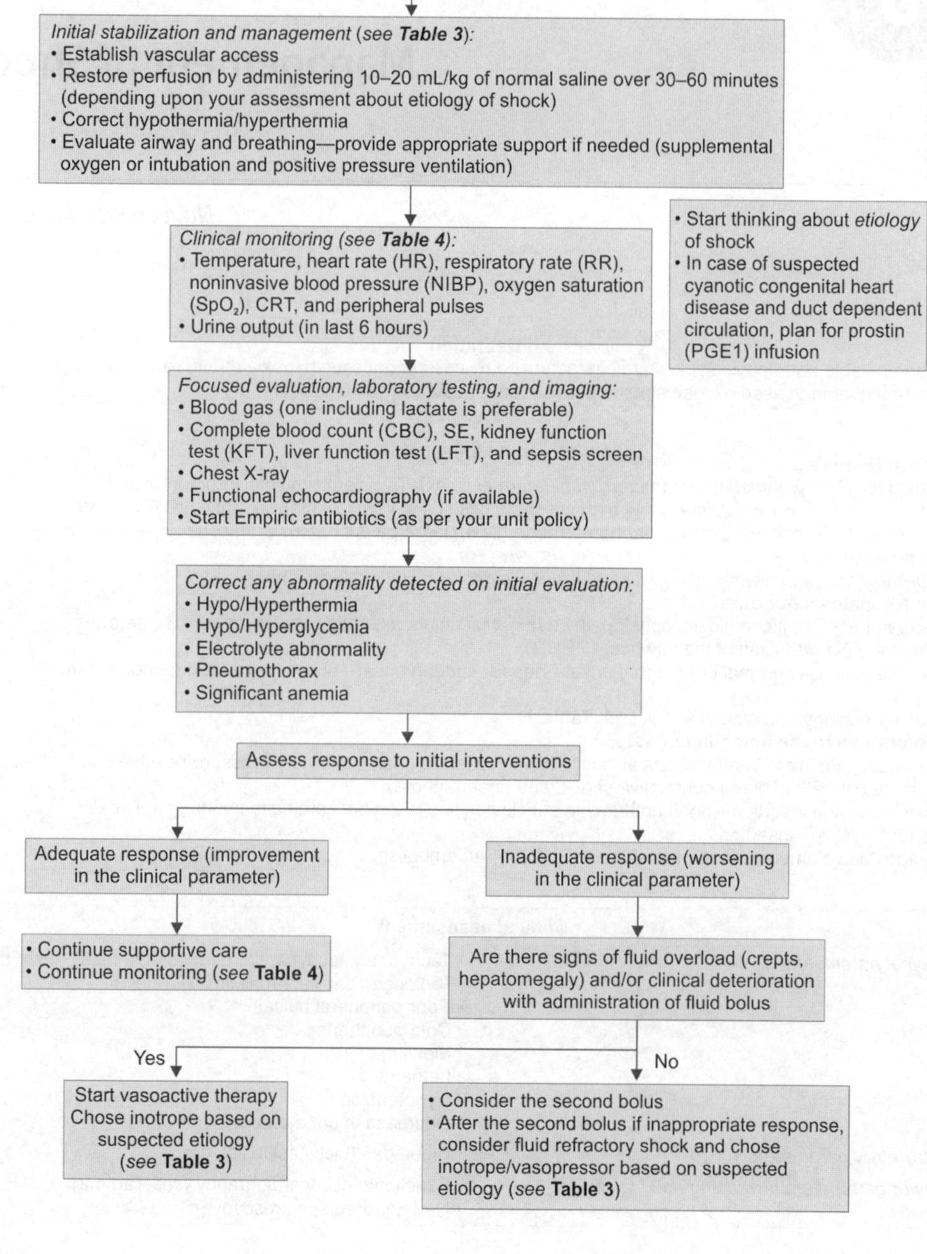

TABLE 1: Type and phase of neonatal shock.

Type of shock	Etiology	Pathophysiology (underlying reason of poor perfusion)
Hypovolemic	• Fluid loss (blood loss in case of abruptio placenta or fetomaternal or fetoplacental hemorrhage) • Capillary leak (sepsis and necrotizing enterocolitis) • Pulmonary hemorrhage, subgaleal bleeding, and intracranial hemorrhage • Diarrhea	Inadequate blood volume
Cardiogenic	• Congenital heart disease—left-sided obstructive lesions such as hypoplastic left heart syndrome, critical aortic stenosis, critical coarctation of aorta, and interrupted aortic arch	Defects of the pump
	• Heart failure, arrhythmia, and cardiomyopathy • Postcardiac surgery • Postpatency of the PDA ligation	
Distributive	• Sepsis • Endothelial injury • Vasodilators	Abnormalities within the vascular beds
Obstructive	• Cardiac tapenade • Pneumothorax • High pulmonary vascular resistance restricting blood flow such as in postpartum hemorrhage (PPH)	Flow restriction
Phase of shock		
Compensated phase	• "Diving reflex" presents blood flow to vital organs maintained • Clinical findings—tachycardia, prolonged capillary refill time (CFT), cold peripheries, decrease urine output but normal blood pressure	
Uncompensated phase	• If not treated in compensated phase, uncompensated phase begins • Blood flow to vital organs also decreases • Clinical features—all features of compensated phase and presence of hypotension	
Irreversible phase	If treatment is not initiated promptly in uncompensated phase, multi organ failure and permanent damage to vital organs ensue; further treatment will not be effective	

TABLE 2: Echocardiography parameters in assessment of shock.

Hypovolemia	• Kissing small LV cavity • RV size • Normal or small RA
Fluid responsiveness	• Inferior vena cava (IVC) collapsibility index > 55% • IVC dispensability index exceeding 18%
LV function	• Left ventricular output (LVO) <150 mL/kg/min suggests decrease LVO • Serial LVO measurements can help in assessing progression of shock/monitoring response to inotropes • Fractional shortening and EF are not so reliable in neonates
Systemic perfusion	• LVO is not a surrogate marker of organ perfusion in first 48 hours of life in preterm very low birth weight infants (when there is left to right shunting happening across foramen ovale and ductus arteriosus) • Superior vena cava flow with some limitations can be considered as surrogate marker of organ perfusion in such circumstances • In absence of any significant shunting, LVO can be considered surrogate marker of organ perfusion

TABLE 3: Treatment options for shock.

Patient group	Clinical issues	Cardiovascular parameters	Suggested management
Extreme preterm during transitional period (first 48 hours of life)	Early low systemic blood flow	• Normal/low BP low blood flow/cardiac output • Large ductus arteriosus • Higher systemic vascular resistance (unless born with chorioamnionitis) • Poor myocardial contractility	• Saline 10–20 mL/kg IV over 1 hour (one bolus is sufficient unless there is documented history of blood loss) • Inotropes • Dobutamine • Dopamine (especially if there is low blood pressure)
VLBW infant with PDA	Low BP ± PDA signs	Low BP; large PDA with left-to-right shunt	• Start NSAIDs as per unit policy to treat hsPDA (IV paracetamol/oral ibuprofen in our settings) • Start inotropes (dopamine) if low blood pressure is there
Neonate with asphyxia	• Myocardial damage • Low systemic blood flow	• Normal/low BP • Poor myocardial contractility	• Saline 10–20 mL/kg IV over 1 hour (care if myocardial function is affected) • Inotropes • Dobutamine • Dopamine or epinephrine (especially if low blood pressure)

Contd...

Contd...

Patient group	Clinical issues	Cardiovascular parameters	Suggested management
Septic shock (high output/vasodilatory shock)	High output cardiac failure secondary to sepsis	• Normal or low BP • High systemic blood flow • Low systemic vascular resistance/capillary leak	• Volume replacement may require >20 mL/kg • Inotropes • Dopamine • Epinephrine
• Septic shock (low output) • Later phase of septic shock (vasoconstriction, poor perfusion, and cold extremities)	Sepsis and poor myocardial function	• Normal or Low BP • Normal or low systemic blood flow • High systemic vascular resistance/capillary leak	• Saline—10–20 mL/kg • Inotropes to maintain blood pressure • Dopamine • Epinephrine • Inotropes to maintain organ perfusion (start once blood pressure is better) • Dobutamine • Milrinone • Do consider steroids (hydrocortisone 1 mg/kg/dose, 8–12 hourly for 2–3 days)
VLBW with acute blood loss (intraventricular/pulmonary hemorrhage)	Acute hypovolemia	Normal or low blood pressure	• Volume replacement may require >20 mL/kg including blood transfusion • Dopamine • Epinephrine
Cardiac etiology	• Suspected heart disease • Cardiomyopathy • Arrhythmia	• Feeble pulses (if etiology is obstructive cardiac lesion) • Rhythm disturbance (arrhythmia)	• PGE1 infusion (for duct-dependent lesions) • Antiarrhythmics

TABLE 4: Clinical monitoring.

Parameter	Frequency
Temperature	Maintain temperature between 36.5 and 37.5°C
Vitals—HR/RR/CFT/peripheral pulses/SpO$_2$/BP	Hourly
Urine output	6–8 hourly
Blood dextrose	6 hourly; confirm any abnormal reading with RBS sample since peripheral blood flow compromised
Hematocrit/serum calcium and electrolytes/renal function tests	At least once daily or more frequently as per the treating physicians discretion
Arterial pH/lactate/other parameters of blood gas	Depending on clinical status
Echocardiography	Depending on clinical status

■ VASOACTIVE AGENTS AND MECHANISM OF ACTION

Dopamine	• Dosage—10–20 µg/kg/min • Mechanism—dopaminergic receptor (<2 µg/kg/min; endocrine and renal effects—decreased thyrotropin, thyroxine, and renal vasodilatation); β1 receptor (2–6 µg/kg/min; increased myocardial contractility); a1 receptor (>6 µg/kg/min; vasoconstriction) • Indirect action on α1, β1 receptors via release of catecholamine • Side effects—pulmonary vasoconstriction at all doses (can be detrimental PPHN); arrhythmia, and endocrine effects
Dobutamine	• Dosage—10–20 µg/kg/min • Mechanism—direct action on dopaminergic, β1 (myocardial contractility), β2 receptor (peripheral vasodilatation) at dose of up to 10 µg/kg/min; at doses of 10–20 µg/kg/min—vasoconstriction • Better agent to improve blood flow • Side effects—arrhythmias and hypotension • Not to be started in babies with severe hypotension (<3rd centile)
Adrenaline	• Dosage—for improving myocardial contractility and decreasing after load—0.1–0.3 µg/kg/min; for increasing BP—0.3–1.5 µg/kg/min • Mechanism—α1, α2, β1, and β2 receptor actions • Side effects—lactic acidemia, hyperglycemia, tachycardia, and pulmonary vasoconstriction (at high doses only)
Noradrenaline	• Dosage—Similar to adrenaline • Mechanism—α1, α2, β1 (no β2 action) • Used in catecholamine refractory septic shock (warm shock) in pediatric population—improves outcome, limited studies in neonates
Milrinone	• Dosage—Loading—50–75 µg/kg over—followed by 0.5–1.5 µg/kg/min • PDE-III inhibitor, inotropic, lusitropic, and inodilatory effects • Use—postcardiac surgery myocardial dysfunction, PPHN-related myocardial dysfunction • Side effects—hypotension, tachycardia, tachyarrhythmia, and thrombocytopenia
Vasopressin	• Dosage—low dose preferred (0.0007 IU/kg/min); high dose—0.001–0.02 IU/kg/min); high dose is associated with significant side effects • V1, V2 receptor—increases vasomotor tone and increases cortisol release • Side effects—cutaneous schema, necrosis, and hyponatremia at high doses • Used in catecholamine refractory shock, warm shock, and PPHN (selective pulmonary vasodilator and systemic vasoconstrictor)

■ HOW TO MAKE INOTROPES/VASOACTIVE AGENTS

Drug	Dose	How to make it
Dopamine (1 mL = 40 mg)	5–20 µg/kg/min	Take 1.5 mL/kg of dopamine and add 5% dextrose to it. Final volume 50 mL. 1 mL/h of this solution is equivalent to 20 µg/kg/h
Dobutamine (1 mL = 50 mg)	5–20 µg/kg/min	Take 1.2 mL/kg of dobutamine and add 5% dextrose to it. Final volume 50 mL. 1 mL/h of this solution is equivalent to 20 µg/kg/h
Adrenaline (1 mL = 1 mg)	0.05–0.5 µg/kg/min	Take 1.5 mL/kg of epinephrine and add 5% dextrose to it to make final volume of 50 mL. 1 mL/h of this solution is equivalent to 0.5 µg/kg/min

Contd...

Contd...

Drug	Dose	How to make it
Noradrenaline (1 mL = 1 mg)	0.05–0.5 µg/kg/min	Take 1.5 mL/kg of epinephrine and add 5% dextrose to it to make final volume of 50 mL. 1 mL/h of this solution is equivalent to 0.5 µg/kg/min
Milrinone (10 mL = 10 mg)	• Loading 50 µg/kg IV over 30 min • Maintenance 0.3–0.75 µg/kg/min	*Dilution (prepared solution)* • Dilute 10 mL of milrinone with 90 mL of NS/D5 (resultant 1 mL = 100 µg) *Loading dose* • Take 0.5 mL/kg (50 µg/kg) of prepared solution and add D5 to it to make total volume 5 mL. Give it over 30 minutes at rate of 10 mL/h *Maintenance* • Running rest of prepared solution at 0.3 mL/kg/h is equivalent to 0.5 µg/kg/min
Sildenafil (10 mg = 12.5 mL)	• Loading 0.4 mg/kg over 3 hours • Maintenance 1.6 mg/kg/day (0.067 mg/kg/h)	*Strength 0.8 mg/mL* • Prepared solution—to 10 mL of sildenafil, add 90 mL of normal saline. Resultant concentration = 0.08 mg/mL *Loading* • Take 5 mL/kg of prepared solution and give it over 3 hours *Maintenance* • Run rest of prepared solution at 0.8 mL/kg/h (1.6 mg/kg/day)
PGE1 (Prostin) 1 mL = 500 µg	0.05–0.1 µg/kg/min	Dilute 1 mL of drug with 49 mL NS to give final concentration of 10 µg/mL and then 0.3 × wt = …. mL/h (0.05 µg/kg/min) 0.6 × wt = …. mL/h (0.1 µg/kg/min)

Key Points to Remember

- Restoring perfusion is the mainstay in shock management.
- Shock and hypotension are not synonyms as hypotension is a late signs of shock.
- Monitor all sick neonates for early signs of shock and treat immediately.
- Supportive care, fluid resuscitation, and inotropes are mainstay of therapy.
- If signs of poor perfusion persist despite two fluid blouses, start vasopressor.
- *Assessment of improvement:*
  - Improvement in CRT
  - Decrease in HR by at least 10 bpm
  - Improvement in pulse volume and increase in urine output next 4–6 hours
- If Hb is <12 g% consider blood transfusion.

Tapering Inotropes

- Start tapering if the baby remains stable for a period of at least 4–6 hours after inotrope initiation.
- Mean blood pressure can be taken as a marker for tapering inotropes. Keep target mean blood pressure 5 mm Hg above the threshold for starting inotropes. Start tapering, if the mean blood pressure is above your target.

- No set protocol for how much to decrease, try to decrease slowly.
- Inotrope added last should be tapered first and omitted, followed by the previous one.

Therapeutic End Points

- Normal pulse volume and capillary refilling time <3 seconds
- Normal heart rate 110–160 bpm
- Warm extremities
- Blood pressure—Between 10th and 90th centile for gestational and postnatal age
- Urine output ≥1 mL/kg/h (valid only beyond 48 hours of life)
- Improvement in mental status
- Difference in pre-post ductal SpO_2 <5%
- Echocardiographically—superior vena cava (SVC) flow >50 mL/kg/min, ejection fraction (EF) >50%, left ventricular output (LVO) >150 mL/kg/min (if PDA has closed) or right ventricular output (RVO) (PV maximum >2 m/s; if PDA is patent).

■ FURTHER READING

1. Rennie JM. Rennie and Roberton's Textbook of Neonatology, 5th edition. Edinburgh: Churchill Livingstone Elsevier. London, UK; 2012.
2. Fanaroff and Martin's Neonatal-Perinatal Medicine, 11th edition; 2019.

Management of Patent Ductus Arteriosus

Kiran More, Atif Majit

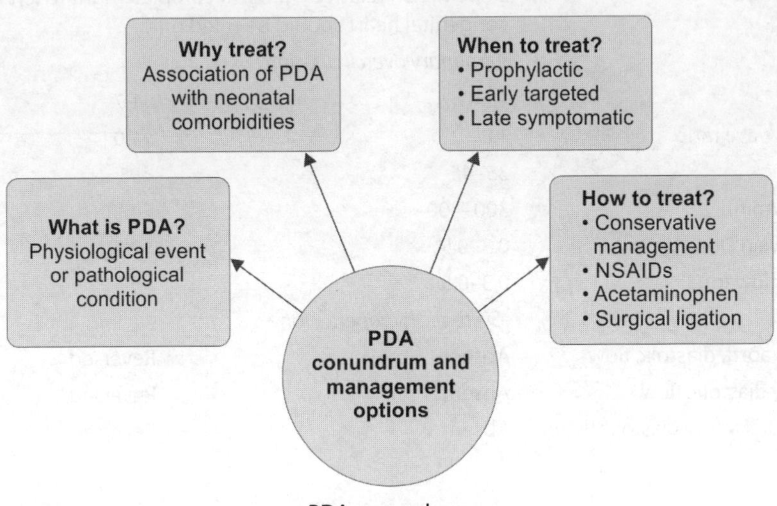

PDA conundrum.

■ PATENT DUCTUS ARTERIOSUS DIAGNOSIS

1. Clinical Signs

- Bounding peripheral pulses
- Hyperactive precordium
- Tachycardia
- Wide pulse pressure (15–25 mm Hg)
- Crescendo systolic murmur
- Episodes of desaturation, bradycardia, or apnea
- Feeding intolerance
- Unexplained metabolic acidosis or hypercarbia
- Signs of congestive cardiac failure
- Episodes of apnea
- Increased ventilatory requirement
- Ventilator dependence

2. Echocardiography Assessment

Timing of performing echo screening: When clinically symptomatic or signs of PDA are present or in the first 72 hours.

ECHO parameters to assess significance of PDA.		
Measurement	*Moderate PDA*	*Large PDA*
Ductus arteriosus		
Diameter (mm)	1.5–3.0	>3.0
Ductal velocity (m/s)	1.5–2.0	<1.5
Flow pattern	Pulsatile unrestrictive	Pulsatile unrestrictive
Direction of flow	Depends on relative Qp:Qs, (if complete right to left flow then congenital heart should be ruled out)	
Pulmonary overcirculation		
LA:Ao ratio	1.5–1.7	>1.7
E wave to A wave ratio	1.0	>1.0
IVRT (ms)	35–45	<35
LVO (mL/kg/min)	300–400	>400
Pulmonary vein Doppler (m/s)	0.3–0.5	>0.5
PA diastolic flow (m/s)	0.3–0.5	>0.5
Systemic hypoperfusion		
Descending aorta diastolic flow	Absent	Reversed
Celiac artery diastolic flow	Absent	Reversed
Middle cerebral artery diastolic flow	Absent	Reversed

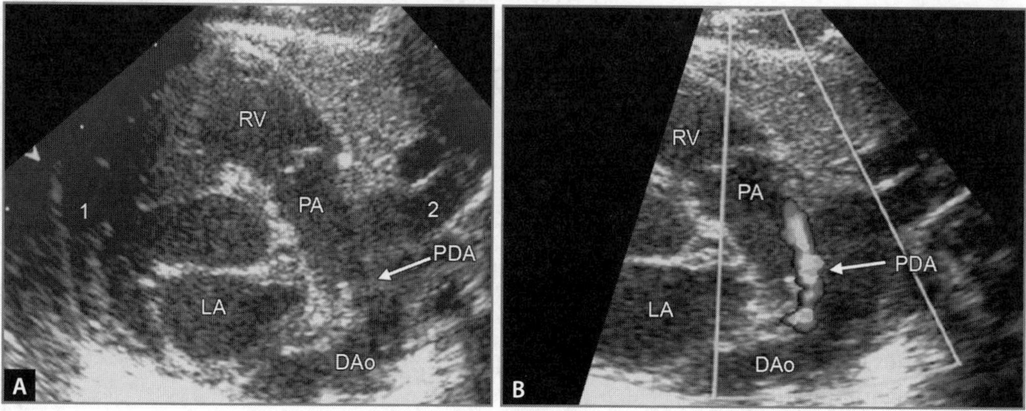

2D and color Doppler of ductal flow.

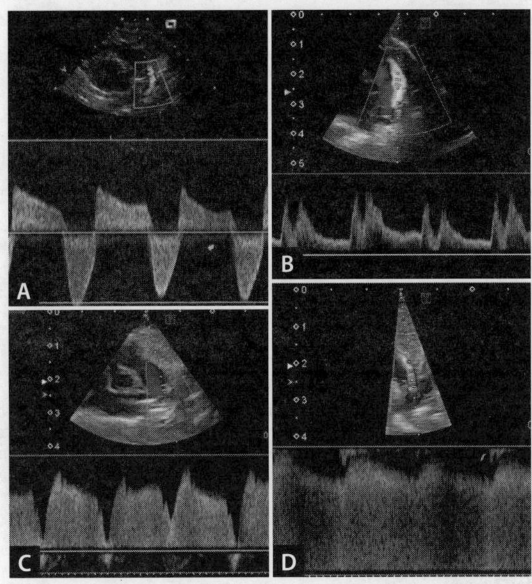

Various ductal flow patterns. (A) Bidirectional shunting in pulmonary hypertension; (B) Pulsatile pattern in unrestrictive hemodynamically significant duct; (C) Growing pattern in transitional circulation; and (D) Closing or continuous pattern in constricting ductus.

3. Biomarkers at Point of Care

Table 1 summarizes utility of these biomarkers for assessing hsPDA.

TABLE 1: Utility of biomarkers assisting diagnosis of PDA.

Biomarkers	Time of testing	Relevance
Plasma N-terminal pro-B type natriuretic peptide (NT-proBNP)	Day 3	May correlate with size and high value may predict hsPDA
Urinary NT-proBNP	Day 2	May correlate with ductal patency
Serum troponin T	48 hours	May correlate with patency, diameter, left atrial-to-aortic diameter ratio, and descending aortic end-diastolic velocity

All markers currently of research interest and not recommended routinely.

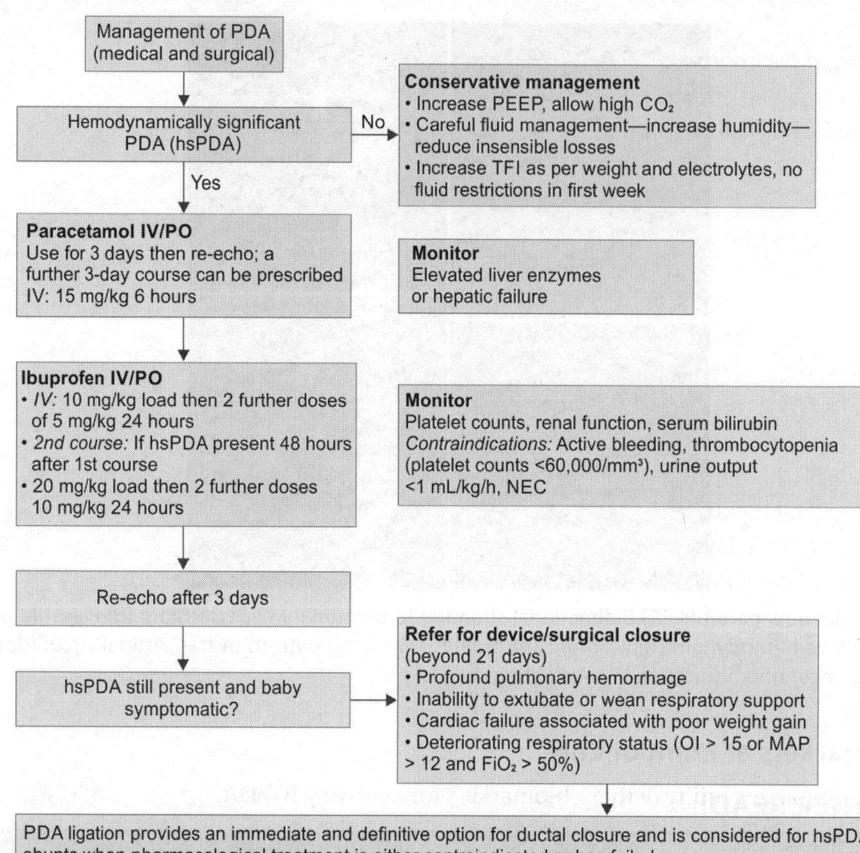

Key Points to Remember

- In the fetus, ductus arteriosus (DA) is an indispensable for fetal survival but clinicians have struggled to understand the significance of a patent ductus arteriosus (PDA) and debated whether to treat it or not.
- Incidence of PDA in very preterm babies varies inversely proportional to gestation and depends on age of babies at assessment.
- A significant PDA is associated with increase in morbidity in preterm infants such as death, and/or severe morbidity, intraventricular hemorrhage (IVH), bronchopulmonary dysplasia (BPD), necrotizing enterocolitis (NEC), and an increased risk of adverse neurodevelopmental outcomes at 2–3 years of age.

- *Conservative approach:* Utilizing strategies to decrease the shunt volume and or the hemodynamics effects of PDA which includes increasing PEEP, careful fluid management, and judicious use of diuretics.
- *Restrictive versus liberal fluids:* Fluid restriction may compromise tissue perfusion in presence of aortic steal and low volumes before surgical closure of PDA could increase the postsurgical complications, so routine fluid restriction not recommended.
- *Furosemide* use could delay its spontaneous closure due to increasing prostaglandin responsiveness of ductus.
- *Choice of respiratory support:* No evidence suggests that noninvasive respiratory support reduces the incidence of PDA.
- *Use of caffeine affects PDA:* Reported a reduction in the rates of death or BPD and PDA and also significant reduction in PDA requiring medical or surgical closure.
- *Indomethacin (Indo) therapy—treatment regimens:* Standard initial dose of 0.2 mg/kg followed by two 0.1 mg/kg daily for 3 days, slow infusion. Prophylaxis 0.1 mg/kg once a day for up to 5 days.
- Transcatheter surgical closure is an emerging technique that could potentially reduce the side effects of surgical closure and offer definitive closure of persistent PDA.
- The genetics and better understanding of pharmacodynamics of drugs would help in dose optimization to provide effective treatment dose while minimizing the side effect profile.

■ FURTHER READING

1. More K, Gupta S. (2020) Patent Ductus Arteriosus: The Conundrum and Management Options. In: Boyle E, Cusack J (Eds). Emerging Topics and Controversies in Neonatology. Cham, Switzerland: Springer; 2020.
2. Morville P, Douchin S, Bouvaist H, Dauphin C. Transcatheter occlusion of the patent ductus arteriosus in premature infants weighing less than 1200 g. Arch Dis Child Fetal Neonatal Ed. 2018;103(3):F198-F201.
3. Singh Y, Fraisse A, Erdeve O, Atasay B. Echocardiographic Diagnosis and Hemodynamic Evaluation of Patent Ductus Arteriosus in Extremely Low Gestational Age Newborn (ELGAN) Infants. Front Pediatr. 2020;8:573627.
4. Weisz DE, More K, McNamara PJ, Shah PS. PDA ligation and health outcomes: A meta-analysis. Pediatrics. 2014;133(4):e1024-46.

Management of Persistent Pulmonary Hypertension

Ashok C

When to suspect PPHN?
- *Hypoxemic respiratory failure* with $AaDO_2 > 200$, $OI > 10$, hyperoxia test $PaO_2 < 150$
- *Differential cyanosis* (higher saturations in preductal—right upper limb than postductal)
  - Saturation difference >5%/PaO_2 difference of >10 mm Hg
  - Coarctation of aorta, HLHS, interrupted arch has differential cyanosis
- *Labile saturations:*
  - During routine handling/nursing care/light sound baby saturation level drops
  - Unlike, in cyanotic CHD saturations are fixed
- *Secondary lung parenchymal condition:* MAS, RDS, TTN, CDH, pneumonia, effusion, and air-leak

Confirm by echocardiography and rule out structural anomalies

Mild PPHN:	*Moderate PPHN:*	*Severe PPHN:*
- OI 10–15 - TR peak velocity <2 m/s and SPAP < 20 mm Hg [$4*TR^2 +5$] - LV in short-axis view "O" shaped—RV pressure <50% of LV - PDA left to right shunt - Atrial shunt (PFO) left to right - Tricuspid annular plane systolic excursion—TAPSE normal - Doppler pulmonary artery acceleration time (PAAT)—normal - Normal LV function	- OI 15–20 - TR 2–4 m/s and SPAP 20–40 mm Hg - LV "D" shaped—RV pressure 50–100% LV - PDA bidirectional flow - PFO bidirectional - RV dilated - RV systolic function normal TAPSE > 8 mm - PAAT: 40–90 ms - LV—ejection fraction unreliable if RV dilated - LV assessed by LVO, LV Tei index, biplanar EF and tissue Doppler	- OI > 20 - TR > 4 m/s and SPAP > 60 mm Hg - LV 'crescent shaped'—RV pressure ≥100% LV - PDA right to left shunt - PFO bidirectional, if right to left R/O TAPVC - RV dilated - RV systolic dysfunction TAPSE < 6–8 mm - PAAT: <40 ms - LV function impaired in LV Tei (myocardial performance index), biplanar EF, tissue or speckle-tracking Doppler

Short-axis view: Left ventricle configuration and severity of PPHN

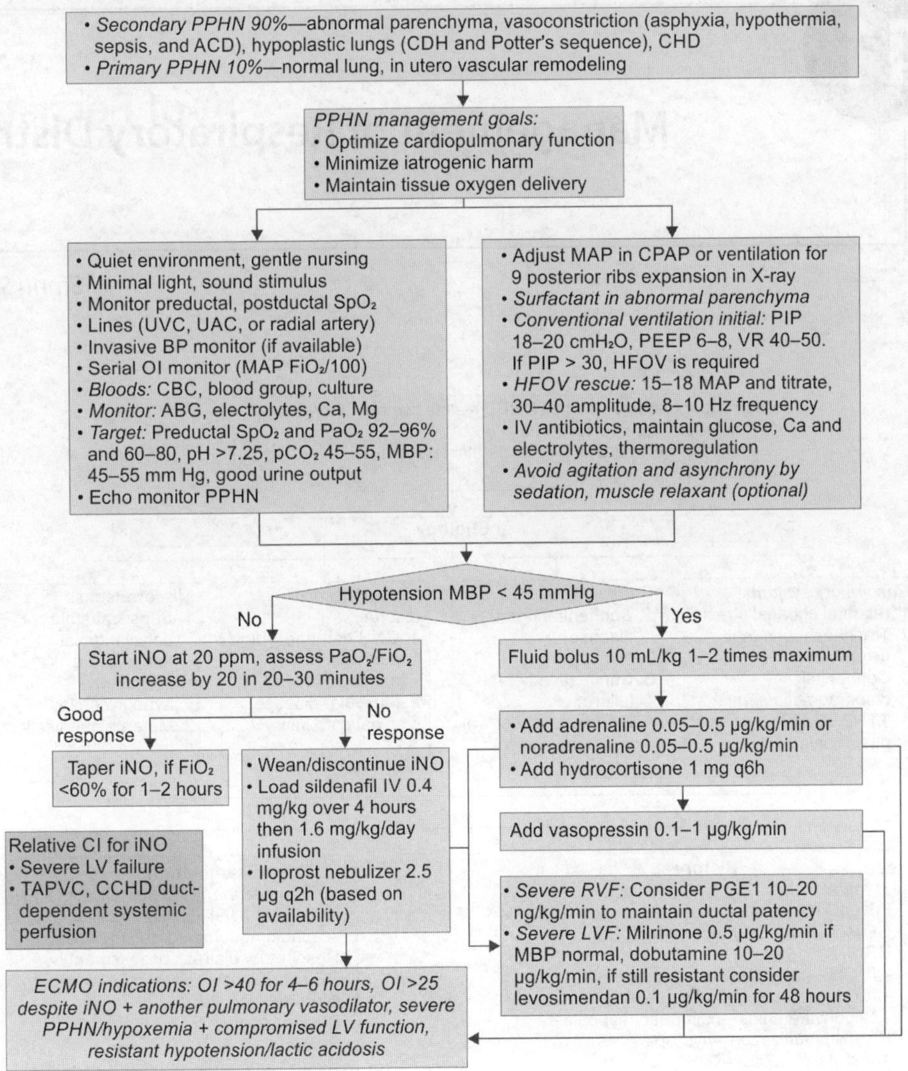

Key Points to Remember

- Confirm diagnosis and PPHN by ECHO.
- Correction of underlying metabolic abnormalities (hypothermia, acidosis, hypocalcemia, hypoglycemia, and polycythemia) is very important before going for iNO therapy.
- Consider tolerating postductal SpO₂ >75%.
- Avoid hyperventilation, CO₂ washout and bicarbonate therapy.

Chapter 11

Management of Respiratory Distress

Smriti Saryan

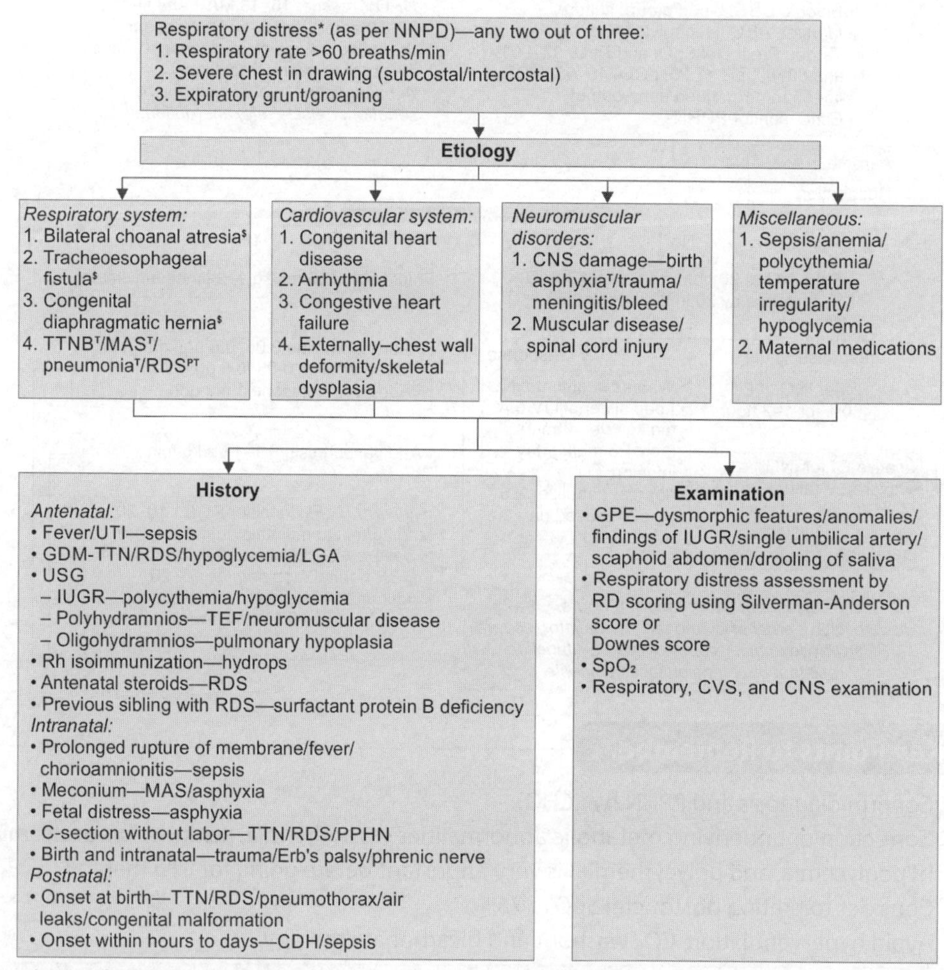

*According to facility-based newborn care module for respiratory distress and 1 out of 4 criteria should be present. The first 3 criteria are same as NNPD but the fourth criteria apnea or gasping has been added.

$Common surgical causes

^{T}Common causes of RD in term baby

^{PT}Common causes of RD in preterm baby

Contd...

Contd...

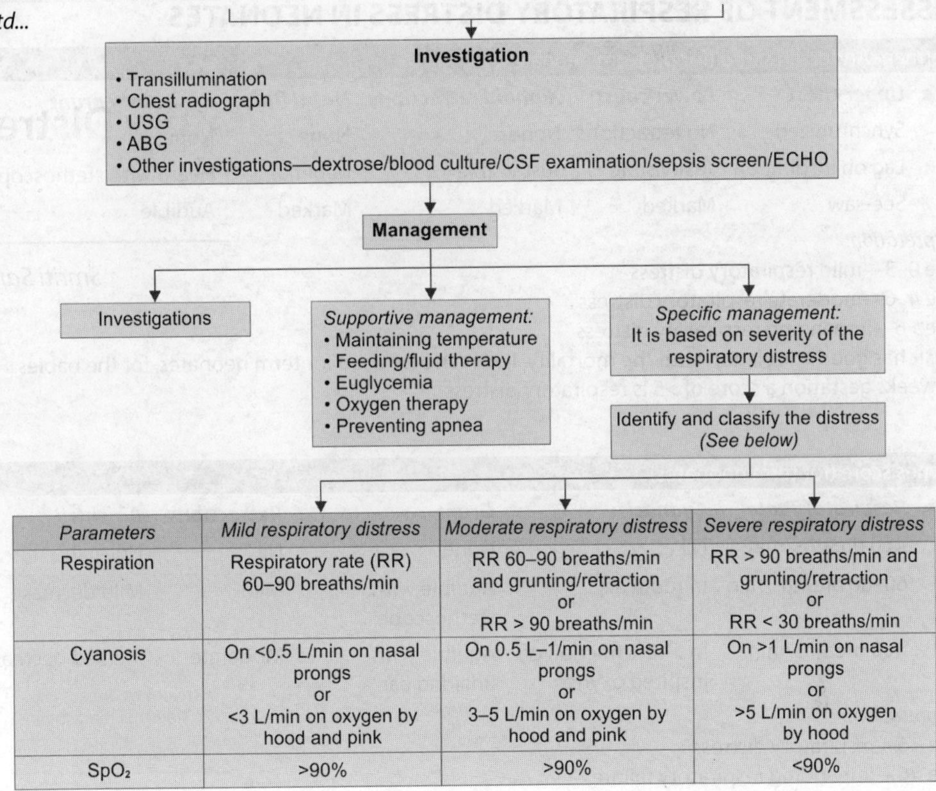

Parameters	Mild respiratory distress	Moderate respiratory distress	Severe respiratory distress
Respiration	Respiratory rate (RR) 60–90 breaths/min	RR 60–90 breaths/min and grunting/retraction or RR > 90 breaths/min	RR > 90 breaths/min and grunting/retraction or RR < 30 breaths/min
Cyanosis	On <0.5 L/min on nasal prongs or <3 L/min on oxygen by hood and pink	On 0.5 L–1/min on nasal prongs or 3–5 L/min on oxygen by hood and pink	On >1 L/min on nasal prongs or >5 L/min on oxygen by hood
SpO_2	>90%	>90%	<90%

▮ SPECIFIC MANAGEMENT PROTOCOL

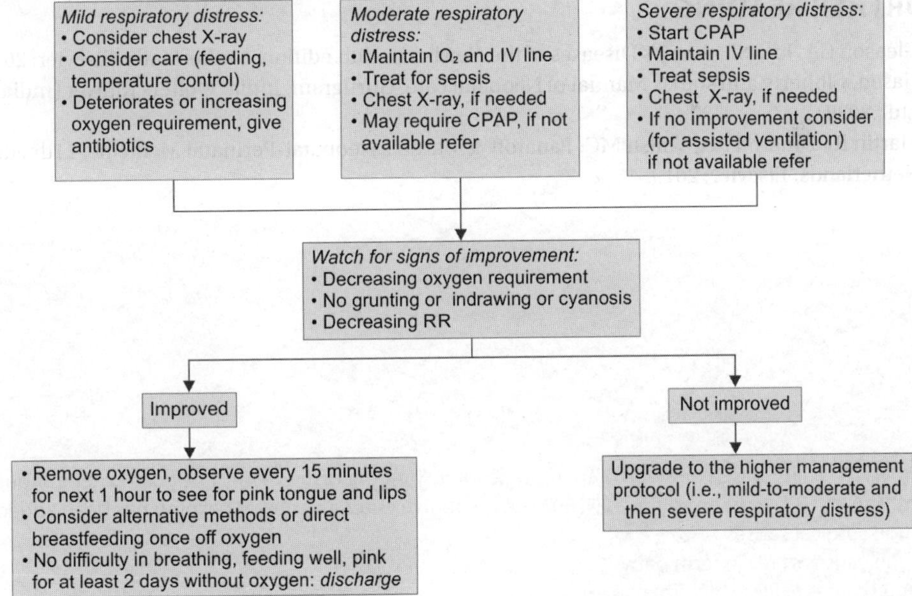

■ ASSESSMENT OF RESPIRATORY DISTRESS IN NEONATES

Silverman–Andersen score (for preterm neonates)

Score	Upper chest	Lower chest	Xiphoid retractions	Nasal flare	Expiratory grunt
0	Synchronized	No retractions	None	None	None
1	Lag on inspiration	Just visible	Just visible	Minimal	Heard with stethoscope
2	See-saw	Marked	Marked	Marked	Audible

Interpretation:
Score 0–3—mild respiratory distress
Score 4–6—moderate respiratory distress
Score >6—impending respiratory distress
Note: It has good correlation with the mortality. It can also be used for term neonates, for the babies >35 weeks gestation a score of >5 is respiratory distress

Downes score (for term neonates)

Score	Respiratory rate	Cyanosis	Grunt	Retractions	Air entry
0	<60 breaths/min	Nil	None	Nil	Normal
1	60–80 breaths/min	In room air	Audible with stethoscope	Mild	Mild decrease
2	>80 breaths/min	In >40% fraction of inspired oxygen	Audible with unaided ear	Moderate	Marked decrease

Interpretation:
Score <6—respiratory distress
Score >6—impending respiratory failure
Note: It correlates with physiological parameters (arterial pH, arterial blood gas) and mortality.

■ FURTHER READING

1. Gleason CA, Juul SE. Avery's Diseases of the Newborn, 10th edition. Netherlands: Elsevier; 2018.
2. Hasen. Cloherty and stark's Manual of Neonatal care. Gurugram, India: Wolters Kluwer (India) Pvt. Ltd.; 2020.
3. Martin RJ, Fanaroff AA, Walsh MC. Fanaroff & Martin's Neonatal-Perinatal Medicine, 11th edition. Netherlands: Elsevier; 2019.

Management of Respiratory Distress Syndrome

Arvind Kant Manipal

- *Risk factors for respiratory distress syndrome (RDS):*
  - Prematurity (most common)
  - Male predominance
  - Maternal diabetes
  - Premature rupture of membrane
  - Elective cesarean in absence of labor
  - Genetic abnormalities of surfactant-associated proteins
  - Perinatal asphyxia

- *Clinical features:*
  - Tachypnea
  - Nasal flaring
  - Grunting
  - Retractions (subcostal, intercostal, and suprasternal)
  - Cyanosis
  - Pallor
  - Lethargic
- *Radiological features:*
  - Low lung volume
  - Ground-glass appearance

■ PATHOPHYSIOLOGY

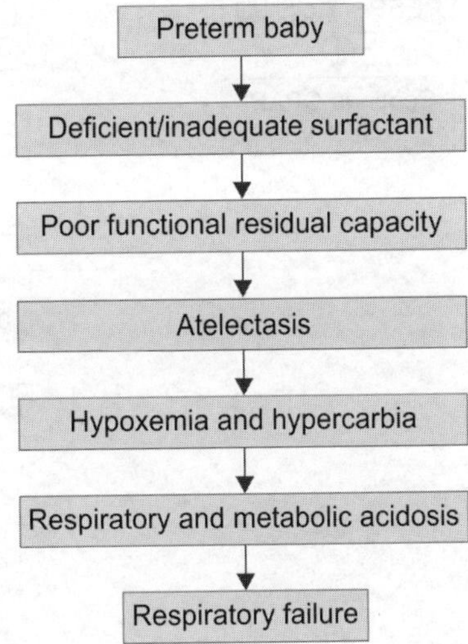

S. No.	Common differential diagnosis	Pointers
1.	Transient tachypnea of newborn	• Common in late preterm and term baby • Chest X-ray—(fluids in fissure)
2.	Sepsis or pneumonia	• Positive sepsis screen • Positive blood culture • Fast deterioration
3.	Meconium aspiration syndrome	• History of MSL • Hyperinflation, patchy opacity
4.	Congenital cardiac disorder	• Not achieve normal saturation level on oxygen support
5.	Perinatal asphyxia	• History of asphyxia
6.	Pulmonary artery hypertension	• Labile oxygen saturation • Pre- and postductal SpO_2 variation >5%
7.	Pneumothorax	• Sudden deterioration • Positive transillumination test
8.	Congenital diaphragmatic hernia	• Severe distress • Scaphoid abdomen
9.	Metabolic	• Hypoglycemia • Hypocalcemia • Polycythemia

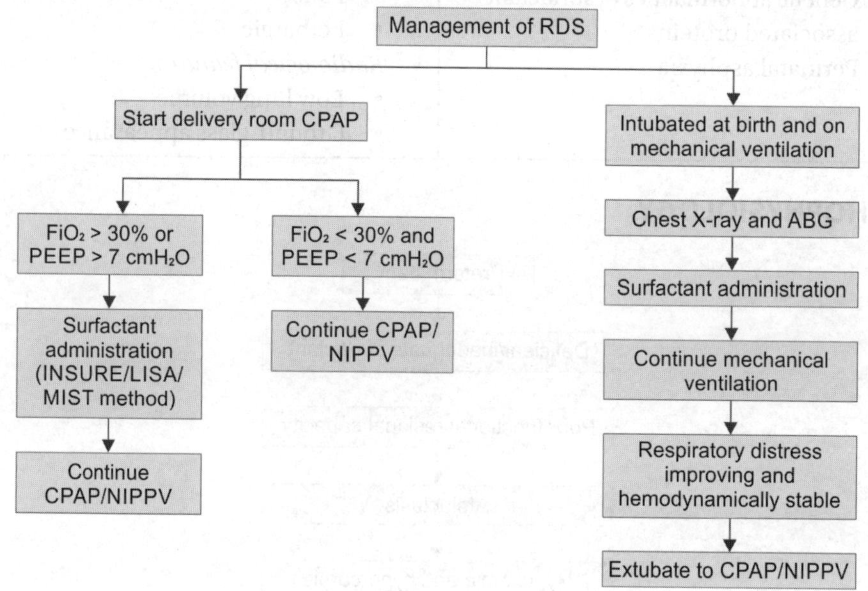

Key Points to Remember

- Respiratory distress syndrome (RDS) is the most common respiratory disorder in preterm newborn (especially in <34 weeks). The incidence of RDS is inversely proportional to gestational age.
- It is because of inadequate surfactant in alveoli that is secreted by type 2 cells in lung, which prevents alveoli to collapse so maintain adequate functional residual capacity (FRC).
- The principal of treatment of RDS is to establish and maintain FRC.
- Newborn with RDS must be started on delivery room continuous positive airway pressure (CPAP) with positive end-expiratory pressure (PEEP) of 5–6 cmH$_2$O and fraction of inspired oxygen (FiO$_2$) as per target saturation.
- Do not do unnecessary investigation [complete blood count (CBC), C-reactive protein (CRP), routine arterial blood gas (ABG)], and routine chest X-ray (perform only when respiratory distress persisting after 6 hours of age, worsening clinical condition and diagnostic dilemma).
- Antenatal corticosteroid to mother to prevent RDS.
- Baby must be spontaneous breathing for CPAP support.
- Noninvasive positive pressure ventilation (NIPPV) may be used for preterm with recurrent apnea.
- Exogenous surfactant administration within 2 hours in preterm with establish RDS who requires PEEP >7 cmH$_2$O or FiO$_2$ >30%.
- Continuous positive airway pressure/NIPPV should be started with caffeine in apnea of prematurity.
- Preterm very low birth weight baby being extubated should be weaned off either to CPAP or NIPPV (preferably).
- Continuous positive airway pressure may be a primary mode of respiratory support in late preterm and term neonate with meconium aspiration syndrome.
- Continuous positive airway pressure should be delivered via nasal mask or binasal prongs and must be snuggly fitted.
- Monitor respiratory distress score to assess improvement/deterioration.
- *Complications of surfactant:* Airway obstruction, bradycardia, hypoxia, and pulmonary hemorrhage.
- *Complications of CPAP:* Pneumothorax, air leak, and nasal trauma.

■ FURTHER READING

1. Gleason CA, Juul SE. Avery's Diseases of the Newborn, 10th edition. Netherlands: Elsevier; 2018.
2. Hasen. Cloherty and Stark's Manual of Neonatal Care. Gurugram, India: Wolters Kluwer (India) Pvt. Ltd.; 2020.
3. Martin RJ, Fanaroff AA, Walsh MC. Fanaroff & Martin's Neonatal-Perinatal Medicine, 11th edition. Netherlands: Elsevier; 2019.
4. Sweet DG, Carnielli V, Greisen G, Hallman M, Ozek E, Te Pas A, et al. European consensus guidelines on the management of respiratory distress syndrome-2019 Update. Neonatology. 2019;115(4):432-50.

Management of Meconium Aspiration

Vivek Choudhury

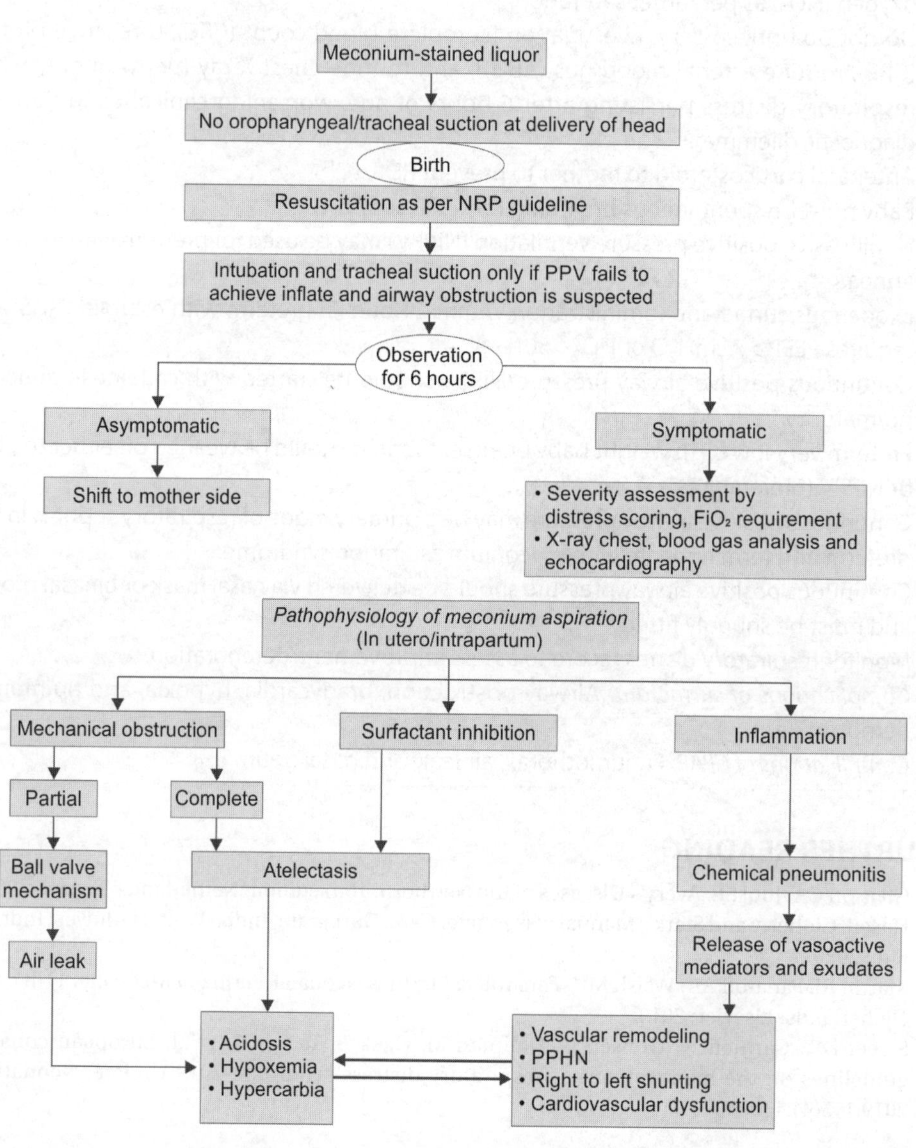

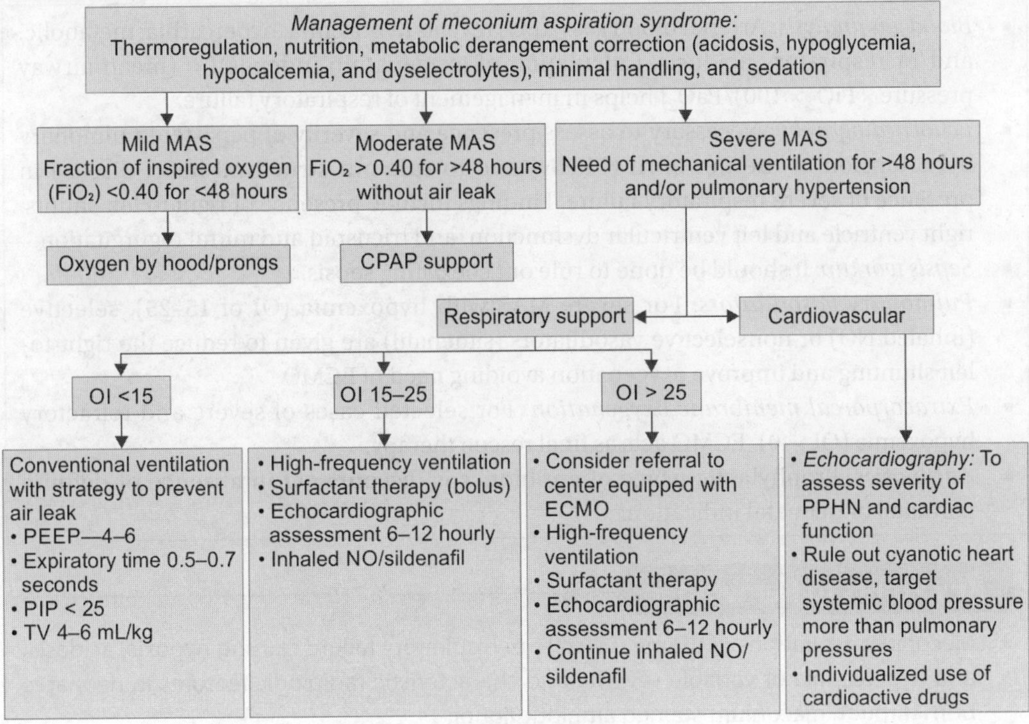

MANAGEMENT

Delivery room management: As per latest NRP recommendation—

Neonatal intensive care unit strategy:

- *General management:* Supportive treatment includes thermoregulation, minimal tactile or auditory stimulation, correction of metabolic abnormalities if any, and maintenance of perfusion.

- *Respiratory support:* Degree of respiratory failure is assessed by respiratory distress scoring, FiO_2 requirement, and oxygenation index. Target preductal oxygen saturation is 90–95%.

- *Ventilation strategy:* Aim is to prevent hypoxemia with minimizing risk of air leak.
  - In absence of severe hypoxemia/PPHN, ventilation should target to achieve PaO_2 between 60 and 80 mm Hg and a $PaCO_2$ of 40–50 mm Hg with PIP not exceeding 25 cmH_2O, PEEP of 4–6 cmH_2O and adequate expiratory time to prevent air trapping.
  - In presence of severe PPHN, high-frequency ventilation is preferred to conventional ventilation with higher setting to recruit lung parenchyma with minimal barotrauma and air leak.

- *Surfactant therapy:* Evidence from meta-analysis suggests surfactant therapy reduces the severity of respiratory distress and need of extracorporeal membrane oxygenation (ECMO) in neonates with invasive ventilation and high FiO_2 requirement. Threshold cut offs suggested are different, for example oxygenation index more than 15 (by NNF-CPG 2021), FiO_2 > 50% on invasive ventilation (Canadian Pediatric Society).

- *Blood gas analysis:* Arterial blood gas (ABG) reveals hypoxemia, hypercarbia, metabolic, and/or respiratory acidosis. Calculation of oxygenation index [OI = (mean airway pressure × FiO_2 × 100)/PaO_2] helps in management of respiratory failure.
- *Echocardiography:* Necessary to assess presence and severity of persistent pulmonary hypertension of the newborn (PPHN) and to rule out structural heart disease in presence of severe respiratory failure. Findings include presence of right to left shunts, right ventricle and left ventricular dysfunction, and tricuspid and mitral regurgitation.
- *Sepsis workup:* It should be done to rule out coexisting sepsis.
- *Pulmonary vasodilators:* For severe MAS with hypoxemia (OI of 15–25), selective (inhaled NO) or nonselective vasodilators (sildenafil) are given to reduce the right-to-left shunting and improve oxygenation avoiding need of ECMO
- *Extracorporeal membrane oxygenation:* For selected cases of severe and refractory hypoxemia (OI >40). ECMO acts as final rescue therapy.
- *Antibiotics:* Prophylactic usage of antibiotics is discouraged in absence of definite perinatal or neonatal indication.

Key Points to Remember

- Meconium aspiration syndrome is a state of respiratory failure causing hypoxia, acidosis, and hypercapnia of variable severity and characteristic radiologic features in neonates born through meconium-stained amniotic liquor.
- Incidence of meconium aspiration syndrome is 3–12% among all deliveries through meconium-stained amniotic fluid. Probability of meconium-stained liquor increases as gestation increases like 3–5% in 37–38 weeks, 10–15% at 39–41 weeks, and 20–30% in gestation >42 weeks.
- Risk factors for developing meconium aspiration include gestational age >40 weeks, moderate or thick meconium stained, need of resuscitation at birth, and low cord pH, maternal tobacco use.
- Among babies with meconium aspiration, approximately half of them require advance ventilator support and mortality rate is 10–12%.

■ FURTHER READING

1. Delivery of a newborn with meconium-stained amniotic fluid. Committee Opinion No. 689. American College of Obstetricians and Gynecologists. Obstet Gynecol. 2017;129:e33-4.
2. Monfredini C, Cavallin F, Villani PE, Paterlini G, Allais B, Trevisanuto D. Meconium Aspiration Syndrome: A Narrative Review. Children (Basel). 2021;8:230.
3. Nangia S, Chandrasekharan P, Lakshminrusimha S, Rawat M. Approach to Infants Born Through Meconium Stained Amniotic Fluid: Evolution Based on Evidence? Am J Perinatol. 2018;35:815-22.
4. Weiner, Gary M, Jeanette Zaichkin J. Textbook of Neonatal Resuscitation, 8th edition. Elk Grove Village, IL: American Academy of Pediatrics; 2021.

14

Management of Apnea

Richa Malik

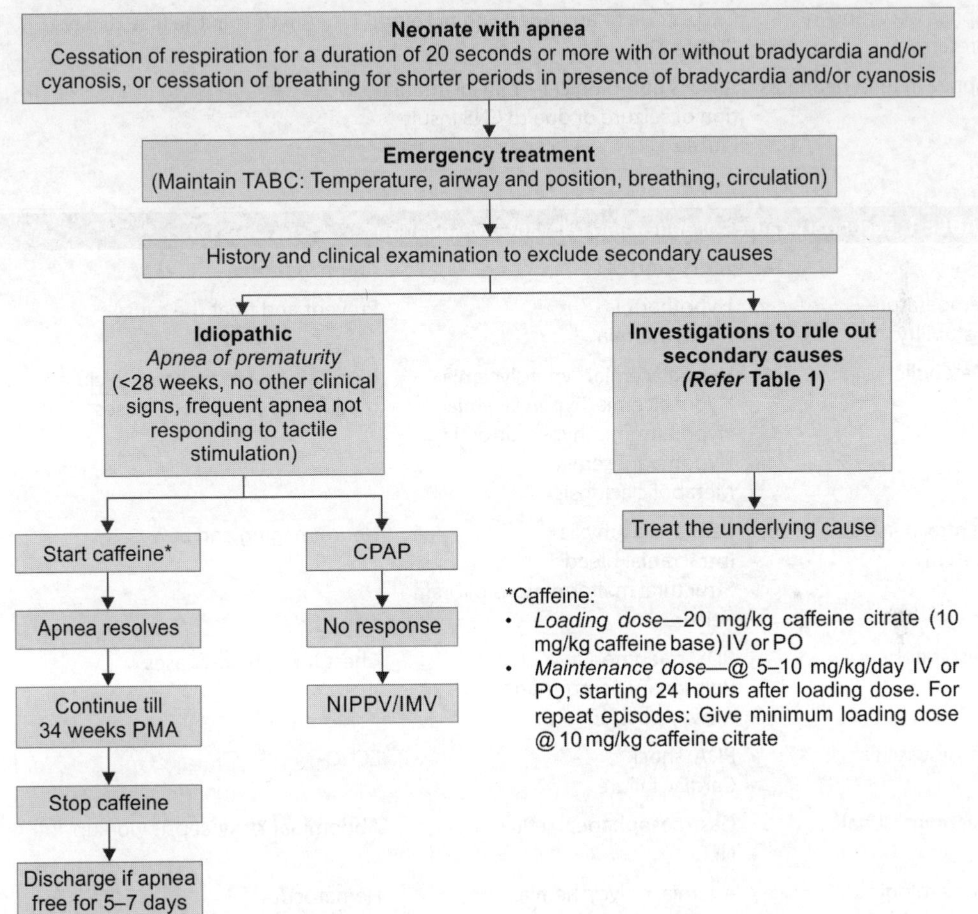

■ CLASSIFICATION

Type	Pathology
Central apnea (40%)	Total cessation of inspiratory efforts with no evidence of obstruction
Obstructive (10%)	Obstructive apnea occurs due to upper airway block and decreased laryngeal and pharyngeal reflexes
Mixed (50%)	Combination of both

Classification based on etiology		
Apnea of prematurity (AOP)	Occurs due to immaturity of respiratory system	Usually, 2–7 days of postnatal life
Apnea occurring in preterms	Occurs due to an underlying problem **(Table 1)**	Anytime in the first 28 days
Apnea in term neonates	Always pathological—may be manifestation of seizure or due to CNS insult **(Table 1)**	

TABLE 1: Secondary causes of apnea and relevant investigations.

	Secondary causes	Investigations
Temperature instability	• Hypothermia • Hyperthermia	Prevent and treat the cause
Metabolic	• Hypoglycemia/hyperglycemia • Hypocalcemia/hypercalcemia • Hyponatremia/hypernatremia • Hypomagnesemia • Metabolic acidosis	Blood sugar, electrolytes, calcium, magnesium, and blood gases
Central nervous system	• Perinatal asphyxia • Intracranial bleed • Structural malformations of brain • Seizures	Neuroimaging and EEG
Respiratory	• RDS, pneumonia • Pulmonary hemorrhage • Airway obstruction	Chest X-ray, blood gases
Cardiovascular	• PDA, shock • Cardiac failure	ECHO
Gastrointestinal	• Gastroesophageal reflux • NEC	Abdominal X-ray, sepsis workup
Hematological	• Anemia, polycythemia	Hematocrit
Infections	• Septicemia, meningitis	Sepsis screen, blood culture, and CSF examination
Miscellaneous	• Inborn errors of metabolism (IEM) • Improper neck posture	IEM workup

Respiratory irregularity seen in REM sleep in preterms	Decrease in carotid body chemoreceptor sensitivity
Pathogenesis: Central apnea	
Decreased ventilator response to hypercapnia and hypoxia	Upregulation of inhibitory neurotransmitters like GABA and adenosine

MANAGEMENT

Immediate Measures

- Stimulating the neonate
- Correcting any obvious causes [maintain temperature, airway and position, breathing, and circulation (TABC)]
- Providing oxygen, if there is persistent desaturation (target SpO_2 90–95%)
- Positive pressure ventilation with bag and mask if no response to stimulation

Treatment of the underlying cause: Antibiotics for sepsis, correction of polycythemia, hypoglycemia or hypocalcemia, and transfuse packed cells (according to guidelines).

Pharmacotherapy

Caffeine is preferred over aminophylline owing to wide therapeutic index and long half-life (Refer to Neonatal Medication chapter).

Mechanism of action:
- Caffeine is a nonspecific inhibitor of adenosine receptors A1 and A2A, located at multiple sites in brain
- Increases CO_2 sensitivity
- Improves minute ventilation
- Decreases hypoxic depression of breathing
- Enhances diaphragmatic activity

Ventilation

- Nasal intermittent positive pressure ventilation (NIPPV) and continuous positive airway pressure (CPAP) can be considered if significant apneic episodes persist despite optimal caffeine therapy. Consider stopping CPAP/NIPPV if no episodes of apnea/ desaturation for 24–48 hours.
- *Mechanical ventilation:* Used if above therapies fail to improve apnea.

> ## Key Points to Remember
>
> - Apnea of prematurity is a diagnosis of exclusion and should be considered only after secondary causes of apnea have been excluded.
> - It is inversely proportional to gestation age (10–20% in neonates <35 weeks to 60–80% among neonates <28 weeks of gestation).
> - It usually resolves by 36–37 weeks' postmenstrual age (PMA) in those born at 28 weeks of gestation or more. In infants born before 28 weeks, spells may persist beyond 40 weeks' PMA.
> - Repeated episodes can result in long-term neurological sequelae and retinopathy of prematurity.

■ FURTHER READING

1. Eichenwald EC, AAP Committee on Fetus and Newborn. Apnea of prematurity. Pediatrics. 2016;137(1):e20153757.
2. Eichenwald EC. National and international guidelines for caffeine use. Are they evidence based? Semin Fetal Neonatal Med. 2020;25(6):1011.
3. Schmidt B, Roberts RS, Davis P, Doyle LW, Barrington KJ, et al. Caffeine for Apnea of Prematurity Trial Group. Caffeine therapy for apnea of prematurity. N Engl J Med. 2006;354(20):2112-21.
4. Schmidt B, Roberts RS, Davis P, Doyle LW, Barrington KJ, M Ohlsson A, et al. Long-term effects of caffeine therapy for apnea of prematurity. N Engl J Med. 2007;357(19):1893-902.

Management of Pulmonary Hemorrhage

Gaurav Jawa, Aheed Khan

Pulmonary hemorrhage in neonates

Incidence
1 to 12 per 1000 live births

↓

Risk factors
- Prematurity
- Perinatal asphyxia or bleeding disorders
- Patent ductus arteriosus (PDA)
- Erythroblastosis fetalis
- Breech delivery
- Hypothermia, infection
- Respiratory distress syndrome
- Administration of exogenous surfactant
- Thrombocytopenia

↓

Presentation: Typically, preterm with frothy pink secretions from endotracheal tube

↓

Increased work of breathing/ventilator requirements/fraction of inspired oxygen (FiO$_2$) needs
Progression to apneas, pallor, and bradycardia with drop in blood pressure

↓

Investigations
- Chest X-ray (CXR) with nonspecific fluffy opacities/white-out lungs
- ECHO to rule out PDA left to right shunt
- Blood gas/complete blood count (CBC), prothrombin time (PT), activated partial thromboplastin time (aPTT), fibrinogen, and D-dimer levels
- Sepsis screen

↓

Management
- *Supportive therapy:* Increased ventilator settings with positive end-expiratory pressure (PEEP) 6–8 cm to splint the blood vessels, higher FiO$_2$. High-frequency oscillatory ventilation (HFOV) has shown better results in studies for pulmonary hemorrhage resolution
- Intravenous (IV) fluids, inotropes, and blood products based on CBC report
- Blood products mostly used as adjunctive therapy
- Vitamin K can be given as second dose
- Fresh frozen plasma (FFP) and platelets for coagulopathy
- Prothrombin complex concentrate (PCC)/whole blood for correction of anemia
- Surfactant administration: Shown to impair platelet aggregation and improve PT. Recent review shows improved mortality with no change in long-term pulmonary morbidities.
- *ET adrenaline* (1:1,000) in the dose of 0.05–0.1 mL/kg has shown benefit
- Recombinant factor VIIa increases thrombin activity and shown to decrease mortality
- *Tolazoline,* nonselective α-adrenergic agonist, given to extremely low birth weight (ELBW) baby as 1–3 mg/kg intravenous stat and if needed as continuous infusion of 2 mg/k/h has shown to mitigate severe respiratory compromise in PH
- Hemocoagulase has been reported as a new effective treatment for PH. It is a purified mixture of enzymes derived from the venom of the Brazilian snake Bothrops atrox and has a thromboplastin-like effect by converting prothrombin to thrombin and fibrinogen to fibrin. Recommended dose of 0.5 KU every 4–6 hours till bleeding stops

---

Key Points to Remember

- A total of 60% of premature infants who survive PH will develop bronchopulmonary dysplasia (BPD).
- An increased incidence of CP and cognitive delay (odds ratio 2.86 and 2.4, respectively) has been reported.
- PH is also associated with an increased risk of seizures and periventricular leukomalacia (PVL) in survivors at 18 months of age.

FURTHER READING

1. AlKharfy TM. High-frequency ventilation in the management of very-low-birth-weight infants with pulmonary hemorrhage. Am J Perinatol. 2004;21(1):19-26.
2. Aziz A, Ohlsson A. Surfactant for pulmonary hemorrhage in neonates. Cochrane Database Syst Rev. 2008;(2):CD005254.
3. Barnes ME, Feeney E, Duncan A, Jassim S, MacNamara H, O'Hara J, et al. Pulmonary haemorrhage in neonates: Systematic review of management. Acta Paediatr. 2022;111(2):236-44.

Management of Bronchopulmonary Dysplasia

Utkarsh Sharma, Vishal Kaushik

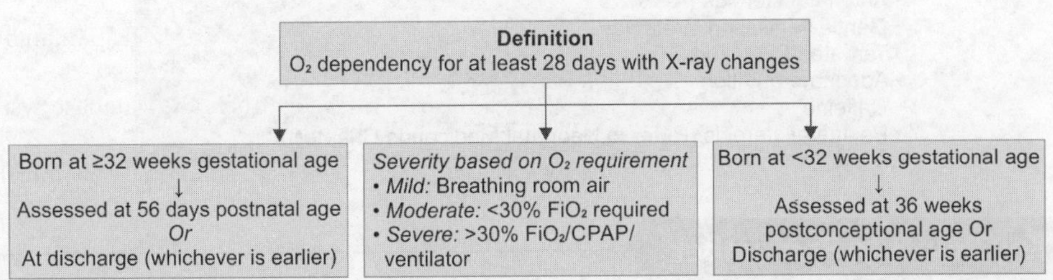

NICHD BPD definition for premature infants <32 weeks requires the following FiO_2 to main SpO_2 in the range of 90–95% for ≥3 consecutive days

Grades	I	II	III
Invasive ventilation		21	>21
n-CPAP, NIPPV or nasal cannula ≥3 L/min	21	22–29	≥30
Nasal cannula 1 to <3 L/min, O_2 by hood	22–29	≥30	
Nasal cannula flow of <1 L/min	22–70	>70	

◾ PATHOGENESIS

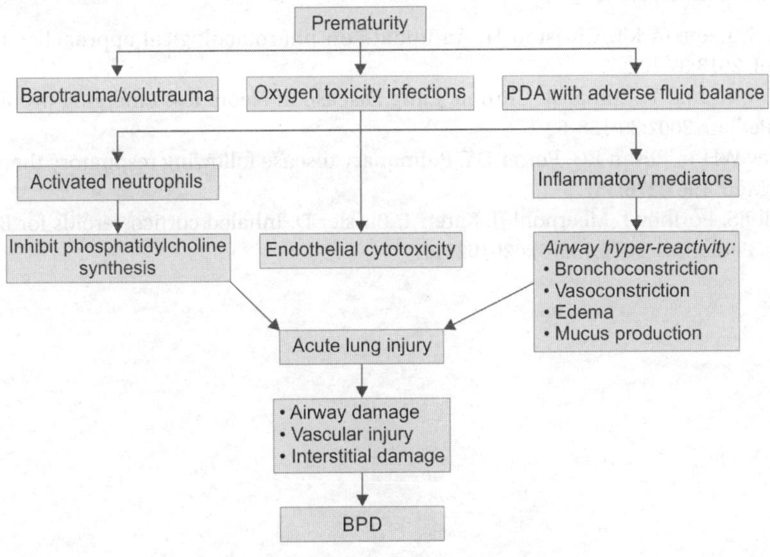

Clinical presentation

- Signs of respiratory distress and increased work of breathing
- Rales and coarse rhonchi on auscultation
- Aspiration along with feeding difficulties is common.
- Four distinct radiographic appearances as described by *Northway et al.*:
  - *Stage 1*—Indistinguishable from severe RDS (1–3 days)
  - *Stage 2*—Marked radiopacity of lungs (4–10 days)
  - *Stage 3*—Cystic, bubbly pattern (10–20 days)
  - *Stage 4*—Hyperexpansion, streaks of abnormal density, areas of emphysema and variable cardiomegaly (from 1 month)

Management

Established strategies
- Antenatal steroids (ANS)
- Gentle ventilation strategies
- Targeted SpO_2 and FiO_2
- Adequate nutrition
- Caffeine
- Postnatal steroids (Refer to Neonatal Medication Chapter)

Key Points to Remember

- Affects 15–50% of very low birth weight babies worldwide.
- Incidence is inversely related to gestational age and birth weight.
- Increased rates have been observed in some parts of the world due to improved survival of immature infants.
- For all oxygen-dependent babies, bronchopulmonary dysplasia (BPD) is now being used as an umbrella term instead of chronic lung disease (CLD) of prematurity.
- In a prospective Cohort study in India, incidence of BPD in infants <32 weeks gestation was found to be 33%.

■ FURTHER READING

1. Ghanta S, Leeman KT, Christou H. An update on pharmacological approaches to BPD. Sem Perinatol. 2013;37:102-7.
2. Narang A, Kumar P, Kumar R. Chronic Lung Disease in Neonates: Emerging problem in India. Indian Pediatr. 2002;39:158-62.
3. Northway WH Jr, Rosan RC, Porter DY. Pulmonary disease following respiratory therapy of HMD. N Eng J Med. 1967;276:357.
4. Shinwell ES, Portnov I, Meerpohl JJ, Karen T, Bassler D. Inhaled corticosteroids for BPD: A meta-analysis. Pediatrics. 2016;138(6):e20162511.

Management of Congenital Diaphragmatic Hernia

Manan Parikh, Preetha Joshi, Vinay Joshi

DEFINITION

Developmental defect in the diaphragm that allows abdominal viscera to protrude into the chest.

EPIDEMIOLOGY

- Incidence is 1:3,000 live births.
- More common in male, two-thirds cases of all
- Ninety percent hernia are left sided.
- Sixty percent congenital diaphragmatic hernia (CDH) are isolated, 40% are complex, associated with other structural abnormalities and syndromes.
- Despite advances in neonatal care, CDH is associated with a high risk of mortality and morbidity.

TYPES

Posterolateral defect (95%)	Anterior or central defect (4%)	Absence of diaphragm (1%)
Known as Bochdalek congenital diaphragmatic hernia (CDH)	Known as Morgagni hernia	Most severe form
85% left sided	Less commonly associated with lung hypoplasia	Worst prognosis
13% right sided		
2% bilateral		

PATHOPHYSIOLOGY

The abnormal communication between the peritoneal and pleural cavities allows herniation of abdominal content into the pleural space compressing the mediastinal structures.

Resultant growth of mediastinal structures, especially lungs, depends on three factors:

(1) Time of herniation	*(2) Size of the defect*	*(3) Site of the defect*
Herniation in early gestation, does not allow lung to grow much as compared to herniation occurring in third trimester and later	More the defect, more the herniation of abdominal contents into pleural cavity → causing more compression on developing lung	Posterolateral defect allows more herniation than anterior or central herniation →

Primary insult occurs during early stages of morphogenesis resulting in poor development of lung.

Congenital diaphragmatic hernia affects the lung and its vasculature in many ways, also causing effects on the heart and ribcage. The "two-hit" theory is believed to be responsible for all the structural, morphological, and functional effects of CDH.

"Two-hit" theory

CDH also affects on lung maturity and surfactant synthesis.

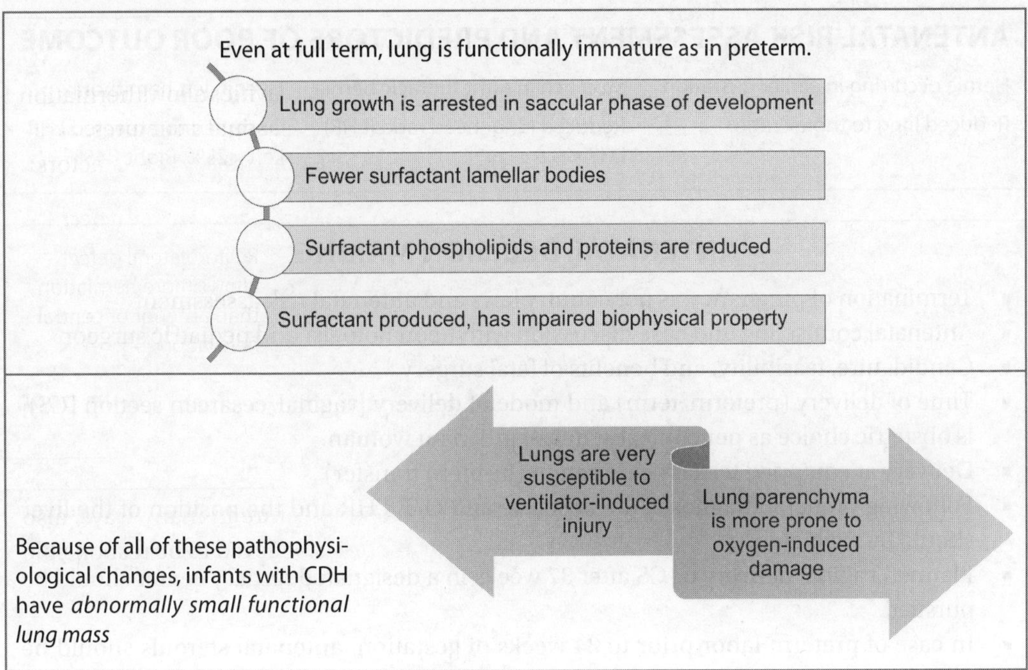

ANTENATAL DIAGNOSIS

With the increased use of prenatal ultrasound, many cases of CDH are now detected before birth. After diagnosis, a more detailed evaluation should be performed to determine the location of the defect, the absolute and observed/expected lung-to-head ratio (O/E LHR), the position of the liver and the presence or absence of other associated congenital anomalies or syndromes.

Pregnant women with fetus having CDH has:	Antenatal USG:	Amniocentesis with cell culture and chromosomal analysis:
• Low alpha fetoprotein • Polyhydramnios	• Absent abdominal stomach bubble • Thoracic stomach bubble • Mediastinal shift • Fetal hydrops	• Trisomy 13 and 18 • 3p microdeletion • 12p tetrasomy
Right side hernia more difficult to detect		*Normal scan does not rule out CDH*

ANTENATAL-ASSOCIATED FINDINGS

Cardiac	Noncardiac	Syndromes
• Hypoplastic left heart • Atrial septal defect • Ventricular septal defect • Coarctation of aorta • Ebstein's anomaly	• Esophageal atresia • Choanal atresia • Omphalocele • Hydronephrosis • Hydrocephalus	• Trisomy 13 • Trisomy 18 • Fryns syndrome • Beckwith-Wiedemann • Pierre Robin sequence

ANTENATAL RISK ASSESSMENT AND PREDICTORS OF POOR OUTCOME

Hernia occurring in earlier gestation	Stomach in right thoracic hernia	Liver in left hemithorax
Reduced lung to thorax ratio	Reduced lung–head ratio (LHR) LHR < 0.6	Observed to expected LHR Left <25%, Right <45%

ANTENATAL DECISION MAKING

- Termination of pregnancy as per country laws and antenatal risk assessment
- Antenatal counseling and case discussion with neonatologist and pediatric surgeon
- Candidature, feasibility, and benefits of fetal surgery
- Time of delivery (preterm/term) and mode of delivery [vaginal/cesarean section (CS)] is obstetric choice as per clinical status of pregnant woman.
- Delivery at equipped tertiary care center (in-utero transfer)
- Following prenatal diagnosis, the absolute and O/E LHR and the position of the liver should be evaluated.
- Planned vaginal delivery or CS after 37 weeks in a designated tertiary center should be pursued.
- In case of preterm labor prior to 34 weeks of gestation, antenatal steroids should be given.

DELIVERY ROOM MANAGEMENT

When CDH is diagnosed antenatally	
Anticipate	**Prepare**
• Stillbirth	• Resuscitation kit, T-piece resuscitator
• Extensive resuscitation with early intubation and no/minimal bagging	• Pulse oximeter, suction
• Pneumothorax	• Big bore nasogastric tube
• Associated cardiac issues	• Intravenous (IV) access, umbilical vein catheter (UVC) preparation
• Congenital deformities, anomalies	• Volume expanders, inotropes, and sedation
• Failure to revive despite resuscitation	• ICD kit, surfactant (in preterm)

SUSPECTING/DIAGNOSING CDH IN DELIVERY ROOM

On examination:	*On auscultation:*
• Barrel-shaped chest	• Absent breath sounds
• Scaphoid abdomen	• Displaced heart sounds

When CDH is not detected antenatally

At birth:	*On treatment:*
• Unexplained respiratory distress	• Difficult resuscitation
• Unexplained asphyxia	• Worsening on bag and mask intermittent positive pressure respiration (IPPR)

CONGENITAL DIAPHRAGMATIC HERNIA RESUSCITATION IN DELIVERY ROOM

Avoid distending gastrointestinal (GI) tract	*Minimize factors precipitating persistent pulmonary hypertension of the newborn (PPHN)*	*Avoid pulmonary air leaks*
• No bag and mask ventilation • Intubate and ventilate as early as possible • Place a big bore nasogastric tube immediately • Decompress stomach and bowel frequently	• Adequate sedation as needed • Gentle suctioning when required • No vigorous stimulation • Intubate and oxygenate early • Measure preductal and postductal SpO_2	• Gentle ventilation • Use t-piece resuscitator • Low peak inspiratory pressure (PIP), low positive end-expiratory pressure (PEEP) while resuscitating • No overzealous correction of hypoxemia • Target preductal $SpO_2 > 85\%$ in first hour of life

NICU MANAGEMENT

The combination of pulmonary hypoplasia and abnormal morphology of the pulmonary vasculature leads to severe respiratory insufficiency in over 90% of cases in the first hours after birth.

Infants who are not diagnosed antenatally, but present soon after delivery with respiratory distress should have been managed with strategies aiming to minimize PPHN and avoid gaseous distension of the bowel.

Stabilization of the clinical condition takes precedence over immediate surgical correction.

DIAGNOSIS AND ASSESSMENT OF SEVERITY

X-ray chest	*Echocardiography*	*Supportive IX*
• Confirms diagnosis, extent • Excludes air leaks • Verify ET endotracheal (ET) tube	• Rule out CHD • Volume status, PPHN • Ventricular dysfunction	• Arterial blood gas (ABG) • Random blood sugar (RBS) • Electrolytes

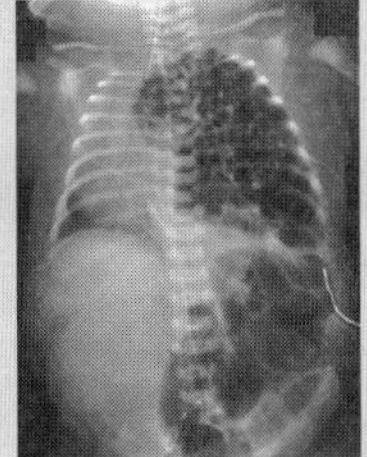

CDH with air and fluid filled bowel loops in chest

CDH with stomach shadow in thorax

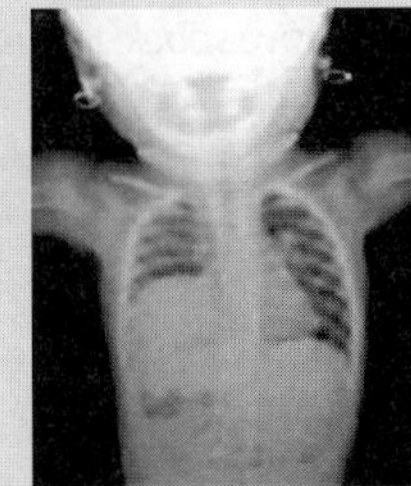

Right-sided CDH with herniation of liver

VENTILATORY CARE

Goal	Mode	Weaning

• Gentle ventilation with permissive hypercapnia
• *Preductal targets:*
  – *SpO_2:* >90%
  – *PaO_2:* 60–80 mm Hg
  – *$PaCO_2$:* 45–60 mm Hg
  – *pH:* 7.25–7.40
• Sufficient oxygenation to prevent metabolic acidosis
• Sufficient CO_2 removal to avoid respiratory acidosis
	• Initial
	• *Conventional ventilation,* pressure controlled
	• *Initial settings:*
	  – *PIP:* 20–25 cmH_2O
	  – *PEEP:* 3–5 cmH_2O
	  – *Rate:* 40–60/min
	• *High-frequency oscillatory ventilation (HFOV)*
	• As rescue mode if PIP > 25
	• Maintain inflation of contralateral lung till 8th rib
	• Can also be used as an elective mode
		• Avoid sudden changes in ventilatory settings
		• *Start weaning after postoperative stabilization*
		• After stabilization, FiO_2 should be weaned if preductal SpO_2 > 95%
		• Reduce PIP/MAP first followed by rate/amplitude/frequency

HEMODYNAMIC MANAGEMENT

Shock	Dysfunction	PPHN

• *Goal*: Achieving appropriate end-organ perfusion determinants:
  – *Heart rate:* Normal
  – Capillary refill <3 seconds
  – Urine output >1 mL/kg/h
  – Lactate levels <3 mmol/L
• In case of hypovolemia, isotonic fluid therapy 10–20 mL/kg NaCl 0.9% and early inotropes should be considered to maintain systemic pressure > pulmonary pressure
	• CDH causes cardiac malposition with decreased LV mass and function
	• While PPHN causing RV dysfunction
	• ECHO-guided approach to determine inotrope for cardiac dysfunction
	• Avoid liberal fluid therapy and boluses to prevent pulmonary edema and volume overload
		• *ECHO to evaluate:*
		  – RV dysfunction
		  – RV overload
		  – Degree of R → L shunt
		• *Line of management:*
		  – Proper lung recruitment
		    - HFOV/± surfactant
		  – Adequate vascular volume
		  – Optimizing systolic BP
		  – Pulmonary vasodilators
		    - Sildenafil, iNO
		  – ECMO (if OI > 40 or intractable PPHN)

Choice of inotrope: As per clinical condition and Echo parameters—
- *Maintaining systolic BP*: Dopamine and/or epinephrine
- *In presence of myocardial dysfunction*: Dobutamine/milrinone
- *Refractory hypotension*: Vasopressin and/or norepinephrine and early consideration of ECMO
- *Unresponsive shock*: Hydrocortisone

Supportive care		
Beneficial	**Cautious**	**Avoid**
Adequate sedation	Gentle suctioning	Gaseous distension
Minimal handling		Muscle relaxants
Proper hydration, nutrition and IVF		Alkalinization
Euthermia		Hypercapnia

MONITORING

Clinical	Bedside	Lab parameters
Sensorium	Arterial BP	Hb, TC, platelets
Perfusion, UOP	ABG, RBS	Septic markers
Preductal and postductal SpO_2	Echo	Electrolytes
Heart rate		Calcium, creatinine

NUTRITION

Restrictive fluid management	Enteral feeding earliest	Medication
Fluid and caloric intake should be increased as per clinical condition	Glucose, lipids, and proteins should be given according to unit policy	Diuretics in case of a positive fluid balance, aim for diuresis of 1–2 mL/kg/h

SURGICAL MANAGEMENT

Better outcomes by delaying surgical repair until hemodynamic and respiratory stability are achieved for 24–72 hours.

Timing	Surgical options

• *Criteria to be met before surgical repair:*
  – Urine output >1 mL/kg/h
  – FiO_2 < 50%
  – Preductal SpO_2 85–95%
  – Normal mean arterial pressure
  – PA pressure < systemic pressure
  – Lactate <3 mmol/L
  – Decannulation, if neonate on ECMO but surgery can be done on ECMO too
  – Failure to meet above criteria in 2 weeks
	• *Type:* Open thoracotomy is preferred over minimally invasive surgical repair
	• Transabdominal repair using subcostal incision with gentle reduction of liver, spleen, viscera into abdominal cavity and closure of defect is performed
	• Large defects are closed with prosthetic Gore-Tex patches

POSTOPERATIVE CARE

- After surgery of large left CDH, there will be an *inevitable pneumothorax* as small left lung cannot fill the whole thoracic cavity, for which a drain is usually placed intraoperatively.
- Postoperative phase is very labile for hemodynamic and respiratory stability.
- Clinical condition to be *managed as per the scenario* keeping in mind all the principles employed in the preoperative care.
- *Gastroesophageal reflux* is common after CDH repair. Proper nutrition with antireflux medications should be employed whenever needed.
- Failure to wean the respiratory support following surgery, suggest *lethal pulmonary hypoplasia.*

<table>
<tr><td colspan="2" align="center">OUTCOME</td></tr>
<tr><td>Morbidities</td><td>Follow-up</td></tr>
<tr><td valign="top">

- *Failure to thrive:*
  - Despite caloric optimization
  - Due to increased work of breathing
- Esophageal dilatation
- Esophageal dysfunction
- Gastroesophageal reflux
- Intestinal obstruction due to volvulus and adhesions
- Chronic bronchitis
- Aspiration pneumonia
- Bronchopulmonary dysplasia
- Scoliosis
- Recurrent diaphragmatic hernia
  - After several weeks or months
- Neurodevelopmental disabilities
- Hearing loss

</td><td valign="top">

- Multidisciplinary approach
  - *Immediate:*
    - Surgical site care
    - Weight gain adequacy
    - Reflux component assessment and care
  - *Long term:*
    - Growth monitoring
    - Feeding adequacy
    - Hearing assessment
    - Ophthalmic evaluation
    - Neurodevelopmental assessment
    - Pulmonary function
    - Adherence to vaccination schedule
    - Vitamin and mineral supplementation
- If associated syndrome—multidisciplinary approach

</td></tr>
</table>

Key Points to Remember

- In infants with CDH, pulmonary vascular resistance (PVR) remains elevated after birth, resulting in right-to-left shunting of blood and severe PPHN which might need management with gentle high-frequency ventilation and inhaled nitric oxide.
- Infant may need volume expansion, umbilical catheterization, pressor support, and even chest tube placement (in case of pneumothorax) in delivery room.
- The key principles of successful delivery room resuscitation and stabilization are the *avoidance of high airway pressures and the establishment of an adequate preductal arterial saturation.*
- Once stabilized in delivery room, on transport:
  - Trained and skilled team
  - Gentle ventilation
  - Maintain stable hemodynamic status, early inotropic support

■ FURTHER READING

1. Bagolan P, Casaccia G, Crescenzi F, Nahom A, Trucchi A, Giorlandino C. Impact of a current treatment protocol on outcome of high-risk congenital diaphragmatic hernia. J Pediatr Surg. 2004;39:313.
2. Frenckner BP, Lally PA, Hintz SR, Lally KP. Prenatal diagnosis of congenital diaphragmatic hernia: how should the babies be delivered? J Pediatr Surg. 2007;42:1533.
3. Jeandot R, Lambert B, Brendel AJ, Guyot M, Demarquez JL. Lung ventilation and perfusion scintigraphy in the follow up of repaired congenital diaphragmatic hernia. Eur J Nucl Med. 1989; 15:591-6.
4. Reiss I, Schaible T, van den Hout L, Capolupo I, Allegaert K, van Heijst A, et al. Standardized postnatal management of infants with congenital diaphragmatic hernia in Europe: The CDH EURO Consortium Consensus. Neonatology. 2010;98(4):354-64.
5. Rottier R, Tibboel D. Fetal lung and diaphragm development in congenital diaphragmatic hernia. Semin Perinatol. 2005;29:86-93.

Oxygen Therapy

Sweta Kumari

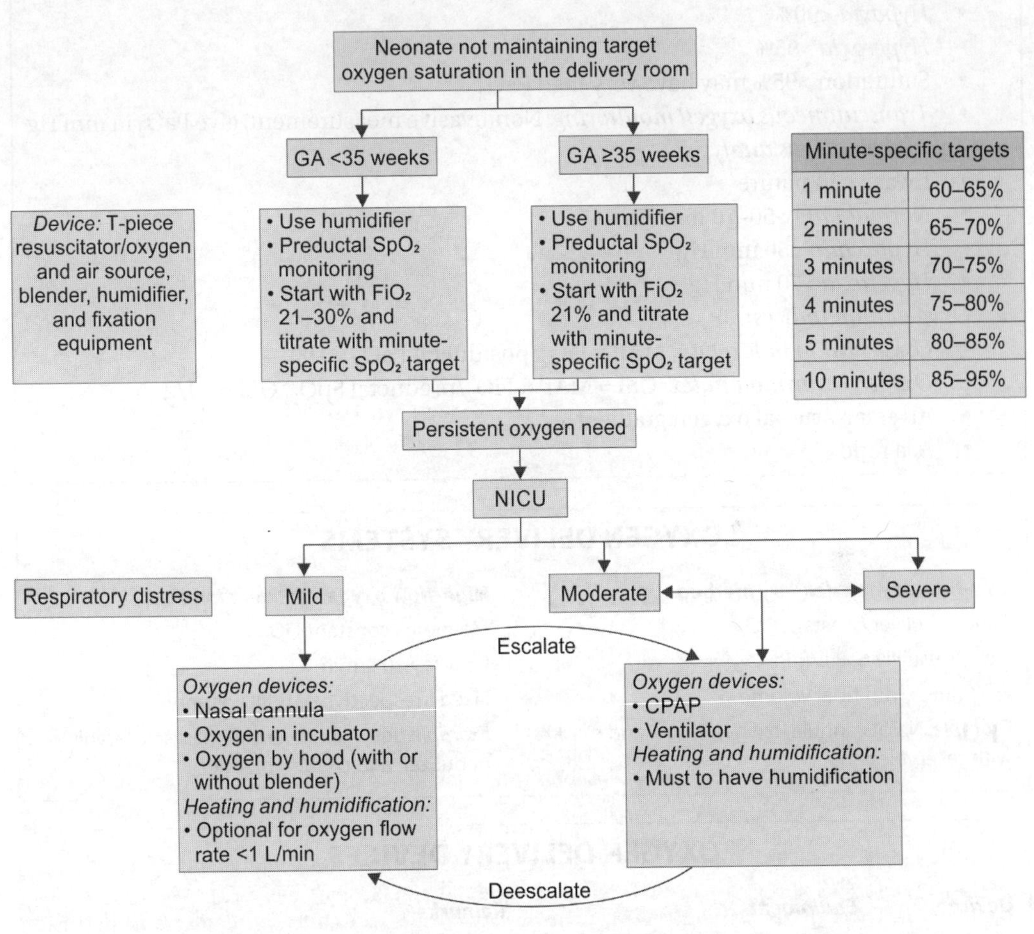

MONITORING OF OXYGENATION

- Measurement of oxygen delivered is done in fraction of oxygen (FiO_2) 0.21–1.00.
- Oxygen level in body is expressed in:
  - Partial pressure of oxygen (PaO_2)—pressure exerted by dissolved oxygen in blood
  - Saturation of oxygen (SpO_2)—percent of Hb totally bound to oxygen
- *Clinical monitoring*: Imprecise and unreliable. One can detect severe hypoxemia from presence of central cyanosis.
- *Pulse oximetry:*
  - Noninvasive and continuous monitoring
  - Normal oxygen saturation—90–95%
  - *Hypoxia <90%*
  - *Hyperoxia >95%*
  - Saturation >95% may have very high PaO_2.
  - *Transcutaneous oxygen monitoring:* Noninvasive measurement, give PaO_2 in mm Hg
- *Arterial blood gas analysis:*
  - Invasive in nature
  - *Normal PaO_2:* 50–70 mm Hg
  - *Hypoxemia <50 mm Hg*
  - *Hyperoxia >70 mm Hg*
- *Oxygenation indices:*
  - *Oxygenation index:* OI = MAP × FiO_2/postductal PaO_2 × 100
  - *Oxygen saturation index:* OSI = MAP × FiO_2/preductal SpO_2, OSI = OI/2
  - Alveolar-arterial oxygen gradient
  - A/a ratio

OXYGEN DELIVERY SYSTEMS

Low-flow oxygen delivery method	High-flow oxygen delivery method
Cannot deliver constant FiO_2	Maintains constant FiO_2
Flow is usually 6–8 L/min	Flow is >10 L/min
FiO_2 varies with tidal volume	Fixed irrespective of tidal volume
Example: Nasal cannula, oxygen hood, and mask with reservoir bags	*Example:* Jet-mixing venturi masks, reservoir nebulizer, and oxygen blender

OXYGEN DELIVERY DEVICES

Device	Equipment	Remarks
Oxygen without blender	Oxygen source, air source, flow meter, humidifier, T piece, nasal prongs, fixating material, and pulse oximeter	• Ensure right connection • Humidification and warming • FiO_2 adjustment according to SpO_2 $$FiO_2 = \frac{\{(0.21 \times \text{Air flow}) + O_2 \text{ flow}\}}{\text{Air flow} + O_2 \text{ flow}}$$

Contd...

Contd...

Device	Equipment	Remarks
Oxygen by nasal prongs	Oxygen source, flow meter, humidifier chamber, nasal prongs, and fixating material	• Flow set at 0.5–1 L/min • Nasal prongs appropriate size
Oxygen by hood	Oxygen source, flow meter, humidifier chamber, distill water, oxygen hood, and pulse oximeter	• Flow set at 4–6 L/min (Not <2 L/min) • Humidification bottle filled with distill water • Hood should not be tight sealed

Key Points to Remember

- Target SpO_2 for all the neonates is 90–95%.
- In neonates born at >34 weeks of gestation and with mild respiratory distress, nasal cannula with low flow rate (0.5–1 L/min) should be used for delivering oxygen in preference to oxygen by hood or incubator oxygen.
- Warming and humidification may be necessary when flow rate through nasal cannula is high-flow rate (>1 L/min).
- Use of oxygen in optimal concentration is lifesaving by rescuing cells where oxygen level is low at tissue level.
- Oxygen is used in approximately 2% of all live births, 97% for babies under 28 weeks. Requirements of oxygen decrease as gestation increases to term.
- Risk factors for need of oxygen supplementation are extreme prematurity, lack of antenatal corticosteroid, and very low birth weight.
- Restricted use of oxygen increases the mortality and necrotizing enterocolitis (NEC) whereas liberal use of oxygen increases the incidence of bronchopulmonary dysplasia (BPD) and retinopathy of prematurity.
- Evidences from multiple randomized controlled trials (RCTs) and prospective meta-analyses suggest that adopting saturation target between 91 and 95% for preterm ≤34-week gestation achieves the critical balance between competing adverse outcome like death/NEC and retinopathy of prematurity (ROP)/BPD.
- For neonates >34 weeks' gestation and neonates with evolving or established BPD, the saturation target remains same.
- Continuous noninvasive monitoring by pulse oximetry with signal extraction technology (SET) is recommended.
- Alarm limit is set at 89% for lower limit and 96% at higher limit. Alarm limit is chosen keeping balance between alarm fatigue and oxygen toxicity.

■ FURTHER READING

1. NNF. (2021). Clinical Practice Guideline 2021 for oxygen therapy in neonates. [online] Available from https://www.nnfi.org/assests/upload/usefull-links-pdf/Oxygen_therapy_in_neonates_NNFI_CPG_Dec2021.pdf [Last accessed August, 2022].
2. Vento M. Oxygen therapy. In: Goldsmith JP, Karotkin EH, Keszler M, Suresh GK (Eds). Assisted Ventilation of the Neonate. Netherlands: Elsevier; 2017. pp. 153-61.
3. Weiner, Gary M, Zaichkin J. Textbook of Neonatal Resuscitation, 8th edition. Elk Grove Village, IL: American Academy of Pediatrics; 2021.

Management of Asphyxia

Deepika Rustogi, Ankit Gupta

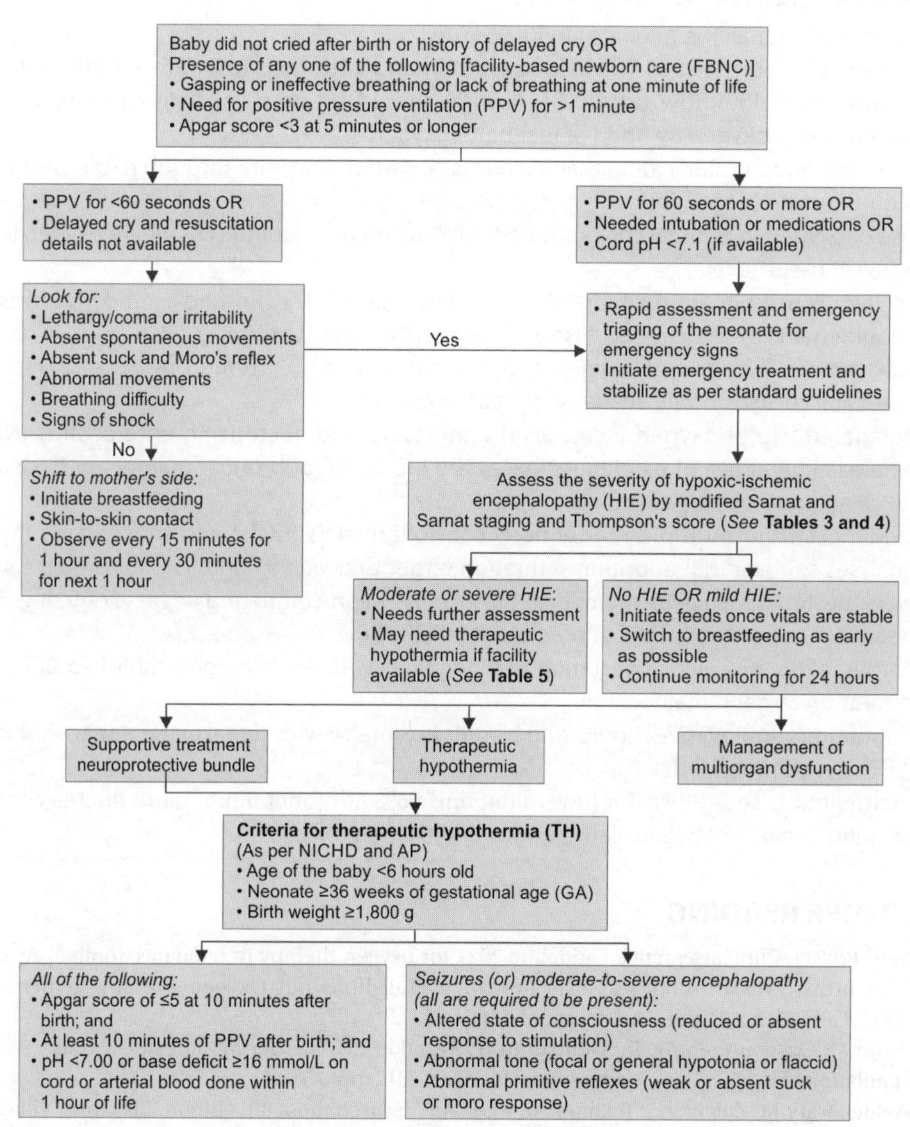

NEUROPROTECTIVE CARE BUNDLE

- Delivery room management as per the Neonatal Resuscitation Program (NRP).
- Hemodynamic support—securing an airway, promoting adequate oxygenation, ventilation, and cardiovascular management
- Baseline investigations followed by serial monitoring of laboratory tests **(Table 1)**.
- Correction of metabolic derangements
- *Avoid hyperthermia:* Risk of death or moderate-to-severe disability is increased 3.6–4-fold for every 1°C increase in body temperature
- *Serial neurological examination:* Hourly till 6 hours, then 12 hourly till 24 hours, and thereafter daily
- Monitoring for multiorgan dysfunction including seizure diagnosis and management **(Table 2)**
- Ongoing developmentally supportive care (DSC)
- Steroids, mannitol, and furosemide have no role in the management of asphyxia.

TABLE 1: Serial laboratory monitoring in HIE and during TH.

Timing	Measurement	Comment
Baseline labs	Complete blood count (CBC), electrolytes, ionized calcium, blood glucose, arterial blood gas, and lactate	
At 24 hours	CBC, serum electrolyte, creatinine, and blood sugar	Liver enzymes (ALT and AST)—desirable
Subsequent sample as per clinical condition of the baby	• Blood glucose • Electrolytes (Na, K, and P) • Blood gas • Renal function test	As clinically indicated
Neuroimaging: • The first MRI is done on days 4–5 (if cooled) and around day 3 (if not cooled) • The second MRI around days 10–14	• It is a useful predictor for long-term outcomes • For prognostication and counseling of parents regarding goals of care	Brain MRI is the gold standard imaging *Pattern of brain injury:* • Selective neuronal necrosis • Parasagittal cerebral injury • Periventricular leukomalacia • Focal ischemic brain necrosis

TABLE 2: Management of multiorgan dysfunction.

System involvement	Signs and symptoms	Pathophysiology	Assessment and tools	Management
Central nervous system (CNS)	Altered consciousness, abnormal tone, and abnormal primitive reflexes	Hypoxia, diminished cerebral perfusion, oxidative injury, and neuronal apoptosis	• Detailed neurological assessment • Modified Sarnat examination • Amiel–Tison Neurologic Assessment at term • Thompson score	MRI is the gold standard technique to detect patterns of cerebral damage
Seizures 50%	Focal, multifocal, tonic, and clonic seizures		Identification and monitoring using amplitude integrated EEG (aEEG)	As per standard protocol
Cardiovascular system (CVS) 62%	• Hypotension, • Arrhythmias • Pre- and postductal saturation split of >5–10%	Attributed to hypoxia, ischemia, metabolic acidosis, multiorgan injury, and coexisting persistent pulmonary hypertension of the newborn (PPHN)	Hemodynamic assessments—vital signs, biochemical parameters, and Echo is the best diagnostic tool	Management of shock and PPHN
Respiratory 23–86%	Oxygen requirement, respiratory support, signs of PPHN	Hypoxia, disruption of the physiological fall in pulmonary vascular resistance	• Interpretation of altered blood gas • Chest X-ray • ECHO	• Tight control of CO_2, avoidance of hypoxia • Respiratory support with aim to maintain pH > 7.25 and a normal to high $PaCO_2$ 37.5–52.5 mm Hg
Renal 22–70%	Oliguria (<1 mL/kg/h)	Acute kidney injury (AKI), syndrome of inappropriate antidiuretic hormone secretion (SIADH), and nephrotoxic medications	• Renal profile (creatinine), fluid balance, urinary electrolytes, and acid-base balance • Cystatin C • Neutrophil gelatinase-associated lipocalin (NGAL)	Urinary catheterization, optimal fluid Management—no role of diuretics

Contd...

Contd...

System involvement	Signs and symptoms	Pathophysiology	Assessment and tools	Management
Hepatic 80%	Transaminitis, alanine aminotransferase/aspartate aminotransferase (ALT/AST) >100 [1.5 times upper limit of normal (ULN)]	Hypoxic injury	Liver function test, prothrombin time, international normalized ratio (LFT, PT, and INR)	Supportive monitoring and caution against use of hepatotoxic drugs
Gastrointestinal tract (GIT) and nutrition	Gastric residues, vomiting, distension, and bleeding	Compromised splanchnic circulation	Clinical monitoring Lack of evidence from randomized controlled trials (RCTs) regarding enteral nutrition	Early minimal enteral nutrition (MEN) with mother's milk, progressed cautiously as per clinical condition
Metabolic 50%	• Electrolyte abnormalities—hyponatremia, hypokalemia, hypocalcemia • Metabolic acidosis • Hyperlactatemia	• SIADH • AKI • Anaerobic metabolism	• Serum electrolytes, blood gas • Rule out inborn errors of metabolism (IEM) if clinically indicated	Optimal fluid and electrolyte management
Glucose metabolism	Hypoglycemia	Anaerobic metabolism	Glucose monitoring every 30–60 minutes until the glucose is normal, then every 4–6 hours	Initiate glucose infusion rate (GIR) of 6–8 mg/kg/min, with 2 mg/kg/min increases in GIR if hypoglycemia occurs
Infection 24%	Elevated inflammatory markers, positive cultures	• Chorioamnionitis is a risk factor • Sepsis can present as perinatal asphyxia	Inflammatory markers, blood cultures	Broad-spectrum antibiotic therapy until sepsis has been excluded
Hematology 40%	Bleeding manifestations, need for blood products	Hypoxia-ischemia, blood loss, and disseminated intravascular coagulation (DIC)	Deranged coagulation profile, elevated nucleated red blood cell (nRBC), and thrombocytopenia	• Blood product transfusion • Relative indication for discontinuation of TH
Skin	Acute, nodular, erythematous, tender eruption, and sclerema	Inflammation and necrosis of subcutaneous fat	Daily skin examination, calcium monitoring	Hydration, diuretic treatment

TABLE 3: Modified Sarnat staging for neonatal encephalopathy.

Severity	*Stage 1: Mild*	*Stage 2: Moderate*	*Stage 3: Severe*
Level of consciousness	Hyperalert	Lethargic	Stupor/coma
Activity	Normal	Decreased	Absent
Neuromuscular control: • Muscle tone • Posture • Tendon reflexes	• Normal • Mild distal flexion • Overactive	• Mild hypotonia • Strong distal flexion • Overactive	• Flaccid • Intermittent decerebration • Decreased or absent
Neonatal reflexes: • Suck • Moro • Tonic neck	• Weak • Strong • Slight	• Weak/absent • Weak, incomplete • Strong	• Absent • Absent • Weak
Autonomic nervous system: • Pupils • Heart rate • Respiratory rate	• Dilated pupils • Tachycardia • Regular	• Constricted pupils • Bradycardia • Periodic breathing	• Variable, unequal • Variable • Apnea
Seizure	None	Common, focal, or multifocal	Uncommon

TABLE 4: Thompson's score for neonatal encephalopathy.

Sign	*0*	*1*	*2*	*3*
Tone	Normal	Hyper	Hypo	Flaccid
LOC	Normal	Hyperalert, stare	Lethargic	Comatose
Fits	None	<3 per day	>2 per day	
Posture	Normal	Fisting, cycling	Strong distal flexion	Decerebrate
Moro	Normal	Partial	Absent	
Grasp	Normal	Poor	Absent	
Suck	Normal	Poor	Absent ± bites	
Respiration	Normal	Hyperventilation	Brief apnea	Apnea requiring IPPV
Fontanel	Normal	Full, not tense	Tense	

Score 1–10: mild HIE, 11–14: moderate HIE, 15–22: severe HIE

TABLE 5: Facility has written protocol for TH and level-3 intensive care.

- Initiate whole body cooling using a servo-controlled mattress/phase-change material (PCM)-based device/ice or gel packs
- Whatever the device used, the cooling targets and monitoring are similar
- Continuous rectal temperature monitoring is required from initiation until 8 hours after rewarming.
- Target rectal temperature is 33–34°C for 72 hours
- *Induction:* Aim to attain target temperature in the first 30 minutes
- *Maintenance:* Continue to maintain target temperature for 72 hours after initiation
- *Rewarming:* Increase rectal temperature to 36.5°C over 6–12 hours, at a rate 0.5°C per hours
- *Rationale:* It reduces free radicals and glutamate levels, decreases oxygen demand, and decreases apoptosis
- *Number needed to treat (NNT):* 7
- Details of techniques of TH see further

CONTRAINDICATIONS FOR THERAPEUTIC HYPOTHERMIA

- Gestational age <36 weeks [confirmed by reliable last menstrual period (LMP) or early antenatal ultrasound or New Ballard scoring system—in this order of importance]
    - Birth weight <1,800 g
    - Postnatal age >6 hours
    - Presence of known chromosomal anomalies
    - Presence of major congenital malformations
    - Active bleeding (bleeding from >2 sites)
- Grade 3 and above intraventricular hemorrhage (IVH) (TH not to be delayed if USG has not been done, but it should be done within 24 hours of birth)
- Moribund neonate.

Stopping Therapeutic Hypothermia

- Identification of a contraindication that was previously undetected.
- Persistent signs of brain death as detected and confirmed by the treating team.
- Parents wish to withdraw the treatment and intensive care (after taking written parental consent).

COOLING DEVICES

- *Whole body cooling devices (more beneficial and preferred):*
    - *High-technology devices:* Automated cooling devices using circulating coolant/fluid.
    - *Low-technology devices:* Example, ice gel packs, phase change material offers a safe and cost effective alternatives in resource limited middle and low income countries.
- *Selective head cooling device:* Examples, cool cap system.

Technique

- Cooling to be done only at the designated tertiary centers with availability of trained staff and resources.
- Once eligible, inform the neonatal intensive care unit (NICU) team, maintain temperature of the baby (skin or axillary) in the range of 36.1–36.5°C while being in the delivery room as well as during transport (do not do passive cooling).
- Bedside ultrasound may be done (if feasible) before starting cooling to rule out intracranial bleed or any gross intracranial anomaly.
- Place the newborn supine with over narrower portion of the cooling mattress and trunk over the broader portion.
- Insert patient end of the rectal temperature probe 3 cm into the rectum. Secure it with a tape over thigh.
- Attach skin probe to the right flank of the abdomen.
- Attach pulse oximeter sensor to the right hand.
- Attach ECG leads for continuous ECG monitoring.
- Continuous aEEG monitoring (if available)

- Place umbilical venous access in addition to peripheral venous access as obtaining venous access in a cooled baby may be very difficult to obtain.
- Place arterial line (radial or umbilical) for invasive arterial pressure monitoring and for sampling (remember—noninvasive blood pressure monitoring may be difficult, erroneous, and unreliable in cooled babies).
- Switch on the cooling machine in case one is using a "servo controlled" device. For phase changing material, the cooling starts as soon as the baby is placed.
- Switch radiant warmer to manual mode with zero heater output. Alternatively, radiant warmer can be switched off.
- *Provide analgesia during TH:* Morphine (preferred) or fentanyl should be given by infusion.
- Anticipate significant bradycardia (<90/min) once cooling has been initiated.
- Monitor infant's rectal, skin, and axillary temperature every 15 minutes for first 4 hours of cooling, then hourly till 72 hours of treatment.
- Hourly vital signs including blood pressure and capillary refill time, Strict fluid intake and output monitoring.
- Continuous monitoring for seizure activity
- *Skin integrity monitoring:* Assess all skin that contacts the cooling blanket at least every hour, change the infant's position every 2–3 hours.
- Hypothermia treatment should be continued uninterrupted for 72 hours, followed by gradual rewarming over 6 hours by 0.5°C every hour.

Key Points to Remember

Definition as per WHO (Low Resource Setting)

"Failure to initiate or sustain spontaneous breathing at birth".

Mechanisms of Injury

- Interruption of umbilical blood circulation (pathology of umbilical cord)
- Impairment of placental gas exchange (Abruptio placenta and placenta previa)
- Insufficient maternal side placental perfusion (maternal hypo/hypertension, abnormal uterine contractions)
- Impairment of maternal oxygenation (cardiovascular and pulmonary diseases, severe anemia)
- Insufficient pulmonary expansion and persistent fetal circulation (severe PPHN).

Pathophysiology of HIE

- *Primary energy failure:* Immediate cellular energy failure, excitotoxicity, free radical damage, and rise in intracellular Ca^{2+}, cellular necrosis
- *Latent phase:* "Pseudonormalization" of energy levels following reperfusion of the ischemic brain with successful resuscitation of at least 6 hours

- *Secondary energy failure:* It occurs 6–48 hours after the initial injury, oxidative stress, excitotoxicity, and inflammation, cellular apoptosis
- *Tertiary energy failure:* Delayed neuronal death due to ongoing inflammation over days to weeks to months.

Poor Prognostic Markers

- Need for PPV for 5 minutes or longer
- Onset of seizure within 12 hours
- Refractory seizure [uncontrolled with first line anti-epileptic drugs (AED)]
- Severe HIE
- Inability to establish breastfeeding by 1 week
- Altered signal intensities in the posterior limb of the internal capsule (PLIC) and abnormalities of thalami and basal ganglia on MRI
- Abnormal aEEG background activity over the first 6 hours of postnatal life.

Follow-up

- All the neonates with perinatal asphyxia must attend the follow-up clinic for monitoring of their growth, development and long-term neurodevelopmental outcome.
- First follow-up at 2 weeks postdischarge
- Serial neurodevelopmental assessments at 3, 6, 9, 12, and 18–24 months of age (best predictor of long-term neurodevelopmental outcomes), with continued DSC and early intervention where indicated
- Adopting "neuroprotective care bundle," with collaboration of neonatologists, neurologists, trained nurses, and allied health professionals can improve outcome of babies with NE/HIE.
- No single gold standard diagnostic test to determine severity or prognosis.

■ FURTHER READING

1. Abate BB, Bimerew M, Gebremichael B, Kassie AM, Kassaw M, Gebremeskel T, et al. Effects of therapeutic hypothermia on death among asphyxiated neonates with hypoxic-ischemic encephalopathy: a systematic review and meta-analysis of randomized control trials. PLoS One. 2021;16(2):e0247229.
2. Facility Based Newborn Care (FBNC). MoHFW, Government of India; 2022.
3. NNF Working Group. Position Statement and Guidelines for Use of Therapeutic Hypothermia to treat Neonatal Hypoxic Ischemic Encephalopathy in India. New Delhi: National Neonatology Forum, India; 2021.
4. O'Dea M, Sweetman D, Bonifacio SL, El-Dib M, Austin T, Molloy EJ. Management of Multi Organ Dysfunction in Neonatal Encephalopathy. Front Pediatr. 2020;8:239.
5. Sarnat HB, Sarnat MS. Neonatal encephalopathy following fetal distress: a clinical and electroencephalographic study. Arch Neurol. 1976;33(10):696-705.
6. Shankaran S, Laptook AR, Ehrenkranz RA, Tyson JE, McDonald SA, Donovan EF, et al. National Institute of Child Health and Human Development Neonatal Research Network. Whole-body hypothermia for neonates with hypoxic-ischemic encephalopathy. N Engl J Med. 2005;353(15):1574-84.

Management of Seizure

Gurleen Sikka

Neonate with seizure:
Maintain TABC and check blood glucose

↓

Treat acute underlying cause:
- *If hypoglycemia (BG <45 mg/dL):* IV bolus of 2 mL/kg of 10% dextrose followed by maintenance @ 6 mg/kg/min
- *If hypocalcemia (iCa < 1.0 mmol/L);* calcium gluconate diluted in D5/D10/DW slowly IV 2 mL/kg under cardiac monitoring

Seizure persists ↓

Injection phenobarbitone loading dose:
20 mg/kg IV over 20 minutes @ 1 mg/kg/min → *If seizure controlled:* Do not start maintenance

Seizure persists ↓

- Give further 5 mg/kg bolus of injection phenobarbitone over 5–10 minutes. Repeat bolus up to maximum 40 mg/kg, if seizure not controlled. OR
- Injection levetiracetam 50 mg/kg IV bolus followed by 40 mg/kg/day maintenance in two-divided dose
- Phenobarbitone over 5–10 minutes
- Repeat if seizures not controlled up to a maximum of 40 mg/kg

→ *If seizure controlled:* Start maintenance dose of phenobarbitone 5 mg/kg/day in 1–2 divided doses after 24 hours of loading dose

If seizure persist ↓

Give injection phenytoin loading dose 20 mg/kg IV over 20 minutes @ 1 mg/kg/min → *If seizure controlled:* Start maintenance dose of phenobarbitone and phenytoin 5 mg/kg/day in 1–2 divided doses

If seizure persist ↓

- Consider injection lorazepam 0.05–0.01 mg/kg IV infusion over 2–5 minutes
- Injection midazolam 0.1 mg/kg IV bolus followed by continuous infusion 1 µg/kg/min
- Consider giving trial of pyridoxine

→ *If seizure controlled:* Maintenance dose of phenobarbitone 5 mg/kg/day in 1–2 divided doses. Stop antiepileptic drug (AED) once seizure free for 48 hours

DEFINITION

Occurrence of sudden alteration in motor, behavior, or autonomic activity, with or without alteration of consciousness **(Table 1)**.

NEONATES AT RISK FOR SEIZURES

Birth asphyxia:

- Sepsis, meningitis
- Preterm, small for gestational age
- Metabolic or electrolyte abnormalities
- Major bleeding.

HISTORY

- *Antenatal:* First-trimester viral illness, pregnancy-induced hypertension (PIH), diabetes, premature rupture of membrane (PROM)/chorioamnionitis, sexually transmitted infections (STDs), drugs or substance abuse, and decreased fetal movements
- *Intrapartum:* Fetal distress, difficult delivery, cord complications, mode of delivery, and instrumentation
- *Postnatal:* Resuscitation, other organ system involvement, feeding history, seizure details: onset, duration, and description **(Table 2)**
- *Family:* Consanguinity, early neonatal deaths, mental retardation, and epilepsy.

EXAMINATION

- *General*: Pallor, icterus, rash, and skin lesions
- *Vital signs*: Temperature, BP, heart rate (HR), respiratory rate (RR), capillary filling time (CFT), and pulse oxygen saturation (SpO_2)
- *Head to toe*: Head circumference, bulging fontanel, needle marks on scalp, dysmorphism, malformations, petechiae, and ecchymoses
- *Systemic examination:* Level of alertness, cranial nerve and motor examination, and examination of all systems
- *Fundus examination*

DIFFERENTIAL DIAGNOSIS

- *Normal behavior* includes nonspecific random movements especially in preterm babies, e.g., benign sleep myoclonus; in rapid eye movement (REM) sleep and electroencephalogram (EEG) is always normal.
- *Jitteriness:* Provoked by a stimulus, rapid, and shaking tremor like can be stopped when the limb is held, baby fully conscious and no other phenomena like eye deviation, sucking, etc.
- *Neonatal tetanus:* Persistent involuntary contraction of the muscle appears after 48 hours and aggravated by touch and stimuli.

INVESTIGATIONS

In all neonates: Blood glucose, serum electrolytes, hemogram, ionized calcium, blood urea/creatinine, liver function tests, blood gas analysis, and cranial ultrasound

Specific circumstances:
- *Suspected sepsis:* Cerebrospinal fluid (CSF) examination
- *Suspected TORCH infections:* Paired mother and baby serology (for toxoplasma, CMV, rubella), body fluids for polymerase chain reaction (PCR) (urine for CMV), CSF for toxoplasma, CMV, and herpes
- *Suspected intracranial bleed:* Ultrasound or CT or MRI head, platelet count, and coagulogram
- *Suspected IEM:* Serum ammonia, amino acids, lactate, pyruvate, and urine for organic acids
- Electroencephalography.

TABLE 1: Identification of seizures.

Motor manifestations:
- Rhythmic jerks of limb(s) or facial part(s)
- Tonic contraction of limb(s)
- Stereotypical movements of limbs (pedaling, rowing, swimming, cycling, and stepping), face (pouting of lips, mouthing, and repeated sucking), eyes (vacant stare, transient eye deviation, nystagmoid movements, and repeated blinking)

Behavioral manifestations: Sudden change in consciousness or cry characteristic

Autonomic manifestations: Fluctuations in heart rate, sudden change in blood pressure (BP), and sudden appearance of unexplained apneic episodes

TABLE 2: Etiology incidence of neonatal seizure.

	%
Hypoxic-ischemic encephalopathy	30–63 (MC)
Intracranial hemorrhage	7–17
Cerebral infarction	6–17
Cerebral malformations	3–17
Meningitis/septicemia	2–14
Metabolic	
Hypoglycemia	0.1–5
Hypocalcemia and hypomagnesemia	4–22
Hypo-/hypernatremia	
Inborn errors of metabolism (such as pyridoxine dependency, folinic acid-responsive seizures, glucose transporter defect, nonketotic hyperglycinemia, and propionic aciduria)	3–4
Kernicterus	1
Maternal drug withdrawal	4
Idiopathic	2
Benign idiopathic neonatal seizures	1

Key Points to Remember

- The most common neonatal seizure—subtle seizures.
- Hypoxic-ischemic encephalopathy—most common cause of seizures in term infants.
- Late onset hypocalcemic seizures—best prognosis.
- Hypoglycemic seizures-worst prognosis.
- Vast majority occurs on day 1 (first 24 hours), 70% occurs by day 4 of life.
- Seizures can occur with clinical manifestations (clinical seizure) or without clinical manifestations (electrical seizure).
- Phenobarbitone remains mainstay of therapy.
- Start the maintenance dose 24 hours after the loading dose of the respective drugs.
- Phenytoin is incompatible with dextrose, should be diluted with normal saline.
- Do not use diazepam/midazolam for control of convulsions in neonates.
- Intravenous (IV) calcium gluconate (10%) is always administered slowly under cardiac monitoring (infusion withheld if HR < 100).
- After a seizure-free period of 48–72 hours, stop anticonvulsants.
- At discharge, stop phenobarbitone if neurological examination and EEG are normal. If the neurological examination or EEG is abnormal (electrical seizure activity or a burst-suppression background): discharge on maintenance therapy.
- Review at monthly intervals and taper anticonvulsants if neurological examination and EEG become normal.
- If anticonvulsants are required beyond 3 months, consult a neurologist and switch to other drugs.
- A cranial ultrasound scan is recommended as per unit policy.
- The interictal EEG is a good guide to prognosis, especially when performed at 12–48 hours.
- Very depressed background or burst suppression indicates a poor prognosis.
- Pyridoxine causes hypotension and apnea, should be used in a NICU setting.
- A normal neurological examination at discharge provides reassurance.

■ FURTHER READING

1. Management of the seizure in newborn. Clinical practice guideline, NNF; 2010.
2. Volpe JJ. Neonatal seizures. Neurology of the Newborn, 4th edition. Philadelphia: Saunders; 2001.
3. WHO. (2011). Guidelines on neonatal seizures. [online] Available from https://apps.who.int/iris/bitstream/handle/10665/77756/9789241548304_eng.pdf;jsessionid=A17D020B403F4BC6C57E4D0608215013?sequence=1 [Last accessed September, 2022].

Neuroprotective Strategies

Somalika Pal

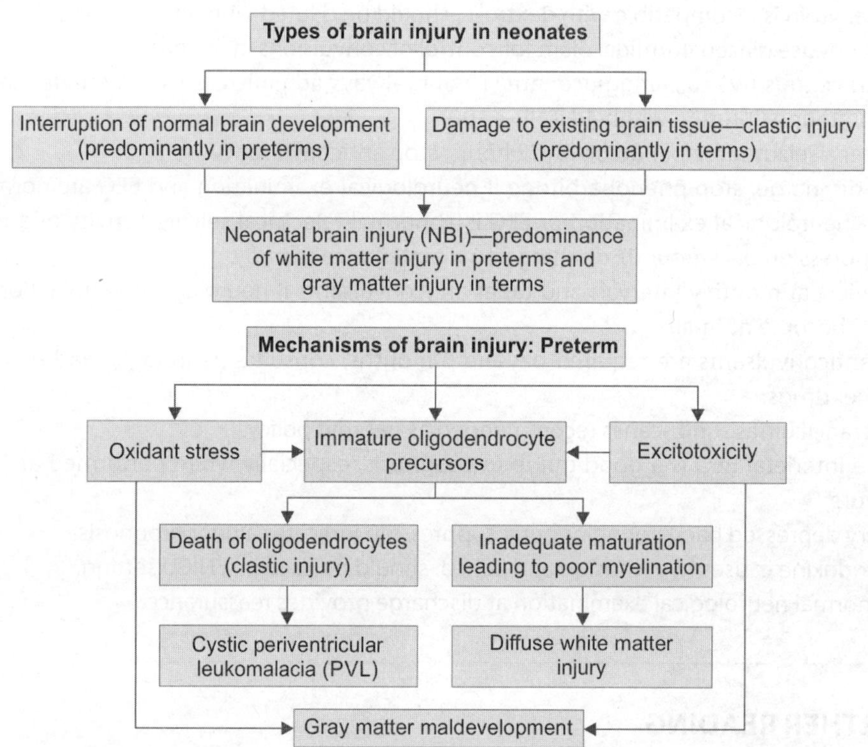

■ NEUROPROTECTIVE INTERVENTIONS FOR PRETERM INFANTS

Antenatal	
Neuroprotective strategies	***Comments***
Strategies for reduction of preterm birth, e.g., iron-folic acid (IFA) and calcium supplementation, appropriate management of maternal conditions predisposing to preterm birth, e.g., hypertension, antiphospholipid antibodies (APLA), cervical incompetence, etc.	• Maternal anemia increases risk of preterm birth • Maternal calcium supplementation results in 12% reduction in risk of preterm birth in developing countries

Contd...

Contd...

Antenatal	
Neuroprotective strategies	**Comments**
In utero transfer of women at risk of preterm delivery	Postnatally transported preterms have significantly higher chances of severe brain injury and lower risk of survival without brain injury

Antibiotics for PPROM (preterm premature rupture of membranes)	• Ascending intrauterine infections significantly increase the risk of fetal brain damage
	• Antibiotics for PROM help in:
	  – About 12% reduction in respiratory distress syndrome (RDS)
	  – About 39% reduction in neonatal sepsis
	  – Decreased neonatal mortality
	  – Decreased IVH (intraventricular hemorrhage)

Antenatal steroids	• Reduced IVH by 45%, RDS by 35%, need for ventilation and surfactant use • Not more than 2 courses to be used evidence of poor fetal head growth with multiple repeated courses
Antenatal magnesium sulfate—most commonly bolus injection of 4–6 g over 30 minutes, followed by maintenance doses of 1–2 g/h for 12 hours. The aim of this procedure is to double the magnesium level in the mother's serum	• *Mechanism of neuroprotection:* Reduces excitotoxic damage [binds to Mg site on N-methyl-D-aspartic acid (NMDA)-glutamate channel)] • A 31% decrease in cerebral palsy (CP) • A 39% decrease in the risk of substantial motor dysfunction
Postnatal	
Neuroprotective strategies	**Comments**
Delayed cord clamping (>30 seconds) in all stable preterm births	Potential 50% reduction in IVH
Caffeine	*Reduction in:* • Apnea • Need for mechanical ventilation • Combined outcome of death or survival with neurodevelopmental impairments (NDI) like CP, cognitive deficit, blindness, and deafness decreased
Gentle ventilation: Noninvasive modes of ventilation—synchronized, volume-targeted ventilation, lower intrathoracic pressures [lower mean airway pressure (MAP)], permissive hypercapnia	Compared to nasal intermittent positive pressure ventilation (NIPPV) both synchronized intermittent mandatory ventilation (SIMV) and high-frequency oscillatory ventilation (HFOV) increased IVH among preterm infants ventilated for RDS
Early initiation of feeding, focus on human milk feeding	Each 10% increase in human milk feeds is associated with about 8–12% lower sepsis/necrotizing enterocolitis (NEC) risk
Minimize use of postnatal steroids	Associated with an increase in CP and neurodevelopmental impairment, especially early steroid use

Contd...

Contd...

Postnatal	
Neuroprotective strategies	*Comments*
Hemodynamic stability—optimal use of inotropes	• Preterm neonatal cerebral circulation is pressure passive, hence the need to prevent fluctuations in BP • Both hypo and hypertension can be detrimental
Timely treatment of jaundice requiring treatment	Preterms are susceptible to bilirubin encephalopathy at a low level of bilirubin
Prevention of sepsis—asepsis protocols, bundling of care, early feeding, judicious use of antibiotics-minimize amikacin usage	Infections are known to adversely affect the developing brain via inflammatory mediators and cytokines
Developmentally supportive care (DSC)—attention to NICU light and sound levels, positioning, pain management, gentle handling, and protected sleep	Pain alleviation and healing environment lowers stress, shown to be neuroprotective
Kangaroo mother care—initiated as early as possible	*Improved:* • Breastfeeding • Growth • Attention and quality of movements • Cognitive development and executive functions for up to 10 years
Focus on postnatal nutrition- early enteral feeding, fortification as needed	Poor postnatal weigh gain is associated with poorer cognitive outcomes

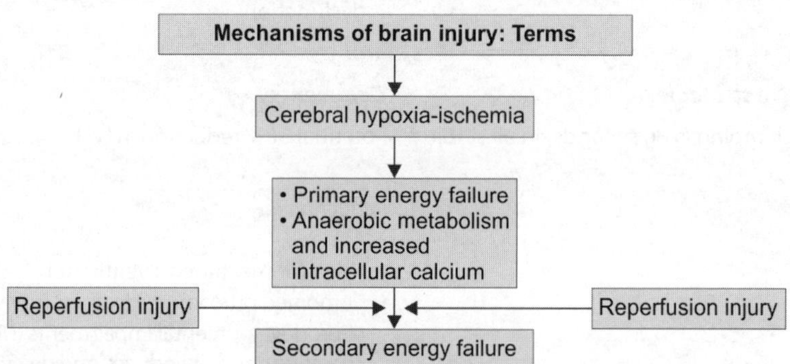

◼ NEUROPROTECTIVE INTERVENTIONS FOR TERM INFANTS

	Approach	*Comments*
Antenatal	Prevention of perinatal asphyxia	
Postnatal	Therapeutic hypothermia (TH) (72 hours of cooling to 33.5 ± 0.5°C followed by slow rewarming, 0.5°C per hour to normothermia) in babies with moderate-to-severe hypoxic–ischemic encephalopathy (HIE)	• Less death and NDI (combined outcome at 18 months) among survivors. RR 0.75 (95% CI 0.64–0.88) • NNT to benefit 7 (95% CI 5–10)

Contd...

Contd...

	Approach	Comments
	Adjunctive therapies with TH on the horizon for term asphyxiated newborns (experimental): • Erythropoietin • Xenon • Argon • Melatonin	

VARIOUS STRATEGIES TO REDUCE BRAIN INJURY IN PRETERM INFANTS: SUMMARY OF EVIDENCE

Antenatal period	In utero transfer for anticipated preterm delivery	Mortality is reduced [OR 0.73 (0.59–0.9)] and morbidity free survival is increased [OR 1.92 (1.02–3.6)]
	Antenatal steroids	• IVH (all grades) is reduced [RR 0.54 (0.43–0.69)] • Developmental delay at 3 years is reduced [RR 0.49 (0.24–1.00)] • Cerebral palsy (all severities) at 2–6 years is reduced [RR 0.60 (0.34–1.03)]
	Magnesium sulfate for pregnant women at risk of imminent preterm birth <34 weeks of gestation	• Cerebral palsy (all severities) at 12–24 months is reduced [RR 0.68 (0.54–0.87)] • Cerebral palsy (moderate to severe) at 12–24 months is reduced [RR 0.64 (0.44–0.92)] • Gross motor dysfunction at 18–24 months is reduced [RR 0.61 (0.44–0.85)]
	Antibiotics following preterm premature rupture of membranes	• Prolongation of pregnancy, reduction in neonatal infection [RR 0.67(0.52–0.85)] and abnormal cranial ultrasound scans [RR 0.81(0.68–0.98)] • At school age, no difference in functional, behavioral or attainment outcomes
Peripartum period	Delayed cord clamping	• Reduction in IVH (all grades) [RR 0.59 (0.41–0.85)] • Reduction in gross motor dysfunction at 18–22 months [RR 0.32 (0.10–0.90)]
Postnatal period	Prevention of hypothermia	• Moderate and severe hypothermia is associated with increased risk of IVH [RR 1.3 (1.1–1.6) for moderate] and death [RR 1.5 (1.3–1.9) for moderate and RR 5.6 (1.1–28.1) for severe hypothermia] • Plastic wraps reduce hypothermia on admission to the nursery or up to 2 hours after birth [RR 0.67 (0.62–0.72)] • Skin-to-skin contact reduces hypothermia at birth for infants with birth weight ≥1,200 and ≤2,199 g [RR 0.09 (0.01–0.64)]
	Judicious management of hypotension	• No evidence for very preterm infants without cardiovascular compromise and insufficient evidence for very preterm infants with cardiovascular compromise regarding routine use of volume expansion for severe disability [RR 0.80 (0.52, 1.23)], CP [RR 0.76 (0.48, 1.20)] • One should be cautious using volume expansion and inotrope in premature infants

Contd...

Contd...

	Prophylactic indomethacin	• Reduction in IVH (grades 3 and 4) [RR 0.66 (0.53–0.82)] • Reduction in ventriculomegaly, PVL or other white matter echo abnormalities [RR 0.80 (0.65–0.97)]
	Caffeine	• Reduction in CP (all severities 12–22 months) AOR 0.58 (0.39–0.87) • Reduction in cognitive delay (18–22 months) AOR 0.81 (0.66–0.99)
	BPD prevention	
	Volume ventilation	Reduction in PVL and IVH (grades 3 and 4) [RR 0.48 (0.28–0.84)]
		Observational studies have shown that hypercapnia ($pCO_2 > 60$ mm Hg) and hypocapnia ($pCO_2 < 35$ mm Hg) can cause brain injury and should be avoided particularly during initial 72 hours after birth (target pCO_2 between 45 and 55 mm Hg, to a maximum of 60 mm Hg)
	Head positioning	Limited evidence
	Nurturing environment and optimizing postnatal growth	
	Prevention of sepsis and NEC	*Postnatal infection and neurodevelopmental outcome:* CP (all types) — Early onset sepsis (EOS)—OR 1.7 (0.84–3.45) Late onset sepsis (LOS)—OR 1.71 (1.14–2.56) EOS + LOS—OR 2.33 (1.02–5.33)
	Restrictive blood transfusion policy	Decrease transfusion associated IVH

■ EXPERIMENTAL NEUROPROTECTIVE STRATEGIES ON THE HORIZON

Anti-inflammatory agents	• Minocycline • Nonsteroidal anti-inflammatory drugs (NSAIDs)	
Anti-excitatory	Topiramate	
Antioxidants	• Melatonin • Allopurinol • N-acetylcysteine	Melatonin also holds promise as a prenatal neuroprotectant that could be administered to pregnant women since it appears safe, crosses the placenta
Prevention of protracted cell death and modulation of plasticity	Erythropoietin	Has remarkable neuroprotective, antiapoptotic, and reparative effects in CNS: • *In terms:* Concern regarding safety, a clinical trial in term neonates with encephalopathy has been placed on hold • *In preterms:* PENUT trial has shown significant benefit on early brain imaging but no benefit on neurodevelopmental scores on follow-up at 2 years of age

Contd...

Contd...

Cell-specific targeting	Microglial activation	
Stem cells	Neuronal, mesenchymal, or hematopoietic stem cells	

Key Points to Remember

- Prematurity and intrapartum complications (perinatal asphyxia) remain the most common causes of neonatal mortality.
- With advances in neonatal intensive care unit (NICU) care, survival of such babies would increase the burden of neurodevelopmental impairments (NDI). Hence, the importance of neuroprotective strategies in managing such neonates.
- Neuroprotection refers to mechanisms and strategies employed to protect the central nervous system (CNS) against injury, both acute as well as long term.
- Ideally, neuroprotection would benefit from multimodal approaches with multiple targets at different stages of neurodevelopment.
- The two most important acquired brain injuries in preterm infants are IVH and PVL, respectively.
- These injuries are commonly seen in very and extreme preterm infants and contribute significantly to the in-hospital mortality and morbidity, as well as it also increases the risk of developing long-term NDI.
- As neonatal care improves overall with reduction in neonatal mortality rates, the burden of survivors with NDIs increases. Hence, the focus should shift from survival to intact survival.
- Established neuroprotective strategies for terms and preterms are now standard of care and should be adopted by all NICUs.

■ FURTHER READING

1. Abate BB, Bimerew M, Gebremichael B, Mengesha Kassie A, Kassaw M, Gebremeskel T, et al. Effects of therapeutic hypothermia on death among asphyxiated neonates with hypoxic-ischemic encephalopathy: A systematic review and meta-analysis of randomized control trials. PLoS ONE. 2021;16(2):e0247229.
2. Gleason CA, Juul SE. Chapter on Neuroprotection strategies of newborn. Averys Textbook of Neonatology, 10th edition. Netherlands: Elsevier; 2018.
3. McGoldrick E, Stewart F, Parker R, Dalziel SR. Antenatal corticosteroids for accelerating fetal lung maturation for women at risk of preterm birth. Cochrane Database Syst Rev. 2020;12(12):CD004454.

Cerebral Function Monitoring

Vishal Gupta

INDICATIONS

- To assess brain activity in near-term or term infants with hypoxic-ischemic encephalopathy to help determine whether therapeutic hypothermia should be initiated.
- Assessment for seizures if a standard electroencephalography (EEG) is not possible at that time.
- Evaluating the pattern of brain activity with amplitude-integrated electroencephalography (aEEG) can be helpful in infants with cerebral insults (e.g., stroke, infarction, and hemorrhage).

TECHNICAL ASPECTS OF aEEG

Number of Electrodes

- In contrast to conventional EEG, an aEEG has fewer electrodes.
- One channel (2 electrodes) or two channels (4 electrodes) are used.

Amplitude-integrated Electroencephalography Electrodes

- To record aEEG, typically, 2 or 4 electrodes and a reference electrode in the midline are used.
- When a single-channel EEG is used, 2 electrodes are placed on the biparietal (P3–P4) region and their voltage potential difference results in an aEEG tracing, as shown in **Figure 1**.
- If a two-channel aEEG is used (i.e., C3–C4), 2 additional electrodes are placed, as shown in **Figure 2**, in addition to the single channel P3–P4 electrodes. The sensitivity for detecting interhemispheric asymmetries and seizures is enhanced with this other channel.

Electrode Placement

- Hydrogel **(Fig. 3)** or subdermal needle electrode **(Fig. 4)** is commonly used in most NICUs.
- The primary determinant of an accurate aEEG recording is to ensure the standard interelectrode distance and that the left and right electrodes are symmetrically placed.
- Careful skin preparation is necessary before electrode placement to avoid high impedance. After shaving (if required), the scalp area where the electrodes will be applied should be cleaned with saline gauze.
- Subdermal needle electrodes are easier to place and have lower impedance.

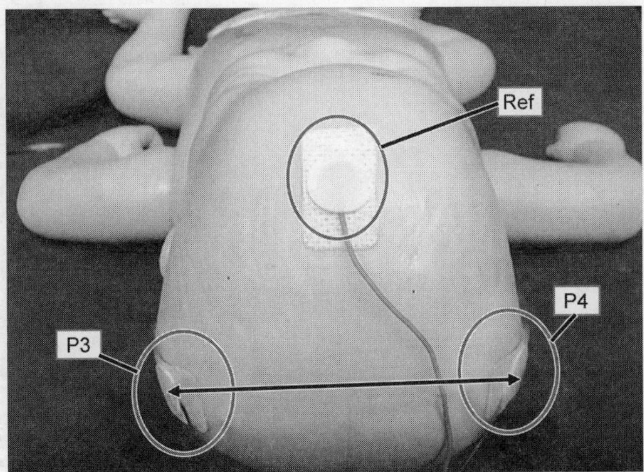

Fig. 1: One-channel aEEG showing electrode placement at locations P3 and P4 along with a reference (ref) or neutral electrode.

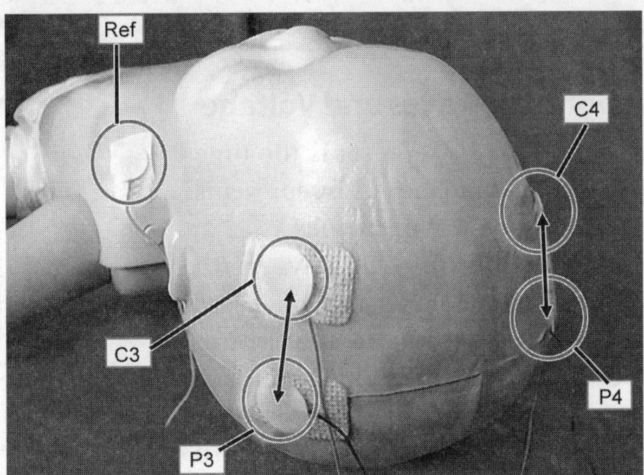

Fig. 2: Two-channel aEEG with electrode placement at C3–C4 and P3–P4 as well as a reference (ref) electrode.

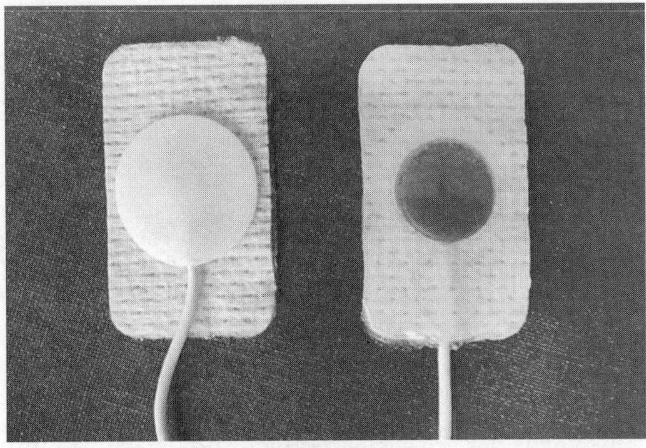

Fig. 3: Hydrogel electrodes.

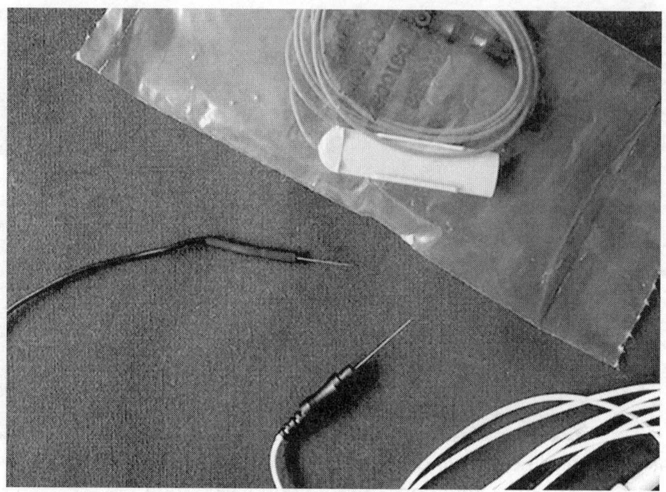

Fig. 4: Needle electrodes.

Amplitude-integrated Electroencephalography Waves and Voltage

- In the aEEG graph, the x-axis represents the time scale measured in seconds, and the y-axis represents voltage (amplitude) measured in microvolts.
- All negative voltages become positive with rectification and time compression of the voltages.
- The resulting minimum and maximum amplitudes are then plotted on an aEEG graph in a semilogarithmic scale every 15 seconds so that voltages of 10–100 mcV are logarithmic and 0–10 mcV are linear **(Fig. 5)**.
- The signals are recorded digitally at a slow speed of approximately 1 mm/min or 60 mm/h (i.e., 6 cm/h), as shown in **Figure 6**.

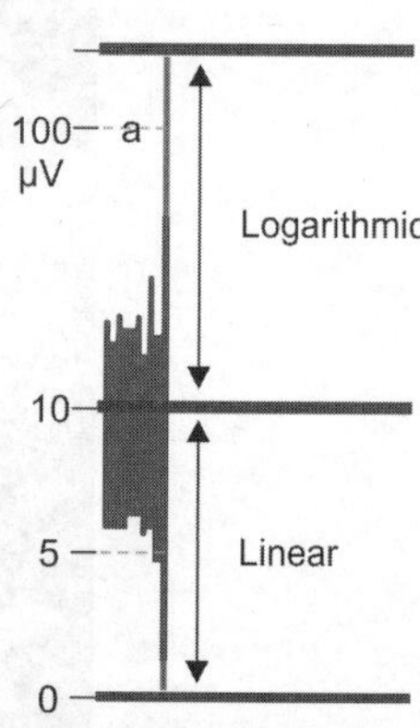

Fig. 5: A semilogarithmic display of amplitude showing voltages that are 10–100 mcV logarithmic and 0–10 mcV linear.

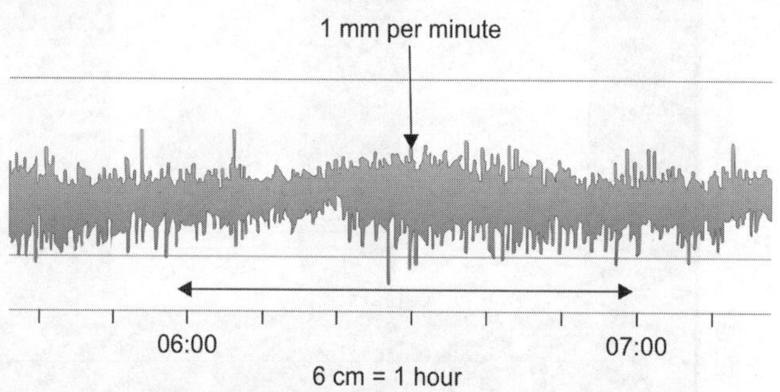

Fig. 6: Time compression in aEEG showing that signals are recorded digitally at a slow speed of approximately 6 cm/h.

- The resultant band-like pattern obtained corresponds to increased or decreased cerebral activity.
- The bandwidth density is directly related to the duration of the aEEG that is recorded.

Impedance

- Impedance is resistance to current flow and reflects the quality of the electrode's contact with the scalp.
- Impedance is measured in Ohms (Ω).
- It should be low (<10 kΩ).

■ INTERPRETATION OF aEEG

The interpretation of aEEG generally includes three categories—(1) classification of the background pattern, (2) sleep-wake cycling, and (3) the presence or absence of seizures.

Background Patterns

There are five basic background patterns:

1. *Continuous pattern:* Continuous background activity with amplitude over 5 mcV in the lower margins and up to 50 mcV in the upper margins **(Fig. 7)**.
2. *Discontinuous pattern:* Discontinuous background with amplitude <5 mcV in the lower margins and >10 mcV in the upper margins **(Fig. 8)**.
3. *Burst suppression:* Discontinuous background with minimum amplitude without variability at 0–1 mcV and burst with high amplitude (>25 mcV) **(Fig. 9)**.
4. *Continuous low voltage:* Continuous background pattern of very low voltage with all voltage <10 mcV **(Fig. 10)**.
5. *Flat or isoelectric tracing:* Mainly inactive background of extremely low voltage (<5 mcV) **(Fig. 11)**.

Sleep-wake Cycling

- Sleep-wake cycle (SWC) on aEEG is characterized by smooth sinusoidal variations, mainly in the lower margin.

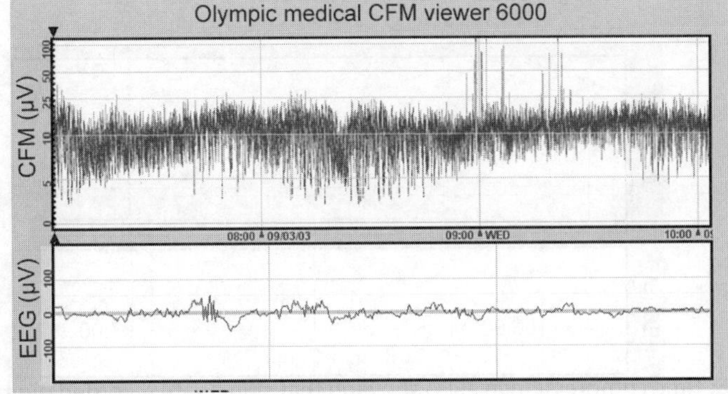

Fig. 7: Continuous pattern normal voltage with sleep-wake cycling.

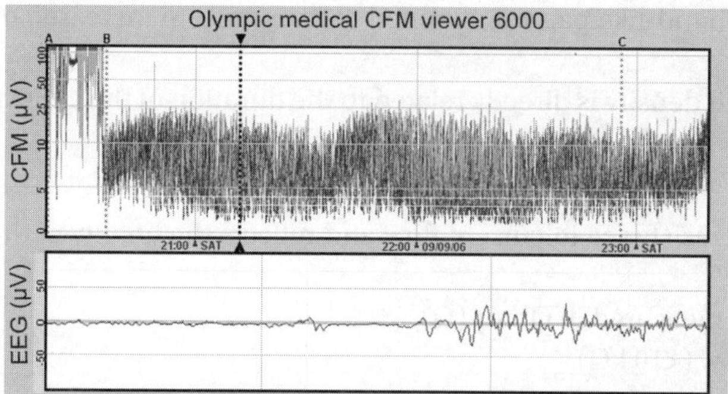

Fig. 8: Discontinuous pattern normal voltage.

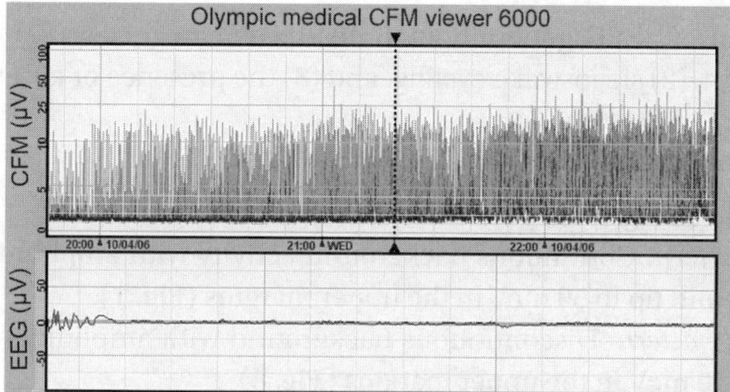

Fig. 9: Burst suppression pattern.

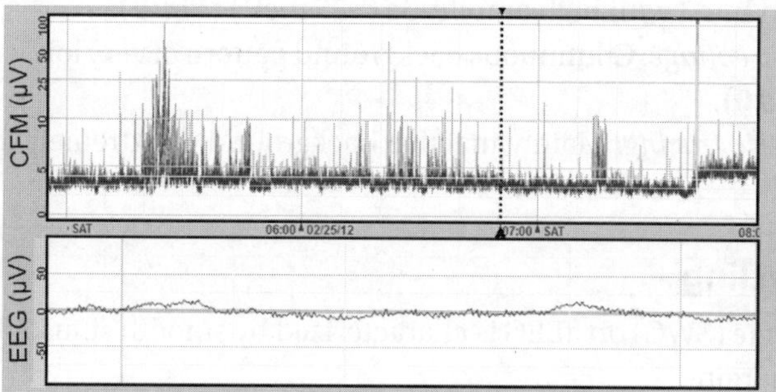

Fig. 10: Continuous pattern with low voltage.

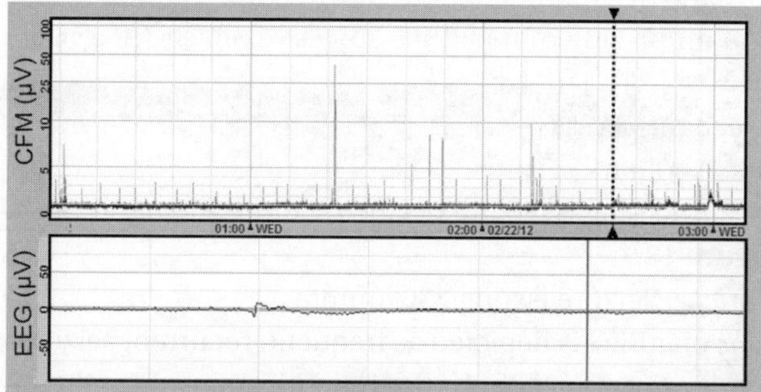

Fig. 11: Flat trace/isoelectric trace.

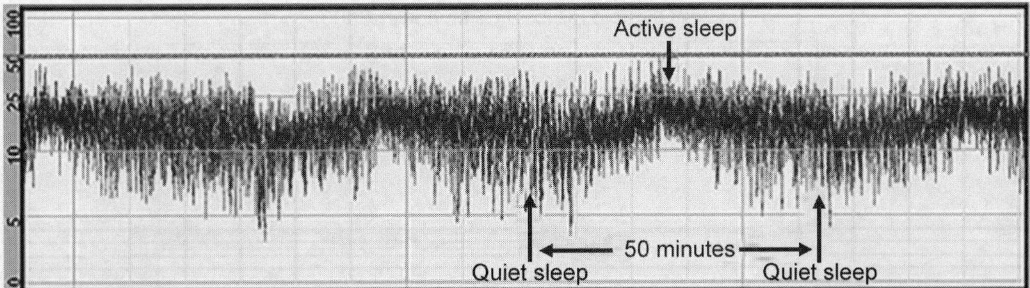

Fig. 12: aEEG trace showing sleep-wake cycle. During quiet sleep, the broader band represents discontinuous background activity and during wakefulness and active sleep, there is a narrow bandwidth and continuous activity.

- The broader bandwidth represents discontinuous background activity during quiet sleep whereas the narrow bandwidth signifies continuous activity during wakefulness and active sleep as shown in **Figure 12**.
- Sleep-wake cycle can be identified as early as 30 weeks' gestation, and its development correlates with postmenstrual age, suggesting better short-term outcomes in preterm infants.
- Term newborns with significant perinatal asphyxia lack SWC. The early return of SWC in these affected infants is thought to be a predictor of good neurodevelopmental outcomes.

SWC is further classified as follows:
- *No SWC:* No cyclic variation of the aEEG background
- *Immature SWC:* Some periods of cyclic variation of the lower amplitude tracings
- *Developed SWC:* Clearly identifiable sinusoidal variations between discontinuous and more continuous background activity, with cycle duration ≥20 minutes.

Detection of Seizure Activity

- Seizures are recognizable on aEEG as an abrupt rise in the lower margin and upper margin, often followed by a short period of decreased amplitude.
- Correct interpretation is greatly improved by simultaneous raw EEG recording available on the modern aEEG machines.
- The simultaneous raw EEG shows seizure activity, with a gradual build-up and then decline in frequency and amplitude of repetitive spikes or sharp-waves with duration of at least 5–10 seconds.
- Seizure can be recognized as:
  - *Single seizure:* A solitary seizure
  - *Repetitive seizures:* Single seizure occurring more frequently in 30 minutes interval as shown in **Figure 13**.
  - *Status epilepticus:* Seizure lasting >30 minutes.
- Status epilepticus on aEEG is depicted as frequent, recurrent seizures; this gives the aEEG tracing a sawtooth appearance, from the repetitive narrowing bandwidth and increased peak-to-peak amplitude **(Fig. 14)**.

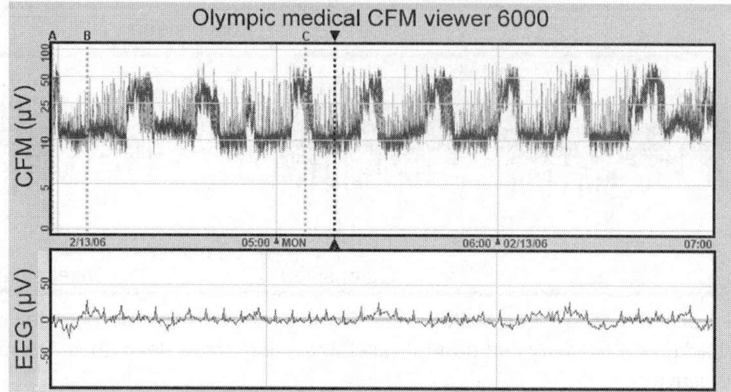

Fig. 13: Repetitive seizures.

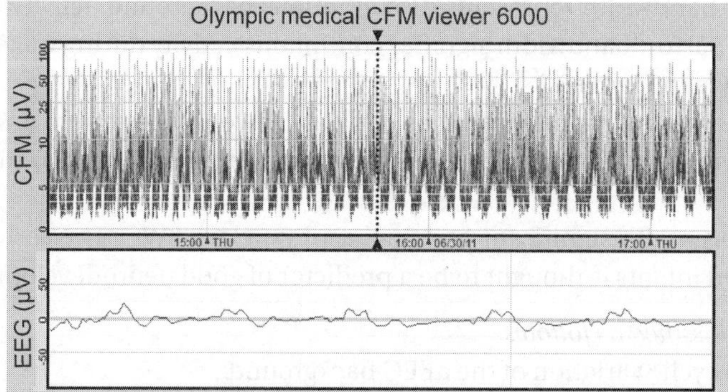

Fig. 14: Status epilepticus (Saw-tooth appearance) of cerebral function monitoring trace.

PITFALLS IN INTERPRETATION aEEG

- Artifacts commonly mistaken for seizures on aEEG.
- A gradual increase and decrease of the upper and lower margins rather than an abrupt rise is suggestive of an artifact.
- *Extracerebral factors*—procedures, handling, and pulsatile respiratory movements from an oscillator causes artifact.
- *Loose electrodes*—impedance will be high if scalp electrodes are loose shown in **Figure 15**. High electrode impedance is very likely to measure such as noise, high frequency ventilation, infusion pumps, and other electrical systems. It, therefore, affects the accuracy of aEEG interpretation.
- *Scalp edema/cephalohematoma*—the amplitude of the electrocortical activity can be decreased by scalp edema or cephalohematoma because the space between the electrode and the brain is increased.
- *Drugs*—morphine, phenobarbital, lidocaine, and midazolam may depress aEEG activity.

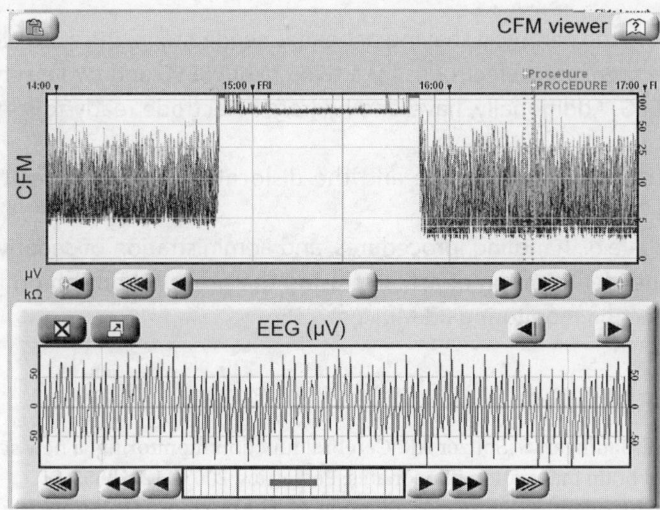

Fig. 15: Example of loose electrode: Impedance is high and a gray bar will appear at the top of the cerebral function monitoring trace.

NEAR-INFRARED SPECTROSCOPY

- Near-infrared spectroscopy is a noninvasive technique that can continuously monitor regional oxygen saturation (rSO_2) which reflects the perfusion status and oxygenation status of underlying tissues at the bedside.
- Near-infrared spectroscopy represents tissue oxygen delivery and consumption.
- Near-infrared light is transmitted and detected by a probe placed on an infant's forehead.
- Near-infrared light at different wavelength is measured and because oxyhemoglobin and deoxyhemoglobin have different absorption spectra, tissue oxygenation can be calculated.
- Near-infrared spectroscopy can be used to estimate cerebral blood volume, cerebral blood flow, and fractional tissue oxygen extraction (FTOE).
- Cerebral rSO_2 is monitored to prevent brain damage in conditions which affect cerebral perfusion and oxygenation. These conditions include hypoxic-ischemic encephalopathy, hypotension, apnea and bradycardia, hemodynamically significant patent ductus arteriosus (hs-PDA), and perioperative status of congenital heart disease.

Key Points to Remember

- Amplitude-integrated electroencephalography (aEEG) is a method for continuous monitoring cerebral function in neonatal intensive care unit (NICU).
- The cerebral function monitor was first developed by Prior and Maynard in 1960s for use in adult patients in intensive care.
- Amplitude-integrated electroencephalography is a limited channel electroencephalography that provides a noninvasive method for continuous observation of cerebral background activity at the bedside.

- Consent from the parents if shaving of head is needed to fix the aEEG electrodes.
- Ensure that there are 4 electrodes for a two-channel EEG and two electrodes for a single channel aEEG. Additionally, have one hydrogel electrode ready to serve as a reference electrode.
- Regularly check for impedance and the dislocation of electrodes to obtain quality recordings.
- Mark events (e.g., handling, procedures, and administration of sedatives or opioids) to facilitate the identification of artifacts using the provided button on the screen of the cerebral function monitoring (CFM).

■ FURTHER READING

1. Burdjalov VF, Baumgart S, Spitzer AR. Cerebral function monitoring: a new scoring system for the evaluation of brain maturation in neonates. Pediatrics. 2003;112(4):855-61.
2. Hallberg B, Grossmann K, Bartocci M, Blennow M. The prognostic value of early aEEG in asphyxiated infants undergoing systemic hypothermia treatment. Acta Paediatr. 2010;99(4):531-6.
3. Lavery S, Shah DK, Hunt RW, Filan PM, Doyle LW, Inder TE. Single versus bihemispheric amplitude-integrated electroencephalography in relation to cerebral injury and outcome in the term encephalopathic infant. J Paediatr Child Health. 2008;44(5):285-90.
4. Maynard D, Prior PF, Scott DF. A continuous monitoring device for cerebral activity. Electroencephalogr Clin Neurophysiol. 1969;27(7):672-73.

Chapter 23

Management of Intraventricular Hemorrhage

Shikha Handa, Kunal S Chawla

TYPES (*SEE* TABLE 1)

- *Extra-axial*: It is defined as bleeding within skull but outside brain tissue. It is further divided into—
  - Epidural hemorrhage
  - Subdural hemorrhage
  - Subarachnoid hemorrhage
- *Intra-axial*: It is defined as bleeding within brain parenchyma. It can be seen as—
  - Intracerebral hemorrhage
  - Intraventricular hemorrhage (IVH)

CLINICAL MANIFESTATIONS

Silent syndrome	• Most common presentation • Clinically silent presentation • Unexplained fall in hematocrit or failure of rise in hematocrit after transfusion can be the only
Saltatory syndrome	• Evolve over hours to days • Alteration in level of consciousness, lethargy • Decreased spontaneous or excitatory motility • Abnormal eye movements or positions or sometimes both • Hypotonia • Respiratory disturbances like apnea • Tight popliteal angle on examination
Catastrophic syndrome	• Rapid evolution from minutes to hours • Altered sensorium • Stupor, coma • Respiratory disturbances like severe apnea • Seizures (generalized tonic-clonic type) • Altered sensorium • Decorticate or decerebrate posturing • Pupils fixed to light • Fixation of eyes to vestibular stimulus • Hemodynamic instability like bradycardia, poor perfusion • Flaccid quadriparesis • Bulging Fontanel

DIAGNOSIS

- A total of 50% of all the IVH occurs within 24 hours (day 1), 25% on day 2, and another 15% on day 3.
- By the end of 96 hours, i.e., day 4, 90% of the IVH can be detected.
- Of all the IVH detected by day 4, 20–40% progress further to more extensive hemorrhages.

Cranial ultrasound: It is the best modality for in-house screening of preterm infants for IVH in neonatal intensive care units throughout hospitalization. Cranial ultrasound has 91% specificity and 100% sensitivity for detection of IVH (*see* **Table 2**).

MRI brain: It helps in better depiction of brain anatomical landmarks and structures, helping in diagnosing small sized lesion, white matter injury, or complications like periventricular hyperechogenecities.

MANAGEMENT

- *Acute phase management*:
  - Ensure airway patency, breathing, and circulation
  - Maintain blood pressure within normal or target range
  - Avoid hypercarbia, acidosis, and events causing to hypoxemia
  - Avoid acidosis, use of hyperosmolar fluids, respiratory distress, or pneumothorax
  - Serial ultrasounds required for regular monitoring of IVH progression and development of its complications
  - Monitoring of signs and symptoms associated with raised intracranial tension (ICT)
  - Alternate day or biweekly monitoring of head circumference
  - Appropriate nutrition—initiation of minimal enteral nutrition and total parenteral nutrition (TPN) (in sick neonates)
- Large IVH should be treated with prompt stabilization to improve long-term outcomes.
- Saltatory syndrome and mainly catastrophic syndrome may require ventilation, inotropic support, antiepileptics support, and volume expansion including blood transfusions.
- DRIFT, drainage, irrigation, and fibrinolytic therapy, activity is an emerging potential therapeutic strategy in treatment of IVH. It has shown positive results in decreasing the need for shunt surgeries, morbidities, and mortalities. This modality is still not adopted as combined risk of therapy is high.
- Other treatment modalities include growth factors like epidermal growth factors and hormones like thyroxine (T4) and stem cell treatment.

Posthemorrhagic hydrocephalus: Two-thirds neonates who develop PHH require serial lumbar puncture (LP) and surgical interventions repeated aspiration through ventricular-assisted device (VAD) or ventriculoperitoneal (VP) shunt.

Lumbar puncture criteria: Presence of two or more indicates the need of LP.

- Increase in HC > 2 mm/day or >14 mm/week
- *Action line:* Levene index exceeding 4 mm above the 97th centile for ventricular index.
- Resistive index >0.85
- Raised ICT features (splayed sutures, bulging fontanel, and neurological features like lethargy, poor feeding, and seizures)
  - *Effective CSF tap:* Start with minimal of 10 mL/kg to maximum of 20 mL/kg at rate of 1 mL/kg/min
  - Ventricular assisted device and ventriculosubgaleal (VSG) shunt is needed when CSF tap exceeds two lumbar puncture or more than one ventricular tap.
  - Interval between VAD insertion and VP shunt should be of minimum 4 weeks or more.
  - Use of carbonic anhydrase diuretic such as acetazolamide and loop diuretic like furosemide is not advisable as they are associated with nephrocalcinosis, electrolyte disturbances and possibility of worse neurological outcomes thus there safety in treating PVHI is still questionable.

TABLE 1: Types of hemorrhages and its clinical features.

Site of hemorrhage	Area involved	Predisposing factor	Clinical features	Management
Subdural hemorrhage (SDH)	Draining veins occupy space between dura and arachnoid membrane. There is rupture of cerebral vein, sinuses, laceration of falx, or tentorium	Traumatic delivery (large baby), difficult instrument (forcep) delivery, breech or brow presentation, rigid pelvis, and rarely bleeding diathesis	Occurs shortly after birth and progresses rapidly. Lethargy, irritability, anemia, asymmetric hypotonia, focal seizures raised ICP, brainstem compression in infratentorial SDH—opisthotonus posture, abnormal extraocular movements, and apnea	• MRI is study of choice • Lumbar puncture contraindicated in large bleeds • Requires prompt stabilization, IV fluid replacement, blood product transfusion, and supportive care with treatment of seizures • Nonsurgical SDH has good outcome
Epidural hemorrhage (EDH)	• Collection of blood between inner skull and dura • Uncommon in older infants	Traumatic instrument delivery causing injury to middle meningeal artery, large cephalohematoma, or skull fractures	Irritability, skull fracture, and excessive crying	• Supportive treatment with possible surgical or needle aspiration • Prognosis is good

Contd...

Contd...

Site of hemorrhage	Area involved	Predisposing factor	Clinical features	Management
Subarachnoid hemorrhage (SAH)	Blood accumulates between arachnoid mater and pia mater	• Local trauma during delivery, ruptured bridging veins of subarachnoid space, small leptomeningeal vessels • Can be seen as extension of SDH	Clinical suspicion arises from neurologic manifestations like irritability, lethargy, focal neurological signs, and seizures may occur in otherwise well-appearing baby	• MRI brain is best modality; lumbar puncture may be required for confirming small SAH. Treatment is symptomatic/supportive • Anticonvulsants, IV fluid therapy needed if seizures/lethargy is seen
Intracerebral hemorrhage (ICH)	Occur within brain tissue after venous infarction. It can be superficial, deep or hemorrhagic infarction	Rupture of aneurysm or AV malformations, coagulation anomalies like DIC, sepsis, shock, or secondary to events like hypoxic ischemic injury	Superficial ICH symptoms may appear during first 48 hours, features of sepsis, focal neurological signs, seizures, asymmetric tone, irritability, decrease consciousness	• Best imaging modality is MRI brain. CT scan can be used if needed for urgent evaluation • Observation and supportive treatment are the mainstay. If midline shift, neurosurgical intervention is needed
Intraventricular hemorrhage: Incidence varies from 20 to 30% **(Table 2)**	*Subependymal germinal matrix:* Highly fragile, vascular network of capillaries located ventrolaterally to lateral ventricle	• *Neonatal factors:* Prematurity (<32 weeks, <1,500 g), sepsis, thrombocytopenia, hypoxic ischemic events, respiratory distress, mechanical ventilation, pneumothorax, rapid volume expansion, air leak, lack of delayed cord clamping, and use of hyperosmolar fluids • *Maternal factors:* Chorioamnionitis, lack of antenatal steroids	• Silent syndrome • Saltatory syndrome • Catastrophic syndrome	

TABLE 2: Grading of intraventricular hemorrhage.

Grade	Volpe grading system (Based on ultrasound findings)	Papile grading system (Based on CT scans findings)
Grade 1	Germinal matrix/subependymal bleed, no or minimal bleed in ventricular lumen (<10%)	Germinal matrix hemorrhage (within subependymal space)
Grade 2	Hemorrhage seen in lateral ventricles, occupying 10–50% ventricular region No ventriculomegaly	Blood starts filling ventricular region
Grade 3	Hemorrhage with occupancy of more than 50% of lateral ventricles Ventriculomegaly seen	Blood starts spreading causing ventriculomegaly
Grade 4	Development intraparenchymal echogenicity called as periventricular hemorrhagic infarction	IVH with intraparenchymal echogenicity seen

PERIVENTRICULAR LEUKOMALACIA/WHITE MATTER INJURY

- It is defined as lesion of cerebral white matter occurring in periventricular region of the brain parenchyma.
- It is focal and diffuse involving loss of premyelinating oligodendrocyte, neurons, and axons.
- Unlike PVHI, it is arterial in nature.
- It develops over weeks with formation of multifocal areas of necrosis which form cyst in deep periventricular cerebral white matter.
- Topographically, it appears patchy with irregular borders and is symmetrical in nature.

Types

- *Cystic:* Rare and most severe form, correlates with spastic diplegia.
- *Noncystic:* Intermediate form, associated commonly with cognitive and behavioral deficits
- *Diffuse:* Mild form, there is impaired myelination in thalamus, cerebral cortex, basal ganglia, and brain stem. It is also associated with cognitive and behavioral defects.

De Vries Grading of Periventricular Leukomalacia

- *Grade I:* Transient echodensities persisting for <7 days
- *Grade II:* Seen as small, localized cyst in frontoparietal area
- *Grade III:* Extensive cystic lesions in periventricular region
- *Grade IV:* Extensive subcortical cyst in deep cerebral white matter

Risk Factors Associated with Periventricular Leukomalacia

- Prematurity
- Monochorionic twins

- Maternal infection including bacterial vaginal infection and chorioamnionitis
- Abnormal placenta or cord insertion
- Hypotension and hypocarbia
- Postnatal use of steroids
- Septicemia

Diagnosis

In brain, MRI is the best imaging modality of choice. It helps in structural evaluation of white matter area and other region of brain parenchyma.

Key Points to Remember

- Most common bleeding in preterm infant arises from subependymal germinal matrix that may result into IVH or its complications like periventricular hemorrhagic infarction (PVHI).
- In term neonates, subdural or subarachnoid hemorrhage is common. It may be related to birth trauma, hypoxic-ischemic encephalopathy (HIE) or coagulopathies, or other undetermined conditions.

Consequences of Intraventricular Hemorrhage

- As the hemorrhage spreads through ventricular system and subarachnoid space, it can cause obliterative arachnoiditis.
- Damage to germinal matrix can lead to disruption of neuronal and glial precursors.
- Particulate matter in hemorrhage leading to ventriculomegaly thus causing obstruction to cerebrospinal fluid (CSF) flow. This is known as posthemorrhagic hydrocephalus (PHH). 12% of neonates with ventriculomegaly (10–50%) and 70% of neonates with severe grade developed PHH.
- Obstruction of terminal vein by large IVH (usually grade III) causes venous infarct, which is also known as PVHI. Its most common sequela is porencephalic cyst. It is mostly asymmetrical fan-shaped and with sharp borders, seen unilaterally.

Outcomes

- Grade I or grade II IVH neonates have high chances of developing cerebral palsy or developmental delay.
- Grade III IVH develops 35% of neurological sequelae.
- Mortality is seen in 20% of neonates with grade III IVH and 50% with grade IV.
- Abnormal DQ and motor deficits are commonly seen in neonates with grade III IVH with percentage of 8% and 54%, respectively.
- Most common outcome of neonates developing PVHI is porencephalic cyst and spastic diplegia of lower limbs.
- There is also risk of neuromotor and cognitive impairment seen with parenchymal hemorrhage.

Preventive Strategy for IVH: Interventions

- *Antenatal period:*
  - Prevent preterm delivery
  - In-utero transport of preterm neonates
  - Antenatal corticosteroids use
  - Magnesium sulfate administration in women with risk of preterm delivery <32 weeks
  - Mothers with premature rupture of membrane (PROM)—administer appropriate antibiotics
- *Postnatal and neonatal intensive care unit (NICU) care:*
  - Warm delivery room and warm resuscitation preventing hypothermia
  - Optimize ventilation strategies, volume targeted
  - Delayed cord clamping for 60 seconds as per recent guidelines
  - Exogenous surfactant administration
  - Caffeine administration for apnea of prematurity
  - Early extubation
  - Minimizing complications like pneumothorax
  - Indomethacin prophylaxis
  - Early nutrition (EBM or TPN)
  - Avoid use of hyperosmolar fluids
  - Prevention of sepsis, necrotizing enterocolitis (NEC)
  - Maintain normal blood pressure range
  - Maintain euglycemic state, hemodynamic stability, and electrolyte balance
  - Prophylactic use of ibuprofen or paracetamol for closure of patent ductus arteriosus (PDA)

■ FURTHER READING

1. Eichenwald EC, Hansen AR, Martin CR, Stark AR. Cloherty and Stark's Manual of Neonatal Care, 8th edition. Gurugram, India; Wolters Kluwer; 2018. pp. 790-811.
2. Lea CL, Smith-Collins A, Luyt K. Protecting the premature brain: current evidence-based strategies for minimizing perinatal brain injury in preterm infants. Arch Dis Child Fetal Neonatal Ed. 2017;102(2):F176-F182.
3. Volpe JJ, Inder TE, Darras BT, de Vries LS, du Plessis AJ, Neil J, et al. Neurology of the Newborn, 6th edition. Philadelphia; Elsevier Saunders; 2018. pp. 637-97.

Management of Hydrocephalus

Jay Kishore

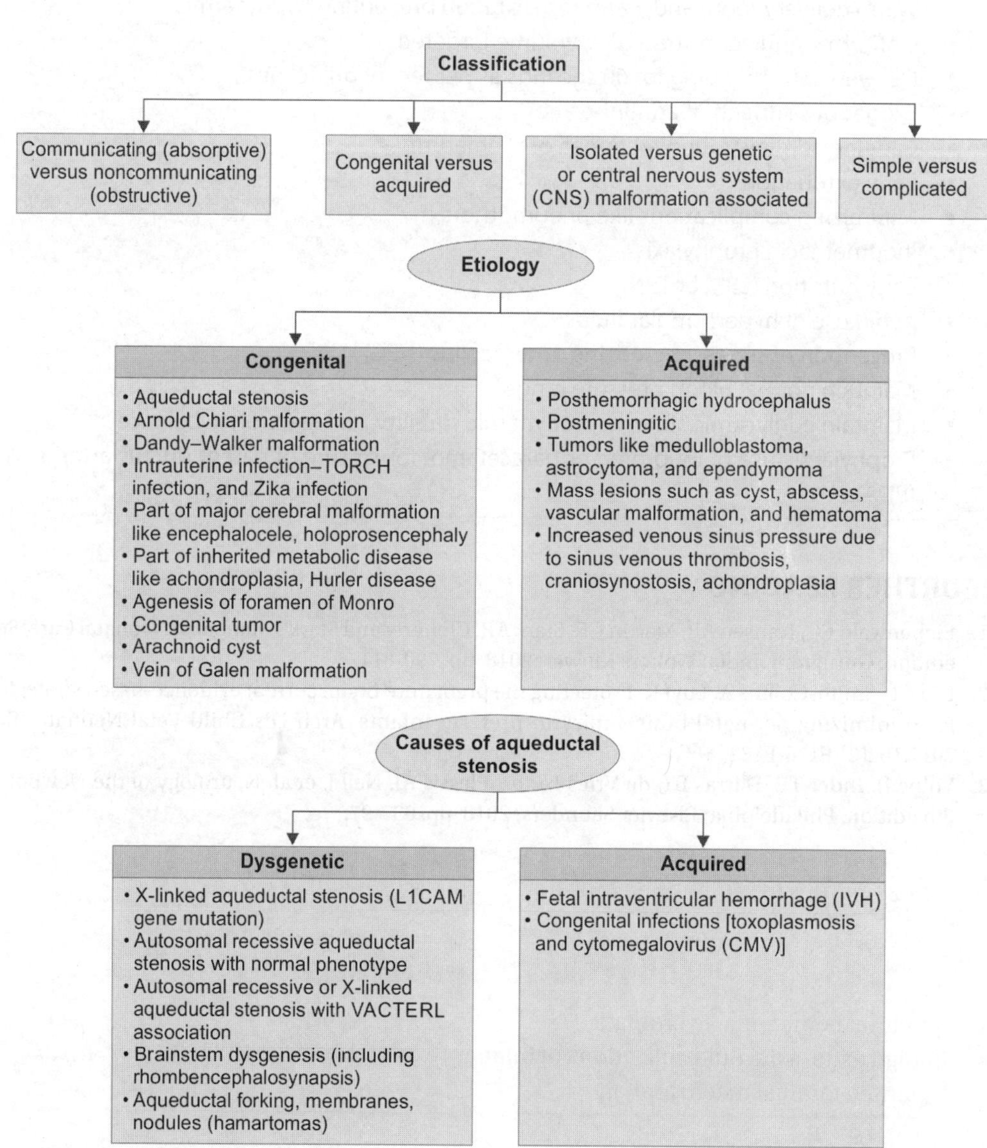

Management algorithm

Elicit antenatal history, history of fetal ventriculomegaly, history of intrauterine infection, and history of alloimmune thrombocytopenia if OFC >2 SD

OFC measurement >2 SD, serial measurement showing >2 mm/day increment, associated malformation, syndrome, and etiology

↓

USG/MRI
Look for progressive ventriculomegaly, periventricular ooze, Levene index (97th centile + 4 mm), anterior horn width (AHW) (3 mm + 1 mm), third ventricle width (2 mm + 1 mm), thalamo-occipital distance (25 mm + 1 mm), resistive index anterior cerebral artery (ACA) (>0.85) with clinical signs

↓

Ventriculosubgaleal shunt (VSG), ventricular access device (reservoir), or external ventricular drain

↓

If ventricular dilation persists
Endoscopic third ventriculostomy (ETV) + choroid plexus coagulation (CPC) (select cases of aqueductal stenosis)
Ventriculoperitoneal shunt (VPS) if weight >1.5 kg and CSF protein <1.5 g/L

CLINICAL FEATURES AND EXAMINATION

- Occipitofrontal circumference (OFC) >2 standard deviation (SD), persistent increase in OFC >2 mm/day
- Bulging tense anterior fontanel
- Bradycardia and apnea
- Poor feeding and vomiting
- Drowsy and irritable
- Scalp vein distended, scalp skin thin and shiny, and cranial sutures splayed
- In advanced cases, craniofacial disproportion, expansion of dome, low set eyes, and ears
- Positive transillumination and epileptic seizure
- Papilledema rare
- Abducens nerve palsy, upward gaze palsy, and sunset sign
- Flexion deformity of the thumbs in X-linked aqueductal stenosis, occipital prominence in Dandy–Walker malformation, myelomeningocele in Arnold Chiari type II malformation
- Chorioretinitis in intrauterine infection.

DIFFERENTIAL DIAGNOSIS

- Subdural hematoma/hygroma
- Benign extra-axial fluid collections of infancy (external hydrocephalus)
- Inherited familial macrocephaly

- Tumors (may or may not be associated with hydrocephalus)
- Fragile X syndrome
- Overgrowth syndromes (e.g., Sotos syndrome and Weaver syndrome)
- Lysosomal storage diseases
- Leukodystrophies
- Hemimegalencephaly/megalencephaly (can be familial or nonfamilial).

Key Points to Remember

Mechanism of Posthemorrhagic Ventricular Dilation (PHVD)

- Obstruction of ventricular system by blood clot.
- Inefficient fibrinolysis of CSF due to low plasminogen and high plasminogen activator inhibitor.
- Chronic obliterative, fibrosing arachnoiditis, and subependymal gliosis involving deposition of extracellular matrix proteins in the foramina of the fourth ventricle and the subarachnoid space.
- Transforming growth factor β-key stimulator of fibronectin and collagen production.

Mechanism of White Matter Injury in PHVD

- Raised intracranial pressure, ischemia, and parenchymal compression
- Free radical mediated injury
- Proinflammatory cytokines
- Loss of gray matter and white matter.

Evidence of Different Therapeutic Interventions in Management of PHVD

- *Repeated lumbar punctures or ventricular taps:* No reduction in the rate of VPS surgery or disability; 7% infection rate in ventriculomegaly trial.
- *Drug treatment to reduce CSF production:* In a large multicenter randomized trial of acetazolamide combined with furosemide, no clinical benefit, worse outcome in terms of shunt surgery, and death or disability.
- *Intraventricular fibrinolytic therapy:* In two small randomized trials, no reduction in VPS surgery and risk of secondary intraventricular bleed.
- *External ventricular drain:* Increased risk of infection.
- *Tapping via an ommaya reservoir:* Most widely used approach, in a multicenter randomized trial, 126 preterm infants ≤34 weeks gestation with ventricular dilatation after grade III-IV hemorrhage were randomized to low threshold (LT) [ventricular index (VI) > p97 and AHW >6 mm] or higher threshold (HT) (VI > p97 + 4 mm and AHW >10 mm), no significant difference in the primary composite outcome of VP shunt placement or death in infants with posthemorrhagic ventricular dilatation (PHVD), at lower threshold—more invasive procedures.

- *Ventriculosubgaleal shunt:* In a review of 95 infants with PHVD treated either with a ventricular reservoir or a subgaleal shunt, no difference in the proportion requiring a permanent VPS.
- *Third ventriculostomy:* Effective in obstructive hydrocephalus, not in PHVD.
- *Choroid plexus coagulation:* Not effective in PHVD.
- *Drainage, irrigation, and fibrinolytic therapy (DRIFT):* In a randomized trial, disability or death significantly less in DRIFT group compared to standard treatment, significantly more secondary IVH in DRIFT group.
- *Stem cell therapy:* Ongoing trial of intraventricular human umbilical cord–derived mesenchymal stem cells in infants with within 7 days of diagnosis of grade III or IV IVH.

Complications of V-P Shunt

- Shunt failure
- Shunt infection
- Slit ventricle syndrome.

Definition

- Increase in cerebrospinal fluid (CSF) space of the brain at high pressure due to imbalance between CSF production and absorption.

1.	• Check for OFC, if more than 2 SD • Check for progressive rise in OFC if >2 mm/day or >14 mm/week
2.	• Elicit antenatal history-fetal ventriculomegaly, TORCH infection, fetal alloimmune thrombocytopenia • Elicit history of IVH in preterm babies
3.	*Detailed examination:* • *Vitals*—look for apnea, bradycardia, and hypertension • *Anthropometry*—OFC measurement, if >2 SD, look for progressive rise (>2 mm/day abnormal) • *General examination (Head to toe)*—bulging anterior fontanel, sutural diastasis, distended scalp vein, thinned scalp skin, facial dysmorphism, red reflex, fundus examination, adducted thumb, back examination for meningomyelocele, or other stigmata of neural tube defect • *Systemic examination*—P/A examination look for hepatosplenomegaly (intrauterine infection)
4.	*Detailed neurological examination:* • *Higher mental function*—level of alertness drowsy/irritable, behavioral state, habituation, consolability, cuddlability, and cry • *Cranial nerve examination*—specially abducens nerve, oculomotor, vagus nerve palsy, upward gaze palsy, and sunset sign • *Motor examination*—quality, quantity and symmetry of movement, passive tone, and active tone • *Reflexes*
5.	*Do cranial USG/MRI*—if ventriculomegaly +, suspect hydrocephalus
6.	Do serial cranial USG, if no progressive increase, arrested hydrocephalus, if progressive ventriculomegaly, follow it

7.	• If progressive ventriculomegaly, is it slow (over weeks) or • Rapid (over days)
8.	• If slow follow for 2–4 weeks, if stops follow for 1 year • If slow and persists beyond 4 weeks, repeated lumbar puncture or CSF drainage q 1–3 days if stops follow for 1 year
9.	If dilation persists in slowly progressive hydrocephalus despite CSF drainage—ventricular drainage device
10.	If rapidly progressive over days, action line—Levene index (97th centile +4 mm), resistive index of ACA > 0.85–ventricular drainage device
11.	If dilation persists despite ventricular drainage device—ETV/CPC in select obstructive cases V-P shunt if weight >1.5 kg and CSF protein<1.5 g/L
12.	If V-P shunt—follow for shunt failure, shunt infection, and slit ventricle syndrome

■ FURTHER READING

1. Mazzola CA, Choudhri AF, Auguste KI, Limbrick DD Jr, Rogido M, Mitchell L, et al. Pediatric hydrocephalus: systematic literature review and evidence-based guidelines. Part 2: Management of posthemorrhagic hydrocephalus in premature infants, Neurosurg Pediatr. 2014;14 (Suppl 1):8-23.
2. Perlman JM. Neurology: Neonatology Questions and Controversies, 3rd edition. Philadelphia: Elsevier; 2018.
3. Swaiman KF, Ashwal S, Ferriero DM, Schor NF, Finkel RS, Gropman AL, et al. Swaiman's Pediatric Neurology, 6th edition. Philadelphia: Elsevier; 2017.
4. Volpe JJ, Inder TE, Darras BT, de Vries LS, du Plessis AJ, Neil J, et al. Volpe's neurology of the newborn, 6th edition. Philadelphia: Elsevier; 2017.
5. Wright Z, Larrew TW, Eskandari R. Pediatric hydrocephalus: current state of diagnosis and treatment. Pediatr Rev. 2016;37(11):478-90.

Management of Acute Kidney Injury

Anunaya Katiyar, Enboklang Suting

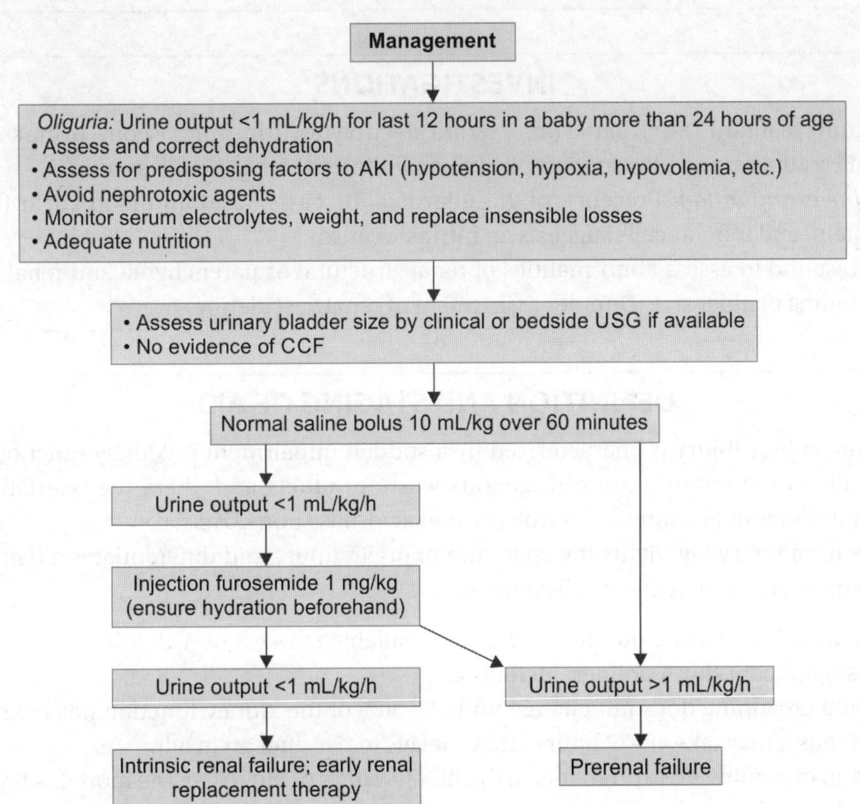

HISTORY

- Antenatal history of drug intake such as indomethacin or enalapril, uncontrolled diabetes, oligohydramnios, or polyhydramnios
- Family history of polycystic kidney disease, renal tubular acidosis, and congenital nephrotic syndrome
- Intrapartum history of perinatal asphyxia, sepsis, shock, and respiratory distress, etc.
- *Urine output:* Few newborns (7%) do not pass urine in the first 24 hours of life.

PHYSICAL EXAMINATION

- Signs of hypovolemia (tachycardia, sunken fontanel, poor skin turgor, and dry mucous membranes)
- Signs of hypervolemia such as clinical edema overdependent areas such as posterior scalp, labia, and scrotum
- Signs of polycythemia, thrombosis, and presence of central catheters
- Blood pressure and peripheral pulses
- Dysmorphic features such as abnormal ears, preauricular pits, hypospadias, ambiguous genitalia, abdominal wall defects, and aniridia which are associated with renal defects
- Palpable abdominal mass in polycystic kidney disease and hydronephrosis.

INVESTIGATIONS

- Serum creatinine (SCr), blood urea, serum electrolytes, urine microscopy, urine sodium and creatinine, and ultrasonography (when indicated) are generally required.
- *Urine examination:* Presence of granular hyaline casts, random blood sugar (RBS), protein, and tubular cells suggests an intrinsic cause.
- Ultrasound to assess abnormalities of renal structural or parenchyma and renal tracts including bladder size. Doppler assessment of renal vasculature.

DEFINITION AND STAGING OF AKI

- Acute kidney injury is characterized by a sudden impairment in kidney function that results in the retention of nitrogenous waste products and alters the regulation of extracellular fluid volume, electrolytes, and acid-base homeostasis.
- The term injury highlights the spectrum of organ injury and differentiates a damaged organ from an organ that has dysfunction.

At present, SCr and urine output are the best available markers of AKI. SCr as a marker of AKI has significant shortcomings, including:

- Serum creatinine does not change until 25–50% of the kidney function has been lost, and thus it may take 48–72 hours for SCr levels to rise after an insult.
- Serum creatinine measurements in the first few days of life reflect the mother's levels.
- At a lower glomerular filtration rate (GFR), SCr will overestimate renal function due to tubular secretion.
- Serum creatinine levels decline at varying rates depending on gestational age. GFR steadily improves from 10–20 mL/min per 1.73 m^2 during the first week of life to 30–40 mL/min per 1.73 m^2 by 2 weeks after birth **(Table 1)**.

TABLE 1: Neonatal modified AKI KDIGO staging.

Stage	Serum creatinine (mg/dL)	Urine output
0	No change in SCr or rise ≤0.3 mg/dL	≥0.5 mL/kg/h
1	SCr rise ≥0.3 mg/dL within 48 h or SCr rise ≥1.5–1.9 times reference SCr[a] within 7 days	<0.5 mL/kg/h for 6–12 h
2	SCr rise ≥2.0–2.9 times reference SCr	<0.5 mL/kg/h for ≥12 h
3	SCr rise ≥3 times reference SCr or SCr ≥2.5 mg/dL[b] or need for dialysis	<0.3 mL/kg/h for ≥24 h or anuria for ≥12 h

KIDIGO: Kidney Disease: Improving Global Outcomes
[a]Reference SCr is defined as the lowest previous SCr value and
[b]SCr value of 2.5 mg/dL represents a GFR of <10 mL/min/1.73 m^2

CAUSES OF ACUTE RENAL FAILURE

Prerenal (75–80%):
- Cautious fluid resuscitation
- Vasopressor support
- Consider diuretics

Intrinsic renal (10–15%):
- Correct electrolyte disturbances
- Stop all nephrotoxic agents
- Strict input-output charting
- Dialysis if indicated

Postrenal obstructive (5%):
- Correct obstruction
- Correct electrolyte disturbances
- Support diuresis

DIAGNOSTIC PARAMETERS TO DIFFERENTIATE PRERENAL FROM INTRINSIC ACUTE KIDNEY INJURY

Indices	Prerenal	Intrinsic
BUN/Cr ratio (mg/mg)	>30	<20
Urine osmolality (mOsm/L)	>400	≤400
Urine–specific gravity	>1.012	<1.014
Urine sodium (mEq/L)	10–50	30–90
Renal failure index*	<3	>3
Fractional excretion of sodium[#] (%)	<0.3	>0.3
Response to fluid challenge	Improved tachycardia Increased urine output >2 mL/kg/h	No effect on tachycardia or urine output

$$\text{*Renal failure index} = \frac{\text{Urine Na}^+ \times \text{Serum creatinine}}{\text{Urine creatinine}}$$

$$\text{\#Fractional excretion of sodium (FENa)} = \frac{\text{Urine Na}^+ \times \text{Serum creatinine} \times 100}{\text{Serum Na}^+ \times \text{Urine creatinine}}$$

■ MANAGEMENT

Treatment of AKI relies on supportive care, fluid and electrolyte balance, acid-base balance, avoidance of nephrotoxins, treatment of complications, and renal replacement therapy whenever required.

- Whenever AKI is suspected, look for distended bladder by palpation or bedside ultrasound. Place an indwelling catheter for accurate urine measurement.
- Stop all nephrotoxic drugs.
- Evaluate for signs of intravascular volume depletion or congestive cardiac failure.
- Start fluid challenge with normal saline 10–20 mL/kg over 60 minutes.
- In absence of urine output, a dose of furosemide can be given @1 mg/kg in a nondehydrated neonate.

Fluid Management

- Fluid restriction to insensible water loss (IWL) along with urinary loss and other measured losses. The IWL in a term neonate is 25 mL/kg/day or 500 mL/m^2/day. IWL can be assumed to be 40 mL/kg/day in preterm infants.
- The fluid should be electrolyte free 10% dextrose water. Replace urine volume for volume with N/5 saline.

Hyponatremia

- Hyponatremia due to dilution secondary to water retention has to be corrected with fluid restriction.
- In most of the cases, there is no sodium deficit and fluid restriction will suffice.
- If symptomatic or hyponatremia is <120 mEq/L, it requires prompt correction with 3% hypertonic saline in a dose of 5 mL/kg over 4–5 hours.

Hyperkalemia

- Stop all potassium in the fluids. If ECG changes are evident, give calcium gluconate 10%.
- This should immediately be followed by methods to decrease the potassium levels.

Medication	Dose	Onset of action
Calcium gluconate	0.5 to 1 mL/kg over 10 minutes	1–5 minutes
Sodium bicarbonate	1 mEq/kg over 10 minutes	5–10 minutes
Glucose and insulin	1 IU insulin/5 g glucose	15–30 minutes
Salbutamol nebulization	2.5 mg by nebulizer over 10 minutes	5 minutes, peak after 90 minutes
Cation exchange resin	1 g/kg intrarectally q6h	1–2 hours
Peritoneal dialysis	Dialysate with low K$^+$ concentration	Immediate

Hypocalcemia

- Symptomatic hypocalcemia should be corrected by infusing calcium gluconate at a dose of 100–200 mg/kg over 10–20 minutes and repeated every 4–8 hours as necessary.

Nutrition

- The goal is to provide 100 kcal/kg/day. Proteins or amino acids can be provided in a dose of 1–2 g/kg/day.
- If on enteral feeds, breast milk can be used.

Acidosis

- Mild metabolic acidosis is common.
- Replacement with bicarbonate or acetate is indicated to treat metabolic acidosis.
- Correction of acidosis can also cause decreased ionized serum calcium concentration, thus correct hypocalcemia before correcting acidosis.

Hypertension

- Basic management constitutes of salt and water restriction, diuretics in higher doses, and/or dialysis.
- Fluid restriction in setting of fluid overload. In severe hypertension, evaluate for renal artery or vein thrombosis.
- Severe hypertension can be managed by continuous infusion of sodium nitroprusside (0.3–10 mcg/kg/min) or labetalol.
- Commonly used oral antihypertensives in newborns are oral amlodipine (0.1–0.3 mg/kg/dose q 12–24 hourly) and enalapril (0.1–0.4 mg/kg/day q 12–24 hourly).

Renal Replacement Therapy

- Indications
- Fluid overload
- Hyperkalemia
- Hyponatremia
- Severe metabolic acidosis which are unresponsive to medical management.
- Renal replacement therapy can be provided by acute peritoneal dialysis (PD), intermittent hemodialysis, or continuous renal replacement therapy (CRRT)

Key Points to Remember

- Examine the baby under the radiant warmer for signs of shock or signs of intravascular volume depletion or congestive cardiac failure.
- Look for dysmorphic features and palpate the urinary bladder.
- Secure IV access and draw blood samples for serum creatinine, blood urea, complete blood count, and serum electrolytes. Stop all nephrotoxic drugs.
- If no signs of CCF and urinary bladder are empty, give IV normal saline @ 10 mL/kg over 60 minutes. Monitor urine output.
- In absence of urine output, give IV furosemide 1 mg/kg in a nondehydrated neonate.
- If urine >1 mL/kg/h after step 2 or 3, treat as prerenal AKI.
- If urine <1 mL/kg/h after step 3, treat as intrinsic renal failure.

- Correct electrolyte imbalance as necessary.
- Continue urine output monitoring.
- Ensure hydration before starting furosemide.
- Correct dehydration before starting fluid challenge.
- Adjusted *drug dosing* as determined by eCCl (estimated creatinine clearance) is required.

◼ FURTHER READING

1. Askenazi DJ, Smith LN, Furth SL, Warady BA. Acute kidney injury and chronic kidney disease. In: Gleason CA, Devaskar SU (Eds). Avery's Diseases of the Newborn, 9th edition. Philadelphia: Elsevier; 2012. pp.1205-21.
2. Jetton JG, Askenazi DJ. Update on acute kidney injury in the neonate. Curr Opin Pediatr. 2012;24(2):191-6.
3. Selewski DT, Charlton JR, Jetton JG, Guillet R, Mhanna MJ, Askenazi DJ, et al. Neonatal Acute Kidney Injury. Pediatrics. 2015;136(2):e463-73.

Anuradha Bansal

Management of Hyperbilirubinemia

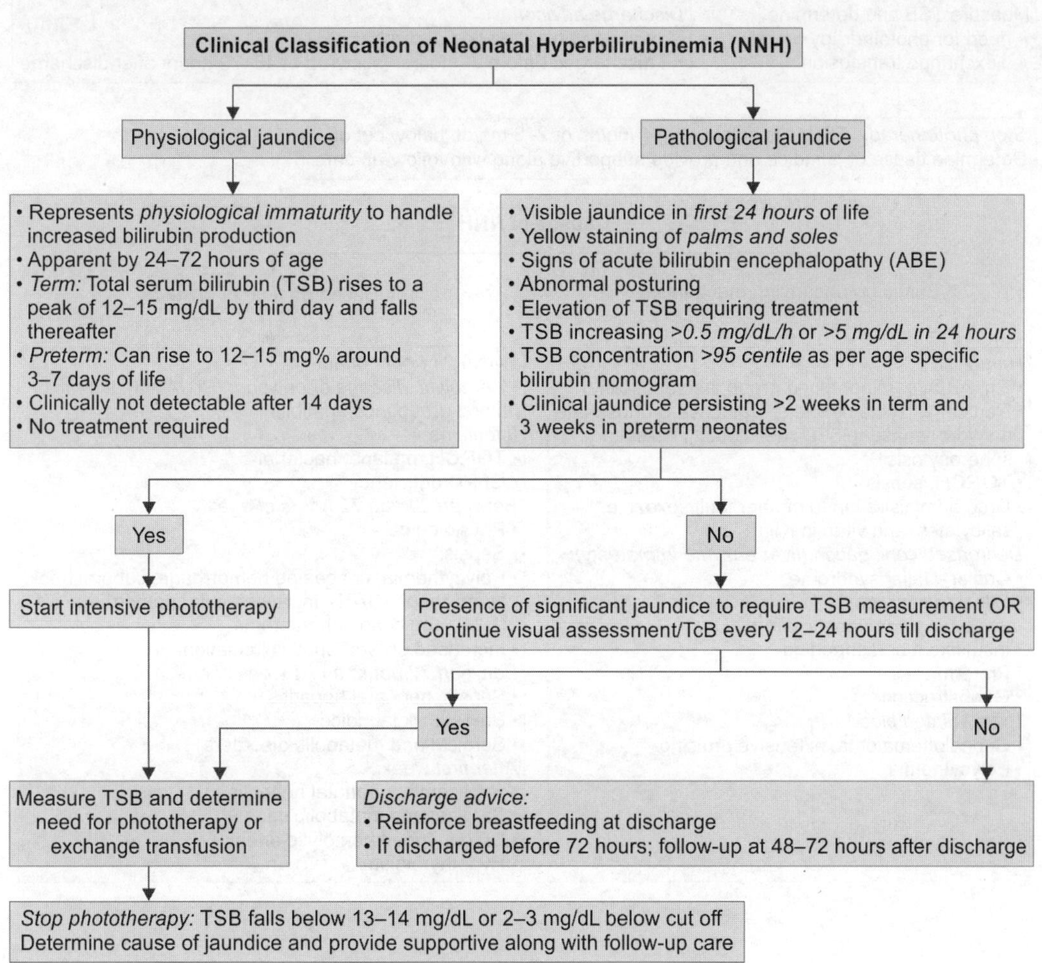

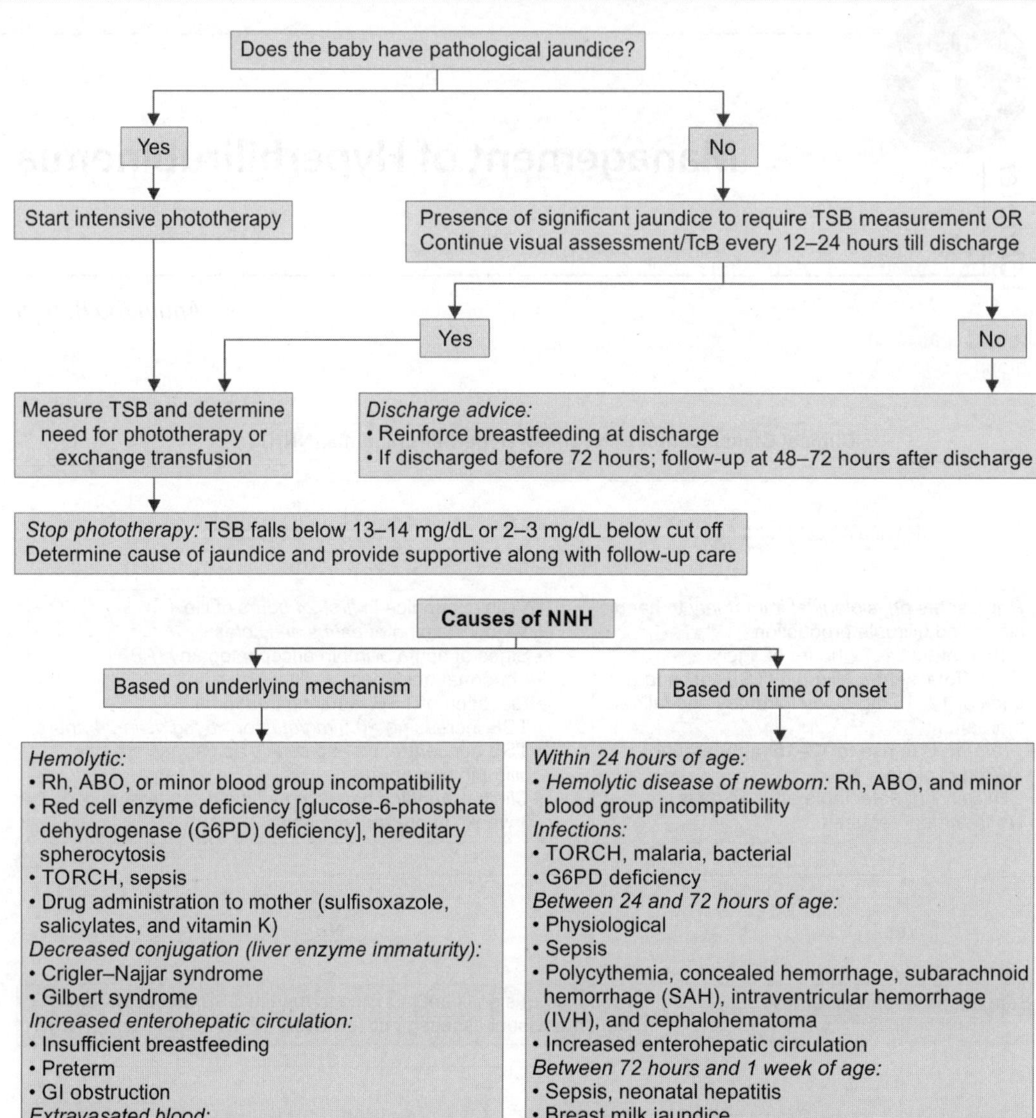
Does the baby have pathological jaundice?
Yes
No
Start intensive phototherapy
Presence of significant jaundice to require TSB measurement OR Continue visual assessment/TcB every 12–24 hours till discharge
Yes
No
Measure TSB and determine need for phototherapy or exchange transfusion
Discharge advice:
• Reinforce breastfeeding at discharge
• If discharged before 72 hours; follow-up at 48–72 hours after discharge
Stop phototherapy: TSB falls below 13–14 mg/dL or 2–3 mg/dL below cut off
Determine cause of jaundice and provide supportive along with follow-up care
Causes of NNH
Based on underlying mechanism
Based on time of onset
Hemolytic:
• Rh, ABO, or minor blood group incompatibility
• Red cell enzyme deficiency [glucose-6-phosphate dehydrogenase (G6PD) deficiency], hereditary spherocytosis
• TORCH, sepsis
• Drug administration to mother (sulfisoxazole, salicylates, and vitamin K)
Decreased conjugation (liver enzyme immaturity):
• Crigler–Najjar syndrome
• Gilbert syndrome
Increased enterohepatic circulation:
• Insufficient breastfeeding
• Preterm
• GI obstruction
Extravasated blood:
• Cephalohematoma, extensive bruising
• Polycythemia
Within 24 hours of age:
• Hemolytic disease of newborn: Rh, ABO, and minor blood group incompatibility
Infections:
• TORCH, malaria, bacterial
• G6PD deficiency
Between 24 and 72 hours of age:
• Physiological
• Sepsis
• Polycythemia, concealed hemorrhage, subarachnoid hemorrhage (SAH), intraventricular hemorrhage (IVH), and cephalohematoma
• Increased enterohepatic circulation
Between 72 hours and 1 week of age:
• Sepsis, neonatal hepatitis
• Breast milk jaundice
• Surgical and metabolic disorders
After first week:
• Septicemia, neonatal hepatitis
• Surgical and metabolic causes
• Drug-induced hemolytic anemia
• Hypothyroidism

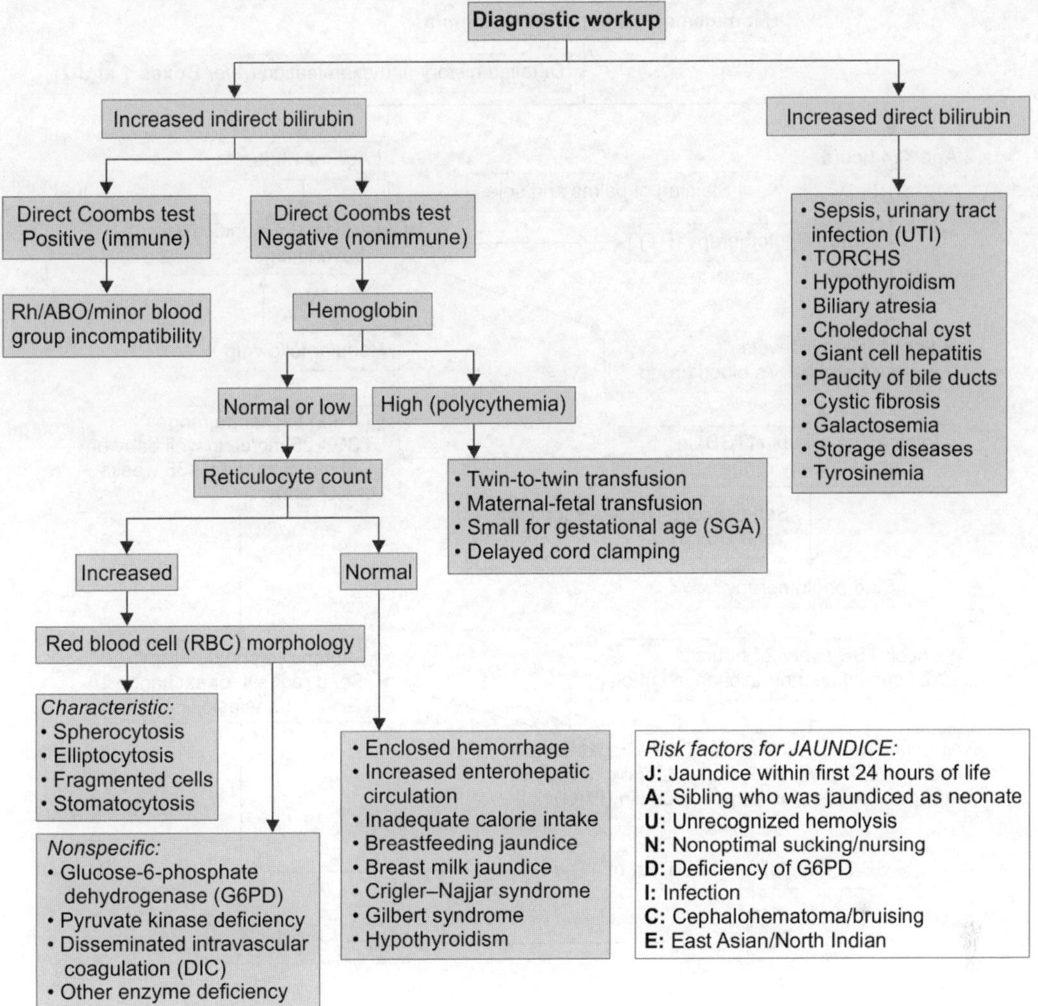
Diagnostic workup
Increased indirect bilirubin
Increased direct bilirubin
Direct Coombs test Positive (immune)
Direct Coombs test Negative (nonimmune)
Rh/ABO/minor blood group incompatibility
Hemoglobin
Normal or low
High (polycythemia)
Reticulocyte count
Increased
Normal
Red blood cell (RBC) morphology
• Sepsis, urinary tract infection (UTI)
• TORCHS
• Hypothyroidism
• Biliary atresia
• Choledochal cyst
• Giant cell hepatitis
• Paucity of bile ducts
• Cystic fibrosis
• Galactosemia
• Storage diseases
• Tyrosinemia
• Twin-to-twin transfusion
• Maternal-fetal transfusion
• Small for gestational age (SGA)
• Delayed cord clamping
Characteristic:
• Spherocytosis
• Elliptocytosis
• Fragmented cells
• Stomatocytosis
Nonspecific:
• Glucose-6-phosphate dehydrogenase (G6PD)
• Pyruvate kinase deficiency
• Disseminated intravascular coagulation (DIC)
• Other enzyme deficiency
• Enclosed hemorrhage
• Increased enterohepatic circulation
• Inadequate calorie intake
• Breastfeeding jaundice
• Breast milk jaundice
• Crigler–Najjar syndrome
• Gilbert syndrome
• Hypothyroidism
Risk factors for JAUNDICE:
J: Jaundice within first 24 hours of life
A: Sibling who was jaundiced as neonate
U: Unrecognized hemolysis
N: Nonoptimal sucking/nursing
D: Deficiency of G6PD
I: Infection
C: Cephalohematoma/bruising
E: East Asian/North Indian

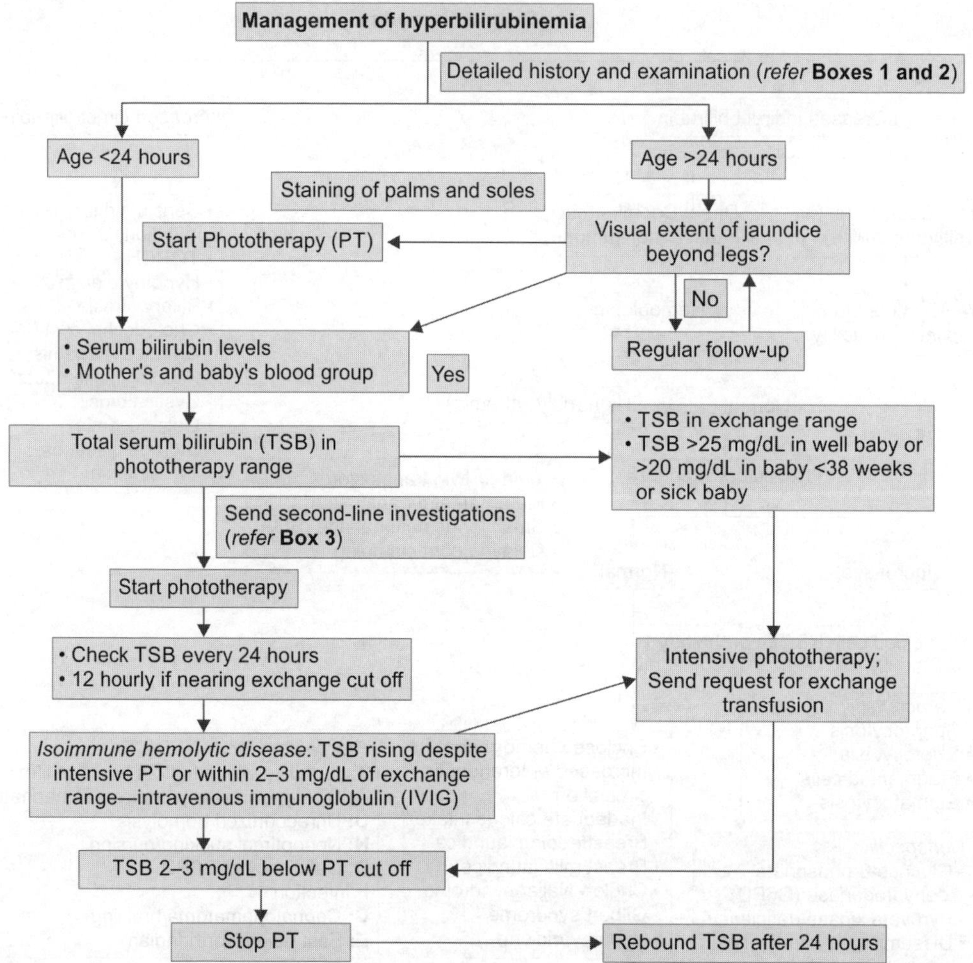

Management of hyperbilirubinemia
Detailed history and examination (refer Boxes 1 and 2)
Age <24 hours
Age >24 hours
Staining of palms and soles
Visual extent of jaundice beyond legs?
Start Phototherapy (PT)
No
Regular follow-up
• Serum bilirubin levels
• Mother's and baby's blood group
Yes
• TSB in exchange range
• TSB >25 mg/dL in well baby or >20 mg/dL in baby <38 weeks or sick baby
Total serum bilirubin (TSB) in phototherapy range
Send second-line investigations (refer Box 3)
Start phototherapy
• Check TSB every 24 hours
• 12 hourly if nearing exchange cut off
Intensive phototherapy; Send request for exchange transfusion
Isoimmune hemolytic disease: TSB rising despite intensive PT or within 2–3 mg/dL of exchange range—intravenous immunoglobulin (IVIG)
TSB 2–3 mg/dL below PT cut off
Stop PT
Rebound TSB after 24 hours

BOX 1: History.

- Age in days and gestational age
- Birth weight
- Mother and baby blood group
- Feeding history (breastfed/top fed, frequency of feeding)
- History of jaundice in previous sibling (suggestive of blood group incompatibility)
- History of maternal fever with rash during pregnancy (points toward intrauterine infection)
- Traumatic delivery
- Stool frequency (constipation increases enterohepatic circulation of bilirubin and hence worsens jaundice)
- Symptoms suggestive of neonatal sepsis such as poor feeding, fever, fast breathing, lethargy, or irritability
- High-colored urine or pale-colored stool (conjugated hyperbilirubinemia)

BOX 2: Examination.

- Modified Kramer's staging for extent of yellow staining
- Pallor/petechiae/purpura/rash
- Current weight and hydration status
- Examine the scalp for cephalohematoma or subgaleal bleed
- Hepatosplenomegaly on abdominal examination
- Signs of bilirubin-induced neurological damage (BIND)—irritability, high-pitched cry, seizures, neck retraction, opisthotonos, lethargy, and poor feeding
- Measurement of head circumference (microcephaly for intrauterine infections)
- Fundus examination for chorioretinitis

BOX 3: Investigations.

- *First line:*
  - Total serum bilirubin (TSB)
  - Mother and baby's blood group (if not done earlier)
- *Second line:*
  - Serum albumin (with high bilirubin levels)
  - Reticulocyte count, peripheral smear, and direct Coombs test (DCT)
- *Prolonged jaundice:*
  - Sepsis screen
  - Urine routine and culture
  - Galactosemia screen
  - TORCH (Toxoplasmosis, Other agents, Rubella, Cytomegalovirus, and Herpes simplex syndrome)
  - Glucose-6-phosphate dehydrogenase (G6PD) levels and thyroid-stimulating hormone (TSH)

Management of prolonged neonatal jaundice

Visibly detectable jaundice beyond 2 weeks of age in a term and beyond 3 weeks of age in a preterm infant

History

- Mode of feeding, adequacy of feeding—pattern of weight (including birth weight and current weight), number of wet nappies
- Color of stool and history of delayed passage of meconium
- Urine color
- Activity and behavior during sleep/waking up
- Any abnormal body movements
- Any bleeding/bruising
- Family history of blood or liver disorders
- Mother's blood group, baby's blood group

Examination

- Plot available weights on a growth chart (the majority of healthy infants should have regained their birth weight by 10–14 days of age). There are special charts for plotting postnatal weights to see whether the weight loss is acceptable or excessive *(refer www.newbornweight.org)*
- *Anthropometry:* To rule out microcephaly
- *Head-to-toe examination:* Look for cataracts, jaundice, pallor, petechiae/purpura, and hydration status
- *Abdominal examination:* Look for hepatosplenomegaly
- *CNS examination:* Any feature of bilirubin-induced encephalopathy

Investigation

Get total serum bilirubin, direct and indirect bilirubin levels

Total bilirubin and bilirubin fractions

Conjugated bilirubin >20% of the total bilirubin
(if the total bilirubin is >5 mg/dL) or >1 mg/dL (if the total bilirubin is <5 mg/dL)

Yes

Neonatal cholestasis (conjugated hyperbilirubinemia)

See next chapter

No

Prolonged unconjugated hyperbilirubinemia

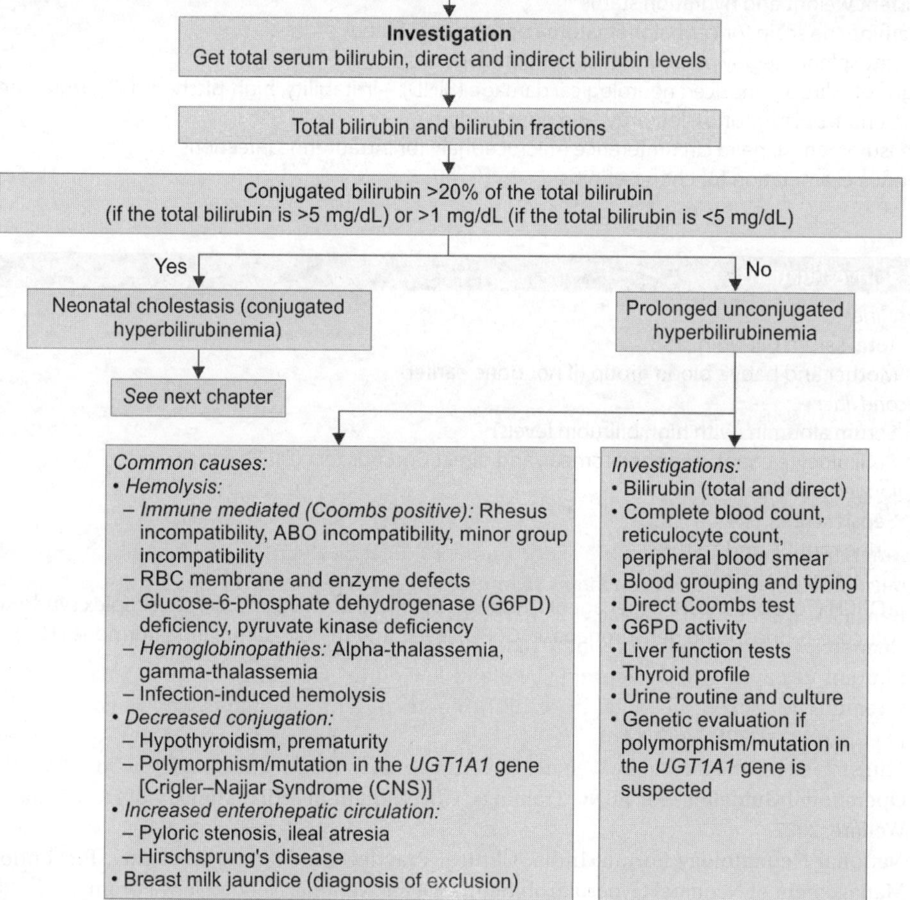

Common causes:
- *Hemolysis:*
  - *Immune mediated (Coombs positive):* Rhesus incompatibility, ABO incompatibility, minor group incompatibility
  - RBC membrane and enzyme defects
  - Glucose-6-phosphate dehydrogenase (G6PD) deficiency, pyruvate kinase deficiency
  - *Hemoglobinopathies:* Alpha-thalassemia, gamma-thalassemia
  - Infection-induced hemolysis
- *Decreased conjugation:*
  - Hypothyroidism, prematurity
  - Polymorphism/mutation in the *UGT1A1* gene [Crigler–Najjar Syndrome (CNS)]
- *Increased enterohepatic circulation:*
  - Pyloric stenosis, ileal atresia
  - Hirschsprung's disease
- Breast milk jaundice (diagnosis of exclusion)

Investigations:
- Bilirubin (total and direct)
- Complete blood count, reticulocyte count, peripheral blood smear
- Blood grouping and typing
- Direct Coombs test
- G6PD activity
- Liver function tests
- Thyroid profile
- Urine routine and culture
- Genetic evaluation if polymorphism/mutation in the *UGT1A1* gene is suspected

TREATMENT OF UNCONJUGATED JAUNDICE

- Try to identify an underlying cause and treat accordingly
- *Phototherapy/exchange transfusion:* There are no separate guidelines for prolonged unconjugated jaundice. The thresholds in American Academy of Pediatrics (AAP) charts at day 6–7 of age can be used for babies more than a week old as the curves flatten after day 6.
- Breast milk jaundice is a diagnosis of exclusion and should be made only after other causes have been ruled out. Interruption of breastfeeding for treatment of jaundice is not recommended.
- Refer to a pediatric gastroenterologist if there is conjugated hyperbilirubinemia or a suspicion of underlying liver disease [unconjugated jaundice with deranged liver function tests (LFTs)].

Key Points to Remember

- Neonatal hyperbilirubinemia (NNH) refers to yellowish discoloration of skin in a newborn baby.
- It is the most common neonatal morbidity in first week of life. Nearly 60% term and 80% preterm newborn may develop some jaundice in first 7 days of life.
- It is important to distinguish between physiological and pathological jaundice.
- Although benign in most cases, pathological jaundice if not treated well in time can lead to transient or permanent neurological damage.
- *Treatment of NNH:* Phototherapy and exchange transfusion are the mainstay of therapy (*See* **Annexure 1**).
- Postdischarge follow-up of newborns with pathological jaundice:
  - Babies needing exchange or those with serum bilirubin >20 mg/dL should be kept under follow-up in the high-risk clinic for neurodevelopmental outcome.
  - Brainstem evoked response audiometry (BERA) at 3 months of corrected age

■ FURTHER READING

1. American Academy of Pediatrics Subcommittee on Hyperbilirubinemia. Management of hyperbilirubinemia in the newborn infant 35 or more weeks of gestation. Pediatrics. 2004;114: 297-316.
2. Bansal A, Mathur NB. Neonatal Hyperbilirubinemia. In: Mathur NB (Ed). Mathur's Essential Neonatology. Delhi: Noble Vision; 2018.
3. Bhutani VK, Stark AR, Lazzeroni LC, Poland R, Gourley GR, Kazmierczak S, et al. Predischarge screening for severe neonatal hyperbilirubinemia identifies infants who need phototherapy. J Pediatr. 2013;162(3):477-82.e1.
4. Ministry of Health and Family Welfare, Government of India. Facility Based Newborn Care (FBNC): Operational Guidelines for FBNC Trainings. Government of India: Ministry of Health and Family Welfare; 2022.
5. National Neonatology Forum, India. Clinical Practice Guidelines: Screening, Prevention and Management of Neonatal Hyperbilirubinemia. Delhi: National Neonatology Forum, India; 2020.

Management of Cholestasis

Bikrant Bihari Lal, Vikrant Sood

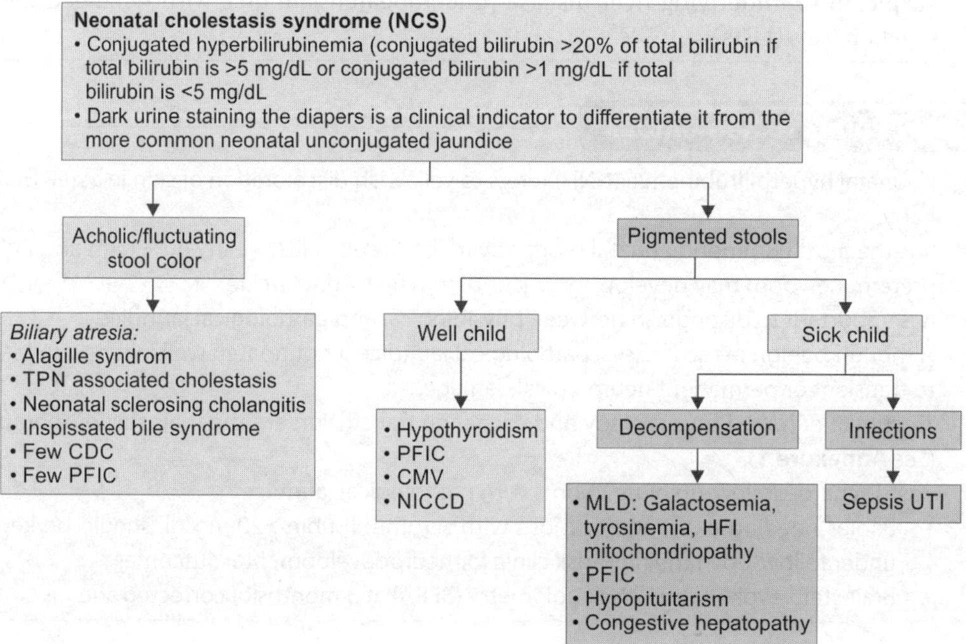

■ HISTORY AND CLINICAL EXAMINATION

Clinical pointers	*Relevance*
History	
Dark urine with diaper staining	Conjugated hyperbilirubinemia
Acholic stools	Possible obstruction to biliary tree/structural biliary disorders
Vitamin K responsive bleeds	Cholestasis
Stormy perinatal course, parenteral nutrition	Suggests total parenteral nutrition (TPN)-associated cholestasis, multifactorial
Pointers toward metabolic liver diseases	• Consanguinity, abortions, and previous sib deaths • Failure to thrive, diarrhea, and vomitings • Recurrence during periods of catabolic stress (*fatty acid oxidation defects*) • Seizures, early morning irritability, and lethargy • Developmental delay, hypotonia, and cataract (*galactosemia*) • Aversion to sugars [hereditary fructose intolerance (HFI)] or proteins (*urea cycle defects*)
Antenatal history	• Intrahepatic cholestasis of pregnancy in progressive familial intrahepatic cholestasis type 3 • Hyperemesis, preeclampsia in fetal very long chain fatty acid oxidation defects • Fever, rash, and lymphadenopathy in early pregnancy in congenital infections
Examination	
Facial dysmorphism	Alagille syndrome, Zellweger syndrome, and other trisomies like Down's syndrome
Eye examination	• Cataract in galactosemia, congenital rubella syndrome • Posterior embryotoxon (on slit lamp), optic nerve drusen in Alagille syndrome • Fundus (cherry red spot in Niemann–Pick disease, chorioretinitis in cytomegalovirus, and optic nerve hypoplasia in hypopituitarism)
Hearing	Affected in congenital rubella infection and progressive familial intrahepatic cholestasis type 1
Visible acholic stools/ per rectal	Strong likelihood of biliary atresia
Genitalia	Hypogonadism, midline defects in hypopituitarism
Skin	Pruritus marks, excoriations, and shiny nails in intrahepatic cholestasis; ecchymosis in cholestatic bleed; and xanthomas in Alagille syndrome
Rickets, Renal enlargement	Tyrosinemia, hereditary fructose intolerance, Caroli syndrome
Firm liver with splenomegaly	Portal hypertension
Palpable lump in right hypochondrium	Choledochal cyst
Congenital heart diseases	Associated with Alagille syndrome, biliary atresia, congenital infections, and trisomies

DIFFERENTIAL DIAGNOSIS

- *Obstructive causes:* Biliary atresia and choledochal cysts
- *Hepatocellular causes:* Idiopathic giant cell hepatitis, infections (sepsis, TORCH, malaria, urinary tract infection), metabolic causes (galactosemia, alpha-1-antitrypsindeficiency, tyrosinemia, storage disorders, and hemochromatosis), and miscellaneous
- Ductal paucity (syndromic or nonsyndromic)
- Undifferentiated

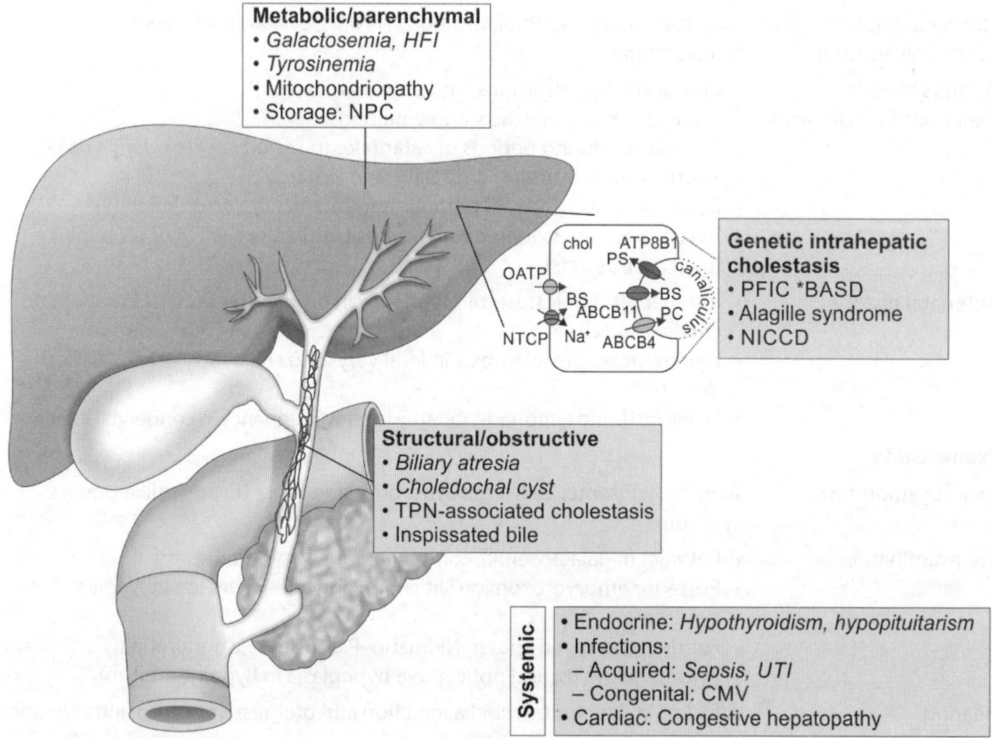

Common causes of neonatal cholestasis

TREATMENT

Nutritional support: Calories 125% of recommended dietary allowance (RDA). Supplement fat soluble vitamins

- Treatment of underlying cause
- In infants with pruritus due to severe cholestasis, the group recommended, in the following order: Ursodeoxycholic acid (UDCA) (20 mg/kg/day), rifampicin (5–10 mg/kg/day), and phenobarbitone (5–10 mg/kg/day)
- Liver transplantation, the standard therapy for decompensated cirrhosis due to any cause.

Key Points to Remember

- Never do total serum bilirubin levels alone in a neonate or infant with jaundice. Do not ignore mildly elevated direct bilirubin levels → repeat till normal levels are achieved.
- Always ask for stool and urine color to diagnose cholestasis early. Do not advise sunlight exposure without detailed history: it gives false reassurance to parents unless cholestasis has been fully investigated.
- Always exclude biliary atresia first in any child with presenting with NCS, especially in a well looking child with/without pale stools.
- Serum gamma glutamyl transpeptidase (GGTP) levels should always be done at baseline to help guide the etiological work up of NCS (e.g., if high levels according to age, think of biliary atresia, etc.).
- TORCH profile testing limited practical relevance in a case with NCS. It should only be considered in cases where there are clinical stigmata of intrauterine infections (like low birth weight, microcephaly, etc.).
- Hepatobiliary iminodiacetic acid (HIDA) scan has poor limited role in evaluation of NCS. It should be avoided unless indicated. It has poor sensitivity for diagnosis of biliary atresia (it cannot diagnose biliary atresia but can only exclude it, if study is excretory) and inadvertently delays the diagnosis. It should not be done in cases with pale stools since in all likelihood, result would be a nonexcretory study. Only indication in current era is where there is a need to exclude biliary atresia (e.g., fluctuating stools color, borderline high or normal serum GGTP levels, noncontributory ultrasound examination, etc.).
- Avoid sending viral markers [(like hepatitis B surface antigen (HbsAg), antihepatitis C virus (HCV), human immunodeficiency virus (HIV), etc.], autoimmune markers, and Wilson disease tests (serum ceruloplasmin, etc.) in cases of NCS.
- Always check prothrombin time-international normalized ratio (PT-INR) in all cases (after giving vitamin K) to exclude underlying liver failure.
- Early referral to a pediatric gastroenterologist or hepatologist is necessary for optimum evaluation.
- Biliary atresia is the most common cause of NCS and requires expedited diagnosis followed by Kasai portoenterostomy surgery.
- Early diagnosis and surgery are the key as success rates are good when Kasai surgery is performed early before advanced fibrosis sets in the liver.
- Hepatobiliary iminodiacetic acid scan is time consuming, does not give any additional information, and has very low specificity, yet continues to be used at several centres delaying the diagnosis.
- Percutaneous cholecysto-cholangiogram is a good tool in hands of experienced intervention radiologist in cases with equivocal histopathological findings.
- When in doubt, intraoperative cholangiogram should be done which is the gold standard for diagnosis and should proceed to Kasai surgery if dye injected through gallbladder doesn't opacify the distal or the proximal bile ducts.

■ FURTHER READING

1. Fawaz R, Baumann U, Ekong U, Fischler B, Hadzic N, Mack CL, et al. Guideline for the evaluation of cholestatic jaundice in infants: joint recommendations of the North American Society for Pediatric Gastroenterology, Hepatology, and Nutrition and the European Society for Pediatric Gastroenterology, Hepatology, and Nutrition. J Pediatr Gastroenterol Nutr. 2017;64(1):154-68.
2. Kumar R, Lal BB, Sood V, Khanna R, Kumar S, Bharathy KGS, et al. Predictors of successful kasai portoenterostomy and survival with native liver at 2 years in infants with biliary atresia. J Clin Exp Hepatol. 2019;9(4):453-9.
3. Rastogi A, Krishnani N, Yachha SK, Khanna V, Poddar U, Lal R. Histopathological features and accuracy for diagnosing biliary atresia by prelaparotomy liver biopsy in developing countries. J Gastroenterol Hepatol. 2009;24(1):97-102.

Management of Bleeding

Ravinder Yadav

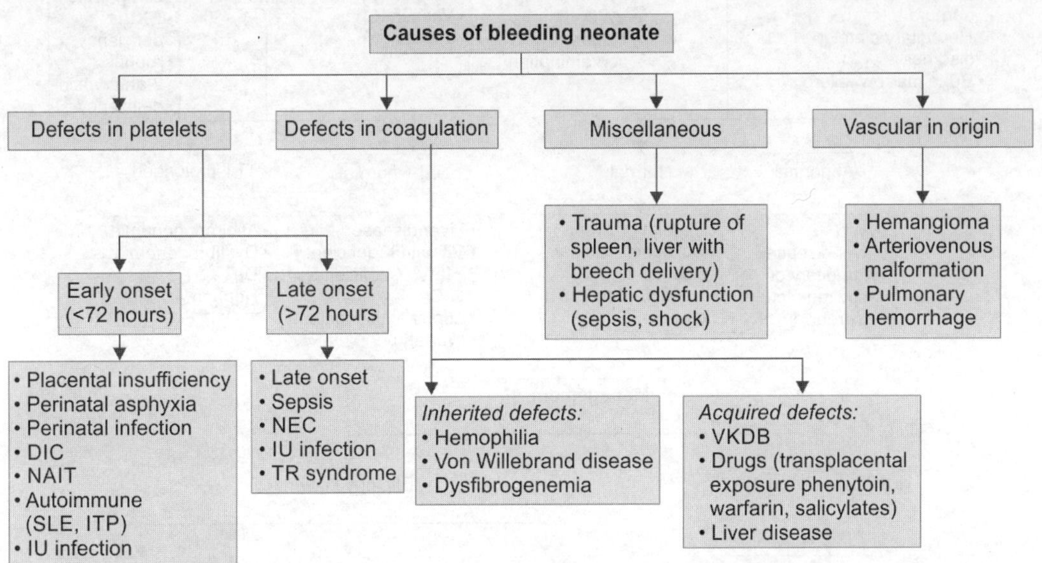

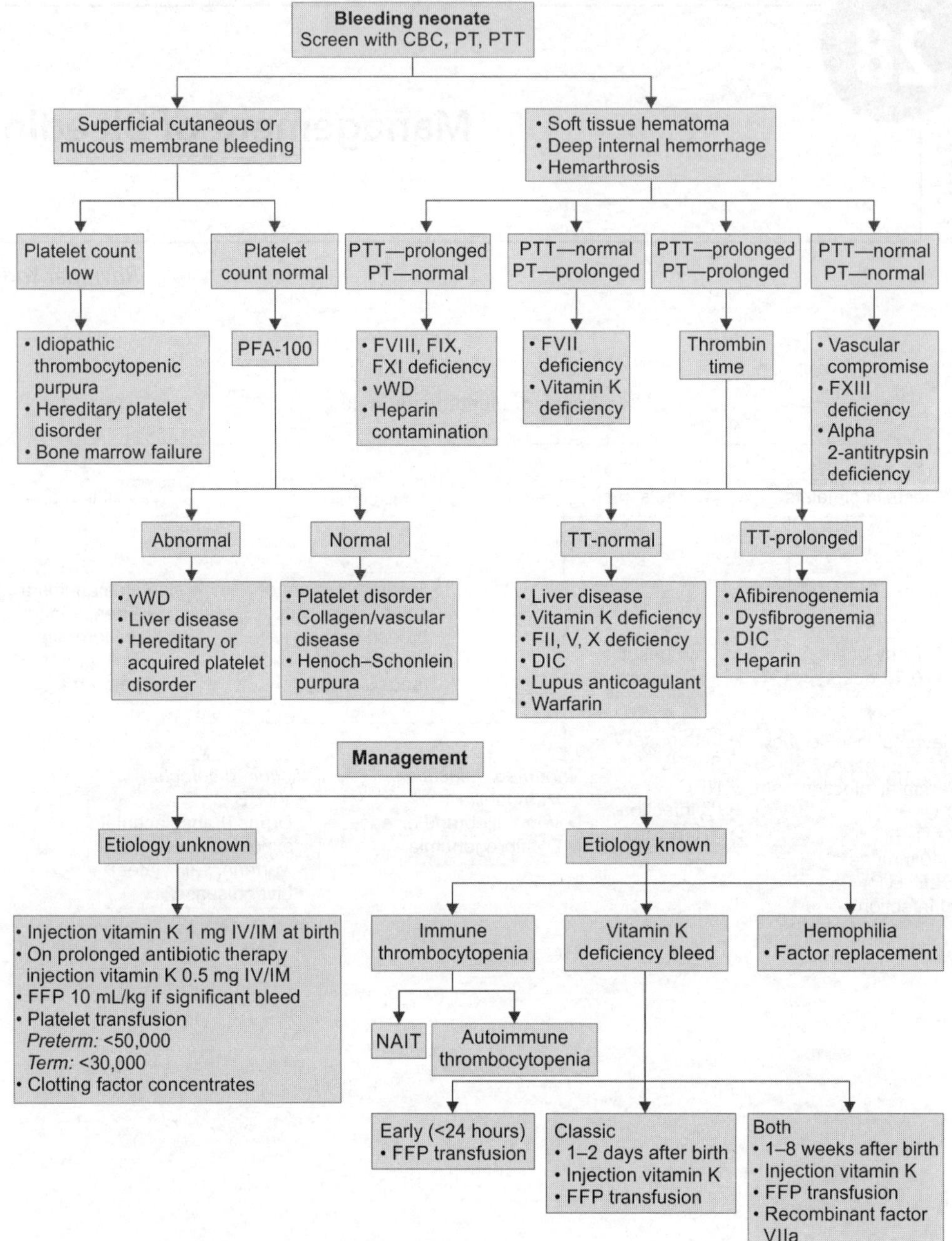

■ FURTHER READING

1. Eichenwald EC, Hansen AR, Martin C, Stark AR. Bleeding. Cloherty and Starks's Manual of Neonatal Care, 8th edition. Philadelphia: Wolters Kluwer; 2017.
2. Manco-Johnson MJ. Bleeding disorders in the neonate. Neo Rev. 2008;9:e162-9.
3. McMillian D, Wu J. Approach to the bleeding newborn. Paediatric Child Health. 1998;3:399-401.

Chapter 29

Management of Polycythemia

Kritika Famra

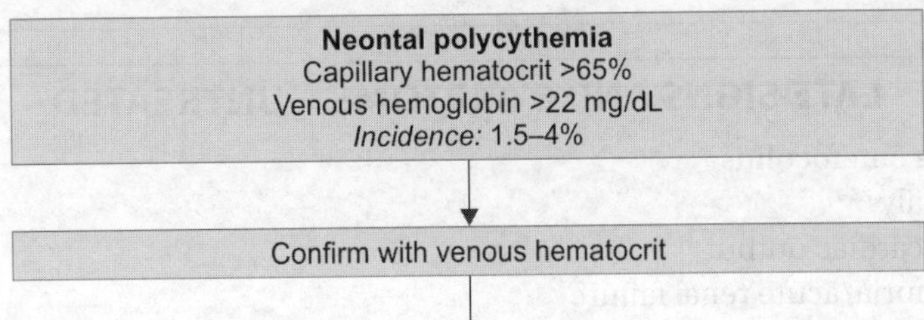

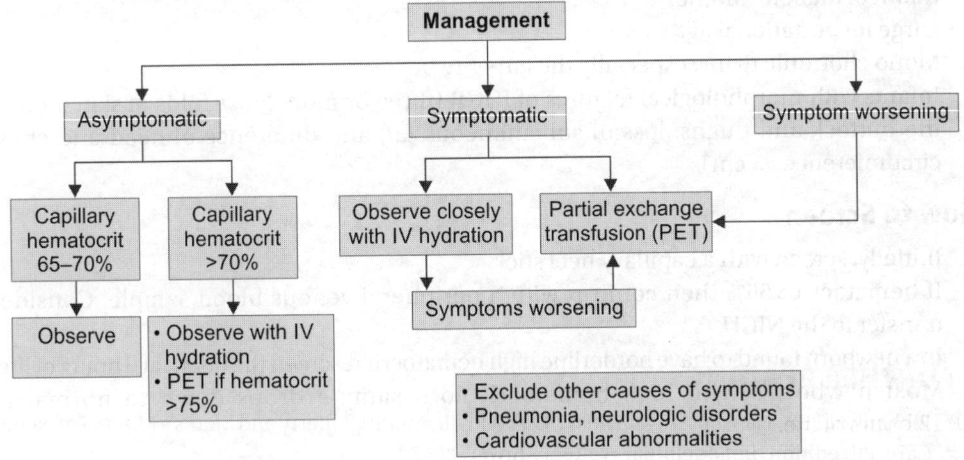

EARLY SIGNS AND SYMPTOMS

Hyperviscosity may affect all organ systems:
- Poor feeding/suck and vomiting
- Jitteriness/irritability
- Hypotonia
- Ruddy complexion or cyanosis
- Tachycardia/tachypnea
- Respiratory distress
- Priapism in males
- Hypoglycemia symptoms and sequelae
- Jaundice.

LATE SIGNS AND SYMPTOMS—UNTREATED

- Necrotizing enterocolitis
- Cardiomegaly
- Decreased cardiac output
- Oliguria/anuria/acute renal failure
- Renal vein thrombosis
- Stroke with neurologic sequelae
- Necrotic fingers/toes/penis
- Adrenal insufficiency
- Testicular/ovarian infarcts and subsequent infertility.

SCREENING FOR POLYCYTHEMIA

Whom to Screen

- Small for gestational age
- Infant of diabetic mother
- Large for gestational age
- Mono chorionic twins, especially the larger twin
- Infants with morphological features of IUGR (three or more loose folds of skin around the buttock and thighs, loss of subcutaneous fat, and difference of head and chest circumference >3 cm).

How to Screen

- Initially, screen with a capillary heel stick.
- If hematocrit >65% then confirm with a peripheral venous blood sample. Consider transfer to the NICU.
- In a newborn found to have borderline high hematocrit rescreen the infant at 6 hours of life.
- Most newborn's with high hematocrit cord sample drops down to normal at 12 hours of life.

When to Screen

- At 2 hours of life, at 6 hours, 12 hours, 24 hours, and 48 hours.

MANAGEMENT

- Asymptomatic infants with venous hematocrit between 65 and 70% are observed for symptoms. IVF hydration and closed monitoring of symptoms hematocrit is repeated after 4–6 hours.
- Symptomatic infants with venous hematocrit of >70% are usually undertaken for partial exchange transfusion (PET).
- Partial exchange transfusion at hematocrit of >70% in the absence of symptoms is controversial.
  - Remember to rule out dehydration
  - Also check, serum bilirubin, glucose, and thyroid-stimulating hormone (TSH) if indicated.

Rawlings chart for estimating the blood volume: 80–90 mL/kg in term babies and 90–100 mL/kg in preterm babies. Blood is usually taken from, umbilical vein, and replaced with 5% albumin or normal saline in peripheral vein.

- Partial exchange transfusion can be performed using normal saline (in a 1:1 exchange), as clinical advantage has not been found with the use of albumin or fresh frozen plasma.

Volume to be exchanged = Blood volume × weight in kg (Observed hematocrit – Desired hematocrit) ÷ Observed hematocrit

Rule of thumb: Volume to be exchanged is usually 20 mL/kg.

OUTCOME

Partial exchange transfusion for polycythemia: What is the evidence?

- No effect on neonatal mortality
- No difference in developmental delay
- Increased risk of necrotizing enterocolitis (NEC) in infants receiving PET
- No difference in short-term complications including hypoglycemia (two studies) and thrombocytopenia (one study)

Due to the uncertainty regarding the long-term outcomes, PET should be restricted in symptomatic infants with hematocrit of >65% and in asymptomatic neonates with hematocrit of >75%.

Key Points to Remember

- Hematocrit at birth is 53%. The hematocrit peaks at around 2 hours of age and values up to 71% may be normal at this age.
- Hematocrit gradually declines to 68% by 6 hours and usually stabilizes by 12–24 hours.
- Polycythemia, elevated hematocrit, is associated with hyper viscosity of blood. As the blood viscosity increases, there is impairment of tissue oxygenation and perfusion and tendency to form microthrombi.

- Significant damage may occur if these events occur in the cerebral cortex, kidneys, and adrenal glands.
- Viscosity of blood is directly proportional to hematocrit and plasma viscosity, and inversely proportional to deformability of red blood cells.
- Relationship between viscosity and hematocrit is almost linear up to a hematocrit of 65% and exponential thereafter.
- Hematocrit measurement is done by both capillary and venous samples.
- Capillary sample gives 5–15% times higher hematocrit level than venous samples because of rouleaux formation and migration of RBC's along the vessel wall.
- Hematocrit level in peripheral blood sample is higher than central venous sample.
- Gold standard blood sample for diagnosis is venous sample.

End Organ Effects of Microthrombi

Complications:
- Microthrombi can lead to hypoxia, hypoglycemia, and acidosis in the newborn.
- The most vulnerable organs are brain, kidneys, and adrenal glands.
- It can lead to decreased circulation in extremities as well leading to necrosis of finger or toes.
- Necrotizing enterocolitis (NEC), kidney failure, seizure, stroke, and decreased fine motor control.

■ FURTHER READING

1. Malan AF, de VH. The management of polycythemia in the newborn infant. Early Hum Dev. 1980;4:393-403.
2. Remon JI, Raghavan A, Maheshwari A. Polycythemia in the newborn. Neo Reviews. 2011;12:e20-8.
3. Stevens K, Wirth FH. Incidence of neonatal hyper viscosity at sea level. J Pediatr. 1980;97:118-9.
4. Swetnam SM, Yabek SM, Averson DC. Hemodynamic consequences of neonatal Polycythemia. J Pediatr. 1987;110:443-7.

Management of Anemia

Swati Bhayana

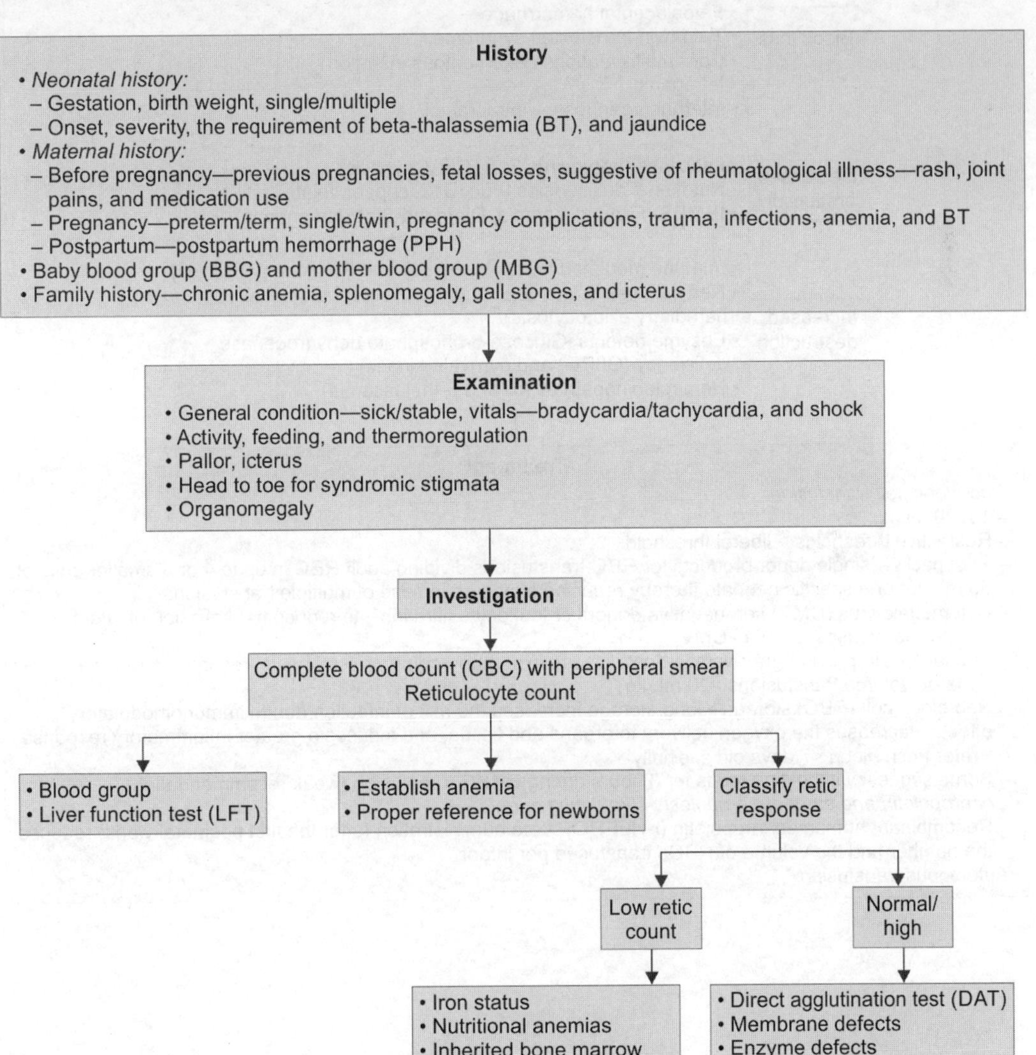

Contd...

Contd...

Differential diagnosis

Anemia with jaundice	Anemia without jaundice
• Immune-mediated hemolysis • Enzyme deficiencies • Membrane defects • Infections, DIC	• Blood loss—fetomaternal, fetoplacental, and twin-twin • Iatrogenic • Intracerebral hemorrhage (ICH) • Congenital—parvovirus

Blood loss
- Fetomaternal hemorrhage [delivery, percutaneous umbilical blood sampling (PUBS), and amniocentesis]
- Fetoplacental hemorrhage
- Twin-twin transfusion syndrome
- Cord malformations (velamentous insertion)
- Iatrogenic
- Internal organ loss— intracranial

Decreased production
- Infections (parvovirus B19, CMV, syphilis)
- Nutritional deficiencies (iron, B12, copper, folate)
- IBMFS (Fanconi anemia, Diamond-Blackfan anemia)

Increased destruction
- Immune mediated hemolysis (ABO and Rh incompatibilities)
- Red cell membrane defects (hereditary spherocytosis, hereditary elliptocytosis)
- Enzyme defects [Glucose-6-phosphate dehydrogenase deficiency (G6PD) and pyruvate kinase]
- Hemoglobinopathies (α- and β-thalassemia)

Treatment
- *Red blood cell transfusion:*
  - 10–20 mL/kg
  - Restrictive thresholds > liberal threshold
  - Pedi packs—single donor products for RBC transfusions dividing adult RBC in up to 4 or 5 smaller units of 50 mL, for one specific neonate thereby reducing exposure in case of multiple transfusions
  - Cytomegalovirus (CMV) seronegative donors or leukocyte filtration—to reduce transmission of latent intracellular viruses, such as CMV
  - Irradiation—to prevent graft-versus-host disease in immune-compromised hosts (recommended, especially for large volume transfusions >20 mL/kg)
  - Red blood cell (RBC) storage—long storage increases the risk of infection due to immunomodulatory effects, decreases the oxygen delivery to organs and tissue, and induces a greater inflammatory response
  - Prefer fresh blood <7 days old specially
  - Some suggest withholding feeds for 3 hours during PRBC transfusion (weak recommendation)
- *Erythropoietin and other erythropoiesis-stimulating agents:*
  - Recombinant human erythropoietin (r-HuEPO)—late administration (after the first postnatal week) reduces the number and the volume of RBCs transfused per infant
- Autologous transfusion

PREVENTATIVE MEASURES

- *Delayed cord clamping (DCC):*
  - At least 30 seconds (up to a maximum of 1–2 minutes after birth) before clamping the umbilical cord
  - Reduce the need for red blood cells (RBCs)
  - Improved circulatory stability
  - Reduction in the rate of intraventricular hemorrhage (IVH) and necrotizing enterocolitis (NEC)
  - Higher hemoglobin (Hb) level at birth and improved iron status at 3–6 months of age
  - Milking the umbilical cord—massaging the cord two to four-times before clamping the cord
  - Smaller trials
  - Reduction of iatrogenic blood loss.
- *Adherence to guidelines:*
  - Adherence to a transfusion guideline
  - Reduction of iatrogenic blood loss—use of microanalysis and transcutaneous instruments, indwelling lines, or catheters.
- *Use of erythropoietin (EPO):*
  - Benefit to prevent in the first weeks of life
  - Studies do support decline in the number of transfusions, decreasing later RBC transfusions.
  - Concerns for retinopathy of prematurity (ROP) after EPO use (controversial).

Key Points to Remember

Developmental Erythropoiesis

- Starts in liver, around 6th week of gestation in the main hematopoietic site
- After the 6th month—bone marrow is the major site
- erythropoietin is the main regulator
- Normal Hb levels

Hemoglobin level			
Week	**Term babies**	**Premature babies (1,200–2,500 g)**	**Small premature babies (<1,200 g)**
0	17.8	16.4	16.0
1	18.8	16.0	14.8
3	15.9	13.5	13.4
6	12.7	10.7	9.7
10	11.4	9.8	8.5

Source: Matthews DC, Glader B. Erythrocyte disorders in infancy. In: Gleason CA, Juul SE (Eds). Avery's Diseases of the Newborn. Philadelphia: Elsevier; 2012. pp. 1080-107.

Physiological Anemia

- All newborn infants have a physiological drop in Hb level—as EPO decreases as a result of a fall in arterial oxygen saturation when the lung replaces the placenta
- 2–3 months after birth
- Preterm infants vulnerable
- More pronounced severity of the developmental postnatal decrease in Hb
- Erythropoiesis in preterm infants impaired due to the low iron stores
- Reduced transplacental transport of iron from mother to fetus—third trimester of pregnancy
- Iatrogenic blood loss due to frequent diagnostic blood tests
- Anemia is a common finding in preterm babies
- Timely diagnosis and appropriate management are essential for optimum growth development of the neonates
- In all neonates below 3 months, blood should be crossed matched before transfusion
- For prevention of late one set anemia, oral iron (dose—2–4 mg/kg elemental iron) should be started from 4 months of age in all term neonates and in preterm from 4 to 6 weeks of life.

■ FURTHER READING

1. Dionisio LM, Dzirba TA. (2021). Neonatal Anemia. [online] Available from https://www.intechopen.com/chapters/78720 [Last accessed September, 2022].
2. Von Lindern JS, Lopriore E. Management and prevention of neonatal anemia: current evidence and guidelines. Expert Rev Hematol. 2014;7(2):195-202.

Blood Transfusion

Nidhi Jain

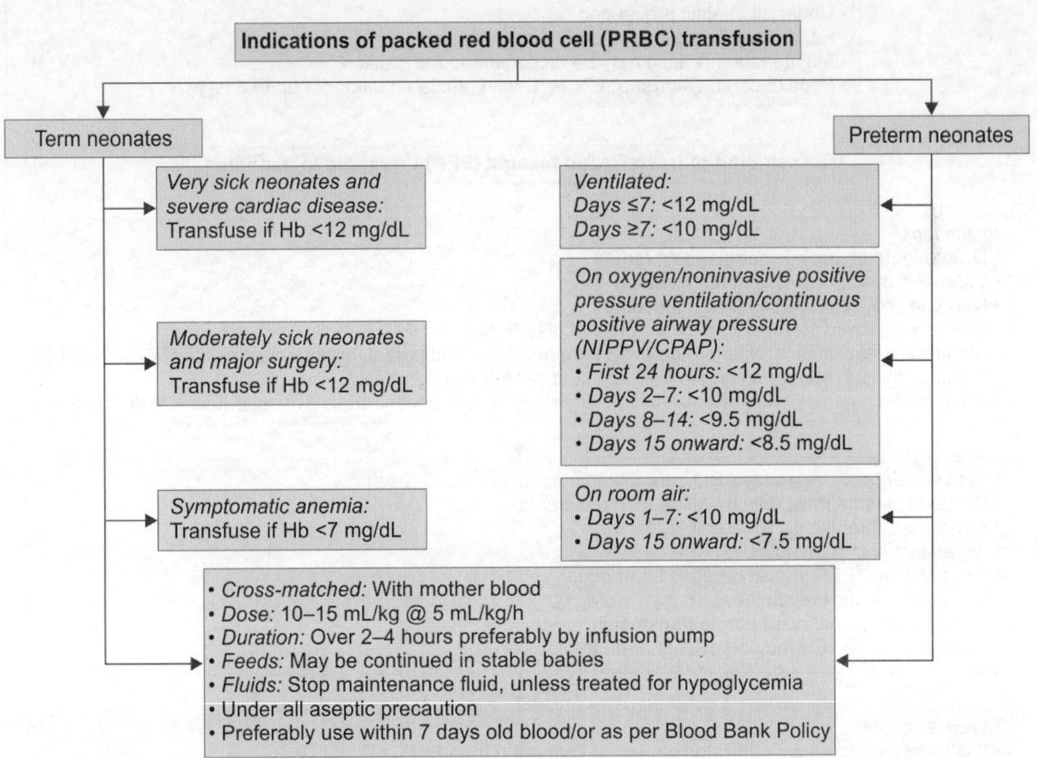

Indications of platelet transfusion threshold in neonates

Neonates with no bleeding [including neonatal alloimmune thrombocytopenia (NAIT)] Transfuse if <25,000	*Neonate with bleeding, current coagulopathy, before surgery and NAIT [If previous sibling with history of intracranial hemorrhage (ICH)* Transfuse if <50,000	*Neonate with major bleeding, before major surgery (neurosurgery)* Transfuse if <100,000

- *Cross-matched:* Not required unless it is a refractory case
- *Dose:* 10 mL/kg @ 10–20 mL/kg/h
- *Duration:* Over 30 minutes
- Transfuse immediately as it received from Blood Bank
- Under all aseptic precaution
- Feeds may be continued during transfusion
- Maintenance IV fluid may be discontinued transfusion
- Platelet can be stored at 22–24°C with gentle agitation for up to 5 days

Transfusion of fresh frozen plasma (FFP) threshold in neonates

Indications:
- Disseminated intravascular bleeding (DIC)
- Vitamin K deficiency associated bleeding
- Neonate with clinically significant bleeding
- Before surgery/invasive procedure with risk of bleeding
- Abnormal coagulation profile [prothrombin time and activated partial thromboplastin time (PT and aPTT) significantly high corresponding to their age and gestational age (GA)]
- Congenital coagulation factor deficiencies where no factor concentrate is available (factor V deficiency)

- *Cross-matched:* Preferably ABO compatible plasma should be used
- Group O plasma must only be given to O recipients
- *Dose:* 10–15 mL/kg @ 10–20 mL/kg/h
- *Duration:* Over 30 minutes
- Once thawed, FFP should be used immediately
- Under all aseptic precaution
- Feeds may be continued during transfusion
- Maintenance IV fluid may be discontinued transfusion

Cryoprecipitate:
- It is used as a more concentrated source of fibrinogen than FFP
- It is primarily indicated when the fibrinogen level is <0.8–1.0 g/L in the presence of bleeding from acquired or congenital hyperfibrinogenemia
- The usual dose is 5–10 mL/kg

Key Points to Remember

- Transfusion of blood components is a common procedure in sick neonates in neonatal intensive care unit (NICU).
- Blood transfusion has potential harm especially in preterm neonates.
- Restrictive threshold PRBC transfusion is recommended in preterm neonates.

- In neonates, smaller volume (10–15 mL/kg) of PRBC is preferred.
- Use of "fresh (<7 days old) PRBC only" is not recommended. Follow the existing protocol by the blood bank for issuing PRBC (oldest first).
- Use of irradiated blood components is strongly recommended. It is more important to use irradiated products only in situations where the volume transfused is quite large (>20 mL/kg).
- Provision of CMV safe blood for transfusion in preterm neonates by using CMV seronegative donors or leukoreduction or a combination of both is strongly recommended.
- Higher threshold (platelet count <25,000/mm^3) should be used for prophylactic platelet transfusions for prevention of major bleeding in preterm neonates.
- In neonatal alloimmune thrombocytopenia, maintaining platelet count >30,000/mm^3 is strongly recommended.
- The routine use of prophylactic FFP in preterm neonates is not recommended.
- Neonates with deranged coagulation parameters and planned for surgical or invasive procedure should receive FFP.

■ FURTHER READING

1. Franz AR, Engel C, Bassler D, Rüdiger M, Thome UH, Maier RF, et al. Effects of liberal vs restrictive transfusion thresholds on survival and neurocognitive outcomes in extremely low-birth-weight infants: the ettno randomized clinical trial. JAMA. 2020;324(6):560-70.
2. National Neonatology Forum of India. (2020). Use of blood components in newborns, Clinical Practice guidelines. [online] Available from http://www.nnfi.org/assests/pdf/cpg-guidelines/Bloodcomponents.pdf [Last accessed September, 2022].
3. New HV, Berryman J, Bolton-Maggs PHB, Cantwell C, Chalmers EA, Davies T, et al. Guidelines on transfusion for fetuses, neonates and older children. Br J Haematol. 2016;175:784-828.
4. Whyte R, Kirpalani H. Low versus high haemoglobin concentration threshold for blood transfusion for preventing morbidity and mortality in very low birth weight infants. Cochrane Database Syst Rev. 2011;(11):CD000512.

Management of Differences of Sex Development

Aaradhana Singh

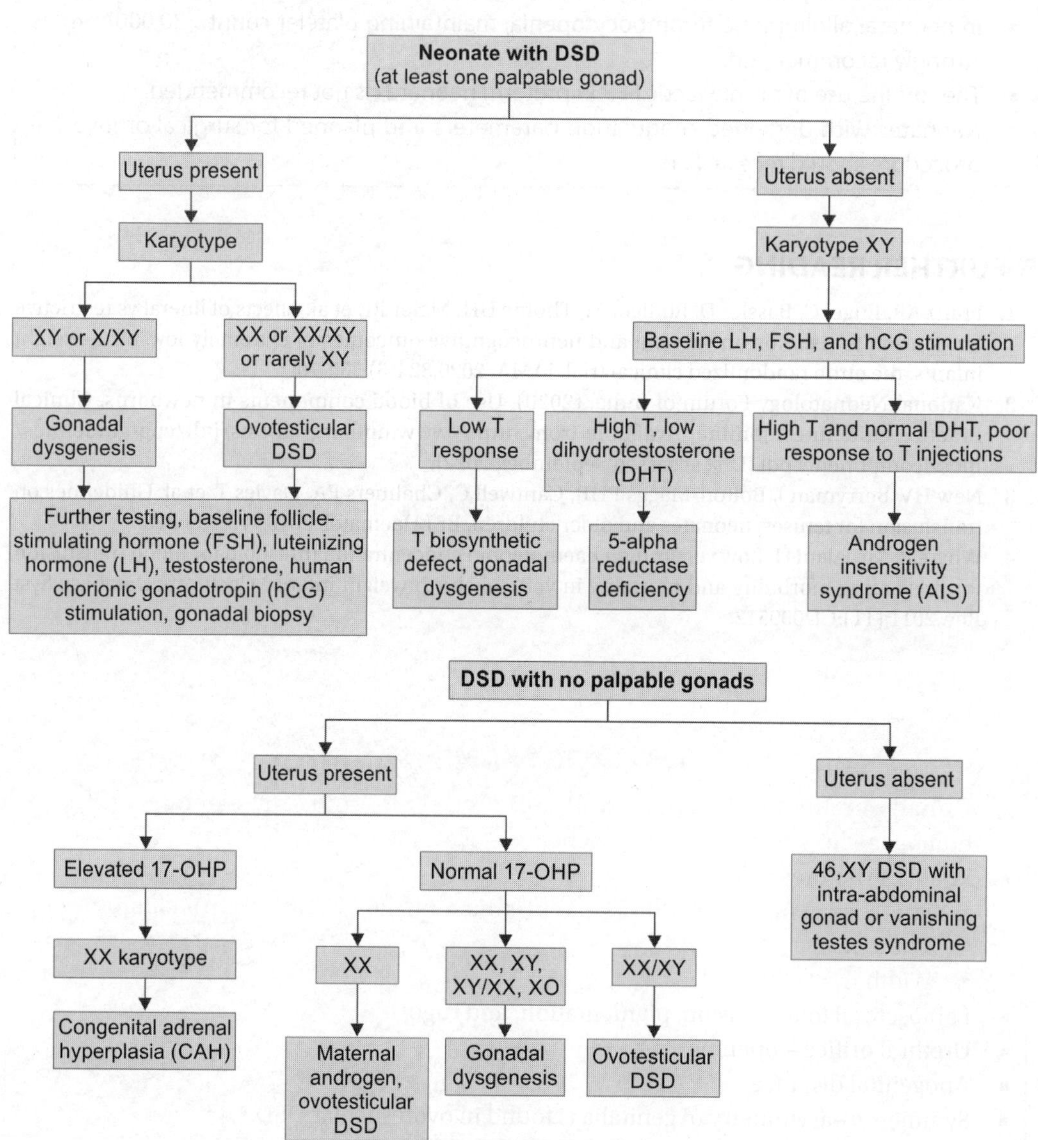

DEFINITION AND CLASSIFICATION
(*See* Annexures 1 and 2)

Differences of sex development (DSD) are a condition in which development of chromosomal, gonadal, and anatomical sex is atypical and incongruent to each other.

HISTORY

- Parental consanguinity [autosomal recessive disorders like congenital adrenal hyperplasia (CAH) and adrenal steroid synthesis defects]
- Genital anomalies in siblings (autosomal recessive disorders)
- Previous neonatal deaths, primary amenorrhea/infertility, recurrent miscarriages, still birth, and delayed puberty in other members
- Maternal exposure to androgens like androgenic progestin, danazol, and antiandrogens (virilization of female fetus)
- Failure to thrive, vomiting in neonate (CAH)
- Maternal virilization during pregnancy (virilizing tumors, placental aromatase deficiency)
- Other organ anomalies and developmental delay (syndromic association)

GENERAL PHYSICAL EXAMINATION

- Hydration (dehydration in CAH)
- Weight (poor weight gain or weight loss in CAH)
- Blood pressure (hypertension in 11-beta- and 17-alpha-hydroxylase deficiency)
- Skin and mucosal pigmentation (CAH)
- Skeletal anomalies [SOX9 mutation–campomelic dysplasia; P450 oxidoreductase (POR) deficiency: Antley–Bixler syndrome]
- Dysmorphic features (genetic syndromes)
- Polydactyly (Smith–Lemli–Opitz syndrome)
- Anatomic malformations (VACTERL).

GENITALIA EXAMINATION

- Gonads—palpable/nonpalpable, number, size, and consistency (smooth, homogeneous—testis, and heterogeneous—ovotestis)
- Phallic structure:
  - Stretched penile length (SPL) <2.5 cm is microphallus, clitoris >1 cm is clitoromegaly.
  - Chordee
  - Width
- Labioscrotal folds—fusion, pigmentation, and rugosity
- Urethral orifice—opening
- Anogenital distance
- Symmetry—asymmetry of genitalia is found in ovotesticular DSD.

For detailed genitalia examination *see* **Table 1**.

Examination of external genitalia should be a mandatory part of newborn examination. Timely detection of hyperpigmentation and absence of palpable testis may prevent fatal outcome in CAH.

Investigations
(see Table 2)

- Serum electrolytes, blood gas analysis, and blood sugar
- Serum 17-hydroxyprogesterone (S.17-OHP)
- Karyotype/fluorescence in situ hybridization (FISH)/quantitative polymerase chain reaction (PCR) for Y chromosome
- Serum levels of adrenal androgens and its precursors (*see* **Annxure 3**)
- Serum anti-Müllerian hormone (AMH), S. inhibin
- Ultrasonography pelvis, kidney, ureter, and bladder (KUB), and labioscrotal region
- Genetic tests

Gender assignment
Consider following factors:
- Diagnosis, genital appearance, surgical options
- Need for lifelong replacement therapy potential for fertility, views of family and cultural practices

Surgical correction
- Timing of surgical correction of atypical genitalia is debatable
- Many support postponement of genital surgery until patient can participate in decision
- *Gonadectomy* to be done if risk of malignancy

DSD management

Medical treatment
- CAH—hydrocortisone (10–15 mg/m²/day) and fludrocortisone 0.05–0.1 mg/day
- Salt supplementation in salt wasting CAH
- Hormonal replacement therapy in cases with hypogonadism

Counseling
- Enhance open interactions with parents
- Do not refer child as "IT, HE, or SHE"
- Advice to postpone naming of the baby and birth certificate
- Fully discuss diagnosis, prognosis, and treatment options
- Involve parents in taking the decision of gender assignment

TABLE 1: Genitalia examination.

Prader scoring: Initially created for the assessment of patients with CAH. Appropriate for 46,XX DSD/DSD with nonpalpable gonads
- Stage 1—clitoromegaly without labial fusion
- Stage 2—clitoromegaly and posterior labial fusion
- Stage 3—greater degree of clitoromegaly, single perineal urogenital orifice, and complete labial fusion
- Stage 4—increasingly phallic clitoris, urethra like urogenital sinus at base of clitoris, complete labial fusion
- Stage 5—penile clitoris, urethral meatus at tip of phallus, scrotum like labia

Anogenital ratio: Ratio of distance between anus and posterior fourchette (AF) divided by distance between anus and clitoris (AC)
Normal ratio = 0.37 in infants
Ratio >0.5 is abnormal and suggests possible virilization in early fetal life.

External masculinization score (EMS score)—designed for 46,XY DSD/DSD with at least one palpable gonad. A score of 0–3 is given for four aspects of male external genitalia. Sum of 4 values is the EMS score giving a maximum score of 12. Score of <11 is abnormal and score of <7 is ambiguous genitalia.

Contd...

Contd...

Score	Labioscrotal fusion	Microphallus	Location of urethral meatus	Location of right gonad	Location of left gonad
3	Yes	No	Normal		
2.5					
2.0			Distal		
1.5				Lower inguinal canal/scrotum	Lower inguinal canal/scrotum
1.0			Mid	Inguinal canal	Inguinal canal
0.5				Abdomen	Abdomen
0	No	Yes	Proximal		

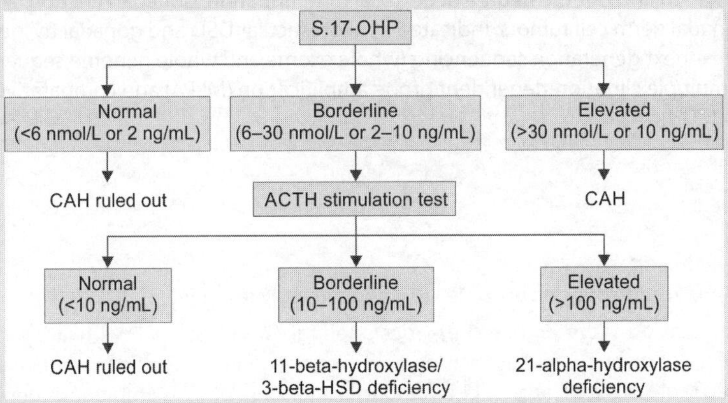

Hypospadias description.

TABLE 2: Details of investigation.

- *Serum electrolytes, blood gases, and blood sugar:*
  - Hyponatremia, hyperkalemia, and metabolic acidosis in salt wasting CAH.
  - Hypokalemia, metabolic alkalosis in hypertensive CAH (11-beta and 17-alpha-hydroxylase deficiency)
- 17-OHP
  - To be done in all cases of DSD after 48 hours of life to rule out CAH.
  - 17-OHP interpretation:

Contd...

Contd...

- *Define sex chromosome (karyotype):*
  - Most commonly—peripheral blood
  - Rarely—skin and gonadal biopsies
  - FISH using X and Y specific probes (24–48 hours)
- *Serum levels of adrenal androgens and precursors:*
  - Testosterone, dihydrotestosterone, serum androstenedione, serum dehydroepiandrosterone sulfate, serum luteinizing hormone, follicle-stimulating hormone at mini puberty (1 week to 3 months of postnatal life). Beyond mini puberty hCG stimulation test is required
  - S. testosterone level of:
    - <50 ng/dL—gonadal dysgenesis, steroidogenic defects
    - 50–300 ng/dL—requires further evaluation by hCG stimulation test
    - >300 ng/dL—testosterone action defects
  - Gonadotropins levels (serum Luteinizing hormone and serum Follicle stimulating hormone)—after 7 days of birth
  - T: DHT ratio >8.5–30 is suggestive of 5-alpha-reductase deficiency
  - T: androstenedione ratio of <0.8 is suggestive of 17-beta-HSD deficiency
- *Serum anti-Müllerian hormone (AMH) and inhibin B:*
  - Anti-Müllerian hormone is secreted by Sertoli cells and inhibin is secreted by other testicular cells too.
  - Anti-Müllerian hormone and inhibin B are low at birth. Levels rise until second year of life.
    - Low anti-Müllerian hormone—gonadal dysgenesis, absent testis
    - Normal anti-Müllerian hormone—steroidogenic defects, leydig cell hypoplasia
- *Radiological assessment:*
  - Ultrasonography
    - First-line imaging modality
    - Adrenals, kidneys, pelvis, inguinal, and labioscrotal
  In neonate, the uterus, ovaries, and adrenals are identifiable.
  - Magnetic resonance imaging (MRI)—reserved for cases where ultrasonography has failed. Should include pelvis and perineum and can identify extra-abdominal ectopic testes
  - *Voiding Cystourethrogram and genitography*—defines internal anatomy of urethra, vagina, cervix, and urethrovaginal confluence
  - *Endoscopic* examination of the urinary tract
  - Exploratory *laparotomy* to localize and characterize/biopsy the gonads
  - Endoscopic examination of the genital tract (*genitoscopy*)—to localize gonads, determine nature and structure of the internal sex organs, and detect any communication with external genital structures.
- *Gonadal biopsy*—to find out the degree of gonadal differentiation, gonadal function, and to identify the risk of gonadal germ cell tumors. Indicated in ovotesticular DSD and gonadal dysgenesis.
- *Genetic testing*—next generation sequencing (whole exome and whole genome sequencing), microarrays, multiplex ligation-dependent probe amplification (MLPA) and comparative genomic hybridization (CGH).

■ ANNEXURE 1

Sex Development in Humans

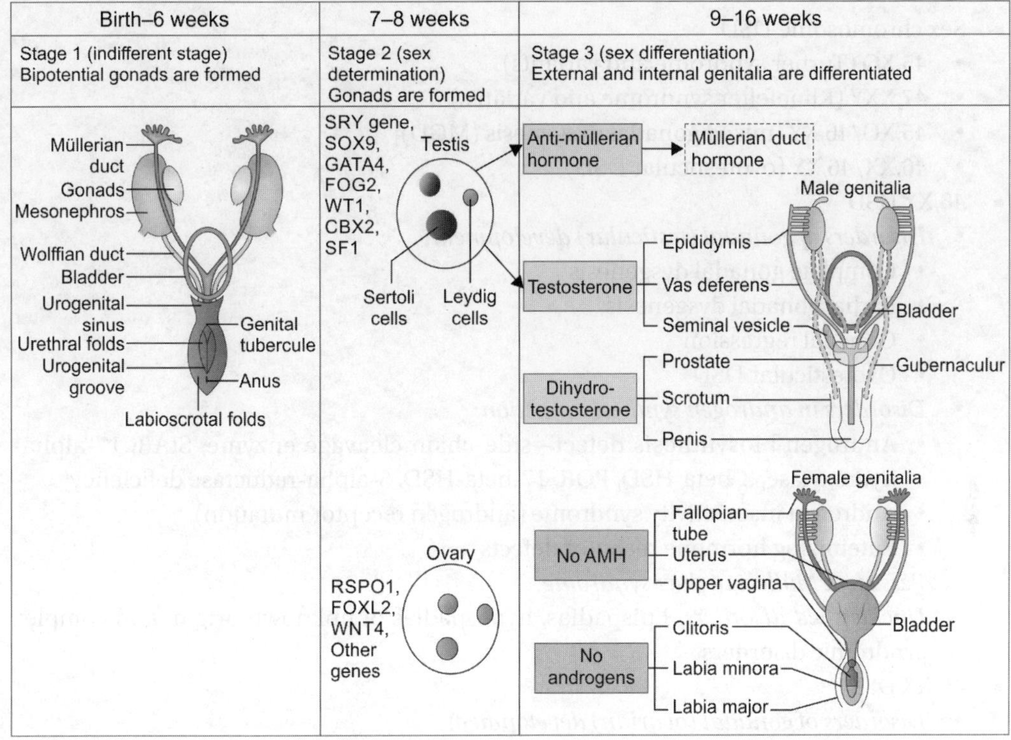

■ ANNEXURE 2

DSD Classification (Chicago Classification 2006)

- Sex chromosome DSD
  - 45,XO (Turner syndrome and variants)
  - 47,XXY (Klinefelter syndrome and variants)
  - 45,XO/46,XY [mixed gonadal dysgenesis (MGD)]
  - 46,XX/46,XY (ovotesticular DSD)
- 46,XY DSD
  - *Disorders of gonadal (testicular) development:*
    - Complete gonadal dysgenesis
    - Partial gonadal dysgenesis
    - Gonadal regression
    - Ovotesticular DSD
  - *Disorders in androgen synthesis or action:*
    - Androgen biosynthesis defect—side-chain cleavage enzyme, StAR, 17-alpha-hydroxylase, 3-beta-HSD, POR, 17-beta-HSD, 5-alpha-reductase deficiency
    - Androgen insensitivity syndrome (androgen receptor mutation)
    - Luteinizing hormone receptor defects
  - *Persistent Müllerian duct syndrome*
  - *Unclassified disorders:* Epispadias, hypospadias of unknown origin, and complex syndromic disorders
- 46,XX DSD
  - *Disorders of gonadal (ovarian) development:*
    - Ovotesticular DSD
    - Testicular DSD (e.g., SRY+, duplicate SOX9)
    - Gonadal dysgenesis
  - *Androgen excess:*
    - Fetal (e.g., 21-alpha-hydroxylase, 11-β-hydroxylase, 3-β-HSD deficiency)
    - Fetoplacental (aromatase deficiency and POR deficiency)
    - Maternal (luteoma, exogenous, etc.)

■ ANNEXURE 3

Adrenal Steroid Synthesis Pathway

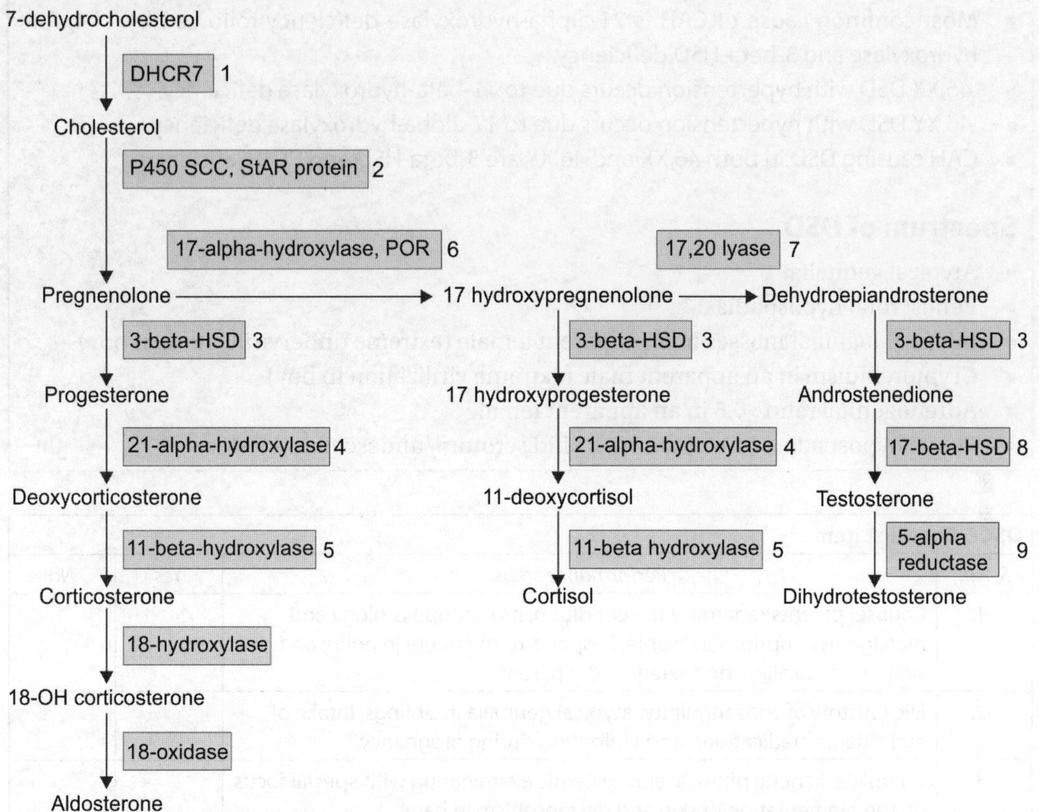

Deficiency of enzymes indicated by numbers 1, 2, 3, 6, 7, 8, and 9 cause 46,XY DSD.
Deficiency of enzymes indicated by numbers 3, 4, and 5 cause 46,XX DSD.

Key Points to Remember

- Most common cause of DSD is CAH.
- Most common cause of CAH is 21-alpha-hydroxylase deficiency followed by 11-beta-hydroxylase and 3-beta-HSD deficiency.
- 46,XX DSD with hypertension occurs due to 11-beta-hydroxylase deficiency.
- 46,XY DSD with hypertension occurs due to 17-alpha-hydroxylase deficiency.
- CAH causing DSD in both 46,XX and 46,XY are 3-beta-HSD and POR deficiency.

Spectrum of DSD

- Atypical genitalia
- Penoscrotal hypospadias
- Bilateral inguinal masses in an apparent female (extreme undervirilization in boy)
- Cryptorchidism in an apparent male (extreme virilization in boy)
- Adrenogenital ratio >0.5 in an apparent female
- Penile hypospadias associated with bifid scrotum/undescended testes.

OSCE/Checklist item

S. No.	Performance steps	Yes	No
1.	Counsel parents regarding the condition, its pathophysiology and management options available. Respond to the query in polite and simple way to allay the anxiety of the parents		
2.	Elicit history of consanguinity, atypical genitalia in siblings, intake of androgenic medications, and virilization during pregnancy		
3.	Complete general physical and systemic examination with special focus on the pigmentation of skin and dysmorphism in baby		
4.	Complete genitalia examination. Identify whether gonads are palpable or not		
5.	Send 8 AM morning sample for 17-OHP after 48 hours of life		
6.	Monitor hydration status, blood pressure, weight, serum electrolytes, and blood sugar especially in second week of life		
7.	If dehydration and dyselectrolytemia, correct it		
8.	Send sample for karyotype/FISH or quantitative PCR for Y chromosome		
9.	Ultrasonography of labioscrotal folds and inguinal region for gonads, pelvis for Müllerian structures and KUB region for renal anomalies and adrenal hyperplasia		
10.	If CAH, start hydrocortisone, fludrocortisone, and salt supplementation		
11.	If CAH ruled out, plan other test like hormonal evaluation and genetic testing		

■ FURTHER READING

1. Ahmed SF, Achermann JC, Arlt W, Balen A, Conway G, Edwards Z, et al. Society for Endocrinology UK guidance on the initial evaluation of an infant or an adolescent with a suspected disorder of sex development (Revised 2015). Clin Endocrinol (Oxf). 2016;84(5):771-88.

2. Lee PA, Nordenstrom A, Houk CP, Ahmed SF, Auchus R, Baratz A, et al. Global disorders of sex development update since 2006: perceptions, approach and care. Horm Res Paediatr. 2016;85(3):158-80.

3. León NY, Reyes AP, Harley VR. A clinical algorithm to diagnose differences of sex development. Lancet Diabetes Endocrinol. 2019;7(7):560-74.

Management of Congenital Adrenal Hyperplasia

Pinky Meena

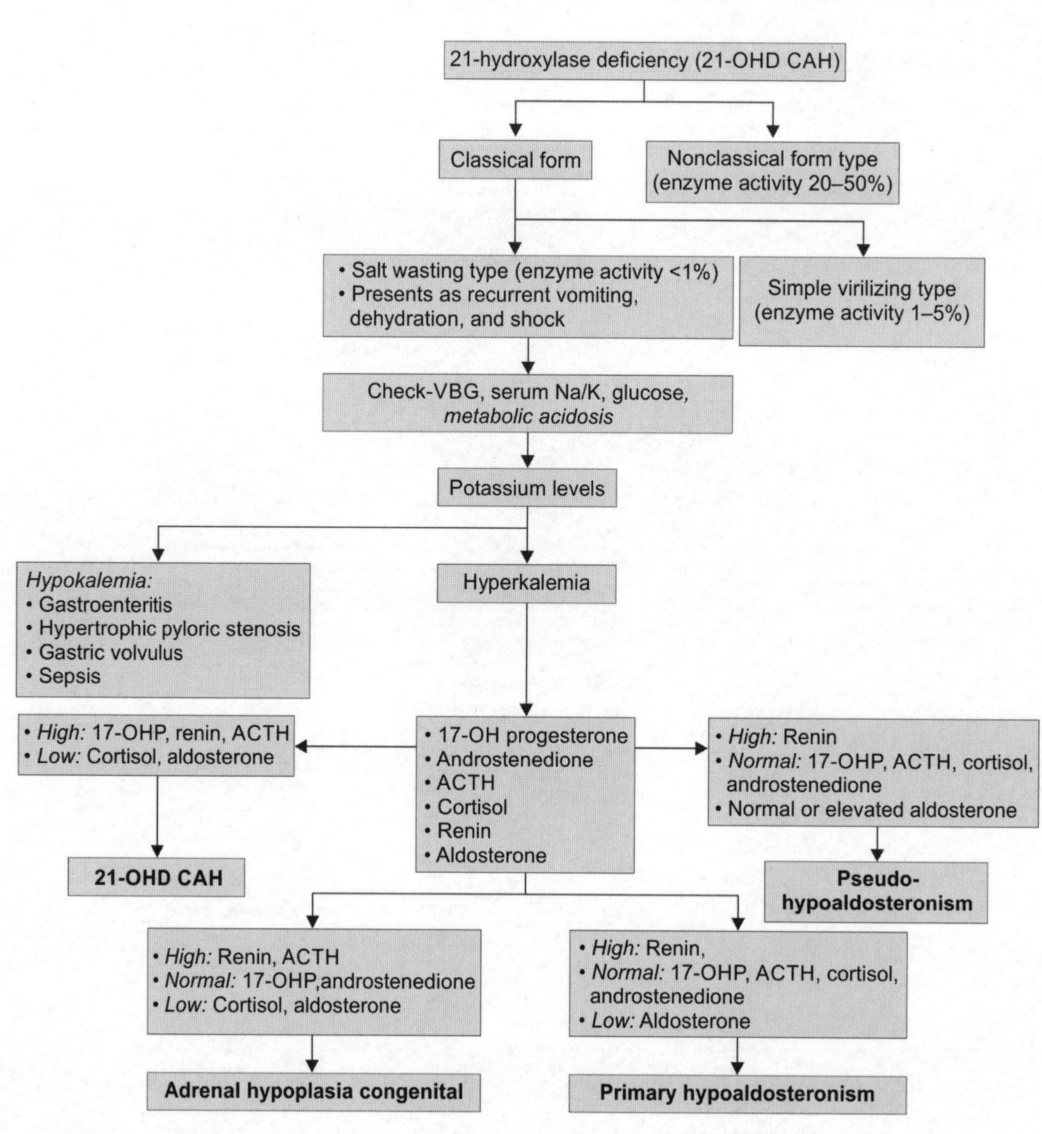

PRESENTATION OF CAH: 21-HYDROXYLASE DEFICIENCY

- In the neonatal period, the *classical variety of CAH* presents with virilization of genitalia in girls, due to hyperandrogenism.
- Girls with mild virilization and boys escape clinical detection at birth.
- These neonates present with *salt wasting crisis congenital adrenal hyperplasia (SW-CAH)* at 1–2 weeks of age, and manifest with failure to thrive, lethargy, poor feeding, recurrent vomiting, pain abdomen, dehydration, and hypotension with metabolic acidosis, hyponatremia, hyperkalemia, and hypoglycemia.
- *Simple virilizing congenital adrenal hyperplasia (SV-CAH)* girls have adequate aldosterone production and present with signs of prenatal virilization without salt wasting. In boys, simple virilizing variant presents as precocious puberty.
- *Nonclassical form congenital adrenal hyperplasia (NCCAH)* of the disorder present in adolescence or later with features of hyperandrogenism in females causing polycystic ovary syndrome (PCOS) morphology or infertility.

Phenotypic and biochemical characteristics of three most common causes of CAH other than 21-OH deficiency.

Subtypes	Phenotype	Elevated metabolites
11β-hydroxylase deficiency	Female virilization	Deoxycorticosterone, 11-deoxycortisol
17α-hydroxylase deficiency	Male undervirilization Female virilization +/-	Deoxycorticosterone, corticosterone
3β-hydroxysteroid dehydrogenase deficiency	Male undervirilization Female virilization +/-	Dehydroepiandrostenedione, 17-OH pregnenolone

CONFIRMATION OF DIAGNOSIS OF 21-HYDROXYLASE DEFICIENCY CAH

- Symptomatic infants should be screened with an early-morning (before 8 AM) baseline serum 17-hydroxyprogesterone (17-OHP) levels by liquid chromatography-mass spectrometry (LC-MS).
- Cosyntropin stimulation test should be done in those with borderline 17-OHP levels, to differentiate 21-hydroxylase deficiency from other enzyme defects.

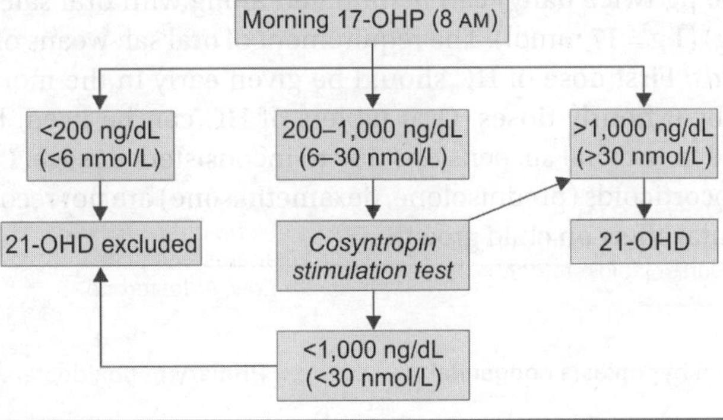

- Tandem mass spectrometry for steroid profiling can be done to differentiate various subsets of CAH.
- Genotyping is recommended only when results of the adrenocortical profile after a cosyntropin stimulation test are equivocal, or cosyntropin stimulation cannot be accurately performed (i.e., patient receiving glucocorticoid), or for purposes of genetic counseling.

MANAGEMENT OF ACUTE ADRENAL CRISIS

- Maintain airway, breathing, and circulation.
- Restore intravenous hydration by intravenous route using a wide bore needle.
- Infuse isotonic saline at 20 mL/kg over 10 minutes if signs of shock are present (maximum up to 60 mL/kg).
- Further fluid replacement to be guided by clinical signs of shock or over-hydration.
- Newborns should be continued on 1.5–2 times fluid as maintenance therapy (half normal saline in 5% dextrose solution).
- Check and correct hypoglycemia. Administer 2 mL/kg of 10% dextrose if low blood sugar is detected. Start glucose infusion rate (GIR) if required and titrate further as per the sugar levels.
- Administer intravenous hydrocortisone (HC) at 50–100 mg/m^2 bolus followed by 50–100 mg/m^2/day in four divided doses (6 hourly). Usual dose in newborn babies is approximately 25 mg bolus followed by 5–6 mg every 6 hourly. Gradually, decrease HC dose by 50% each day to bring to maintenance dose if hemodynamically stable.
- Manage hyperkalemia by calcium gluconate infusion, insulin dextrose infusion, and salbutamol nebulization. In most instances, it corrects with institution of glucocorticoid therapy in high doses.
- Continue intravenous route till patient is fit to consume orally.
- Check and correct any dyselectrolytemia.
- Monitor vitals, intake, output, and sensorium.

Maintenance Therapy

- Gradually, taper HC by 50% each day and once hemodynamically stable start maintenance therapy with oral HC (10–15 mg/m^2 in three divided doses) and fludro-cortisone (100 µg twice daily) can be initiated along with oral salt supplementation (4–8 mmol/kg) (1 g = 17 mmol). The requirement of oral salt weans off after infancy.
- *Glucocorticoids:* First dose of HC should be given early in the morning with waking up followed by 6 hourly doses. Oral tablets of HC can be used; however, it is not recommended to use oral suspensions due to inconsistent dosage. Long-acting potent forms of glucocorticoids (prednisolone, dexamethasone) are not recommended as they have detrimental effect on child growth.

- *Mineralocorticoids (MCs):* Fludrocortisone should be supplemented in all babies with classical CAH including those with SV-CAH as it reduces requirement of corticosteroid and optimizes final height outcomes. The requirement for MCs is higher during infancy at 0.05–0.2 mg/day and decreases as the child grows. The drug should be started at a lower dose initially and titrated according to serum electrolytes (K) and blood pressure. Monitor for hypertension, edema, and hypokalemia.

Stress Dosing

- To cope with stressful situations like febrile illness (>38.5°C), gastroenteritis with dehydration, major surgery accompanied by general anesthesia, and major trauma the glucocorticoid dosage should be increased to two to three times of maintenance dose till the time of illness and brought down to normal dose as event subsides.
- However, no dose increment is required to cope with daily mental and emotional stress and minor illness and/or before routine physical exercise.
- The immediate caregivers and relatives of such infants should be educated for adrenal crisis prevention and giving intramuscular dose of HC.

Monitoring

- Follow-up monthly till 3 months of life thereafter at 3 monthly duration.
- Regular assessment of growth velocity, weight, blood pressure, physical examination, and annual bone age in addition to obtaining biochemical measurements (17-OHP) to assess the adequacy of glucocorticoid therapy.

Surgical Treatment

- A multidisciplinary team with competence in disorders of sex development (DSD) management is recommended. In all pediatric patients with CAH, particularly minimally virilized girls (Prader I–II) and mildly undervirilized boys (EMS 7–11), parents must be informed about surgical options, including delaying surgery and observation until the child is older.
- Usually, the sex assignment in 46,XX newborns with CYP21A2-D or CYP11B1 is female, and genital surgery may be necessary, but the timing of the surgery remains controversial.
- In male newborns with severe hypospadias, urological surgery is certainly indicated for functional repair. It is advisable to refrain from invasive surgery that is not essential for health and to encourage patient participation and decisions in the choices regarding the sexual sphere.

> ### Key Points to Remember
>
> - Congenital adrenal hyperplasia (CAH) is an autosomal recessive disorder with an incidence ranging from 1:10,000–1:20,000 births.
> - It is caused by enzymatic defect in adrenal and gonadal steroidogenesis.
> - The most common defect in CAH is deficiency of enzyme 21-hydroxylase caused by mutation in CYP21A2 gene (95% of all forms of CAH).
> - The block in corticosteroid and mineralocorticoid enzymatic pathway causes deficit production of corticosteroid and aldosterone, and the intermediate products are diverted to androgen synthesis.
> - Primary adrenal insufficiency to produce cortisol leads to secondary increase in adrenocorticotropic hormone (ACTH) production from pituitary, further causing adrenal hyperplasia.
> - Ensure DBS sample for CAH screening is sent for all newborns before discharge, preferably after 24–72 hours of life.
> - Follow the DBS 17-OHP levels and activate quick action for follow up.
> - Examine all babies for genital ambiguity at birth.
> - Keep high index of suspicion for adrenal crisis in neonates presenting with dehydration, shock, and poor weight gain.
> - Institute HC therapy urgently after storing critical sample for hormonal profile.

■ FURTHER READING

1. Claahsen-van der Grinten HL, Speiser PW, Ahmed SF, Arlt W, Auchus RJ, Falhammar H, et al. Congenital adrenal hyperplasia-current insights in pathophysiology, diagnostics, and management. Endocr Rev. 2022;43(1):91-159.
2. Dabas A, Bothra M, Kapoor S. CAH newborn Screening in India: challenges and opportunities. Int J Neonatal Screen. 2020;6(3):70.
3. Speiser PW, Arlt W, Auchus RJ, Baskin LS, Conway GS, Merke DP, et al. Congenital adrenal hyperplasia due to steroid 21-hydroxylase deficiency: An Endocrine Society Clinical Practice Guideline. J Clin Endocrinol Metab. 2018;103(11):4043-88. doi: 10.1210/jc.2018-01865.

Management of Hypoglycemia

Sonali Verma

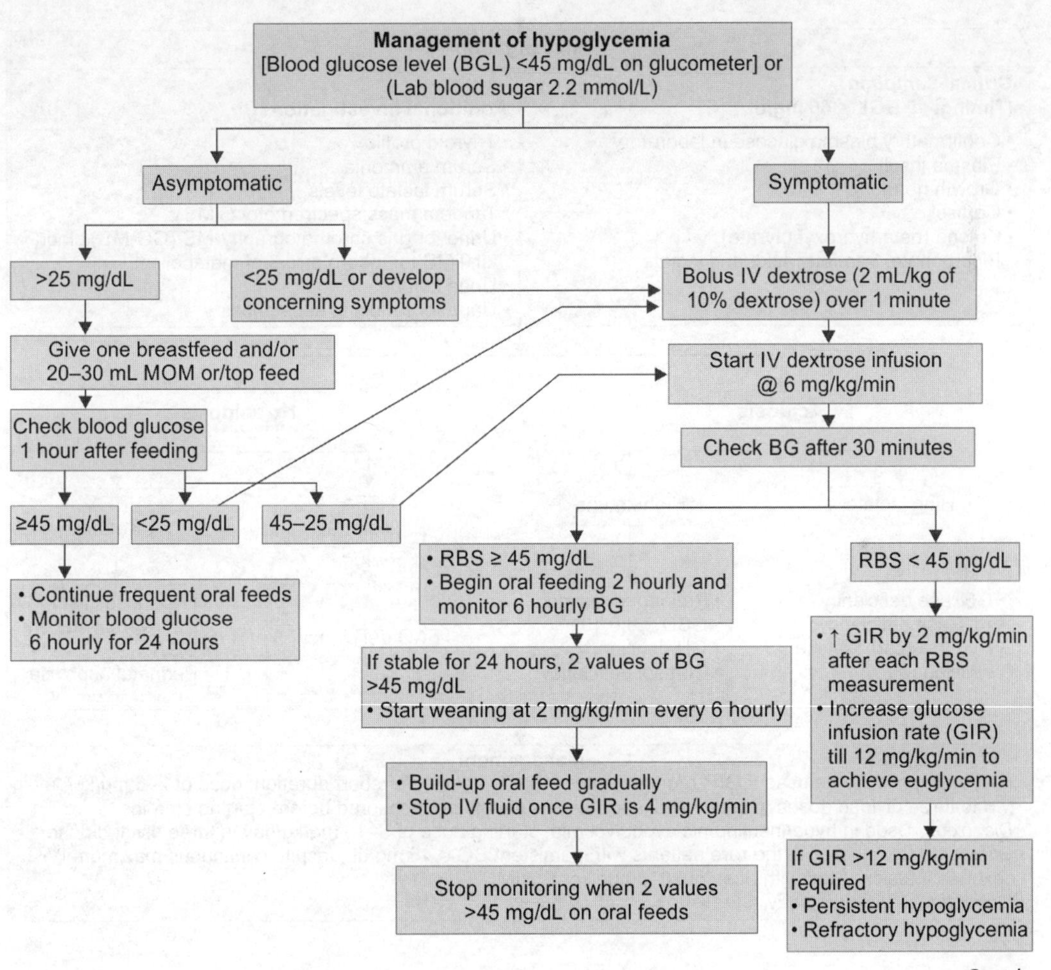

Contd...

Contd...

Management of persistent hypoglycemia
• Persistent >7 days
• Retracting >12 mg/kg/day
• Defined as when normal BS is not attained even on GIR of 12 mg/kg/min or requirement of GIR for 7 days

Causes
Congenital
PSHI (perinatal stress-induced hyperinsulinemia)
(Cause: SGA/IUGR/asphyxia and cesarean delivery)
• Hyperinsulinemia
• Hypopituitarism (ACTH deficiency and GH deficiency)
• Cortisol deficiency
• Glycogen storage disease
• Disorders of gluconeogenesis
• Fatty acid oxidation defect

Investigation

Critical sampling:
(Timing: @ BGL < 45 mg/dL)
• Confirmatory plasma glucose in laboratory
• Plasma insulin
• Growth hormone
• Cortisol
• Ketone (beta-hydroxybutyrate)
• Bicarbonate, free fatty acid, and lactate

Additional investigations
• Thyroid profile
• Serum ammonia
• Serum lactate levels
• Tandem mass spectrometry (TMS)
• Urine for gas chromatography-MS (GC-MS)/blood for TMS for inborn errors of metabolism
• Urine ketones
• Urine for reducing substances

Acidosis
No acidosis

High lactate
High ketone
↑ FFA ↓ Ketone
↓ FFA ↓ Ketone

• G6Pase deficiency
• FDPase deficiency
• Pyruvate carboxylase deficiency

• Prolonged fasting
• GSD 3,6,9,10
• GH deficiency
• Cortisol deficiency

FAO deficiency

• Hyperinsulinism
• Panhypopituitarism
• SGA
• Perinatal asphyxia

Management
• Hydrocortisone: To be used if GIR requirement is >12 mg/kg/min; for short duration; dose of 2–6 mg/kg/day in two to three divided doses. Cortisol and insulin levels should be measured before starting steroids
• Diazoxide: Used in hyperinsulinemic hypoglycemia; starting dose of 5–10 mg/kg/day in three divided dose
• Glucagon: Considered in the rare patients with persistent BG < 45 mg/dL despite continuous maximum IV dextrose infusion. Start with dose of 20–30 µg/kg, SC/IM
• Octreotide: 2–10 µg/kg/day, SC

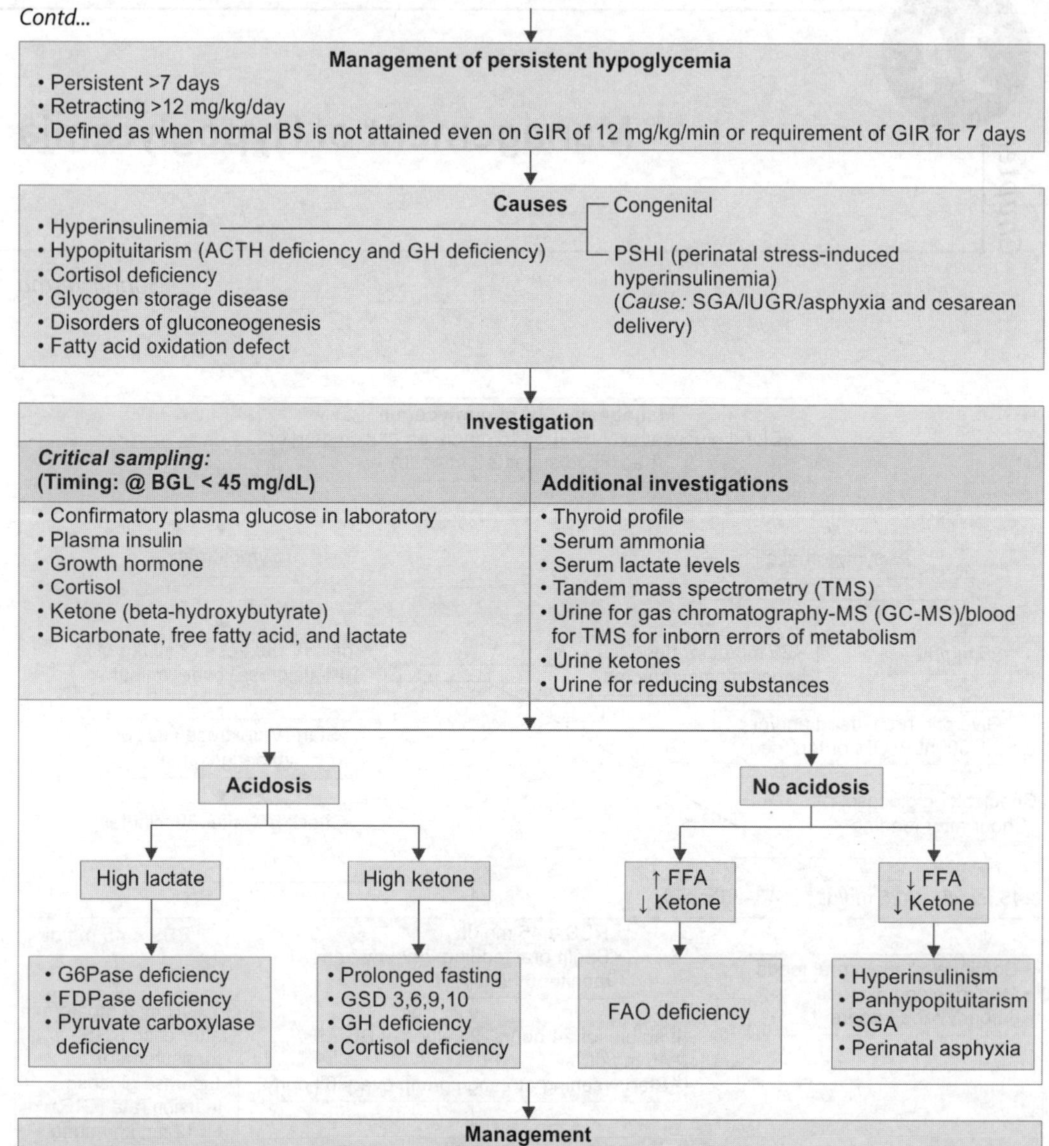

WHOM TO SCREEN FOR HYPOGLYCEMIA?

At risk neonates	*Neonates with*
<ul><li>Premature infants [<37 weeks gestational age (GA)]</li><li>Low birth weight (LBW) infants (<2,500 g)</li><li>Small for gestational age (SGA) (birth weight <10th percentile)</li><li>Large for gestational age (LGA) (birth weight >90th percentile)</li><li>Infant of diabetic mother</li><li>Mother is on propranolol and labetalol</li><li>Infants on intravenous (IV) fluid and on parenteral nutrition</li><li>Sick infants (sepsis, perinatal asphyxia respiratory distress, shock, polycythemia, and seizure)</li><li>Family history of neonatal hypoglycemia/inborn error of metabolism</li></ul>	<ul><li>Hemihypertrophy</li><li>Macroglossia</li><li>Omphalocele</li><li>Ambiguous genitalia</li><li>Hyponatremia</li><li>Hypokalemia</li><li>Hepatomegaly in storage disorder</li><li>Midline defects, micropenis in hypopituitarism</li></ul>

WHEN TO SCREEN?

Clinical conditions	*Time schedule*
Routine screening for high-risk newborn	2, 6, 12, 24, 48, and 72 hours of life
Sick neonates (sepsis, asphyxia, polycythemia, and shock)	Every 6–8 hours

CLINICAL MANIFESTATIONS OF HYPOGLYCEMIA

Neurogenic	*Neuroglycopenia*
<ul><li>Shakiness, trembling, and jitteriness</li><li>Tachycardia</li><li>Pallor</li><li>Hypothermia</li></ul>	<ul><li>Lethargy, floppiness</li><li>Irritability, weak/high-pitched cry</li><li>Poor feeding</li><li>Seizures, eye-rolling</li><li>Tachypnea, cyanosis</li><li>Lip smacking, twitching, and convulsions</li></ul>

Key Points to Remember

- *Definition*: WHO defines hypoglycemia as BGL < 45 mg/dL.
- *Transitional neonatal hypoglycemia*: BGL as low as 30 mg/dL within 1–2 hours of birth are common in normal newborns.
- *Refractory hypoglycemia*: GIR > 12 mg/kg/min for 24 hours and persistent hypoglycemia: for >7 days.
- Neonatal hypoglycemia is a preventable cause of brain injury.

- Early initiation of breastfeeding within 1 hour and frequent breastfeeding can prevent hypoglycemia.
- Hypoglycemia is common problem in PT/LBW, sick neonates and infants of diabetic mother.
- Neonates at risk of hypoglycemia should be screened using glucometer. However for confirmation send blood sample in fluoride vial
- Symptoms of hypoglycemia are nonspecific and can be confused with neonatal disease such as sepsis, hypothermia, and apnea.
- Asymptomatic hypoglycemia can causes brain injury therefore should be treated urgently.
- $$\text{GIR (mg/kg/min)} = \frac{\%\text{dextrose being infused} \times \text{IV rate (mL/kg/day)}}{144}$$
- GIR (mg/kg/min) = Total fluid (mL/kg/day) _____ × _____ % dextrose × 0.07.
- Initiate and continue breastfeeding or MOM at earliest.
- Always quantify MOM before starting breastfeeding.
- If an IV line can not be established quickly, give 2 mL/kg of 10% dextrose by orogastric tube.
- Avoid fluctuations in blood sugar level.
- Avoid >15% dextrose infusion through a peripheral vein.
- Use a syringe/infusion pump to deliver glucose.
- Avoid frequent dextrose boluses.
- Send blood in fluoride or oxalate vial for laboratory glucose estimation.
- Always search for an underlying cause—polycythemia, sepsis, meningitis, hypothermia, and intrauterine growth restriction (IUGR).
- Do not give antibiotics unless sepsis is suspected.
- Babies who had hypoglycemic episodes whether symptomatic or asymptomatic are at risk of neurological sequelae such as seizure, developmental delay, and cognitive deficit.
- The outcome is determined by factors such as duration, severity of hypoglycemia, and comorbidities.
- Long-term follow-up is required for their neurodevelopmental assessment and visual defect.

■ FURTHER READING

1. Edwards T, Harding JE. Clinical Aspects of Neonatal Hypoglycemia: A Mini Review. Front Pediatr. 2021;8:562251.
2. Facility Based Newborn Care, Training Module for Doctors and Nurses, MoHFW, GOI; 2022.
3. Sweet CB, Grayson S, Polak M. Management strategies for neonatal hypoglycemia. J Pediatr Pharmacol Ther. 2013;18(3):199-208.

Management of Hypocalcemia

Seema Rai

Neonate with hypocalcemia
Definition
- Hypocalcemia in term and preterm newborns with >1,500 g is defined as total serum calcium <8 mg/dL (2 mmol/L) or ionized calcium <4.4 mg/dL (1.1 mmol/L)
- Hypocalcemia in preterm infants weighing <1,500 g is defined as total serum calcium <7 mg/dL (1.75 mmol/L) or ionized calcium <4 mg/dL (1 mmol/L)

Early-onset hypocalcemia (<72 hours of life)
- Infants of mother with preeclampsia
- Prematurity (ELBW and VLBW neonate)
- Sepsis
- Intrauterine growth restriction (IUGR)
- Perinatal asphyxia (Apgar score <4 at 1 minute)
- Infants of diabetic mother (IDM)
- Maternal vitamin D deficiency

Late-onset hypocalcemia (>72 hours of life)
- Increased phosphate load (cow milk, parenteral nutrition)
- Primary hypoparathyroidism (DiGeorge syndrome, CASR mutation)
- Secondary hypoparathyroidism
- Hypomagnesemia
- Vitamin D deficiency
- Pseudohypoparathyroidism

Clinical features
- The clinical features usually depend on the day of presentation as in early onset is mostly asymptomatic and late-onset hypocalcemia is usually symptomatic
- The symptoms of hypocalcemia are irritability jitteriness, lethargy, poor feeding, muscle twitching, tetany, seizures, and cardiac arrhythmias

Investigation
- Serum calcium, phosphorous, SALP, magnesium, serum albumin, creatinine, ECG showing prolonged Qtc interval, QRS, and ST segment changes
- Serum parathyroid hormone (PTH), vitamin-D level, chest X-ray (look for thymic shadow in DiGeorge syndrome) rarely knee X-ray

Contd...

Contd...

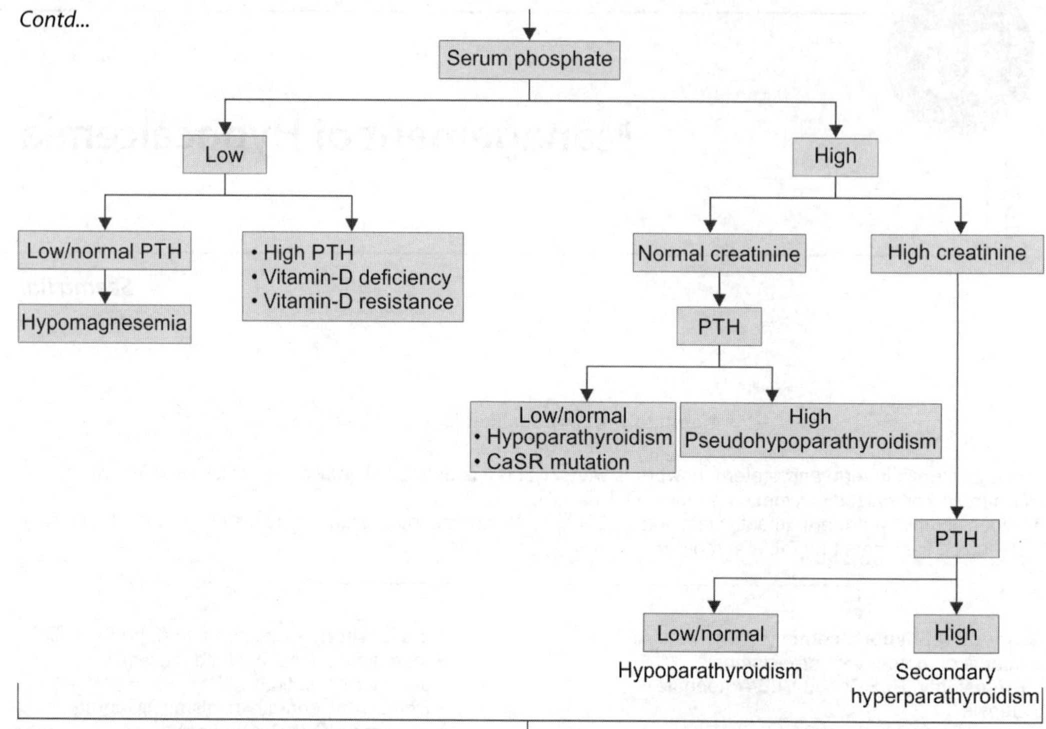

Treatment
- The treatment of hypocalcemia will depend on the symptoms present and extent of hypocalcemia, generally <7 mg/dL in term and <6 mg/dL in preterm requires treatment
- In asymptomatic newborns to treat with 40–80 mg/kg/day of calcium supplementation
- In symptomatic newborns, 2 mL/kg of 10% calcium gluconate. Over 10 minutes followed by 2.5 mL/kg/day of continuous infusion, gluconate, under ECG monitoring
- Vitamin D may be needed for long-term management

Key Points to Remember

- Calcium is essential for skeletal integrity and plays very vital role in neuromuscular and cellular function.
- The full-term infant contains approximately 27 g of calcium, most of it acquired during the last trimester; the net transfer of calcium across the placenta is 300–400 mg/day at term and due accretion in last trimester preterm newborn will be more prone to hypocalcemia.
- Each 1 g/dL fall of serum albumin below 4 g/dL leads to fall in serum calcium by 0.8 mg/dL and pH (alkalosis decreases the ionized serum calcium and acidosis effect is vice versa)
- Extravasation of calcium can lead to intense tissue necrosis and dedicated intravenous line should be ensured.
- Inj. calcium gluconate is diluted in equal amount of distilled water and administered slowly under cardiac monitoring by an infusion pump (withhold infusion if HR < 100 BPM).
- Do not add calcium to maintenance IV fluid instead give if as a low slow bolus using syring infusion pump.

■ FURTHER READING

1. Allgrove J. Shaw NJ. Calcium and bone disorders of children and adolescents. Endocrine Development. Basel: Karger; 2015.
2. Taylor-Miller T, Allgrove J. Endocrine diseases of newborn: epidemiology, pathogenesis, therapeutic options, and outcome "Current insights into disorders of calcium and phosphate in the newborn". Front Pediatr. 2021;9:600490.
3. Vuralli D. Clinical approach to hypocalcemia in newborn period and infancy: who should be treated? Int J Pediatr. 2019;2019:4318075.

Chapter 36

Management of Congenital Hypothyroidism

Smita Ramachandran

Flowchart 1: Management of congenital hypothyroidism by ISPAE.

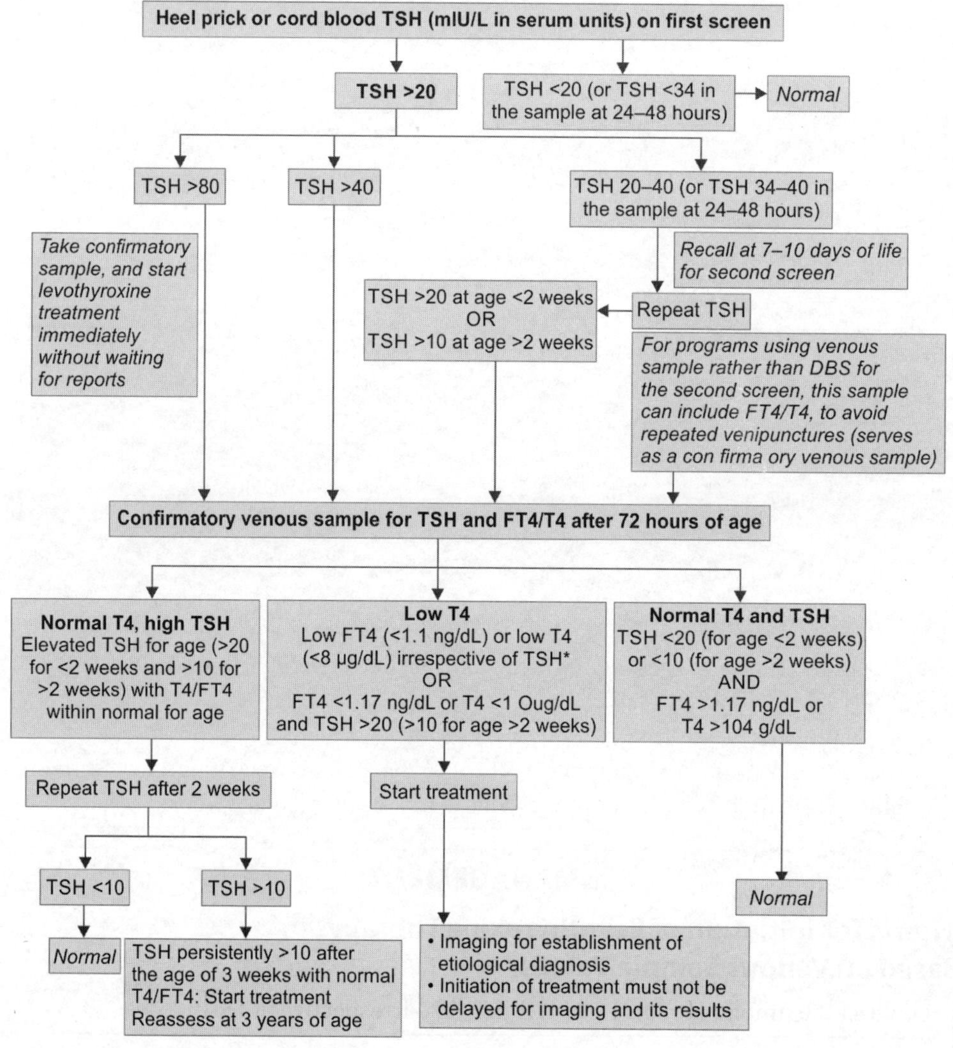

CLINICAL FEATURES

The neonate may present with:

- Delay in skeletal maturation (absence of femoral and tibial epiphyses)
- Hypothermia, jaundice, lethargy/decreased activity, and poor feeding
- Macroglossia and macrosomia
- Umbilical hernia, wide anterior fontanel, and open posterior fontanel.

During infancy they may present with:

- Constipation, hoarse cry, and decreased muscle tone
- Coarse skin and brittle hair
- Delayed milestones
- Failure to thrive and poor linear growth.

DIAGNOSIS

Management for workup for congenital hypothyroidism by Indian Society for Pediatric and Adolescent Endocrinology (ISPAE) is shown in **Flowchart 1**.

- *Thyroid function test:*
  - Venous sample for serum thyroid-stimulating hormone (TSH), total/free T4 is sent.
  - Low T4/FT4 with increased TSH is labeled as primary hypothyroidism.
  - Low T4/FT4 with low TSH is likely to be secondary or central CH.

- *Neonatal screening:*
  - Neonatal screening should be done using either serum or filter paper assays.
  - Primary TSH assay is recommended for screening purpose.
  - Cord blood or sample taken after 48–72 hours of life can be used for screening.
- *Imaging:*
  - Ultrasound of the thyroid gland or Tc-99m can be used together or singly depending upon the availability to aid in the diagnosis.
  - However, initiation of treatment should not be withheld in case of delay in imaging.

Newborn Screening Timing

- 48–72 hours postnatal age—all term, newborns, preterms (PT), low birth weight (LBW), and very low birth weight (VLBW).
- Day 7 of life-sick newborns
- 4 weeks of life—high-risk neonates [VLBW, LBW, PT, and sick neonates in neonatal intensive care unit (NICU), same sex twins, early discharged at 2 weeks]

MANAGEMENT

Criteria for Initiation of Levothyroxine Therapy (Based on Venous Sample Values)

- Low T4 (100 nmol/L) or low FT4 (<1.1 ng/dL)—irrespective of TSH.

- Mild low T4 (128 nmol/L) or FT4 (<1.17 ng/dL) in presence of TSH >20 mIU/L (age <2 weeks) or TSH >10 mIU/L if age >2 weeks.
- Normal T4/FT4 with persistently elevated TSH >10 mIU/L at >3 weeks.

Dosage

- Initial recommended dose in neonatal period is 10–15 µg/kg/day given as single dose.
- Target is to maintain T4/FT4 in upper normal range and TSH in normal range (<5 mIU/L).
- If T4/FT4 are in upper normal range, one should not pursue for a normal TSH.

Follow-up

- Serum T4/FT4 is measured at 2 weeks and TSH with T4/FT4 at 1 month.
- Then T4/FT4 and TSH are measured every 2 months till 6 months of age.
- Every 3 months during 6 month–3 years.
- Every 3–6 months thereafter, till completion of growth and puberty.

Key Points to Remember

- Congenital hypothyroidism (CH) is one of the most common preventable causes of mental retardation, and has an incidence of 1 in approximately 1,000 Indian newborns.
- This may be transient or permanent. The most common cause of permanent CH is thyroid dysgenesis or agenesis followed by thyroid dyshormonogenesis. However, recent evidence indicates an increased incidence of dyshormonogenesis as a cause from India and worldwide.
- *Education:* Universal implementation of newborn screening program.
- *Screening:*
  - Specimen collection at 48–72 hours postnatal age or at birth as per hospital guidelines
  - Specimens are collected from the heel (or the umbilical cord if taken at birth)
- *Early follow-up:* Rapid recall for follow-up for all newborns with TSH >20.
- *Management:*
  - Early thyroxin replacement therapy in a newborn diagnosed with CH
  - Other diagnostic tests—imaging for etiological diagnosis
- *Follow-up:* Regular follow-up of children.

FURTHER READING

1. Desai MP, Sharma R, Riaz I, Sudhanshu S, Parikh R, Bhatia V. Newborn screening guidelines for congenital hypothyroidism in India: Recommendations of the Indian Society for Pediatric and Adolescent Endocrinology (ISPAE)—Part I: Screening and Confirmation of Diagnosis. Indian J Pediatr. 2018;85(6):440-7.
2. Fisher DA. Disorders of the thyroid in the newborn and infant. In: Sperling MA (Ed). Clinical Pediatric and Adolescent Endocrinology, 3rd edition. Philadelphia, PA: Saunders; 2002. p. 164.
3. Sudhanshu S, Riaz I, Sharma R, Desai MP, Parikh R, Bhatia V. Newborn screening guidelines for congenital hypothyroidism in India: Recommendations of the Indian Society for Pediatric and Adolescent Endocrinology (ISPAE)—Part II: Imaging, Treatment and Follow-up. Indian J Pediatr. 2018;85(6):448-53.

Metabolic Bone Disease of Prematurity

Aashish Sethi

Clinical features

Infants with MBDP demonstrate few symptoms or sign until late into disease process. They may present with:
- Reduced linear growth with normal head growth (arrested growth velocity)
- Jitteriness, tetany (features of hypocalcemia)
- Abnormally wide cranial sutures, wide splayed metaphysis, and osteopenia (features of rickets)
- Spontaneous fractures of ribs and long bones (pain while handling, tenderness, or deformity)
- Tachypnea, intercostal/subcostal retractions (signs of respiratory distress)
- Difficulty in weaning from ventilator (deranged pulmonary function)

Investigations

- *When:*
  - From 2 to 4 weeks of age
  - 1–4 weekly till 4 months of age or longer depending upon degree of risk
- *What:*
  - *Bone profile:* Total calcium (albumin adjusted)/ionized calcium, serum alkaline phosphatase (ALP), phosphate (PO_4)
  - Plasma iPTH (intact parathormone)

Raised ALP, Low PO_4, Normal/Raised PTH
- *Calcipenic state* (suggested by ↑ PTH)
  - Start oral calcium supplements
  - Optimize 25 (OH) vitamin-D
  - Total enteral calcium to phosphate intake ratio should be kept between 1.5:1 and 1.7:1, on a mg-to-mg basis
  - Optimize calcium supply from parenteral nutrition, if applicable, with molar calcium to phosphate ratio 1.3:1–1.7:1
  - Monitoring 1–2 weekly with plasma PTH and serum ALP, adjusting calcium dose and calcium to phosphate ratios based on iPTH
- *Phosphopenic state* (suggested by normal PTH)
  - Consider starting oral phosphate supplements, while making sure that total enteral calcium to phosphate intake ratio should remain between 1.5:1 and 1.7:1 on a mg-to-mg basis (oral calcium supplements may need to be started concurrently)
  - Optimize phosphate supply from parenteral nutrition, if applicable, while keeping molar calcium to phosphate ratio 1.3:1–1.7:1
  - Monitor 1–2 weekly with plasma iPTH and serum ALP, and adjusting phosphate (also calcium dose if applicable) and adjusting calcium to phosphate ratios based on iPTH and ALP

Management

At risk groups
- *Preterm:* Below 28 weeks gestation
- Birth weight below 1,500 g
- Parenteral nutrition for >2 weeks
- Chronic lung disease
- Bronchopulmonary dysplasia
- Necrotizing enterocolitis
- Prolonged administration of glucocorticoids, antacids, or loop diuretics

PREVENTION

- Breast milk fortification
- Maintain serum 25 hydroxyvitamin D concentration above 20 ng/mL, by providing 400 IU vitamin D daily.
- Enteral or intravenous calcium to phosphate ratios should be maintained.
- Preterm and low birth weight infants should receive 120–200 mg/kg/day of calcium and 60–140 mg/kg/day of phosphorous through enteral feeds as per nutritional consensus guidelines.
- European Society of Pediatric Gastroenterology, Hepatology, and Nutrition (ESPGHAN) and American Society for Parenteral and Enteral Nutrition Board recommended calcium 1.3–3.0 mmol/kg/day and phosphate 1.0–2.3 mmol/kg/day, with a molar calcium to phosphate ratio in the range 1.3:1–1.7:1 in parenteral nutrition.

Key Points to Remember

- Metabolic bone disease of prematurity (MBDP) is characterized by skeletal demineralization of preterm infants arising from multiple factors.
- It is also referred as rickets of prematurity and osteopenia of prematurity.
- 16–40% of extremely low birth weight (ELBW) neonates may develop MBDP, while the age of presentation varies between 6 and 16 weeks of age.
- The prevalence could be higher as there is enhanced survival of sick preterm neonates in both developing and developed countries.
- Burden of the disease—MBDP has a high incidence among neonates born ELBW, which may be higher in view of enhanced sick preterm survival.
- Screening—All ELBW (<1,000 g birth weight) and LBW (<1,500 g birth weight) with risk factors.
- Prevention—Ensure optimal enteral and parenteral calcium to phosphate ratios.
- Management—Calcium and phosphate supplementation in recommended ratios with monitoring 1–2 weekly.

■ FURTHER READING

1. Chacham S, Pasi R, Chegondi M, Ahmad N, Mohanty SB. Metabolic bone disease in premature neonates: an unmet challenge. J Clin Res Pediatr Endocrinol. 2020;12(4):332-9.
2. Chinoy A, Mughal MZ, Padidela R. Metabolic bone disease of prematurity: causes, recognition, prevention, treatment and long-term consequences. Arch Dis Child-Fetal Neonatal Ed. 2019;104(5):F560-6.
3. Koletzko B, Goulet O, Hunt J, Krohn K, Shamir R, Parenteral Nutrition Guidelines Working Group; European Society for Clinical Nutrition and Metabolism, et al. 1. Guidelines on Paediatric Parenteral Nutrition of the European Society of Paediatric Gastroenterology, Hepatology and Nutrition (ESPGHAN) and the European Society for Clinical Nutrition and Metabolism (ESPEN), Supported by the European Society of Paediatric Research (ESPR). J Pediatr Gastroenterol Nutr. 2005;41(Suppl 2):S1-87.

Management of Inborn Errors of Metabolism

Prince Pareek

Neonate with high index of suspicion of IEM

↓

Screening investigations
- Complete blood count (neutropenia and thrombocytopenia seen in organic academia)
- Arterial blood gas and electrolytes (pH, pCO_2, and base excess)
- Blood glucose
- Plasma ammonia
- Plasma lactate
- Liver function tests
- Urine ketones
- Urine nonglucose reducing substances
- Serum uric acid (low in molybdenum cofactor deficiency)

↓

Confirmatory investigations
- Gas chromatography–mass spectrometry (GC-MS) of urine—for organic acidemias
- Tandem mass spectrometry (TMS)—for organic acidemias, urea cycle defects, aminoacidopathies, and FAO defects
- Lactate/pyruvate ratio
- Urinary urea cycle defect metabolites
- *Enzyme assay:* Biotinidase assay, GALT (galactose 1-phosphate uridyltransferase) assay
- *Neuroimaging:* MRI, MRS (magnetic resonance spectroscopy)
- *Electroencephalography (EEG):* To detect specific abnormalities, e.g., comb-like rhythm in Maple syrup urine disease (MSUD), burst suppression in nonketotic hyperglycinemia (NKH), and holocarboxylase synthetase deficiency
- Plasma very long chain fatty acids (VLCFA) levels
- Cerebrospinal fluid (CSF) amino acid analysis
- Mutation analysis

↓

- Approach to lacticemia
- Approach to hyperammonemia
- Approach to hypoglycemia (*See* Endocrine section)

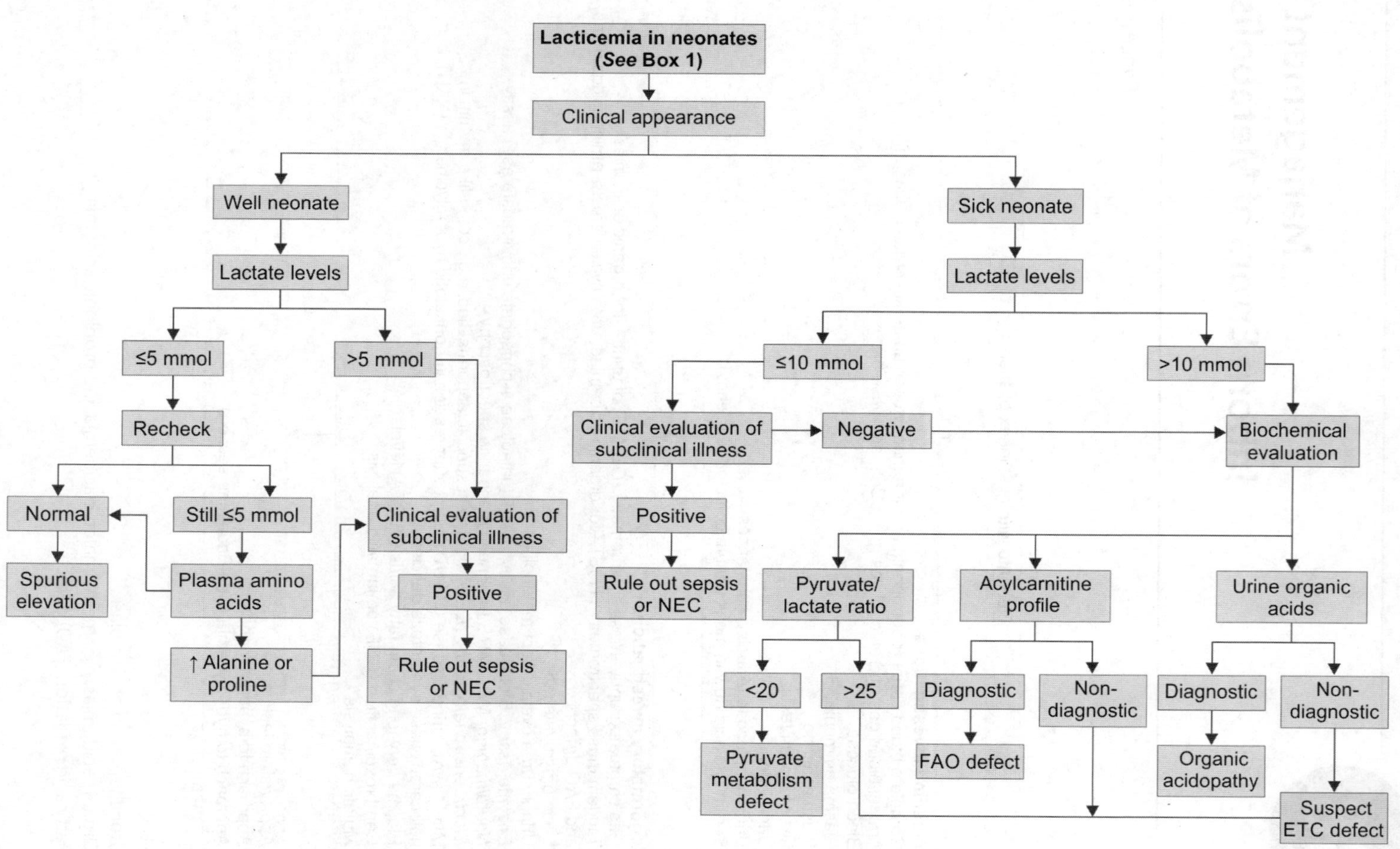

Lacticemia in neonates (See Box 1)
Clinical appearance
Well neonate
Sick neonate
Lactate levels
Lactate levels
≤5 mmol
>5 mmol
≤10 mmol
>10 mmol
Recheck
Normal
Still ≤5 mmol
Clinical evaluation of subclinical illness
Clinical evaluation of subclinical illness
Negative
Biochemical evaluation
Spurious elevation
Plasma amino acids
Positive
Positive
↑ Alanine or proline
Rule out sepsis or NEC
Rule out sepsis or NEC
Pyruvate/lactate ratio
Acylcarnitine profile
Urine organic acids
<20
>25
Diagnostic
Non-diagnostic
Diagnostic
Non-diagnostic
Pyruvate metabolism defect
FAO defect
Organic acidopathy
Suspect ETC defect

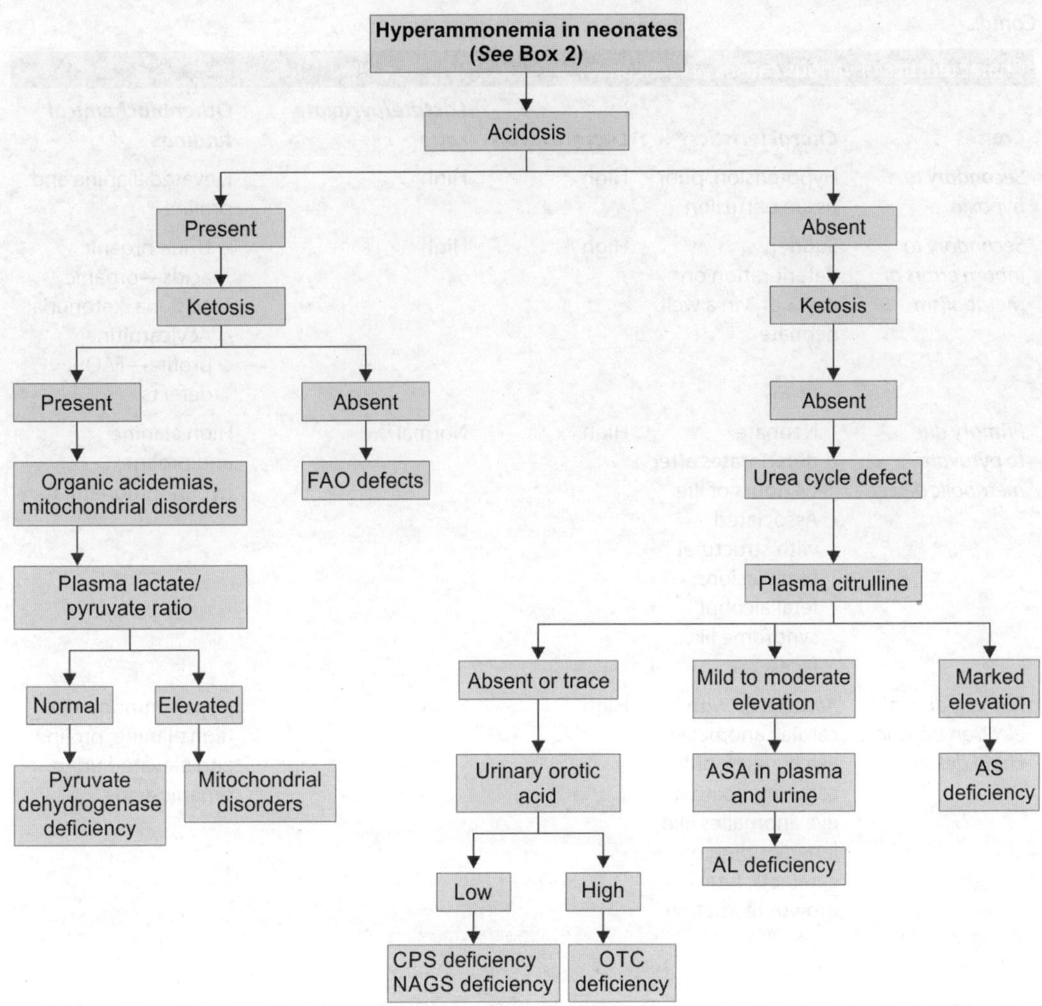

BOX 1: Causes of lacticemia in neonates.

- *Primary causes*:
  - Pyruvate dehydrogenase deficiency
  - Disorders of tricarboxylic acid cycle
  - Disorders of electron transport chain
- *Secondary causes (more common)*:
  - Hypoxic ischemic encephalopathy
  - Neonatal sepsis
  - Necrotizing enterocolitis
  - Shock
  - Bronchopulmonary dysplasia
  - Organic acidemias, e.g., methylmalonic acidemia and propionic acidemia
  - Fatty acid oxidation (FAO) defects

Contd...

Contd...

Characteristics of various causes of lacticemia.

Causes	Characteristics	Lactate levels	Lactate/pyruvate ratio	Other biochemical findings
Secondary to hypoxia	Hypotension, poor tissue perfusion	High	High	Elevated alanine and proline
Secondary to inborn errors of metabolism	Sudden deterioration on day 2 or 3 in a well neonate	High	High	• Urine organic acids—organic aciduria, ketonuria • Acylcarnitine profile—FAO defects
Primary due to pyruvate metabolic defect	• Neonate deteriorates after 24 hours of life • Associated with structural brain lesions; fetal alcohol syndrome like faces	High	Normal	High alanine and proline; hyperammonemia
Primary due to electron transport chain defect	Associated with cardiac anomalies like hypertrophic cardiomyopathy; eye anomalies like lens clouding or cataracts; fetal growth restriction	High	High	Hyperammonemia; high alanine, proline, and elevated urine organic acids

Management of lacticemia.

- *Secondary causes:*
  - Treat the cause
- *Primary causes:*
  - Acidosis correction (24-measured bicarbonate) × (weight in kg) × 0.5 = mEq of bicarbonate
  - Replace half of the deficit in first hour, and the other half over next 24 hours
  - Dialysis has minimum role in lactate clearance
  - Halting catabolism provides intravenous glucose till specific defect is known
  - Acyl carnitine and amino acids profile are required before advancing diet
  - Adequate nutritional support is important to prevent catabolism
  - In stable patients, enteral feeding is less likely to raise lactate levels
  - Provide vitamins that act as cofactors for common enzymatic defects: thiamine for pyruvate dehydrogenase complex and biotin for pyruvate carboxylase
  - Other vitamins such as riboflavin, vitamin C, vitamin E, and coenzyme Q10 act as antioxidants and cofactors for the mitochondrial respiratory chain
  - Treat associated biochemical derangements

BOX 2: Causes of hyperammonemia in neonates.

- *Urea cycle defects*:
  - Carbamoyl phosphate synthetase
  - Ornithine transcarbamylase
  - Argininosuccinic acid synthetase
  - Argininosuccinase
- *Organic acid disorders*:
  - Propionic acidemia
  - Methylmalonic acidemia
  - Isovaleric acidemia
- Pyruvate dehydrogenase deficiency
- Electron transport chain disorders
- Glutaric aciduria type II
- Multiple carboxylase deficiency
- Fatty acid oxidation defects
- Lysine protein intolerance
- Hyperornithinemia, hyperammonemia, and homocitrullinemia (HHH syndrome)
- Transient hyperammonemia of prematurity
- Perinatal asphyxia

BOX 3: Features of hyperammonemia.

- *Clinical features*:
  - Vomiting
  - Poor feeding
  - Lethargic
  - Seizures
  - Hyperventilation
  - Coma
- *Metabolic features*:
  - Hyperammonemia
  - Aminoacidemia
  - Respiratory alkalosis
- *Neuropathological features*
- *Acute*:
  - Cerebral edema
  - Alzheimer type II astrocytes
  - Neuronal injury
  - Spongy white matter
- *Chronic*:
  - Neuronal loss
  - Demyelination

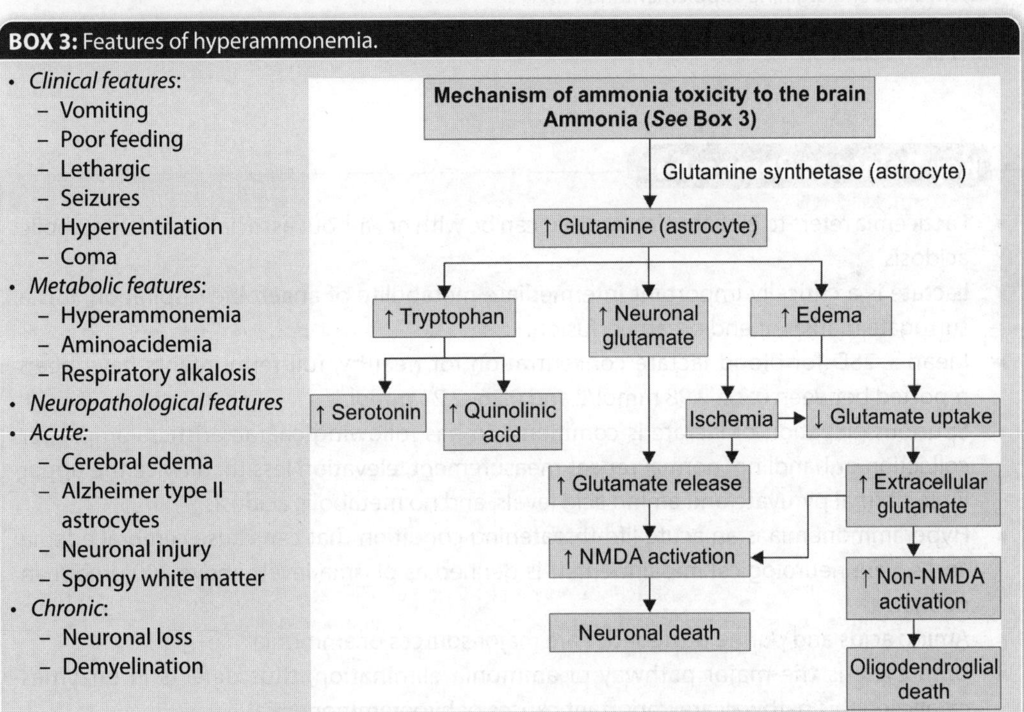

Management of neonatal hyperammonemia.

- *Antenatal diagnosis and prevention*:
  - Measurement of abnormal metabolite in amniotic fluid
  - Analysis of DNA from chorionic villus sampling or cultured amniocytes
  - Enzyme analysis of cultured amniocytes
- *Early neonatal detection*: Early detection and prompt institution of therapy
- *Ammonia removal*:
  - Hemodialysis
  - Peritoneal dialysis
  - Hemofiltration
  - Exchange transfusion
- *Alternate pathways of ammonia excretion*:
  - Sodium benzoate
  - Phenylacetate
  - Phenylbutarate
  - Arginine
- *Dietary therapy*:
  - Low protein diet
  - High nonprotein diet
  - Essential amino acid supplementation
  - Citrulline and arginine supplementation
- *Gene therapy*
- *Liver transplantation*

Key Points to Remember

- Lacticemia refers to elevated lactate that can be with or without associated with metabolic acidosis.
- Lactate is a critically important intermediate metabolite of anaerobic respiration; it is a surrogate marker of end organ perfusion.
- Mean ± 2SD for blood lactate concentration for healthy, full-term infants have been reported between 0.22–2.98 mmol/L and 0.26–2.21 mmol/L.
- Spurious elevation of lactate is common and has following characteristics—improper collection or handling, normal repeat measurement, elevation less than twice the upper limit, normal pyruvate and amino acid levels, and no metabolic acidosis.
- Hyperammonemia is an acute life-threatening condition that can cause cerebral edema and severe neurological impairment. It is defined as plasma levels above 100 µmol/L in neonates.
- Amino acids and purine nucleotides are major sources of ammonia.
- Urea cycle is the major pathway of ammonia elimination; thus defects in enzymes catalyzing this pathway are important causes of hyperammonemia.
- Ammonia arises from amino acid metabolism and by gut bacteria, is transported through the portal circulation to periportal hepatocytes where 90% of ammonia enters the urea cycle and is converted to urea.

- The remaining 10% is carried to perivenous hepatocytes where ammonia is condensed with glutamate to glutamine through the glutamine synthetase (GS). This pathway is present in astrocytes in the brain, kidney, and skeletal muscle.
- Hyperammonemia occurs when there is increased production or reduced elimination, so ammonia levels increase in the blood which crosses the blood brain barrier and causes brain dysfunction.

■ FURTHER READING

1. Ganetzky RD, Cuddapah SR. Neonatal lactic acidosis: a diagnostic and therapeutic approach. Neo Rev. 2017;18(4):e217-27.
2. Savy N, Brossier D, Brunel-Guitton C, Ducharme-Crevier L, Pont-Thibodeau GD, Jouvet P. "Acute pediatric hyperammonemia: current diagnosis and management strategies." Hepat Med. 2018;10:105-15.
3. Volpe J, Inder TE, Darras BT, De vries LS, du Plessis A, Neil J, et al. Volpe's Neurology of the Newborn, 6th edition. Philadelphia: Elsevier; 2017.

ABC of Ventilation

Kumar Ankur

- The goals for ventilations are:
  - *Oxygenation:* Keep oxygen level up
  - *Ventilation:* Keep CO_2 in range

TARGET VENTILATION

- Once we intubate the baby, our target is to prevent ventilation (V) perfusion (Q) mismatch.
- At rest: V is similar to Q and for optimal gas exchange: V/Q is close to 1. However, even in a healthy lung at different ZONES there could be different (regional pattern of gas exchange in different lung zones).
- To achieve this, we target to achieve or tidal volume between 4 and 6 mL/kg (i.e., twice the dead space volume).

V/Q mismatch: Changes in both V/Q can result in changes in V/Q.
- If there is no ventilation then V/Q = 0
- Decreased ventilation V/Q < 1
- If there is no perfusion to an area (dead space)/Q = infinity
- Decreased perfusion V/Q > 1

V/Q < 1 (intrapulmonary shunt effect):
- Low V and normal Q
- Low PaO_2 and high $PaCO_2$

V/Q > 1 (dead space effect):
High PaO_2 and low $PaCO_2$ (normal O_2 and CO_2 content)

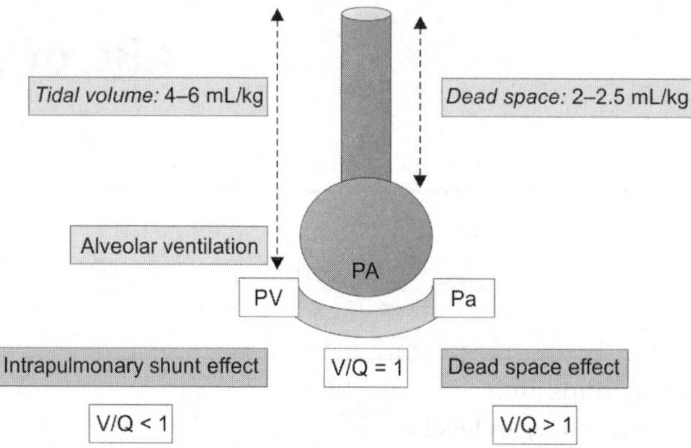

Causes of V/Q mismatch

- *Restrictive disease:* Disease where the lung has the difficulty in expansion or inhalation (problem in alveoli), e.g., transient tachypnea of the newborn/hyaline membrane disease (TTNB/HMD)/pneumonia/mass lesion/acute respiratory distress syndrome (ARDS)/ neuromuscular disease/chest wall and spinal deformity/congenital cystic adenomatoid malformation (CCAM)/late bronchopulmonary dysplasia (BPD) (after fibrosis).
- *Obstructive disease:* Where there is a problem with exhalation, e.g., meconium aspiration syndrome/TTNB/BPD/positive pressure ventilation (PPV) [with high peak inspiratory pressure (PIP)]/congenital lobar emphysema (CLE)/mucus plugging (bronchitis/ infection)/chronic ventilation.

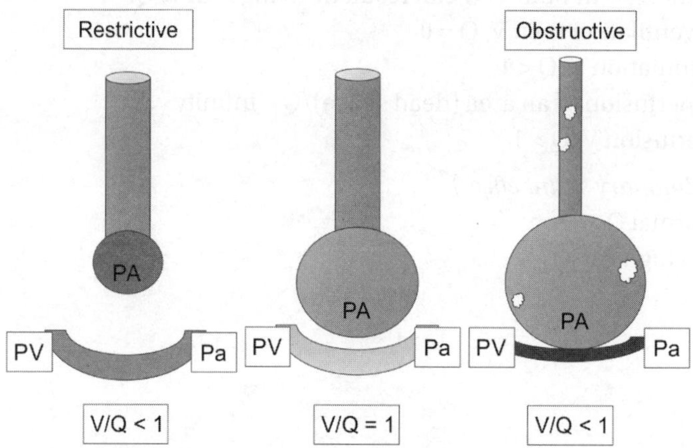

■ WHAT IS A MECHANICAL VENTILATOR?

- A mechanical device that pushes predetermined amounts of mixtures of air O_2 at predetermined pressure/volume into the lungs.
- Gas will go to the area of least resistance.

- In addition, an exhalation valve is added to the system.
- When open, a continuous flow occurs through the system, preventing accumulation of excessive carbon dioxide (CO_2) in the tubing.
- On closure of this valve, pressure increases in chamber, the ventilator tubing, and the infant's airway until the preset pressure level is reached.
- The ventilator is cycled by the opening and closing of the expiratory valve by the solenoid system.
- In conventional ventilation, inspiration is active and exhalation is passive.

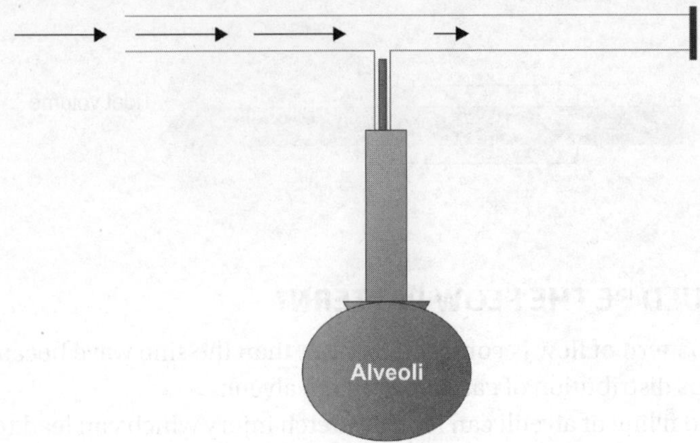

HOW TO SET VENTILATOR PARAMETERS?

- There are six parameters. These are also measured by the ventilator, using a flow sensor.

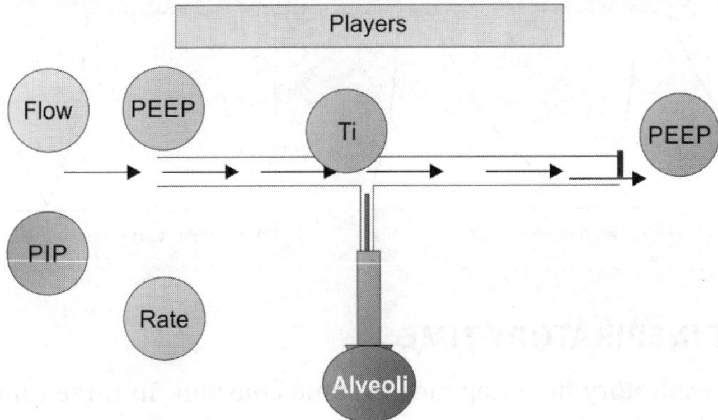

HOW TO SET FLOW RATE?

- Choices are between 4 and 10 L/min
- *Depends on:*
  - Minute ventilation (flow > 3 × MV)
  - Need for square wave versus sine wave
  - Ventilator and tubing characteristics.

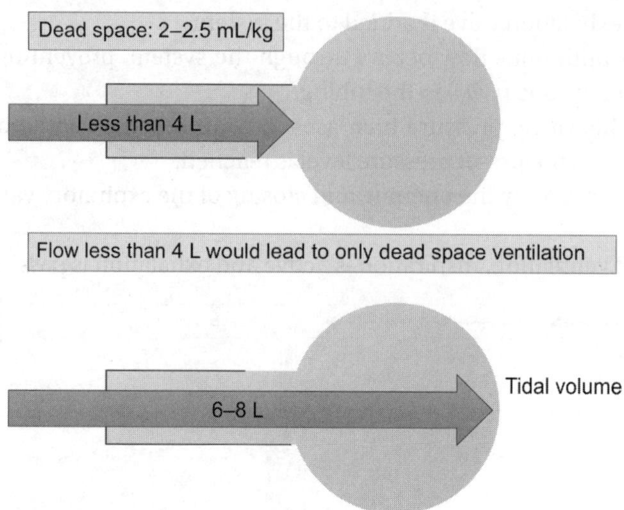

WHAT SHOULD BE THE FLOW PATTERN?

- Square wave pattern of flow is considered better than the sine wave because it would lead to homogenous distribution of gas across all the alveoli.
- However, rapid filling of alveoli can lead to stretch injury which can lead to air leak/BPD.

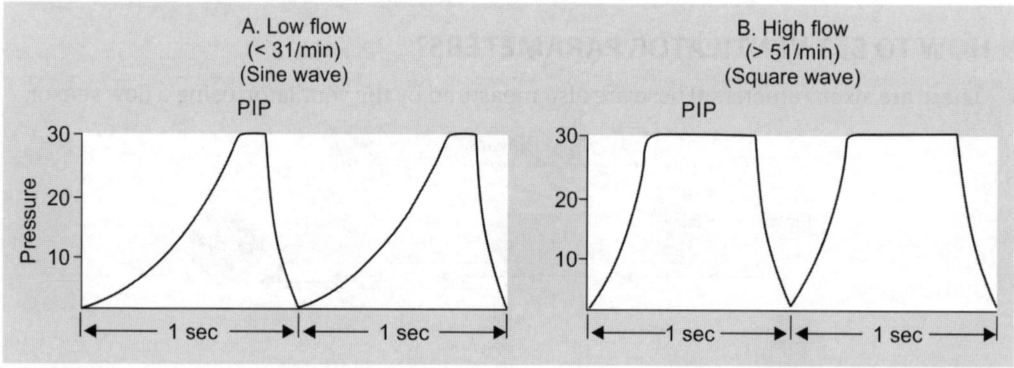

HOW TO SET INSPIRATORY TIME

- Inspiratory or expiratory time depends on time constant. In three time constants, 95% equilibration takes place.

$$\text{Time Constant (TC): C} \times \text{R}$$

C: Compliance
R: Resistance
- Depends on weight and gestational age of neonates
- Choices are between 0.35 and 0.5 seconds

- If inspiratory TC is expected to be:
  - *Normal*: 0.40–0.45 seconds
  - *Short*: 0.30–0.40 seconds
  - *Long*: 0.5 seconds

$$\text{Inspiratory time (Ti)} = 3 \times \text{inspiratory TC}$$
$$\text{Expiratory time (Te)} = 3 \times \text{expiratory TC}$$

- Generally, Te is two to three times the Ti because during inspiration all the airways get dilated however, during exhalation airways collapse.
- If we keep Ti, too short then the target tidal volume will not get delivered and we keep exhalation time too short, this can lead to incomplete exhalation causing air trapping.

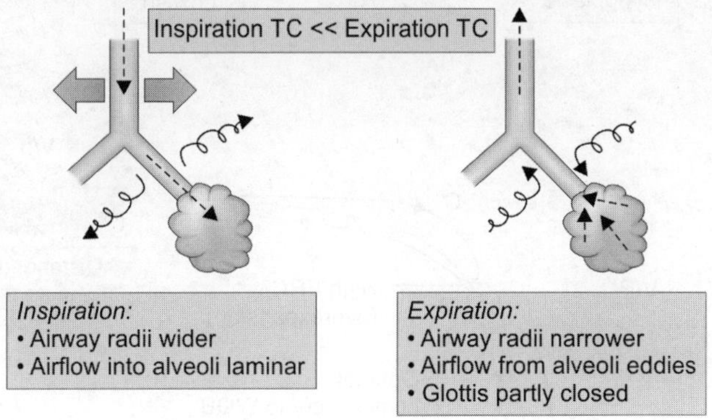

Inspiration and expiration time constants (TC).

HOW TO SET OPTIMUM POSITIVE END-EXPIRATORY PRESSURE

- The level of positive end-expiratory pressure (PEEP) at which static lung compliance is maximized has been termed the best, or optimum, PEEP.
- This is the level of PEEP at which O_2 transport (cardiac output and O_2 content) is greatest.
- If the level of PEEP is raised above the optimal level, dynamic compliance decreases rather than increases.
- Additionally, venous return and cardiac output are compromised by excessive PEEP.
- One hypothesis for this reduction in dynamic lung compliance is that some alveoli become over expanded because of the increase in pressure, which puts them on the "flat" part of the compliance curve.

How to set PEEP

- Choices are between 3–8 cmH₂O
- If FRC is expected to be:

FRC	PEEP	Disease
Normal:	3–4 cm	Apnea
Moderately reduced:	5–6 cm	Mild surfactant
Severely reduced:	6–8 cm	Diffuse alveolar

Deflates   What is optimal PEEP   Overdistended

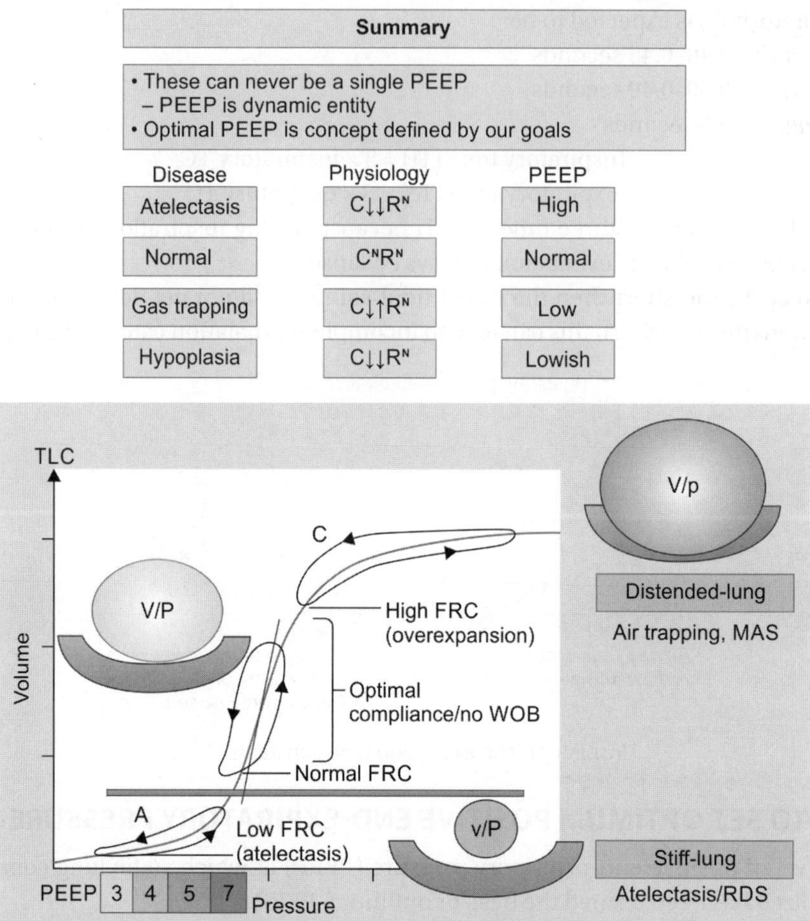

Optimal compliance for ventilation.

■ HOW TO SET PEAK INSPIRATORY PRESSURE

Peak inspiratory pressure (PIP) is the pressure which is required to open the lung. However, after adequate PEEP need for optimum PIP would be less to achieve target tidal volume.

- Choices are between 12–20 cm
- If compliance is normal set 12
- If compliance is less, set appropriate PEEP and observe chest rise
  - *Mildly stiff:* 12–14 cm
  - *Moderately stiff:* 16–18 cm
  - *Severely stiff:* 20+ cm

■ HOW TO SET RESPIRATORY RATE?

- Choices are between 20 and 60 beats/min

- *Considerations are:*
  - Work of breathing (WOB)?
  - Is there asynchrony: need for overdrive?
- WOB   normal   ↑   ↑ ↑
  - Asynchrony   minimal +   + +
  - Pressure need   minimal +   + +
- Respiratory rate (RR)   ~20   ~40–50   ~50–60

▮ WHAT IS MEAN AIRWAY PRESSURE?

- Mean airway pressure (MAP) (P_{aw}) is determined by PIP, the fraction of time devoted to the inspiratory phase (TI /Ttot, where Ttot is total respiratory cycle time), and PEEP.
- MAP is the main factor which affects the oxygenation.

$$P_{aw} = 0.5 \times (PIP - PEEP) \times (TI /Ttot) + PEEP$$

There are five different ways to increase mean airway pressure:

1. Increase inspiratory flow rate, producing a square-wave inspiratory pattern
2. Increase PIP
3. Reverse the inspiratory-to-expiratory ratio or prolong the inspiratory time (I-time) without changing the rate
4. Increase positive end-expiratory pressure; and
5. Increase ventilatory rate by reducing expiratory time without changing the I-time

In practice, increasing PEEP appears to be the safest and most effective way to achieve optimal P_{aw}, in part because normally, the greatest proportion of the respiratory cycle is the expiratory phase.

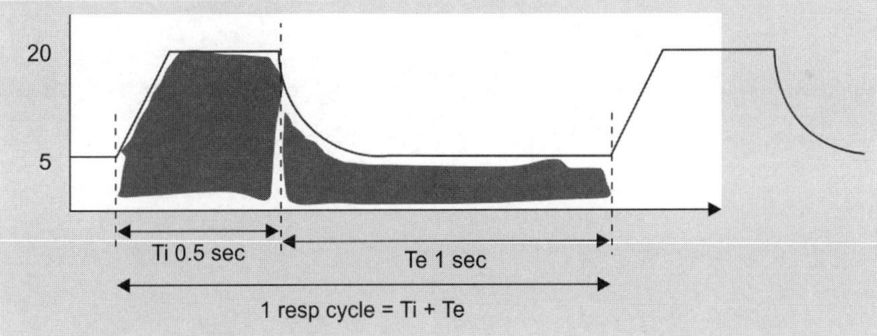

Key Points to Remember

- Breathing requires the expenditure of energy. For gas to be moved into the lungs, force must be exerted to overcome the elastic and resistive forces of the respiratory system. This is mathematically expressed by the following equation:

  Work of breathing = Pressure (force) × Volume (displacement)

  where pressure is the force exerted and the volume is the displacement.

- Work of breathing is the integrated product of the two, or simply the area under the pressure–volume curve.
- Approximately two-thirds of the work of spontaneous breathing is the effort to overcome the static elastic forces of the lungs and thorax (tissue elasticity and compliance).
- Approximately one-third of the total work is applied to overcoming the frictional resistance produced by the movement of gas and tissue components (airflow and viscous).
- Most of the infants can be managed with noninvasive ventilation (NIV) [continuous positive airway pressure/high-flow nasal cannula or noninvasive ventilation (CPAP/HFNC or NIV)], however, few of them may require invasive ventilation.

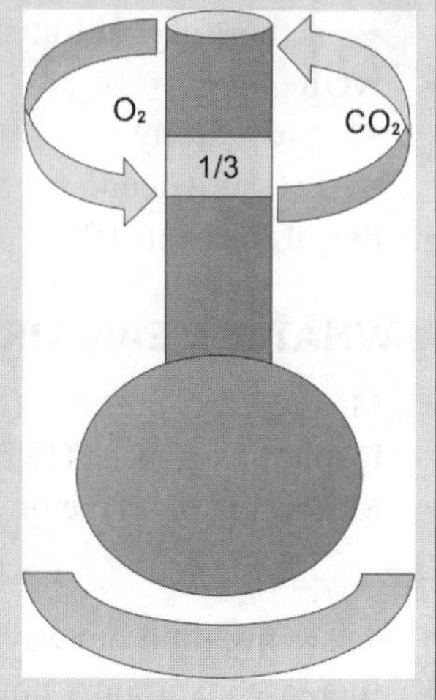

■ FURTHER READING

1. Keszler M, Gautham KS. Goldsmith's Assisted Ventilation of the Neonate: An Evidence-Based Approach to Newborn Respiratory Care, 7th edition; 2022.

Pulmonary Graphics

Lovish Gupta, Sanjeev Chetry

■ BASICS OF PULMONARY GRAPHICS

The pulmonary graphics are broadly classified into two groups:

1. *Scalar or waveforms*
2. *Loops*

The three major waveforms are:

1. *Pressure*
2. *Flow*
3. *Volume.*

These waveforms are displayed against time.

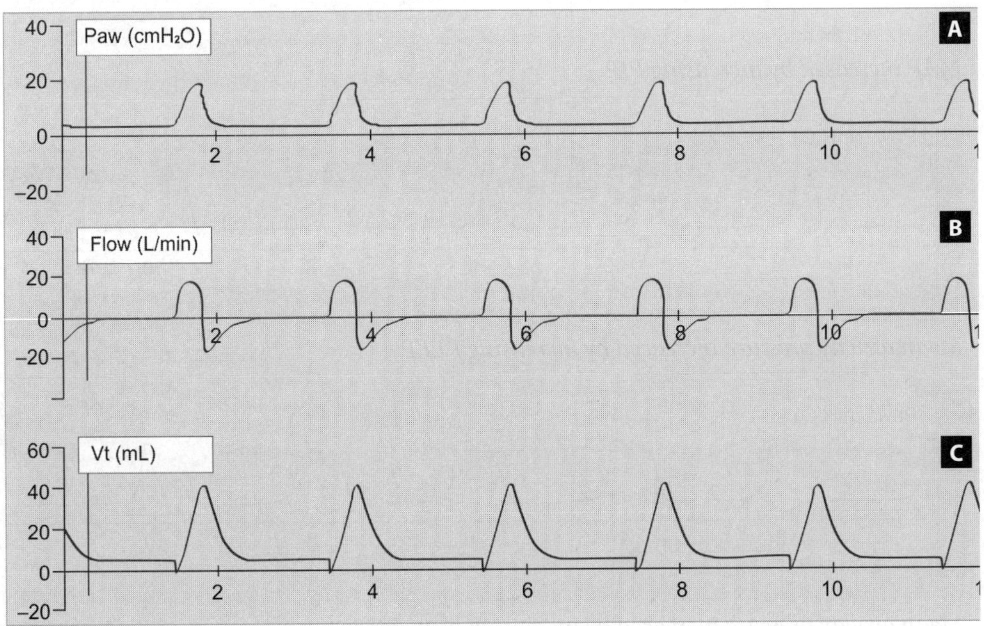

A. Pressure waveform depicts
B. Flow waveform
C. Volume waveform

Pressure Waveform

- The pressure waveform has upward (inspiration) and downward (expiration) scalars.
- The uppermost point of the waveform represents peak inspiratory pressure (PIP).
- Mean airway pressure (MAP) is represented by the area under the curve.
- The inspiratory time can be measured from the point of upward deflection until PIP is reached.
- The expiratory time begins at PIP and lasts until the next positive deflection.
- Ventilation is a product of tidal volume and frequency. The primary determinant of tidal volume is amplitude, the difference between PIP and positive end-expiratory pressure (PEEP) which is referred to as delta P (DP).
- As oxygenation is determined by MAP, increasing the area under the curve will increase the MAP and thus improve oxygenation. This can be done by increase in:
  - Peak inspiratory pressure
  - Positive end-expiratory pressure
  - Inspiratory time
  - Rate

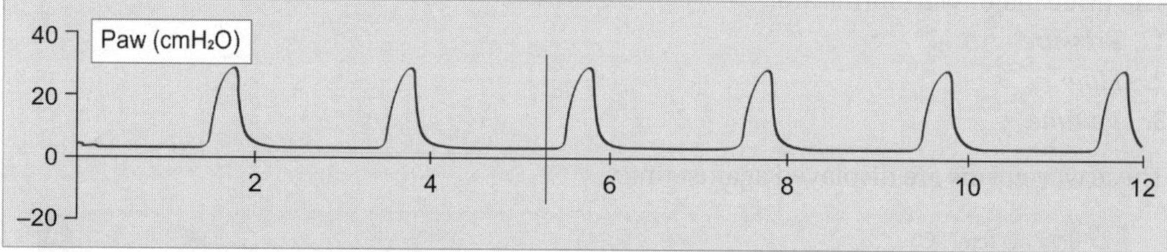

1. *MAP increased by increasing PIP*

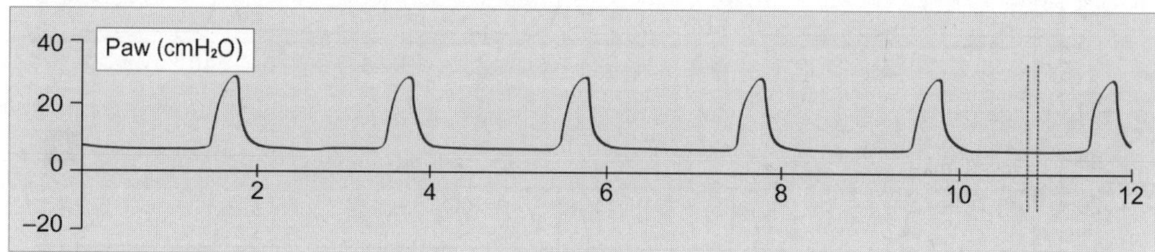

2. *Mean airway pressure increased by increasing PEEP*

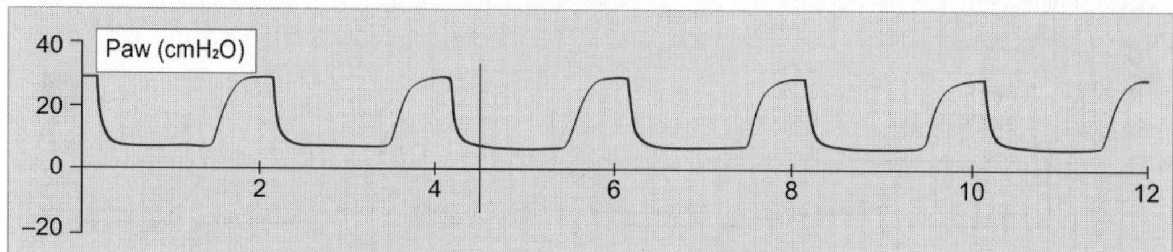

3. *Mean airway pressure increased by increasing inspiratory time*

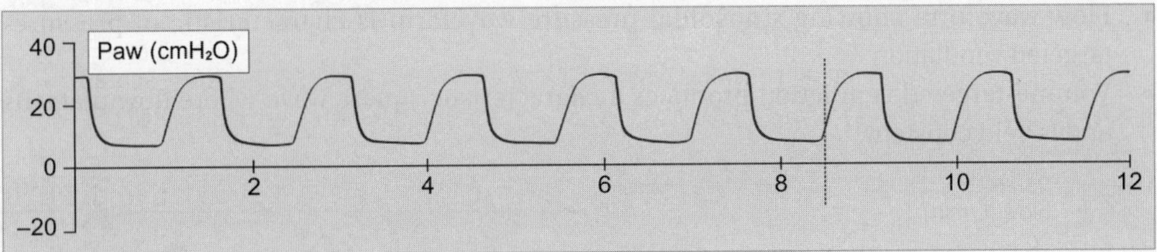

4. *Mean airway pressure increased by increasing rate*

Flow Waveform

The flow waveform has two components:

1. *Positive flow or inspiratory flow (Above the zero baseline):*
   - Accelerating flow (at the start of inspiration)
   - Decelerating flow (velocity slows as the lung approaches capacity)
   - Peak inspiratory flow is represented by the highest positive point of waveform
2. *Negative flow or expiratory flow (Below the zero baseline):*
   - Accelerating flow (at the start of expiration)
   - Decelerating flow (velocity slows as the lung empties to functional residual capacity)
   - Peak expiratory flow is represented by the lowest negative point of waveform.

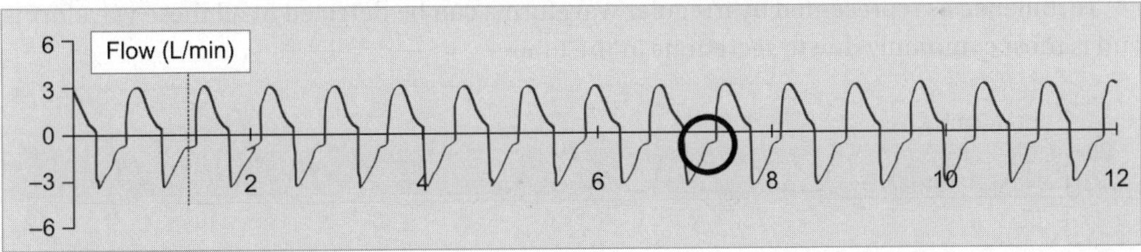

- Flow waveform showing air trappings. The next breath begins to start before decelerating expiratory limb reaches the baseline (circled), which prevents complete emptying of the lung and thereby leading to air trapping.
- Pressure-targeted ventilation typically produces a spiked or sinusoidal waveform.

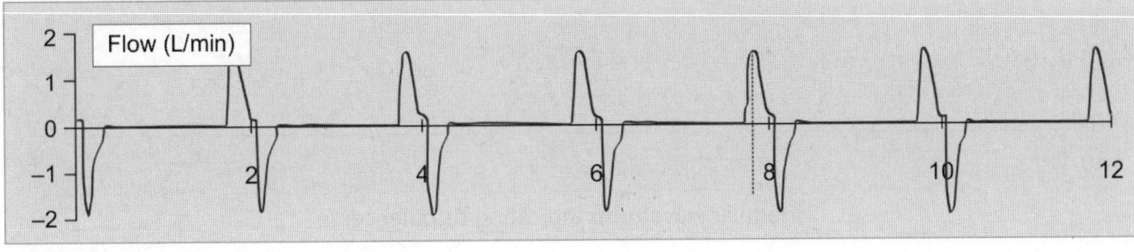

- Flow waveform showing sinusoidal pressure waveform is characteristic of pressure-targeted ventilation
- Volume-targeted ventilation produces a characteristic square wave where flow plateaus and is held constant.

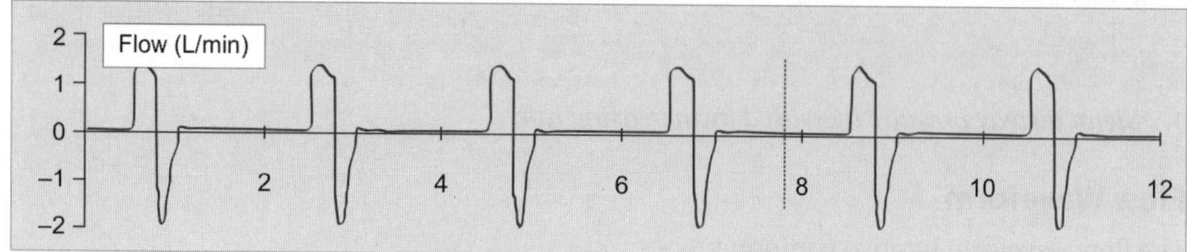

Volume-targeted ventilation produces a square wave.

Volume Waveform

- They are similar in appearance to the pressure waveform, except that it starts and ends on the baseline.
- During pressure-targeted ventilation, peak volume delivery occurs early in inspiration, then decreases.
- Volume-targeted ventilation, which creates a "shark's fin" pressure waveform.
  Turbulence as represented by irregular waveforms can be detected in all these waveforms and is most commonly due to secretions in the tube.

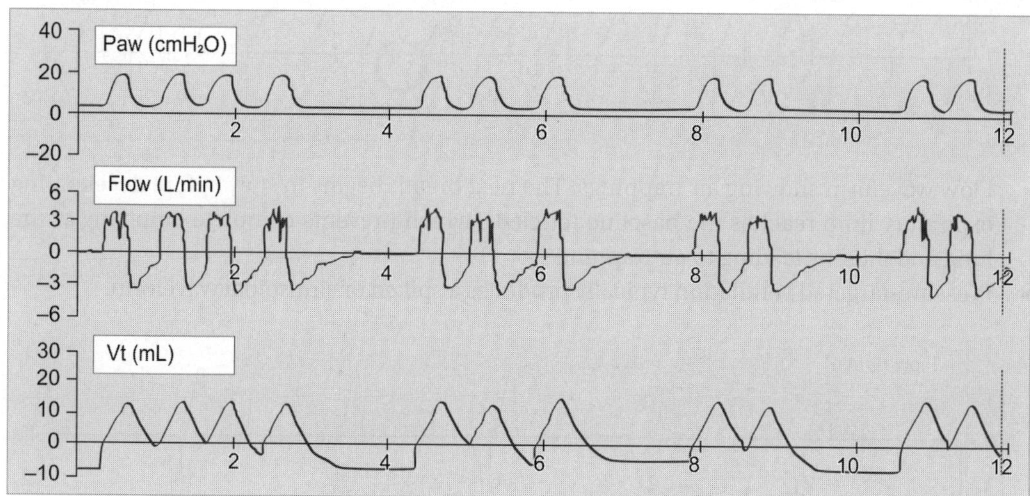

Irregular waveforms indicating turbulence.

Pulmonary Mechanics and Loops

Changes in pressure versus volume or flow versus volume can also be graphed over time and these are called loops.

Pressure–volume Loop

Pressure–volume loop indicates compliance.

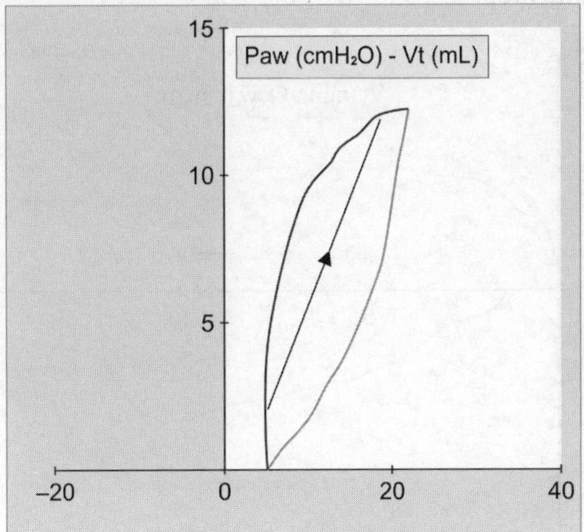

Pressure–volume loop.

- As the pressure in lungs increases, there is progressive increase in the volume of gas in the lung.
- The shape of this loop is hysteresis.
- The shape of pressure volume loop can help to detect hyperinflation or hypoinflation.
- Loop flattening at the upper end, referred to as either a "duck tail" or "penguin beak" indicates hyperinflation.

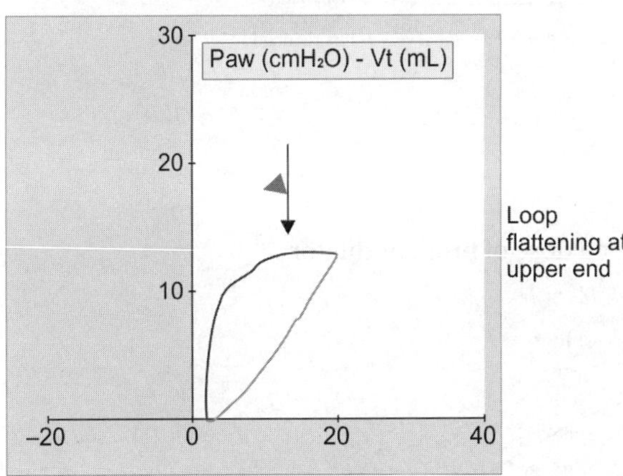

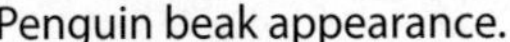

Penguin beak appearance.

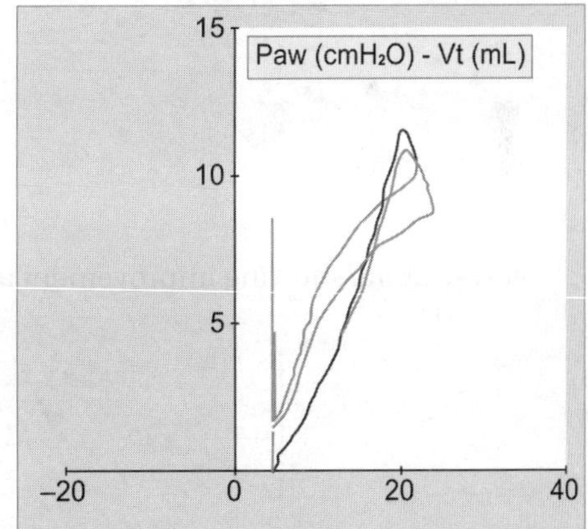

Figure of 8 appearance indicating air hunger.

Inadequate hysteresis, producing a figure of 8 appearance, is indicative of inadequate flow.

Flow–volume Loop

- A normal flow–volume loop is circular or oval in appearance.

- The upper and lower limits, representing peak inspiratory and expiratory flows, respectively, should be nearly equivalent and are like mirror image of each other.
  A normal flow–volume loop.

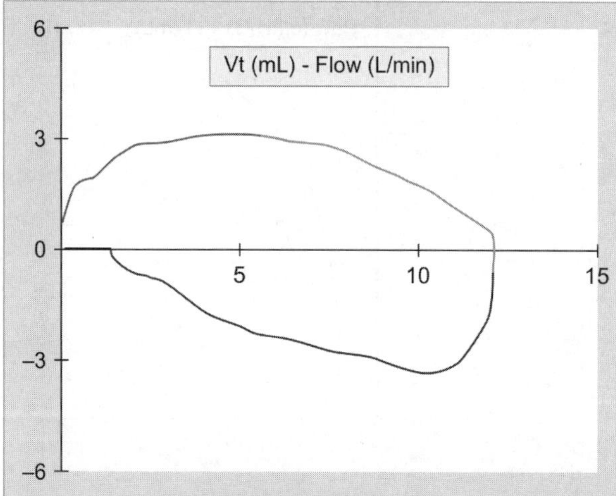

Flow–volume loop with increased airway resistance.

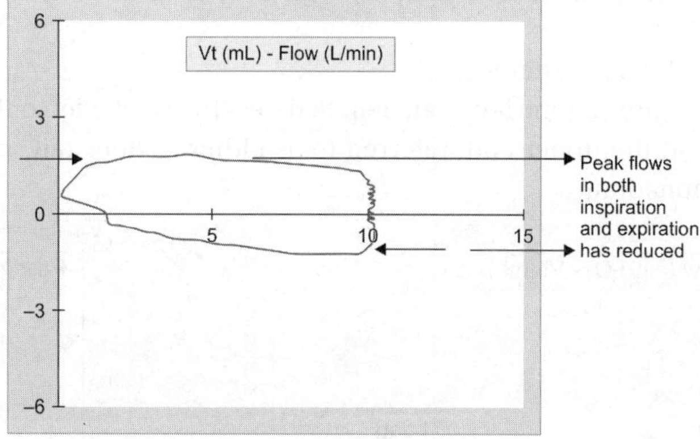

Flow–volume showing improvement after a dose of bronchodilator.

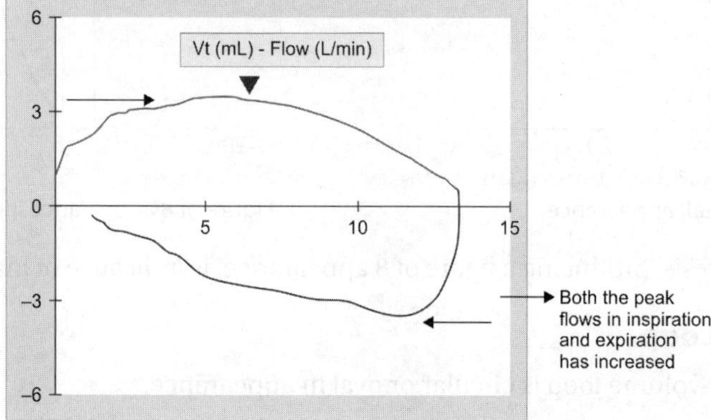

■ CLINICAL SCENARIOS

Pulmonary graphics can also help in diagnosing.

- *Endotracheal tube leak*

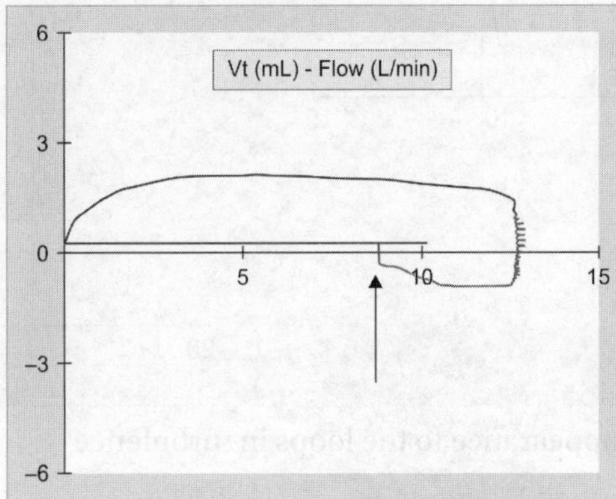

Flow–volume loop showing endotracheal tube leak where the expiratory portion fails to reach the origin.

- *Optimum PEEP*

Graphics can aid in the determination of the best PEEP.

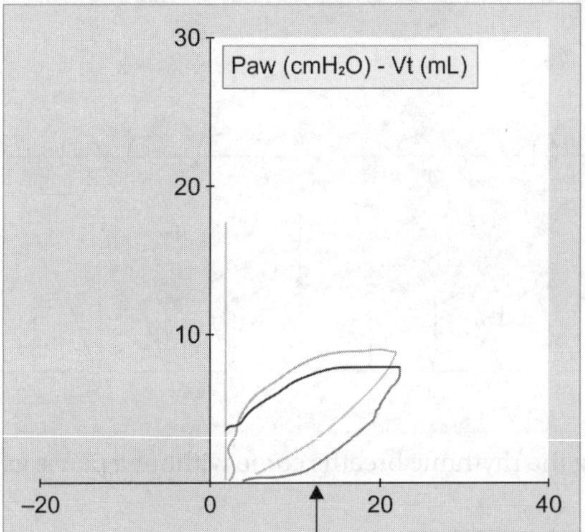

Abnormality in the pressure–volume loop, characterized by a need for a higher opening pressure. The loop looks "box-like" rather than elliptical. There is improvement when the PEEP (and concomitantly the PIP) is raised.

- *Turbulence*

It can be noted in both flow–volume or pressure–volume loop.

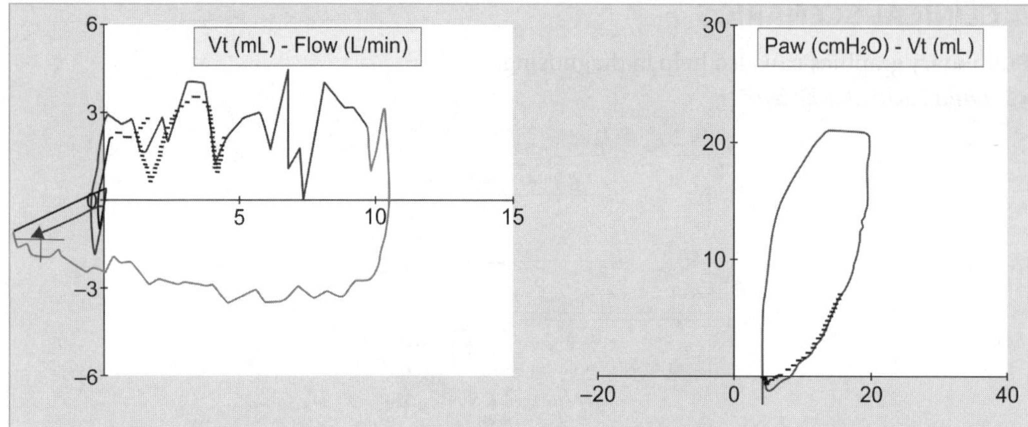

The "noisy," irregular appearance to the loops in turbulence

- *Autocycling*

The pulmonary graphics can also detect autocycling as the graph below shows.

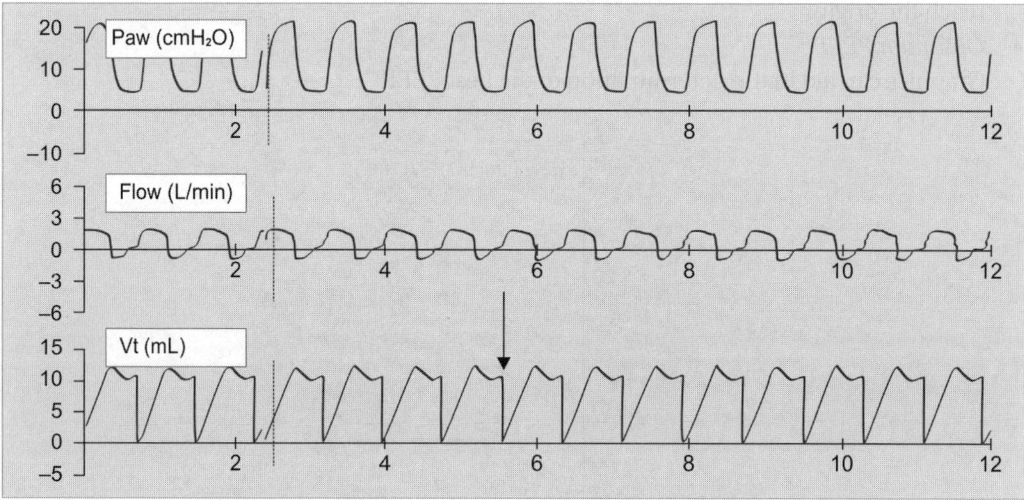

Note: In autocycling the rhythmic breaths come without a pause as well as the large leak.

Key Points to Remember

- The graphical display of measured and derived values captured during the process of mechanical ventilation is known as real time pulmonary graphics.
- It helps in the assessment of the disease and adjusts the ventilator parameters to achieve optimal ventilation and oxygenation.
- It represents interaction between the mechanical ventilator and the baby receiving support for respiratory failure.

- Real-time pulmonary graphics give useful information regarding the breath-to-breath performance of the ventilator and interaction of the baby with the ventilator.
- Complications of mechanical ventilation, such as air trapping and hyperinflation, may be detected by graphics before they are clinically apparent.
- Customization of settings for each baby can be done by fine-tuning of ventilator settings based on pathophysiology and patient response as the loopsdepicts.
- Frequency of blood gas analysis and radiography can be reduced thereby reducing the cost of care and increasing the comfort of the patient.

Principle

- With the advent of new sensor technology, a microprocessor-based technology is integrated with the function of the ventilator.
- The sensor technologies are of two types:
  1. Thermal
  2. Differential pressure type.
- These sensors detect either flow or pressure and convert the signal to a clinically useful analog value.
- The sensor detects patient effort to breathe or "trigger" and achieves synchrony between the patient's own effort and the delivery of a mechanical breath by the ventilator.

Advantages

- Fine-tuning or ventilator parameters can be adjusted.
- The patient's response to pharmacologic agents such as surfactant, diuretics, or bronchodilators can be determined.
- Trend of monitored events over a prolonged period of time can be stored.

Disadvantages

- Many clinical situations are identified at the bedside and may appear confusing as each clinical scenario may be different and have distinct learning curves.
- Understanding of graphs may at times be considered complex.

■ FURTHER READING

1. Becker MA, Donn SM. Real-time pulmonary graphic monitoring. Clin Perinatol. 2007;34(1):1-17.
2. Keszler M, Gautham KS. Goldsmith's Assisted Ventilation of the Neonate: An Evidence-Based Approach to Newborn Respiratory Care, 7th edition; 2022.
3. Mammel MC, Donn SM. Real-time pulmonary graphics. Semin Fetal Neonatal Med. 2015;20(3): 181-91.

Interpretation of Blood Gas Analysis and Change in Ventilatory Strategies

Anup Thakur, Mudita Arora

Interpretation of ABG (*see* Box 1).		
Step 1	What is pH?	• pH <7.35—Acidosis • pH >7.45—Alkalosis
Step 2	Determine whether it is primarily metabolic or respiratory	• HCO_3 <24—metabolic acidosis • HCO_3 >24—metabolic alkalosis • Normal range of $PaCO_2$—35–45 mm Hg • $PaCO_2$ <35—respiratory alkalosis • $PaCO_2$ >45—respiratory acidosis
Step 3	• Determine whether compensated or not compensated • If the pH does not normalize then it is called as uncompensated disorder. If the pH value returns to normal then it is compensated. Partial or complete compensation will depend on the range of pH. A normal range pH points toward well compensation. Rule of the thumb is that body never overcompensates. Hence, pH remains close to 7.4.	• Compensation occurs in same direction • In case of primary metabolic acidosis (HCO_3 <24, $PaCO_2$ will be less for compensation) • Primary metabolic alkalosis (HCO_3 >24, $PaCO_2$ will get accumulated)
	• Is the disorder simple or mixed? – To determine this we need to calculate if the compensation is complete or there is a superadded abnormality. Usually, a normal pH may indicate either a well-compensated disorder or a mixed disorder. Compensation occurs in same direction	• Primary respiratory acidosis ($PaCO_2$ >45, kidneys will retain HCO_3 and HCO_3 will be more) • Primary respiratory alkalosis ($PaCO_2$ <35, HCO_3 will decrease)
Step 4	Calculate PaO_2	
Step 5	Identify possible cause of acid-base imbalance	

Contd...

Contd...

Normal Values	
Arterial Blood Gas	
pH	7.35–7.45
pCO_2	35–45 mm Hg
pO_2	50–70 mm Hg
HCO_3	20–24 mEq/L
BE	±5

Compensation in respiratory and metabolic disorders (*see* Box 2).		
Disturbance	**Response**	**Expected Change**
Metabolic acidosis		
$\downarrow HCO_3$	$\downarrow PaCO_2$	12 mm Hg/10 mEq $\downarrow HCO_3$
Metabolic alkalosis		
$\uparrow HCO_3$	$\uparrow PaCO_2$	8 mm Hg/10 mEq $\uparrow HCO_3$
Acute Respiratory acidosis		
$\uparrow PaCo_2$	$\uparrow HCO_3$	1 mEq/10 mm Hg $\uparrow PaCO_2$
Chronic respiratory acidosis		
$\uparrow PaCO_2$	$\uparrow HCO_3$	4 mEq/10 mm Hg $\uparrow PaCO_2$
Acute respiratory alkalosis		
$\downarrow PaCO_2$	$\downarrow HCO_3$	2 mEq/10 mm Hg $\downarrow PaCO_2$
Chronic respiratory alkalosis		
$\uparrow HCO_3$	$\uparrow PaCO_2$	4 mEq/10 mm Hg $\downarrow PaCO_2$

Note:
- pCO_2 elevation of 10 mm Hg decreases pH by 0.08, while pCO_2 decrease of 10 mm Hg increase pH by 0.08.
- A pH change of 0.15 corresponds to a base change of 10 mEq/L.

If the calculated compensation does not match the measured value then, think of mixed disorder.

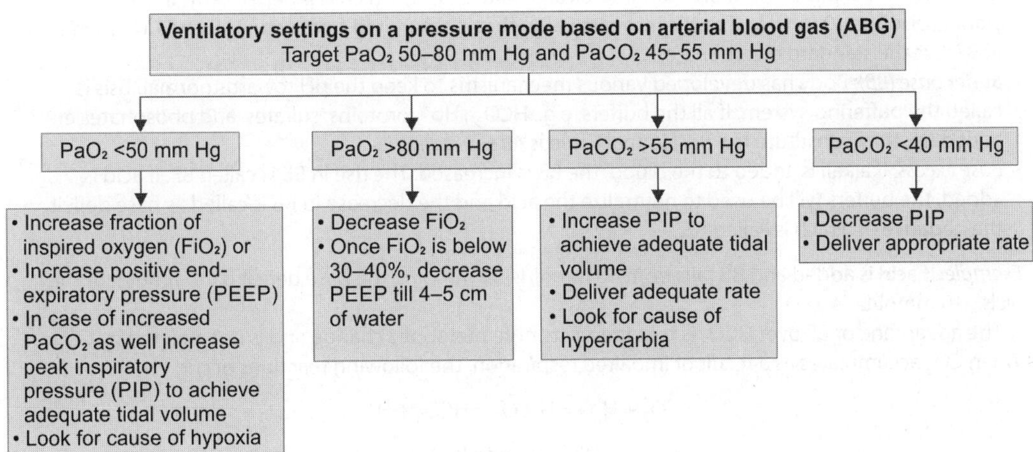

BOX 1: Interpretation.

Arterial blood gas should be interpreted taking into account the clinical history. There are some values which are directly measured in blood gas and some values which are calculated (not directly measured).
- Measured values (pH, pCO_2, and pO_2)
- Calculated values [HCO_3^-, base excess (BE), oxygen saturation, and lactate].

Measured Values

- *pH:* It reflects the concentration of extracellular hydrogen ion.

pH = $-\log [H^+]$; Normal $[H^+]$ is 40 nmol/L; Normal range of pH $-7.35-7.45$

Henderson–Hasselbalch equation: Expresses the relationship among pH, pKa, and the concentrations of an acid and its conjugate base

$$pH = pKa + \log [HCO_3^-]/[H_2CO_2]$$
$$\text{or} \quad pH = pKa + \log [HCO_3^-]/[0.03 - pCO_2]$$

(where 0.03 is the solubility coefficient of carbon dioxide), for each mm Hg pCO_2, 0.03 mL CO_2 is dissolved per 100 mL of plasma. pKa = constant, it is the pH value at which H_2CO_3 is 50% dissociated.

$$PK = 6.1 \text{ for } H_2CO_3$$
$$pH = 6.1 + \log [HCO_3^-]/[H_2CO_2]$$

Normal ratio $HCO_3^-/H_2CO_3 = 20/1$ and hence pH $= 6.1 + \log 20 = 6.1 + 1.3 = 7.4$.
- *H^+:* The proton which is highly reactive cation needs to be in a narrow physiologic range for normal cellular function for which various buffering mechanisms have been developed. Normal value is 40 nmol/L.
- *pCO_2:* Partial pressure of CO_2 in blood (dissolved CO_2 in blood)
- *pO_2:* Partial pressure of O_2 in blood (dissolved oxygen in blood).

Calculated Values

- *HCO_3^- (A):* This is the bicarbonate concentration in the blood.
- Normal value is 22–26 mmol/L. In newborns it may be lower also.
- *HCO_3^- (st):* $CO_2 + H_2O = HCO_3^- + H^+$. This equation shows that bicarbonate concentration is affected by the carbon dioxide. Therefore standard bicarbonate is used which is independent of CO_2 as standardized as 40 mm Hg. The bicarbonate value that is calculated from actual H^+ and CO_2 40 mm Hg at 37°C is the standard bicarbonate.
- *Buffer base (BB):* Body has developed various mechanisms to keep the pH towards normal. This is called the buffering system. If all the buffers, e.g., HCO_3^-, Hb^+, proteins, sulfates, and phosphates are added up, they constitute the BB. Normal value is 48 ± 5 mmol/L.
- *Base excess:* If alkali is added to the blood, the BB is increased. The rise in BB is called BE. If acid is added, the buffers will be used to neutralize the acid and the decrease in BB is called as base deficit, the negative of which is called BE.

Example: If acid is added and BB falls from 48 mmol/L–38 mmol/L, the base deficit is 10 mmol/L or the BE is -10 mmol/L.

The advantage of BE over HCO_3 is that it depicts pure metabolic change and is not affected by CO_2. When CO_2 accumulates as a result of impaired respiration, the following reactions occur:

$$CO_2 + H_2O = H_2CO_3 = HCO_3 + H^+$$
$$Hb^- + H^+ = HHb$$

Contd...

Contd...

The decrease in amount of Hb^- buffer is equal to the amount of HCO_3 released in the reaction. Therefore, total amount of buffer anion content will not change. Therefore, changes in the $paCO_2$ will not change BE.
- *SaO_2:* This is the percentage of hemoglobin saturated with oxygen calculated from the hemoglobin oxygen dissociation curve. SaO_2 is lesser than SpO_2 in neonates, if the machine uses adult hemoglobin oxygen dissociation curve for this calculation as oxygen is more tightly bound to the fetal hemoglobin.

BOX 2: Regulation of acid-base balance.

Regulation is done by various intracellular and extracellular buffer systems which are primarily directed by two main organ systems—lungs and kidney. This important function is mainly done by buffers.

Buffers

Buffers are substances that resist the change in pH when acids and bases are added to the body. These are the first line of defense against any changes in pH.

Different buffer systems prevail in different parts of the body:
- *Extracellular fluid (ECF):*
    - Major buffer is bicarbonate buffer system.
    - Minor buffers are intracellular proteins and phosphates.
- *Blood:*
    - Major buffers are bicarbonate buffer system and hemoglobin.
    - Minor Buffers are plasma proteins and phosphates.
- *Intracellular fluid:* Major proteins and phosphates
- *Urine:* Major ammonia and phosphate.

Carbonate bicarbonate buffer system:

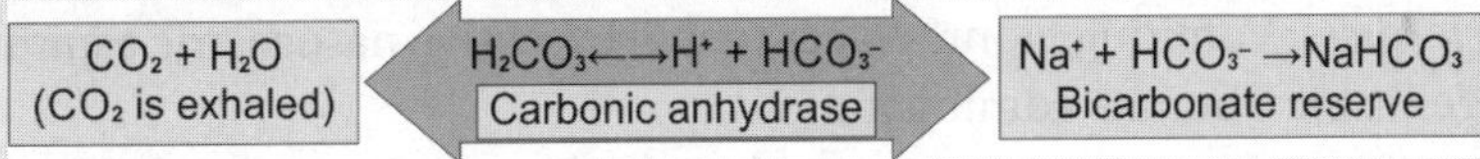

Respiratory Regulation

When chemical buffers alone cannot prevent changes in blood pH, second line of defense starts to work. Lungs eliminate or retain CO_2 causing rapid changes in pCO_2 normalizing the pH. Changes occur within minutes and test can be repeated to see the results.

Renal Regulation

These are the third line of defense mechanism. Their main action is to secrete H^+ or conserve HCO_3^- to keep the pH close to 7.4. Takes hours to days for correction. One must take into account the limited ability of the premature infant to secrete or absorb H^+ and HCO_3^-, respectively.

Anion gap (AG) = Unmeasured anions – unmeasured cations = measured cations – measured anions = (Na + K) – (HCO$_3$ + Cl). Normal value is <16 mmol/L.
- *Normal anion gap:* When there is bicarbonate loss from body or rapid dilution of ECF. Chloride is proportionately increased in these conditions, e.g., gastrointestinal tract (GIT) and renal loss of bicarbonate (renal tubular acidosis).

Contd...

Contd...

- *Increased anion gap:* Addition of strong acid in system, e.g., lactic acidosis, organic acidemias, e.g., lactic academia, ketonemia, renal failure, and excess salt therapy

$$\text{Urinary anion gap (UAG)} = (UA - UC) = [Na^+] + [K^+] - [Cl^-]$$

It is a rough index of urinary ammonium excretion. Ammonium is positively charged so a rise in its urinary concentration will cause a fall in UAG. UAG differentiates between GIT and renal causes of a hyperchloremic metabolic acidosis. Remember GUT (negative), if UAG is negative the HCO_3 losses are from the gut and if positive the loss is from the kidneys.

COMMON CAUSES OF DISORDERS

- *Metabolic acidosis:*
  - *High anion gap:*
    - Lactic acidosis caused by tissue hypoxia—asphyxia, hypothermia, and shock
    - Sepsis
    - Inborn errors of metabolism—organic acidemias/pyruvate carboxylase deficiency/primary lactic acidosis/galactosemias
    - Renal failure
    - Toxins (e.g., benzyl alcohol)
  - *Normal anion gap:*
    - Renal bicarbonate loss—caused by immaturity/renal tubular acidosis/carbonic anhydrase inhibitors
    - Gastrointestinal loses—ileostomy/fistula/diarrhea
    - Aldosterone deficiency.
- *Metabolic alkalosis:*
  - *Gastric losses:* Vomiting, nonreplacement of excessive nasogastric aspirates
  - Iatrogenic bicarbonate administration
  - Persistent vomiting seen in congenital adrenal hyperplasia
  - Inadvertent use of diuretics
  - Urea cycle disorders
  - Following blood transfusion—citrate in blood gets converted to bicarbonate.
- *Respiratory acidosis:*
  - *Lung abnormality:* Respiratory distress syndrome (RDS)/pneumonia/transient tachypnea of newborn/meconium aspiration syndrome
  - *Upper airway obstruction:* Tracheolaryngomalacia/choanal atresia/Pierre Robin sequence
  - *Hypoventilating disorders:* Hypoxic-ischemic encephalopathy (HIE)/encephalopathy/intracranial bleed
  - *Neuromuscular insufficiency:* Congenital myopathy/neuropathies
  - Poor ventilation.
- *Respiratory alkalosis:*
  - *Iatrogenic:* Excessive ventilator settings.

How to Collect Arterial Blood Gas Sample?

- Arterial blood gas (ABG) sample can be collected from artery (radial/umbilical) or from an indwelling catheter, arterialized capillary by a heel prick or venous sample.
- *For heel prick:* Warm the heel to cause local vasodilatation using steam towel or warm water. Avoid squeezing and discard the first drop to fill drop from the oozing tissue. It should be avoided in neonates with shock.
- *For arterial sample:* Follow strict asepsis using alcohol containing sterile solution.
- Allen test is performed to ensure collateral supply from ulnar artery before pricking the radial artery.
- Heparinize 1 mL (25 G) syringe using 0.05 mL of heparin (1,000 units/mL). Practically just flushing the syringe with heparin yields this amount.
- Prick the artery/collect from an indwelling catheter. Collect a free flowing sample and transport immediately on slushed ice for processing.

How to Avoid Errors?

- *Arterial/capillary/venous* blood can be used. Since pulse oximetry can be used to monitor the SpO_2 levels, venous blood gives fairly adequate values. Venous pH is lower than arterial pH and pCO_2 levels are higher.
- *Anticoagulant:* Heparin is used in the strength of 0.05 mL of 1,000 units/mL. Practically, flushing the syringe with heparin yields that amount. Avoid excess heparin as it is acidic and can reduce the PH. It can bind to calcium and potassium and alter their value. Sodium heparin can falsely elevate sodium levels.
- *Avoid air bubble:* Visually inspect the sample after collection and expel all the air and cover the syringe with a cap. Air bubbles can alter the PaO_2 and pCO_2 toward room air. pCO_2 will decrease and PaO_2 can increase.
- *Avoid hemolysis:* Avoid vigorous mixing of the sample and transport on an ice cube if delay in assessment is expected. Temperature can cause PH, pCO_2 and pO_2 to change every 10 minutes.

Quality Improvement Opportunities

- Arterial blood gas sample should be collected in heparinized syringe with immediate processing. If delay in processing is expected, then sample should be transported on crushed ice.
- Decrease time to processing.
- Decrease phlebotomy losses.

Key Points to Remember

- Keep clinical condition, previous ABG and therapeutic interventions in mind while interpreting the ABG report.
- As a dictum, if both pCO_2 and HCO_3 move in the same direction and are in the compensatory range, it is a simple disorder. If they move in the opposite directions, i.e., one is rising and the other is falling (or only one is changing), it is a mixed disorder.
- There is no need to supplement bicarbonate routinely in case of high anion gap metabolic acidosis. In spite, correct underlying etiology like adequate ventilation and circulation in case of lactic acidosis due to hypoxia.
- Complex physiological processes in our body help to maintain a tight regulation of acid-base balance.
- Small changes in hydrogen ions can alter the function of various proteins and affect the metabolic status of the body.
- Maintaining pH in normal range is important for maintaining normal function of cell membranes and proteins.
- pH 6.9–7.6 is not compatible with life.

■ FURTHER READING

1. Rose B, Post T, Stokes J. Clinical Physiology of Acid-base and Electrolyte Disorders, 6th edition. United States: McGraw Hill Lange Publisher; 2022.

Management of Pain

Kaushaki Shankar

Assessment of pain

Acute procedural pain
- Neonatal infant pain scale (NIPS) (*see* **Table 1**)
- Premature infant pain profile—revised (PIPP-R) (*see* **Table 2**)
- Neonatal facial coding system (NFCS)

Postoperative pain
- Neonatal pain, agitation, and sedation scale (N-PASS)
- COMFORT and COMFORTneo scale

Ventilated babies
N-PASS

Prolonged or chronic pain
- N-PASS
- EDIN SCALE (Echelle de la Douleur Inconfort Noveau-Ne-neonatal pain and discomfort scale)

Of these, the PIPP-revised (for acute and procedural pain) and N-PASS (for ventilated babies and for chronic pain) are among the most commonly used (see below)

Management of neonatal pain

General measures
- Use clustering of care, bundling of investigations, and avoid unnecessary handling
- Use noninvasive methods of investigation. Avoid painful procedures
- Using point of care devices
- Avoid bright light, loud noise, and control thermal stress
- Avoid adhesive tapes over hair, moisten tapes before removal
- Skilled and trained personnel should be placing peripheral, central, or arterial lines

Nonpharmacologic measures
- *Breastfeeding:* Direct breastfeeding more effective than maternal holding, maternal skin-to-skin contact, topical anesthetics, music therapy, and expressed breast milk or sucrose
- Non-nutritive sucking (NNS)
- Nesting/swaddling/facilitated tucking (gently maintaining arms and legs in flexed position)
- Skin-to-skin contact [kangaroo mother care (KMC)]
- Sensorial saturation (use of touch, massage, voice, and smell)
- Music and massage therapy

Pharmacological
(*see* **Table 3**)

What measures to choose?	
Procedure	*Suggested pain mitigants*
Heel Prick	Lancet
Venipuncture/IV Cannulation, arterial puncture, retinopathy of prematurity (ROP) assessment, peripheral arterial line, and lumbar puncture	• Nonpharmacologic measures and • Topical local anesthesia (LA) (e.g., EMLA; topical eye drops of proparacaine for ROP assessment)
Central line placement, peripherally inserted central catheter (PICC) line, suprapubic bladder aspiration	• Nonpharmocologic measures and • Topical LA; lidocaine infiltration (+/- IV opioids)
Chronic pain (e.g., postoperative pain, congenital skin disorders such as epidermolysis bullosa)	• IV paracetamol and morphine or fentanyl • Fentanyl reported to be better for postoperative congenital diaphragmatic hernia and other congenital lung malformations with persistent pulmonary hypertension of the newborn (PPHN), due to its vascular stabilizing properties

Noninvasive and invasive mechanical ventilation	• For noninvasive ventilation and continuous positive airway pressure (CPAP):
	  – Nonpharmacologic approach
	On mechanical ventilation:
	  – Routine sedation not preferred
	  – Fentanyl or morphine boluses can suffice for analgesia in both preterm and term neonates
	  – Midazolam should be given only for agitated term neonates (after excluding other causes for agitation) or neonates with PPHN
	• Morphine to be avoided in <27 week GA; midazolam to be used with caution in <35 week GA
	• INSURE: Atropine plus remifentanil/propofol

Umbilical catheterization	IV acetaminophen (10 mg/kg), avoid skin fixation suturing

TABLE 1: Neonatal infant pain scale (N-PASS).

Assessment	Sedation		Normal	Pain/agitation	
Criteria	**−2**	**−1**	**0**	**1**	**2**
Crying irritability	No cry with painful stimuli	Moans or cries minimally with painful stimuli	• Appropriate crying • Not irritable	• Irritable or crying at intervals • Consolable	• High-pitched or silent-continuous cry • Inconsolable
Behavior state	• No arousal to any stimuli • No spontaneous movement	• Arouses minimally to stimuli • Little spontaneous movement	Appropriate for gestational age	• Restless, squirming • Awakens frequently	• Arching, kicking • Constantly awake or • Arouses minimally/no movement (not sedated)
Facial expression	• Mouth is lax • No expression	Minimal expression with stimuli	• Relaxed • Appropriate	Any pain expression intermittent	Any pain expression continual
Extremities tone	• No grasp reflex • Flaccid tone	• Weak grasp reflex • ↓ muscle tone	• Relaxed hands and feet • Normal tone	• Intermittent clenched toes, fists or finger splay • Body is not tense	• Continual clenched toes, fists, or finger splay • Body is tense
Vital Signs HR, RR, BP, and SaO_2	• No variability with stimuli • Hypoventilation or apnea	<10% variability from baseline with stimuli	Within baseline or normal for gestational age	• ↑ 10–20% from baseline • SaO_2 76–85% with stimulation—quick ↑	• ↑ >20% from baseline • SaO_2 ≤75% with stimulation—slow ↑ • Out of sync with vent

Premature neonates pain assessment (points added to compensate for limited ability to communicate pain):
• + 3 if <28 weeks gestation/corrected age
• + 2 if 28–31 weeks gestation/corrected age
• + 1 if 32–35 weeks gestation/corrected age

Sedation assessment	**Pain/agitation assessment**
Score: 0 to −10	Score: 0 to +10
Score 0: Response to stimuli normal for GA	Include pain assessment every time vitals are assessed (pain – the fifth vital)
Light sedation: −2 to −5	Goal of intervention: Score ≤3
Deep sedation: −5 to −10	Pain mitigating actions for painful stimuli/procedures should be carried out prophylactically (before score reaches 3)
Negative score without opioids/sedatives: Neurological depression/sepsis/persistent pain	

TABLE 2: Premature infant pain profile-revised (PIPP-R).

Infant indicator	Indicator score				Infant indicator score
	0	**+1**	**+2**	**+3**	
Change in heart rate (bpm) Baseline: ______	0–4	5–14	15–24	>24	
Decrease in oxygen saturation (%) Baseline: ______	0–2	3–5	6–8	>8 or increase in O_2	
Brow bulge (sec)	None (<3)	Minimal (3–10)	Moderate (11–20)	Maximal (>20)	
Eye squeeze (sec)	None (<3)	Minimal (3–10)	Moderate (11–20)	Maximal (>20)	
Nasolabial furrow (sec)	None (<3)	Minimal (3–10)	Moderate (11–20)	Maximal (>20)	
			***Subtotal score:**		
Gestational age (weeks + days)	>36 weeks	32 weeks–35 weeks, 6 days	28 weeks	<28 weeks	
Baseline behavioral state	Active and awake	Quite and awake	Active and asleep	Quiet and asleep	
			****Total score:**		

Note:
*Subtotal for physiological and facial indicators. If subtotal score >0, add GA and BS indicator scores.
**Total score: Subtotal score + GA score + BS score

Scoring Instructions

- *Step 1:* Observe infant for *15 seconds at rest* and assess vital sign indicators.

  [Highest heart rate (HR) and lowest O_2 saturation (O_2 SAT) and behavioral state]

- *Step 2:* Observe infant for *30 seconds after procedure* and assess *change* in vital sign indicators (maximal HR, lowest O_2 SAT and duration of facial actions observed)
  If infant requires an increase in oxygen at any point before or during procedure, they receive a score of 3 for the O_2 SAT indicator.
- *Step 3:* Score for corrected gestational age (GA) and behavioral state (BS) if the subtotal score >0.
- *Step 4:* Calculate total score by adding subtotal score + BS score

Score	Interpretation	Intervention
0–6	Minimal or no pain	No action
7–12	Mild to moderate pain	*Nonpharmocologic measures:* Reassess in 30 minutes for effectiveness
>12	Severe Pain	*Pharmacologic measures:* Reassess after 15–30 minutes for titration

TABLE 3: Pharmacological measures.

Drug	Dose (Route)

Oral sucrose 24% solution (0.2 mL/kg)	• Preterm—0.5 mL/dose, term—1 mL/dose
	  – 2 minutes before procedure (oral), peak effects occurs at 2 minutes, duration of analgesia is 4 minutes
	  – For intubated patients, sucrose is placed directly on tongue as follows:
	  – 24–26 weeks—0.1 mL; 27–31 weeks—0.25 mL; 32–36 weeks—0.5 mL; 37–44 weeks—1 mL

Fentanyl	0.5–4 µg/kg per dose IV slow push (not faster than 1 µg/kg/min), 5 minutes before procedure, IV infusion 1–3 µg/kg/h
Acetaminophen	• 24–30 weeks GA: 20–30 mg/kg/day • 31–36 weeks GA: 35–50 mg/kg/day • 37–42 weeks GA: 50–60 mg/kg/day • 1–3 months postnatal: 60–75 mg/kg/day
Succinylcholine	1–2 mg/kg IV immediately prior to intubation, repeat dose of 1 mg/kg up to a maximum of 4 mg/kg
Rocuronium	0.3–0.6 mg/kg per dose slow IV push over 5–10 seconds
Midazolam	• 0.05–0.2 mg/kg IV over at least 5 minutes. Repeat as required, usually every 2 to 4 hours. • Continuous IV infusion 0.01–0.06 mg/kg/h (10–60 µg/kg/h) • *Intranasal:* 0.2–0.3 mg/kg per dose
Morphine	• Intermittent 0.05–0.2 mg/kg per dose IV over at least 5 minutes, repeat as required usually every 4 hours • *Continuous infusion:* Loading dose 100–150 µg/kg over 1 hour followed by 10 to 20 µg/kg/h
Topical anesthesia	• Lidocaine-prilocaine mixture (EMLA) in cream base • 4% tetracaine in cream or gel base • 4–5% lidocaine in gel base
Lidocaine (preservative free without epinephrine)	• 0.5 mL/kg subcutaneous infiltration of 1% solution up to 3–5 mg/kg • 0.25 mL/kg subcutaneous infiltration of 2% solution up to 3–5 mg/kg
Propofol	1–2.5 mg/kg IV

Remifentanil	• For intubation
	• *Alone:*
	  – Preterm 29–32 weeks: 2 µg/kg IV bolus over 1 minute (may repeat dose)
	• *Along with midazolam:*
	  – Preterm 28–34 weeks: 1 µg/kg IV bolus over 60 seconds
	• *For mechanical ventilation:*
	  – Full term 0.15–0.5 µg/kg/min, use with midazolam

Dexmedetomidine	0.5-1.5 µg/kg/h IV infusion

Key Points to Remember

- "Pain is an unpleasant sensory and emotional response associated with actual or potential tissue damage, or described in terms of such damage."
- A newborn receives painful stimuli everyday especially during neonatal intensive care unit (NICU) stay.
- By 24 weeks of gestation, lateral spinothalamic tract, which carries pain fibers, develops so a viable preterm can feel pain.
- Painful stimulus has impact on both short- and long-term neurological outcomes.
- Develop unit policy for management of pain (select pain assessment tools that suit your unit and comfort of the nursing staff for better neonatal outcomes).

OSCE/Checklist

S. No.	Performance steps	Yes	No
1.	Sensitive to short- and long-term effects of painful stimuli		
2.	Aware of physiological and behavioral markers of pain in newborn		
3.	Identify and apply a pain scale appropriate to the situation		
4.	Perform general and nonpharmacologic measures before baby handling		
5.	Knows the indications and calculation of dosage for pharmacologic measures		
	Total score		

▪ FURTHER READING

1. Committee on fetus and newborn and section on anesthesiology and pain medicine. Prevention and management of procedural pain in the neonate: An update. Pediatrics. 2016;137(2):e20154271.
2. Witt N, Coynor S, Edwards C, Bradshaw H. A guide to pain assessment and management in the neonate. Curr Emerg Hosp Med Rep. 2016;4:1-10.

Lung Protective Strategies

Sankalp Dudeja

ANTENATAL

- Preventing premature delivery
- *Antenatal steroids in impending premature birth (24–34 weeks)*: Antenatal steroids accelerate the lung maturity and at risk within next 7 days, reduce the chances of respiratory distress syndrome (RDS). The benefit in respiratory distress and mortality is offset by increased survival of preterm newborns and therefore, there is no effect on the incidence of bronchopulmonary dysplasia (BPD).

IN THE DELIVERY ROOM

- In case a preterm baby has respiratory distress, start continuous positive airway pressure (CPAP) early: CPAP is superior to intubation and positive pressure ventilation (PPV).
- There is no role of prophylactic surfactant in preterms.
- Use blender and adjust fraction of inspired oxygen (FiO_2) as per the target oxygen saturation (SpO_2), avoid hyperoxia.
- In case PPV is required, use a T-piece resuscitator especially in preterm infants.

IN THE NEONATAL INTENSIVE CARE UNIT

- If the baby has respiratory distress, start CPAP early.
- No benefit of noninvasive positive pressure ventilation (NIPPV) over CPAP in terms of reduction of BPD or mortality.
- CPAP + early surfactant better than waiting for CPAP failure and then intubating and giving surfactant.
- For surfactant administration, LISA (less invasive surfactant administration) is better than INSURE. Early administration (preferably within first 30–60 minutes is better than late administration).
- Avoid intubation and mechanical ventilation as much as possible. If unavoidable, then only intubate. If mechanical ventilation is initiated, then synchronized mode of ventilation facilitates weaning and shorted duration of ventilation.

- High-frequency ventilation is slightly less damaging as compared to conventional ventilation. It marginally reduces death and BPD as compared to conventional ventilation.
- In conventional ventilation, volume target ventilation (4–6 mL/kg) is better than pressure target ventilation.
- Ventilation strategies for lung protection (based on physiological principles. None based on evidence from large RCTs/meta-analyses):
  - Be liberal with PEEP, while avoiding overdistention.
  - Minimize PIP (ΔP)
  - Permissive hypercapnia, especially after first few days of ventilation.
  - Extubate at the earliest opportunity even if it means high CPAP or high NIPPV settings.
- *Drugs*: Postnatal dexamethasone definitely decreases death/BPD, but at the cost of increased cerebral palsy. Therefore, not routinely recommended. The risk:benefit ratio of giving steroids is in favor of steroids if patient's chances of developing BPD are high, but not otherwise. These should be reserved for ventilation-dependent patients at 2–3 weeks of life.
- Caffeine (preferably started within first 3 days of life) reduces the risk of BPD.
- Vitamin A has some role in mitigating lung injury. Marginal reduction in death/BPD with prophylactic vitamin A, but only when given intramuscularly, which is practically difficult.
- Breast milk feeding is associated with lower incidence of BPD compared to the formula. Although the quality of evidence is low, there are numerous other advantages of breast milk and hence should be promoted.
- Long-chain polyunsaturated fatty acid (LCPUFA) administration—no role.

■ FURTHER READING

1. Bhunwal S, Mukhopadhyay K, Bhattacharya S, Dey P, Dhaliwal LK. Bronchopulmonary dysplasia in preterm neonates in a level III neonatal unit in India. Indian Pediatr. 2018;55(3):211-5.
2. Goldsmith JP, Edward K, Gautham S, Martin K. Assisted Ventilation of the Neonate: An Evidence-based Approach to Newborn Respiratory Care, 6th edition. Philadelphia: Elsevier; 2016.

Ventilatory Strategies in Common Respiratory Disorder

Amanpreet Sethi

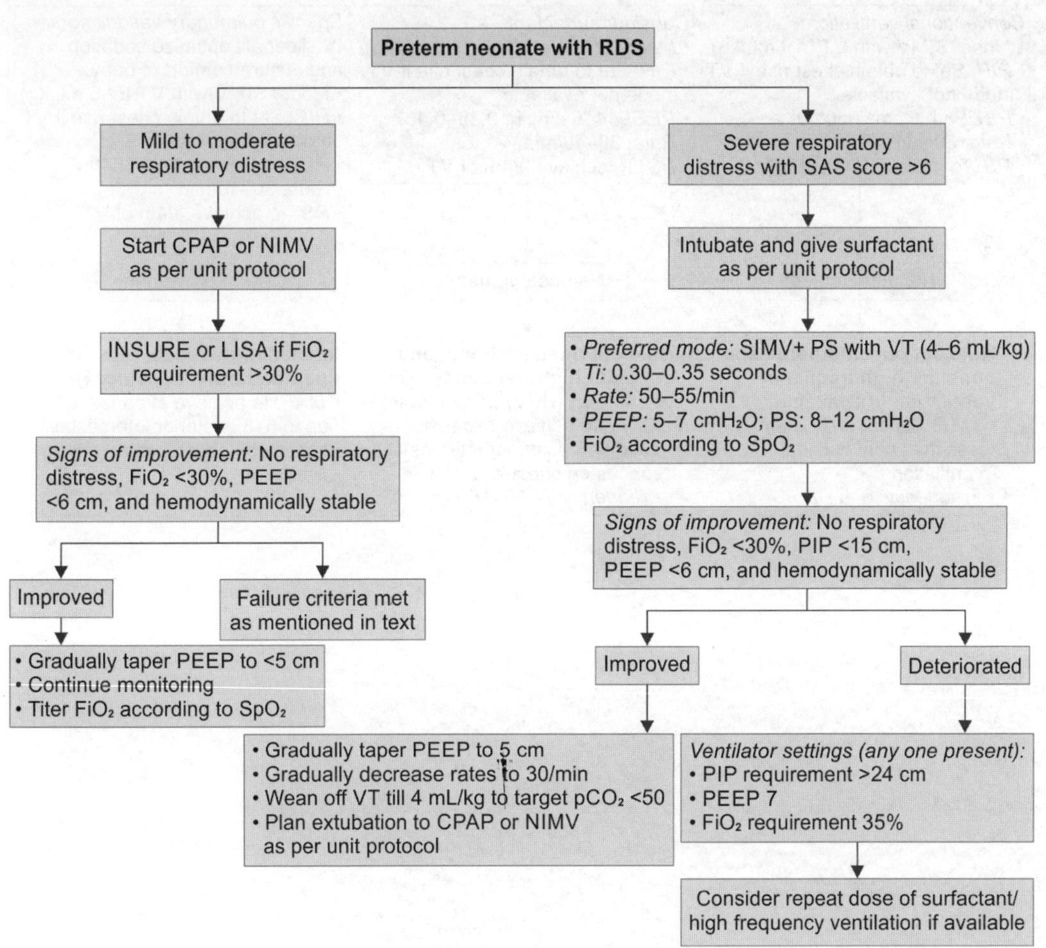

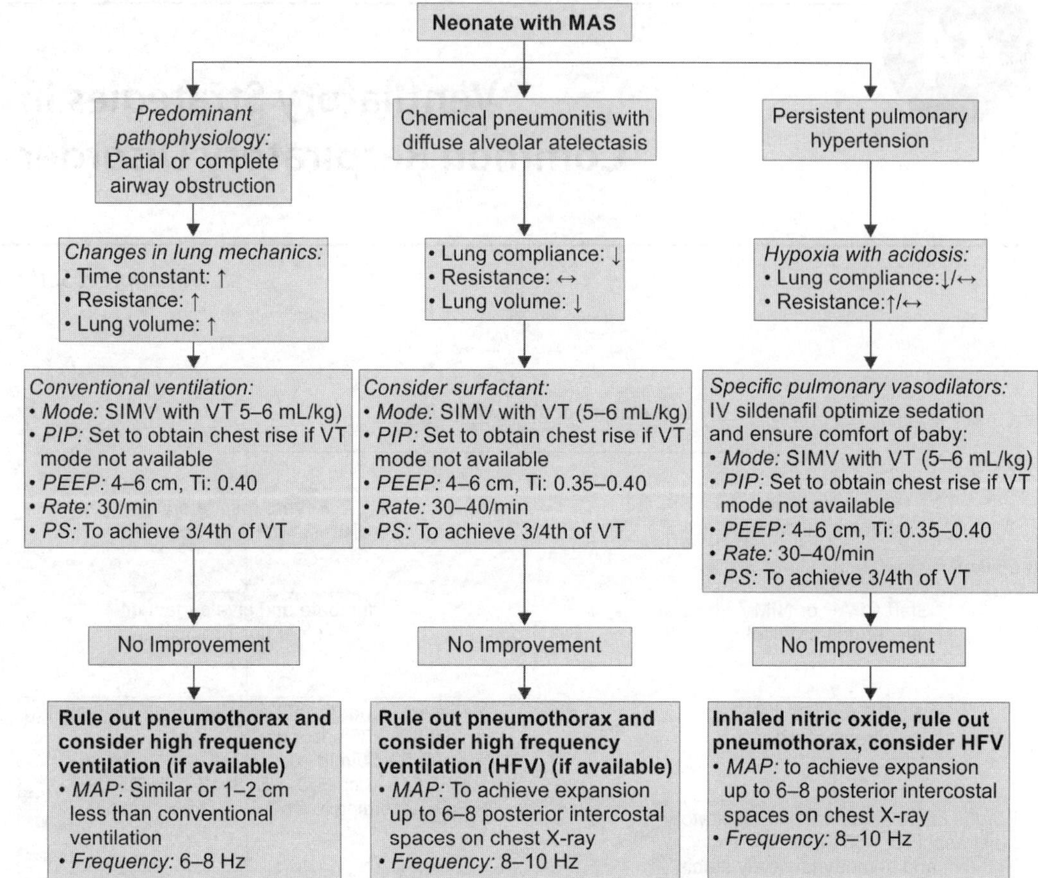

Neonate with MAS

Predominant pathophysiology: Partial or complete airway obstruction

Chemical pneumonitis with diffuse alveolar atelectasis

Persistent pulmonary hypertension

Changes in lung mechanics:
• Time constant: ↑
• Resistance: ↑
• Lung volume: ↑

• Lung compliance: ↓
• Resistance: ↔
• Lung volume: ↓

Hypoxia with acidosis:
• Lung compliance: ↓/↔
• Resistance: ↑/↔

Conventional ventilation:
• Mode: SIMV with VT 5–6 mL/kg)
• PIP: Set to obtain chest rise if VT mode not available
• PEEP: 4–6 cm, Ti: 0.40
• Rate: 30/min
• PS: To achieve 3/4th of VT

Consider surfactant:
• Mode: SIMV with VT (5–6 mL/kg)
• PIP: Set to obtain chest rise if VT mode not available
• PEEP: 4–6 cm, Ti: 0.35–0.40
• Rate: 30–40/min
• PS: To achieve 3/4th of VT

Specific pulmonary vasodilators: IV sildenafil optimize sedation and ensure comfort of baby:
• Mode: SIMV with VT (5–6 mL/kg)
• PIP: Set to obtain chest rise if VT mode not available
• PEEP: 4–6 cm, Ti: 0.35–0.40
• Rate: 30–40/min
• PS: To achieve 3/4th of VT

No Improvement

No Improvement

No Improvement

Rule out pneumothorax and consider high frequency ventilation (if available)
• MAP: Similar or 1–2 cm less than conventional ventilation
• Frequency: 6–8 Hz

Rule out pneumothorax and consider high frequency ventilation (HFV) (if available)
• MAP: To achieve expansion up to 6–8 posterior intercostal spaces on chest X-ray
• Frequency: 8–10 Hz

Inhaled nitric oxide, rule out pneumothorax, consider HFV
• MAP: to achieve expansion up to 6–8 posterior intercostal spaces on chest X-ray
• Frequency: 8–10 Hz

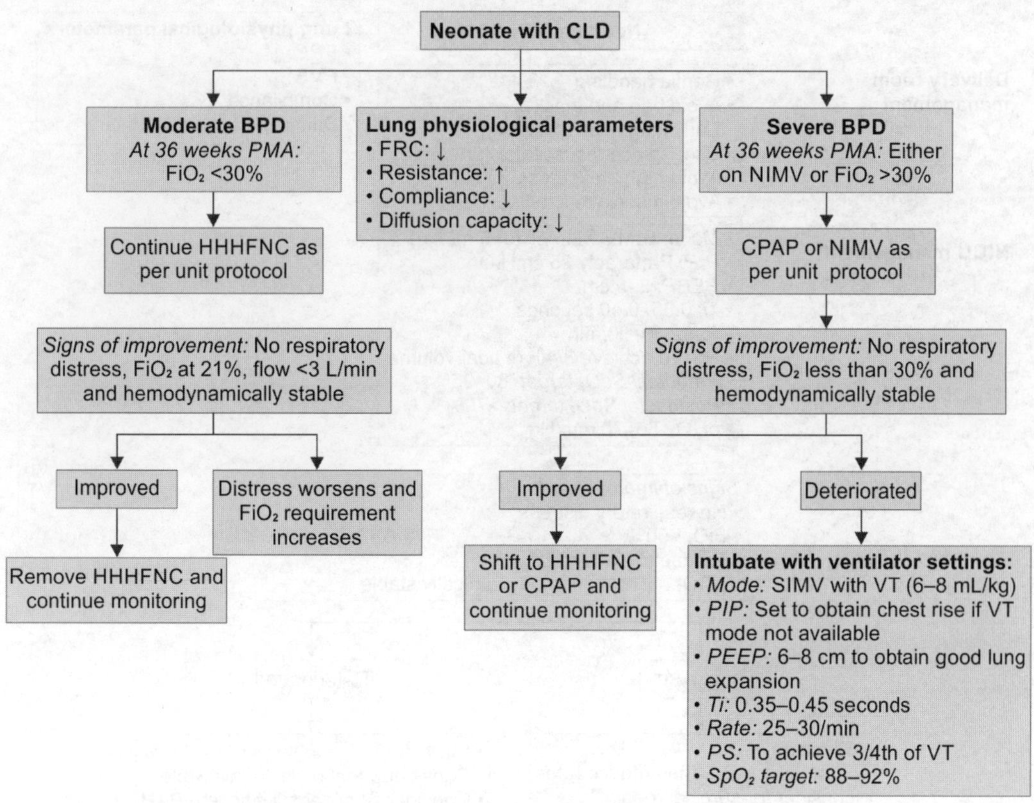

Neonate with CLD
Moderate BPD
At 36 weeks PMA:
FiO₂ <30%
Lung physiological parameters
• FRC: ↓
• Resistance: ↑
• Compliance: ↓
• Diffusion capacity: ↓
Severe BPD
At 36 weeks PMA: Either on NIMV or FiO₂ >30%
Continue HHHFNC as per unit protocol
CPAP or NIMV as per unit protocol
Signs of improvement: No respiratory distress, FiO₂ at 21%, flow <3 L/min and hemodynamically stable
Signs of improvement: No respiratory distress, FiO₂ less than 30% and hemodynamically stable
Improved
Distress worsens and FiO₂ requirement increases
Improved
Deteriorated
Remove HHHFNC and continue monitoring
Shift to HHHFNC or CPAP and continue monitoring
Intubate with ventilator settings:
• Mode: SIMV with VT (6–8 mL/kg)
• PIP: Set to obtain chest rise if VT mode not available
• PEEP: 6–8 cm to obtain good lung expansion
• Ti: 0.35–0.45 seconds
• Rate: 25–30/min
• PS: To achieve 3/4th of VT
• SpO₂ target: 88–92%

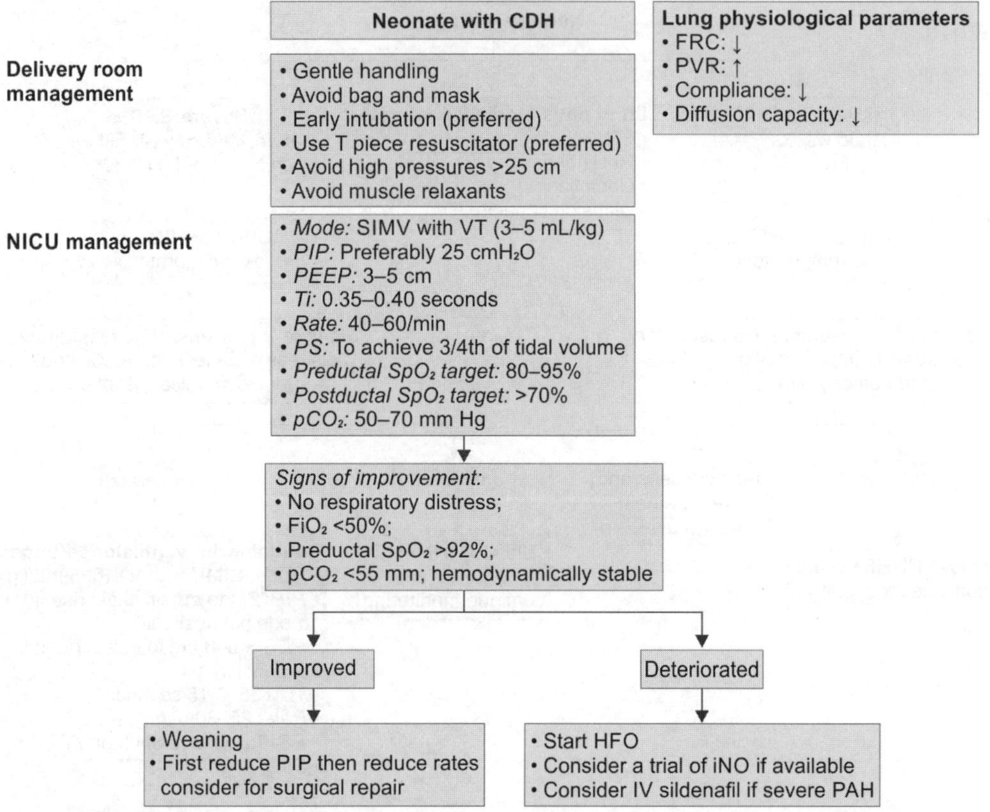

Key Points to Remember

Neonate with ROS

- Respiratory distress syndrome is one of the most important respiratory disorders in premature infants. The following pathophysiological mechanisms are responsible for increased work of breathing in these tiny preterm infants:
  - *Reduced quantity and function of surfactant:* Leading to atelectasis and reduced functional residual capacity (FRC)
  - *Impaired lung fluid clearance:* Leading to reduced compliance and poor response to exogenous surfactant
  - *Mechanical factors such as increased chest wall and airway compliance:* Leading to early collapse of terminal airways during expiration phase and reduced FRC
  - Inflammation leading to augmented surfactant metabolism and pulmonary airway and vascular membrane injury
  - Presence of thickened mesenchymal space in the canalicular and saccular stage of lung development resulting in decreased diffusion of oxygen across the membranes.

Neonate with Meconium Aspiration Syndrome

- Meconium aspiration syndrome occurs in one-third cases of meconium-stained amniotic fluid (MSAF) with around 50% chances of mechanical ventilation. MAS is complicated by unique pathophysiological features as described below:
    - Surfactant dysfunction due to chemical pneumonitis with loss of FRC and white out lung.
    - Complete or partial obstruction of airways leading to heterogeneous lung disease with distinct areas of collapse/atelectasis and hyperinflation.
    - Hypoxia leading to increased pulmonary vascular reactivity leading to persistent pulmonary hypertension of newborn (PPHN).
- So, the clinical spectrum and disease pathophysiology of MAS depend on the relative predominance of one of the above mentioned three features. Therefore, ventilation strategy is also tailored to target the predominant pathophysiology.

Neonate with Chronic Lung Disease

- Chronic lung disease or bronchopulmonary dysplasia (BPD) in premature infants is an emerging problem in India due to improved survival of extreme preterm infants.
- The most commonly used definition of BPD in preterm infants born at <32 weeks of gestation is the need of additional oxygen for ≥28 days assessed at postmenstrual age (PMA) of 36 weeks.
- The incidence of CLD is approximately 40% in preterm infants born at <29 weeks. Large studies on incidence of CLD in India are lacking. A recent study from a tertiary center in India reported 11.2% incidence in survived preterm infants born at <33 weeks of gestation.
- In CLD of prematurity, there is a wide range of pathological changes starting from the upper airway till distal alveoli as mentioned below:
    - *Upper airway:* Glottic edema, subglottic stenosis, tracheomalacia, bronchomalacia, and tracheitis/tracheal stenosis
    - *Lower airway:* Smooth muscle hypertrophy leading to hyper-reactivity; increased mucous gland hypertrophy leading to enhanced mucous production and collapses
    - *Alveoli and pulmonary vascular bed:* Decreased alveolarization leading to decreased surface area for gas exchange; heterogenic areas of localized atelectasis and hyperinflation; decoupling of alveolo-vascular bed leading to impaired gas exchange; increased smooth muscle hypertrophy in pulmonary vessels leading to chronic pulmonary hypertension.

Neonate with Congenital Diaphragmatic Hernia/Lung Hypoplasia Type Disorders

The basic pathological changes complicating the management of CDH are:

- Due to the pressure effect of the herniated bowel, the ipsilateral and contralateral lung becomes hypoplastic. Apart from the abnormal lung development, there are changes in the surfactant metabolism also.

- Due to abnormal lung development, there is impaired growth of the pulmonary vessels with increased smooth muscle hypertrophy and impaired activity of the vascular endothelial growth factors, nitric oxide synthase, and increased activity of phosphodiesterase 5 and expression of endothelin-1 and endothelin-A receptor. Thus, there are high chances of pulmonary hypertension after birth.
- Due to the pressure effect of the herniated bowel, there is impaired development of the heart also sometimes leading to hypoplastic left ventricles thus complicating the management of these sick babies.

Principles of ventilation are: (1) lung protective ventilation; (2) permissive hypercapnia; and (3) permissive hypoxia.

■ FURTHER READING

1. Bhunwal S, Mukhopadhyay K, Bhattacharya S, Dey P, Dhaliwal LK. Bronchopulmonary dysplasia in preterm neonates in a level III neonatal unit in India. Indian Pediatr. 2018;55(3):211-5.
2. Goldsmith JP, Karotkin E, Suresh G, Keszler M. Assisted Ventilation of the Neonate: An Evidence-based Approach to Newborn Respiratory Care, 6th edition. Philadelphia: Elsevier; 2016.
3. Ibrahim J, Bhandari V. The definition of bronchopulmonary dysplasia: an evolving dilemma. Pediatr Res. 2018;84:586-8.

Chapter 45

Sudden Deterioration on Ventilator

Mayank Priyadarshi

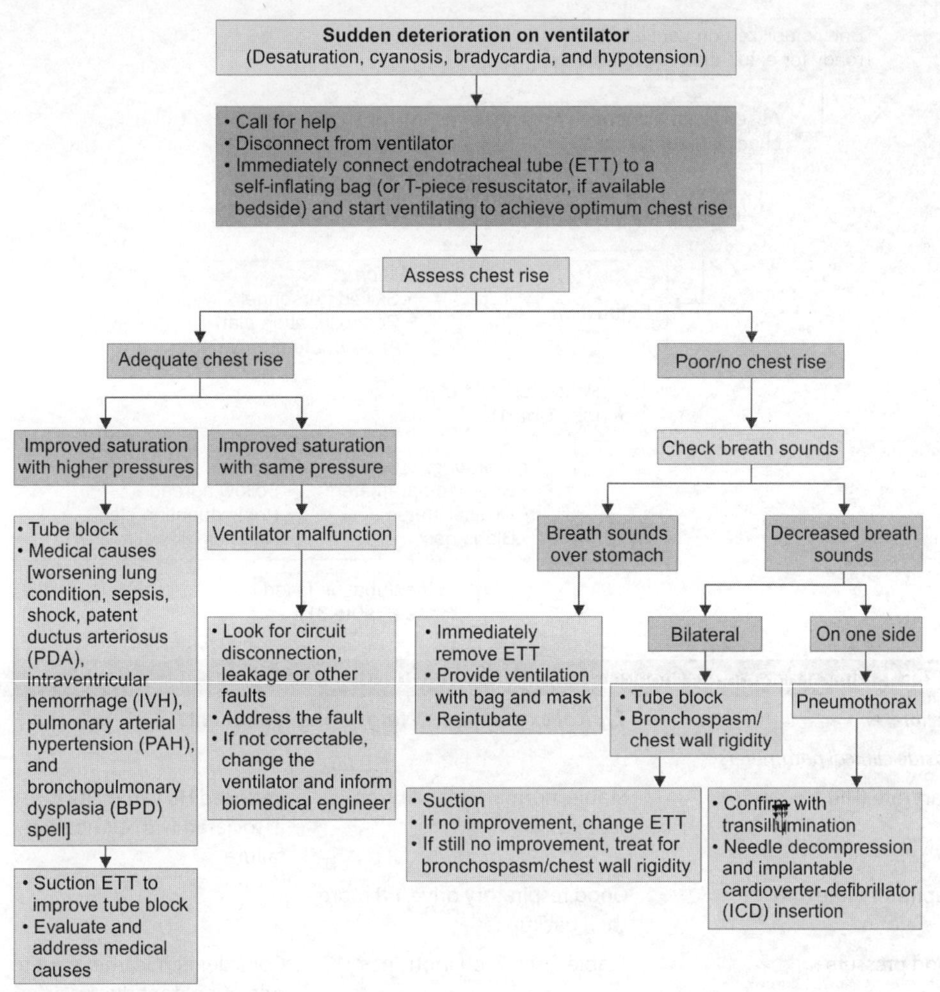

■ FURTHER READING

1. Keszler M, Gautham KS. Goldsmith's Assisted Ventilation of the Neonate: An Evidence-Based Approach to Newborn Respiratory Care, 7th edition; 2022.

Ventilation Weaning Strategies

Mamta Jajoo, Saraswati Kini

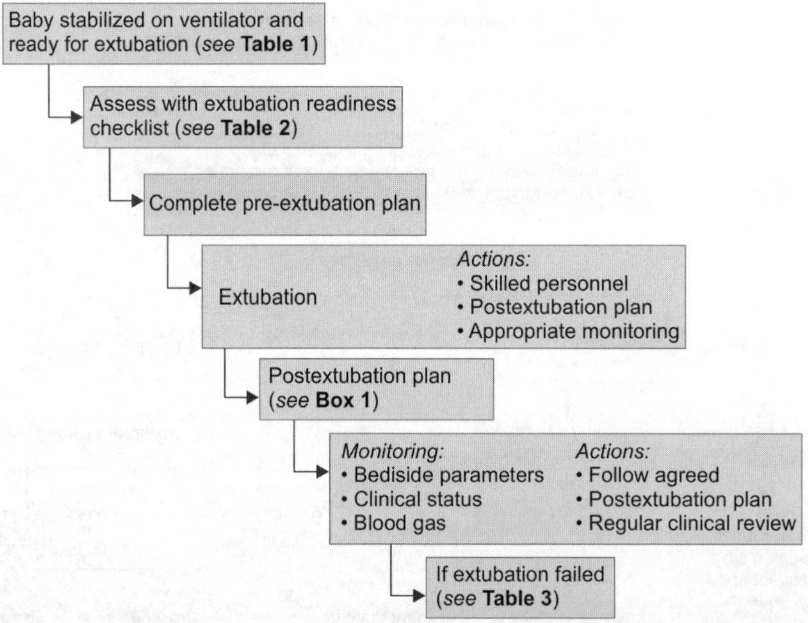

TABLE 1: Clinical parameters should be considered for extubation.

Parameter	Typical extubation settings	Comments
Bedside clinical parameters		
Heart rate (HR)	Stable, normal variability, no bradycardia	Reduced HR variability is associated with extubation failure
Respiratory rate (RR)	Good respiratory drive, RR more than backup rate	
Blood pressure	Stable, usually off inotropes	Consider echocardiogram to rule out patent ductus arteriosus (PDA)
O_2 saturations	Target 90–95%	Less than 90% increases mortality and also ND delay

Contd...

Contd...

Parameter	Typical extubation settings	Comments
Ventilator parameters for extubation		
Mode of ventilation	Pressure control-assist control (PC-AC) or PC-pressure support ventilation (PSV)	
FiO_2	Stable oxygenation at $FiO_2 \leq 0.4$	In infants with established lung disease, extubation may be appropriate from a higher FiO_2
MAP	Consistently $\leq$ 7–9 cmH_2O	May be higher in babies with established lung disease
Backup rate	Below the spontaneous RR typically 20–30	Optimize respiratory drive, consider caffeine
Blood gas parameters		
pH	≥ 7.20	Manage both respiratory and metabolic components of acidosis
$paCO_2$	30–45 mm Hg in first 3–4 days, permissive hypercapnia tolerated subsequently	After first 3–4 days, babies tolerate higher $paCO_2$ and extubation decision should be based on clinical status, $paCO_2$ trend and pH
Lactate	≤ 2.5 mmol/L	If higher, consider the cause and manage as appropriate
Hb	>10 g/dL with hematocrit >30%	Consider higher threshold if higher MAP or need of inotropes
Ventilatory parameters		

- *Conventional ventilation [AC, synchronized intermittent mandatory ventilation (SIMV), and PSV]:*
  - *SIMV:* PIP $\leq$16 cmH_2O, positive end-expiratory pressure (PEEP) $\leq$6 cmH_2O, rate $\leq$20, $FiO_2 \leq 0.30$
  - *AC/PSV, BW < 1,000 g:* MAP $\leq$ 7 cmH_2O and $FiO_2 \leq 0.30$
  - *AC/PSV, BW > 1,000 g:* MAP $\leq$ 8 cmH_2O and $FiO_2 \leq 0.30$.
- *Volume ventilation:*
  - Tidal volume $\leq$4.0 mL/kg (5 mL/kg if <700 g or >2 weeks of age) and $FiO_2 \leq 0.3$

TABLE 2: Checklist for extubation readiness.

Checklist question	Items to check	Pre- and postextubation plan activities
Respiratory history?	Antenatal history [steroids/premature rupture of membrane (PROM)]	Address the cause
Extubation history?	Previous extubation failures	
Did the baby receive surfactant?	Timing, dose, and response	Optimize the total surfactant

Contd...

Contd...

Checklist question	Items to check	Pre- and postextubation plan activities
Evidence of improving or stable lung disease?	Trends in markers of compliance (MAP/PIP/VTe/FiO_2)	Identify MAP to target post-extubation PEEP
Evidence of metabolic compensation to hypercapnia?	Chloride, pH, and pCO_2	Agree a pH lower limit, review chloride intake
Evidence of good respiratory drive?	Baby is breathing above backup rate without significant recessions	Consider a short trial of ET CPAP (spontaneous breathing trial) or low backup rate in patient triggered modes
Stop sedation or analgesia	History of medication and responses	Consider need for ongoing sedation or analgesia after extubation, for example, tolerance of CPAP in an older baby
Would the baby benefit from caffeine?	Use caffeine	Give 24 hours before extubation (if already on caffeine, no extra boluses required)
Will the lung disease or respiratory drive benefit from CPAP/NIV/humidified high flow nasal cannula?	Consider gestational age and severity of current lung disease	Identify MAP required to keep lungs open
Check OG tube		Deflate stomach via NGT
Is baby off inotropes or resolving sepsis or not?	Cardiac status and recent history of sepsis with evidence of resolution (improving lactate and sepsis markers)	Observe period of stability on stopping inotropes
Is there any PDA?	Look for Cardiac status	Clinical and echocardiography assessment
What is the Hb level?	Check optimal Hb level in context of age, clinical status, and degree of ventilatory support	Consider red cell transfusion if Hb < 10 g/dL and MAP > 8 cmH_2O and/or FiO_2 > 0.4
Look for excess tissue fluid?	Recent renal function, weight changes, and nutritional status	Can consider short course of diuretics to improve lung compliance
Are parents informed about status of baby?	Aware of risk of reintubation or complications	Ensure good and consistent communication
Is one experienced nurse available when extubation is done	Skill mix check	Optimize position and device interface Experienced tolerance of initial post extubation instability
What are the reintubation thresholds?	Patient course and physiological markers	Individualize threshold parameters for reintubation

BOX 1: Postextubation management.

- *Respiratory support:* The use of continuous positive airway pressure (CPAP) following extubation of preterm infants has been shown to reduce extubation failure compared to headbox or oxygen hood
- *Adjunctive therapies:*
  - *Caffeine:* Associated with faster weaning, within 2–7 days after initiation of the treatment. 52% less risk of failed extubation dose is 20 mg/kg/day bolus followed by 5 mg/kg/day
  - Caffeine improves functional residual capacity, compliance, outcomes such as extubation failure, number of days on invasive and noninvasive ventilation (NIV), and long-term outcomes like neurodevelopment
- *Nebulized racemic epinephrine* for postextubation stridor
- *Chronic diuretics:* Furosemide has been used in infants who are difficult to wean from ventilator, especially with evidence of fluid overload
- *Inhaled and/or systemic steroids:* For infants who have been intubated for prolonged periods, who have a history of traumatic or multiple endotracheal intubations, or who previously failed extubation owing to subglottic edema
- *Nutritional support:* Good calories, enteral, or parenteral nutrition

TABLE 3: Causes of failed extubation.

Airway/lung problem	Decreased respiratory drive	Muscular dysfunction	Neuromuscular	Cardiac
Mucus plugs and secretions	Excessive sedation	Muscle weakness	Diaphragmatic dysfunction	Hemodynamically significant PDA
Consolidation	Need for caffeine	Severe electrolyte disturbances	Prolonged neuromuscular blockade	Cor pulmonale
Severe cystic bronchopulmonary dysplasia (BPD)	Infection		Myotonic dystrophy	
Nasal obstruction	Central nervous system (CNS) abnormality		Spinal muscular atrophy	
Postextubation stridor (laryngeal edema, subglottic stenosis)	Hypocapnia		Brain anomaly	
Large airway anomalies (tracheomalacia)			Cervical spinal injury	
Congenital lung anomalies (e.g., congenital lobar emphysema)				

> ## Key Points to Remember
>
> ### What is Weaning?
>
> Weaning is the process of slowly decreasing the respiratory support as the condition of the infant improves.
>
> ### Aim of Weaning
>
> - Removing from positive pressure ventilation as soon as possible in line with protective lung strategies, to avoid potential damage from long-term or unnecessary ventilation.
> - "Reduce ventilation time as much as possible"
>
> ### When to Start Weaning?
>
> - Gas exchange is satisfactory and work of breathing is minimal
> - Primary disease is under control
> - Off sedation
> - Inotropes reduced
> - Baby is on patient-triggered ventilation (PTV) (volume-targeted ventilation).
>
> ### Basic Principles of Weaning
>
> - Most harmful parameter to be weaned first
> - Wean one parameter at a time with small decrements
> - Support work of breathing during weaning.
>
> ### How to do Weaning?
>
> - *Wean fraction of inspired oxygen (FiO$_2$):* Decrease 10% at a time, monitor oxygen saturation (SpO$_2$), keep saturation between 90 and 95%.
> - *Reduce peak inspiratory pressure (PIP):* Two at a time: Observe for chest rise, oxygenation, CO$_2$ retention, and Tidal volume: to keep at least 5–6 mL/kg.
> - Fast weaning of PIP leads to inadequate MV and mean arterial pressure (MAP), atelectasis, desaturation, and increased work of breathing which further increases FiO$_2$ and PIP requirement.
> - There is no "one-size-fits-all" protocol for weaning, it depends on experience, clinical, and other parameters.
> - Early weaning and extubation (<24 hours) seems feasible and might be protective for the lung and the brain.
> - Adjunctive therapies may increase success rate of extubation.

■ FURTHER READING

1. Davis PG, Henderson-Smart DJ. Nasal continuous positive airways pressure immediately after extubation for preventing morbidity in preterm infants. Cochrane Database Syst Rev. 2003;(2):CD000143.
2. Sant' Anna G, Keszler M. Weaning from mechanical ventilation. In: Goldsmith JP, Karotkin EH, Keszler M, Suresh GK (Eds). Assisted Ventilation of the Neonate, 6th edition. Philadelphia: Elsevier; 2017. pp. 243-50.

Continuous Positive Airway Pressure

Tejo Pratap

INDICATIONS

Respiratory distress:

- *Preterm infants (<35 weeks):* SAS score >3
- *Term infants (≥35 weeks):* SAS score >5
- Recurrent apneas in a preterm infant
- Postextubation in very low birth weight (VLBW) infant.

CONTRAINDICATIONS

- Poor respiratory efforts
- Nasal seal is poor (cleft palate)
- Tracheoesophageal fistula
- Congenital diaphragmatic hernia
- Pneumothorax and other air leak syndromes.

PRINCIPLES OF WORKING

- Splints upper airway resistance
- Decrease work of breathing
- Conserve surfactant
- Increases functional residual capacity (FRC)
- Increased tidal volume
- Increased lung compliance
- Decrease V/Q mismatch.

PREPARATION OF MACHINE AND INTERFACE

- Assemble the sterile circuit
- Fill distilled water in humidifier and clean water in bubble chamber
- Connect air and oxygen to blender, switch on the humidifier
- Fix the cap to the baby and appropriate size prongs to the cap
- Connect interface to the sterile circuit.

INITIAL SETTINGS

Initial settings depend on the underlying condition of the neonate.

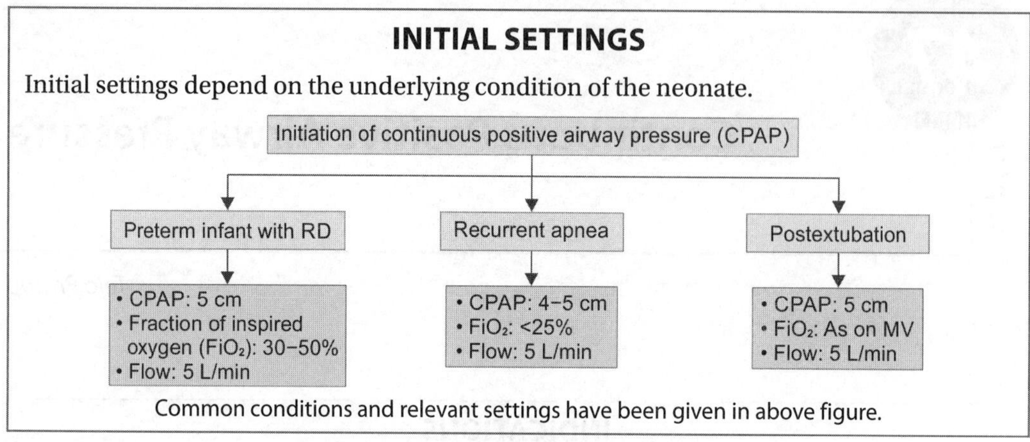

Common conditions and relevant settings have been given in above figure.

ADJUSTMENT OF CPAP PRESSURE AND FiO$_2$

- *Increase CPAP in steps of 1 cm:* If retractions present and SpO_2 < 90%, chest X-ray (half hour after starting) <6 spaces
- *Increase FiO$_2$ in steps of 5%:* If mild or no retractions and SpO_2 < 90%
- For every 10% increase in FiO_2 assess the need for increase in CPAP pressure by 1 cm
- No change in CPAP or FiO_2 is required if baby is comfortable, minimal or no retractions, CFT and BP are normal, SpO_2 between 90 and 95%, bubbling is good and breath sounds are heard.

FAILURE OF CPAP OR NEED FOR MECHANICAL VENTILATION

- SpO_2 < 90% on FiO_2 > 70% and CPAP > 7 cm
- Moderate to severe retractions on CPAP > 7 cm
- Recurrent apneas
- Shock or multiorgan dysfunction
- Poor respiratory efforts or $PaCO_2$ > 60 mm Hg.

NURSING CARE AND MONITORING

- Ensure correct size and function of nasal prongs
- Ensure gap between columella and nasal prongs
- Fix the prongs to the cap and cover ears with cap
- Remove prongs, inspect nostrils, use saline drops if needed, and do gentle massage in each shift
- Ensure water level in bubble chamber and humidifier
- Record depth of immersion of expiratory limb
- Maintain monitoring sheet.

WEANING OF CONTINUOUS POSITIVE AIRWAY PRESSURE

- Reduce FiO_2 if SpO_2 > 95% in steps of 5%
- If FiO_2 reduced by 10% and retractions are mild or absent, reduce CPAP pressure by 1 cm till CPAP is 5 cm and FiO_2 is 50%.
- Subsequently reduce FiO_2 in steps of 5% till FiO_2 < 30% before reducing CPAP pressure from 5 to 4 cm of water
- Remove CPAP if FiO_2 is < 25% and CPAP is 4 cmH_2O.

FURTHER READING

1. Keszler M, Gautham KS. Goldsmith's Assisted Ventilation of the Neonate: An Evidence-Based Approach to Newborn Respiratory Care, 7th edition; 2022.

Heated Humidified High-flow Nasal Cannula

Ashish Jain

INDICATIONS

- Neonates with bronchopulmonary dysplasia [to assist weaning from high fraction of inspired oxygen (FiO_2)]
- Respiratory support postextubation
- Nasal CPAP
- Neonates 34–36 weeks corrected gestational age as primary support
- Neonates not deemed stable enough to be tried self-ventilation in room air
- Postoperative respiratory support
- Babies with nasal trauma from nCPAP
- *Newer indications under trial:* Stabilization in delivery room, during intubation
- *Anesthetic induction:* THRIVE (transnasal humidified rapid insufflation ventilatory exchange).

CONTRAINDICATIONS

- Blocked nasal passage (choanal atresia)
- Trauma/surgery to nasopharynx
- Smaller babies with respiratory distress as the primary therapy
- Severe cardiovascular instability.

PRINCIPLES OF WORKING

- Heated humidified high-flow nasal cannula (HHHFNC) is small (<1 cm), tapered cannulae used to deliver heated, humidified high-flow air and blended oxygen at flow rates of >1 L/min.
- It has evolved as easy and user-friendly alternative to continuous positive airway pressure (CPAP), that proved to be gentler on noses with efficacy similar to CPAP in a significant proportion of babies.

ADVANTAGES

- Washout of nasopharyngeal dead space with better gas exchange
- Decrease in inspiratory resistance in upper airways and reduced work of breathing
- Improved lung compliance with warm and humidified gases
- Reduction of metabolic cost of gas conditioning
- Provision of distending pressure that allow better recruitment and oxygenation.

DISADVANTAGES

- Pressure is highly variable and cannot be measured or regulated
- There are no alarms with most high-flow nasal cannula (HFNC) systems
- Inability to select properly sized prongs could increase risk for lung injury (overexpansion or atelectasis) as well as gastric distention.

RECOMMENDED SETTINGS

- *Prongs:* Must be smaller than 50% of nares
- Flow 4–8 L/min
- FiO_2 usually <40%
- *Operating temperature:*
  - 34–35°C for 5 L/min
  - 36–38°C for >5 L/min
- Use appropriately sized nasal cannula (use manufacturer's weight guides)
- *Weaning:* Variable strategies—
  - It may not be possible to wean flow if $FiO_2 > 0.3$
  - Attempt to reduce by 1 L/min 24 hourly if $FiO_2 <0.25–0.3$ in >1.5 kg
  - Attempt to reduce by 0.5 L/min 12 hourly if $FiO_2 <0.25–0.3$ in <1.5 kg
  - Attempt to stop if requiring 2.0 L/min or less
  - If $FiO_2 > 0.1$ or increased WoB, return to previous settings

Failure: If the baby is requiring $FiO_2 > 0.5$ or has CO_2 retention, acidosis, or apnea, s/he is likely to need alternative support.

Key Points to Remember

- High-flow nasal cannula is an important part of neonatal respiratory care and has role in preterm >28 weeks gestational age in postextubation setting as well as can be applied successfully as primary support, though it is less effective than CPAP which should be readily available as rescue therapy.
- Further research into its use in extremely preterm infants, approach to assess surfactant necessity and optimal pathway to weaning will improve its usability and benefits.

■ FURTHER READING

1. Keszler M, Gautham KS. Goldsmith's Assisted Ventilation of the Neonate: An Evidence-Based Approach to Newborn Respiratory Care, 7th edition; 2022.

Sreedhara MS

49

Chapter

High-frequency Oscillatory Ventilation

PRINCIPLES OF WORKING

- *Turbulent vortices in large airways*: Turbulent vortices easily overcome the dead space of larger airways and transport oxygen during inspiration.
- *Asymmetric inspiratory/expiratory profiles*: During inspiration, there velocity is higher for oxygen-rich gases in the lower airways facilitating oxygen transport to alveoli. During expiration, the velocity is higher for oxygen poor gases in the upper airways facilitating clearing of carbon dioxide.
- *Radial mixing in main bronchi*: Turbulence during inspiration induces a stirring motion of gases predominantly in the right main bronchus causing efficient radial mixing of oxygen.
- *Laminar flow:* A decelerated laminar flow in distal airways allows for optimal diffusive gas transport.
- *Pendelluft*: Different regions of lungs have differences in compliance, this leads to flow between these regions.
- Direct ventilation of central alveoli.

TYPES

- *High-frequency jet ventilators*: Short pulses of high pressure gases are delivered to the upper airways.
- *High-frequency oscillators*: An electronically controlled piston oscillates to create pressure waves in a continuous bias flow.
- *High-frequency flow interrupters*: Inspiratory flows are altered electronically to achieve different peak inspiratory pressures.

INITIAL SETTINGS

- During high-frequency ventilators, alveolar ventilation which determines $pCO_2 = (\text{Tidal volume})^2 \times \text{Frequency}$
- During conventional ventilation, alveolar ventilation = Tidal volume × Respiratory rate.

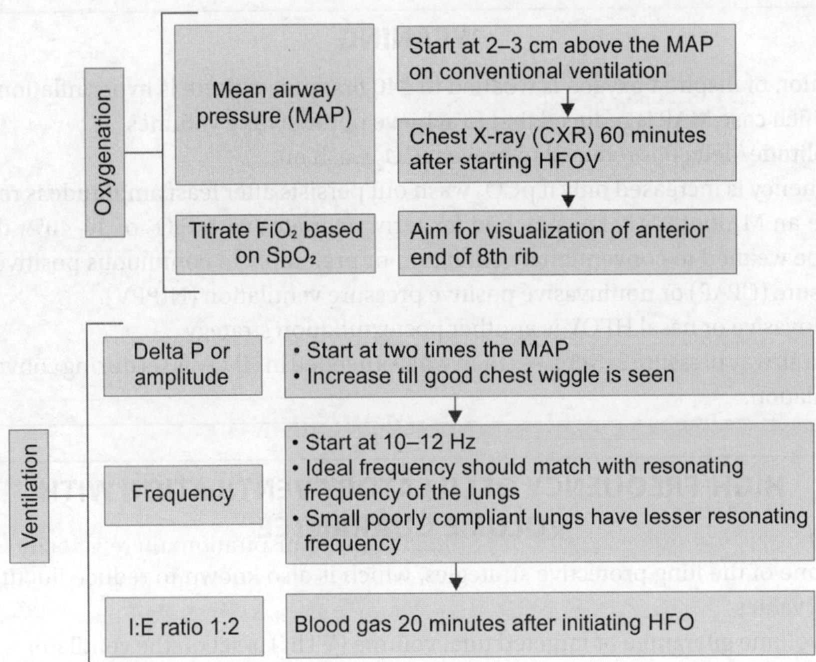

OPTIMIZATION OF VENTILATION

MAP

- Increase MAP in 1–2 cm increments to achieve good lung expansion
- CXR is useful to prevent hyperexpansion
- Excessive MAP increases intrathoracic pressure and decreases venous return causing shock

Delta P

- Increase delta P in 2–4 increments to achieve good chest wiggle
- Increase in delta P washes out pCO_2
- Can be increased to three times the MAP
- Monitor pCO_2 in blood gases frequently till stabilization

Frequency

- Frequency is based on the underlying pathology
- Low volume poorly compliant lungs example preterm RDS may need frequency of 8
- Term neonates with PPHN may need frequency of 12
- Reduction in frequency washes out pCO_2
- Generally frequency is a constant setting is not frequently changed
- When delta P is more than three times the MAP and pCO_2 is still high frequency can be reduced
- When delta P is less than two times the MAP and pCO_2 is low frequency can be increased

WEANING

- Fraction of inspired oxygen is weaned to ≤40 first unless there is hyperinflation in CXR in which case MAP is reduced first to achieve optimal lung volumes.
- Amplitude/delta P is reduced to prevent CO_2 wash out.
- Frequency is increased only if pCO_2 wash out persists after least amplitude is reached
- Once an MAP of 8–10, i.e., reached for term neonates with FiO_2 of 30–40%, the baby can be weaned to conventional ventilation or preferably to continuous positive airway pressure (CPAP) or noninvasive positive pressure ventilation (NIPPV).
- Noninvasive or nasal HFOV is another postextubation strategy.
- Mean airway pressure 2–3 cm less than what is needed in HFOV is set during conventional ventilation.

HIGH-FREQUENCY OSCILLATORY VENTILATION WITH VOLUME GUARANTEE

- It is one of the lung protective strategies, which is also known to reduce fluctuation in pCO_2 values
- The volume guarantee or targeted tidal volume (VThf) is set on the ventilator
- The VThf is usually around 1.5–3 mL per kg. It is decided based the pCO_2 in blood gases.
- The amplitude limit ($Ampl_{max}$) is set at 10–15% above the average amplitude required to reach the target tidal volume
- The ventilator changes the delta P or the amplitude to deliver the set tidal volumes.

■ FURTHER READING

1. Keszler M, Gautham KS. Goldsmith's Assisted Ventilation of the Neonate: An Evidence-Based Approach to Newborn Respiratory Care, 7th edition; 2022.

Inhaled Nitric Oxide

Anil Batra

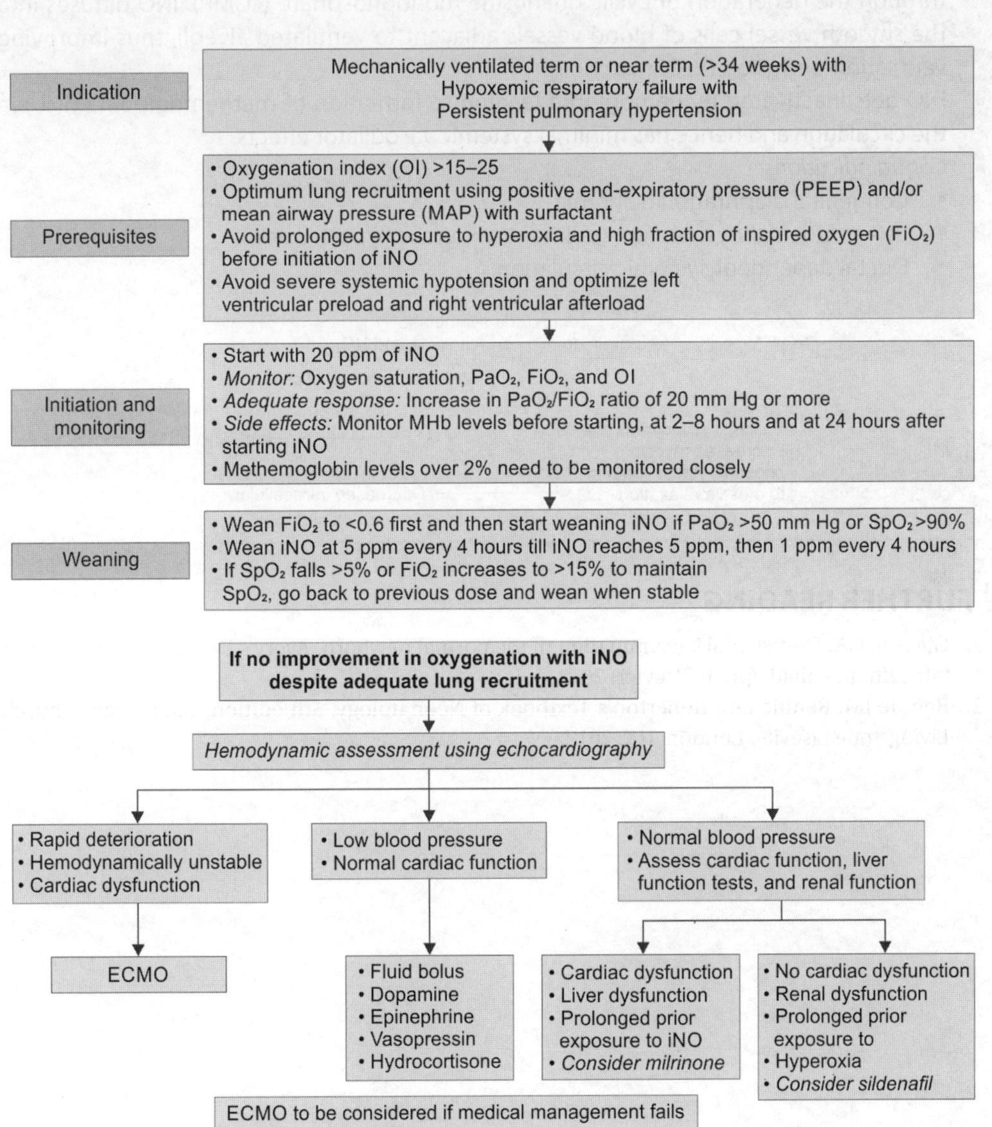

Key Points to Remember

- Inhaled nitric oxide (iNO) is the only United States Food and Drug Administration (US FDA) approved selective pulmonary vasodilator indicated in treatment of term and near term infants (>34 weeks gestational age) with hypoxemic respiratory failure with pulmonary hypertension.
- Inhaled nitric oxide reduces the need for extracorporeal membrane oxygenation (ECMO) and outcome of death in term neonates with persistent pulmonary hypertension of the newborn (PPHN).
- Endogenous NO is produced by endothelial cells and causes pulmonary vasodilation through the generation of cyclic guanosine monophosphate (cGMP). iNO diffuses into the smooth vessel cells of blood vessels adjacent to ventilated alveoli, thus improving ventilation-perfusion (V/Q) matching.
- iNO gets inactivated by hemoglobin leading to formation of methemoglobin (MHb) in the circulation and hence has minimal systemic vasodilator effects.
- *Contraindications:*
  - Congenital diaphragmatic hernia
  - Left ventricular dysfunction (pulmonary venous hypertension)
  - Ductal dependent systemic circulation.

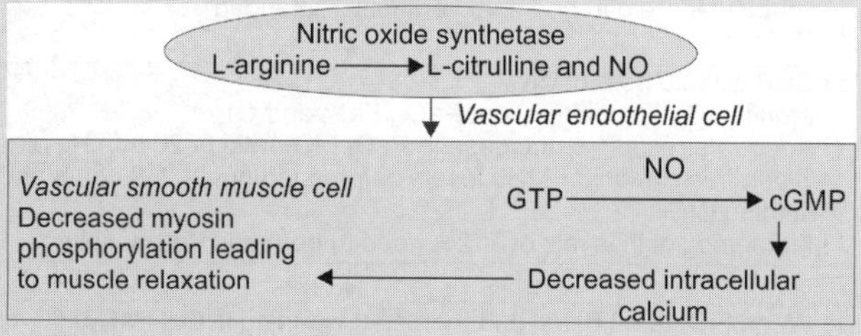

■ FURTHER READING

1. Gleason CA, Devaskar SU. Examination of the normal newborn. Avery's Diseases of the Newborn, 9th edition. Philadelphia: Elsevier; 2012.
2. Rennie JM. Rennie and Roberton's Textbook of Neonatology, 5th edition. Edinburgh: Churchill Livingstone Elsevier. London, UK; 2012.

Rachit Mehta, Vinay Joshi, Preetha Joshi

Extracorporeal Membrane Oxygenation

51

Chapter

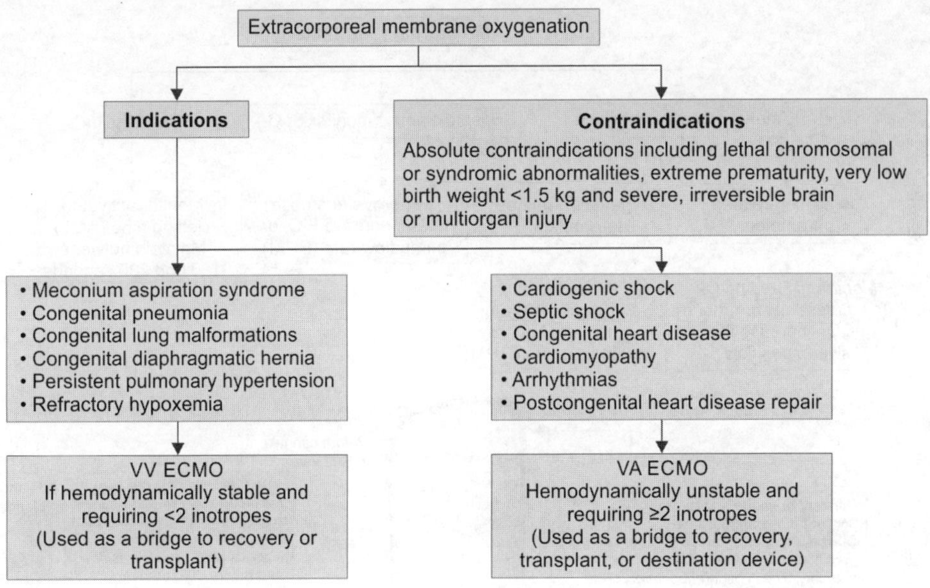

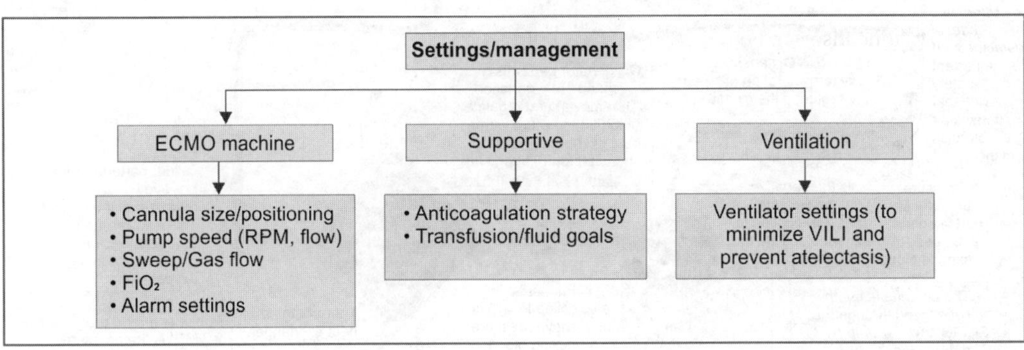

INITIAL SETTINGS

- Flow is usually set at 70–100 mL/kg/min but titrated to normalize lactate, mean arterial pressure, capillary refill time, and stable hemodynamics.
- For neonates, the whole circuit contains approximately 250 mL priming volume
- *Sweep gas:* 1–2 L/min
- *Fraction of inspired oxygen (FiO$_2$):* Based on pO$_2$ and saturations.
- Bolus heparin 50–100 unit/kg (maximum 5,000 units) for cannulation as indicated. Patients who are bleeding may require a smaller dose and titrate heparin infusion to maintain desired range as per institutional guidelines and institutional specific assay for maintaining anticoagulation (10–30 units/kg/h).

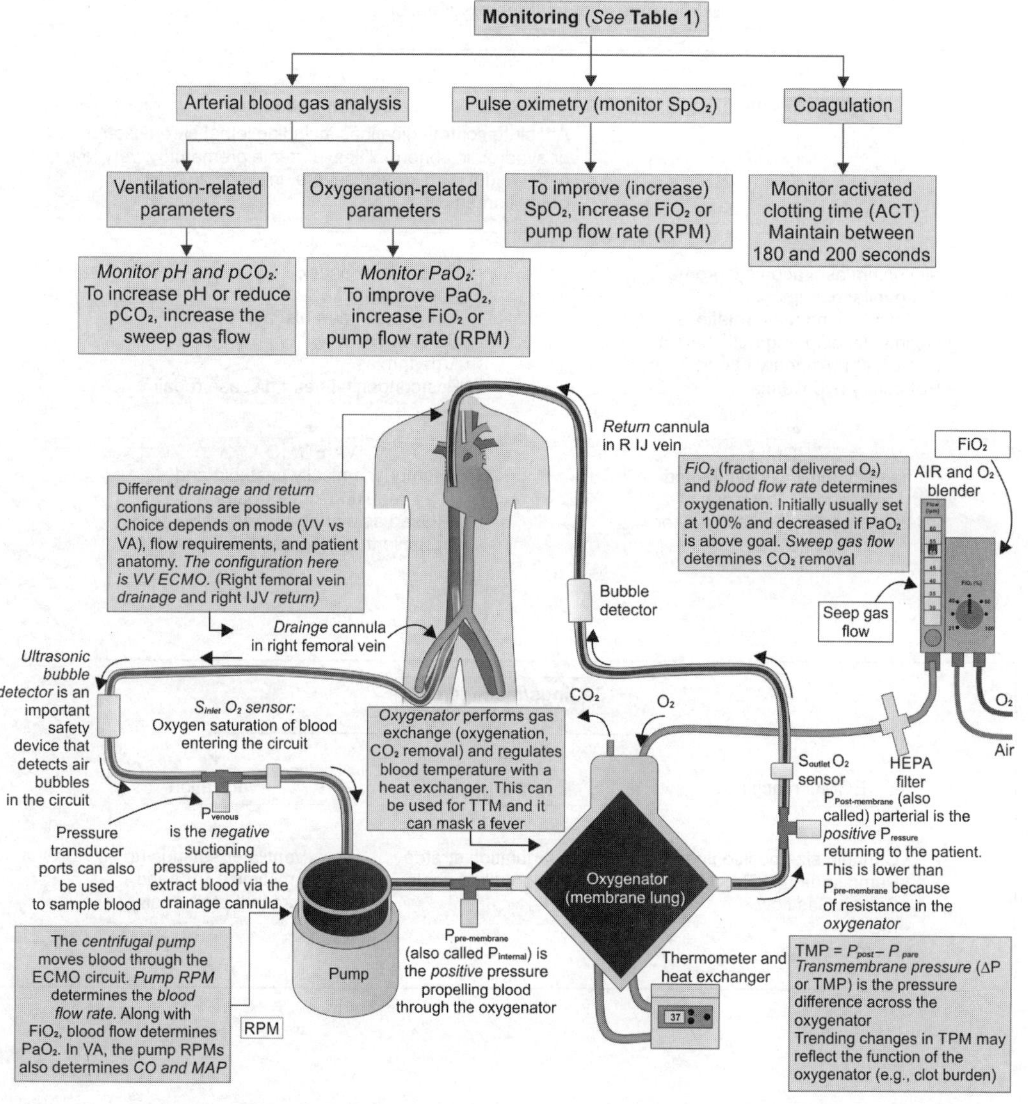

TROUBLESHOOTING

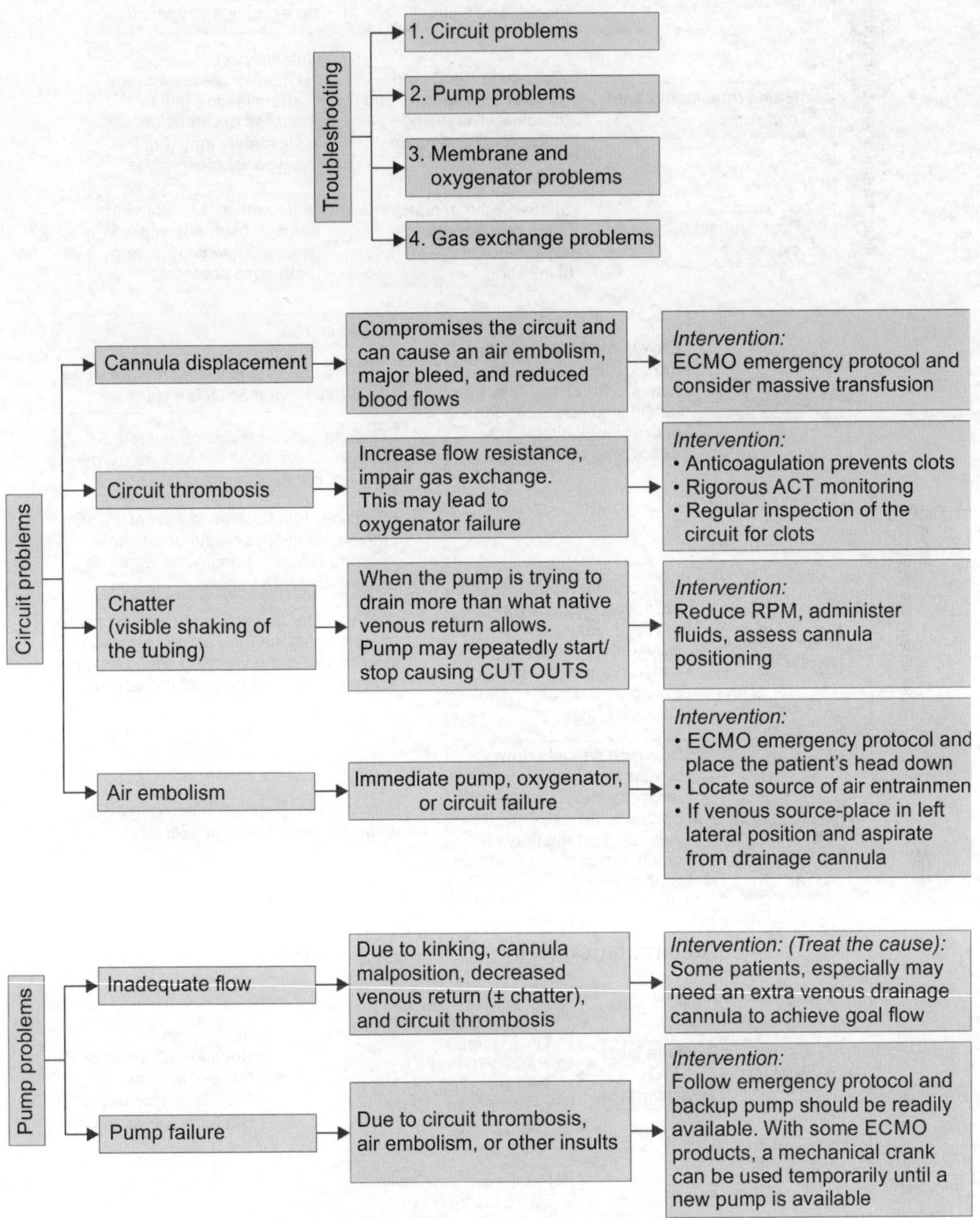

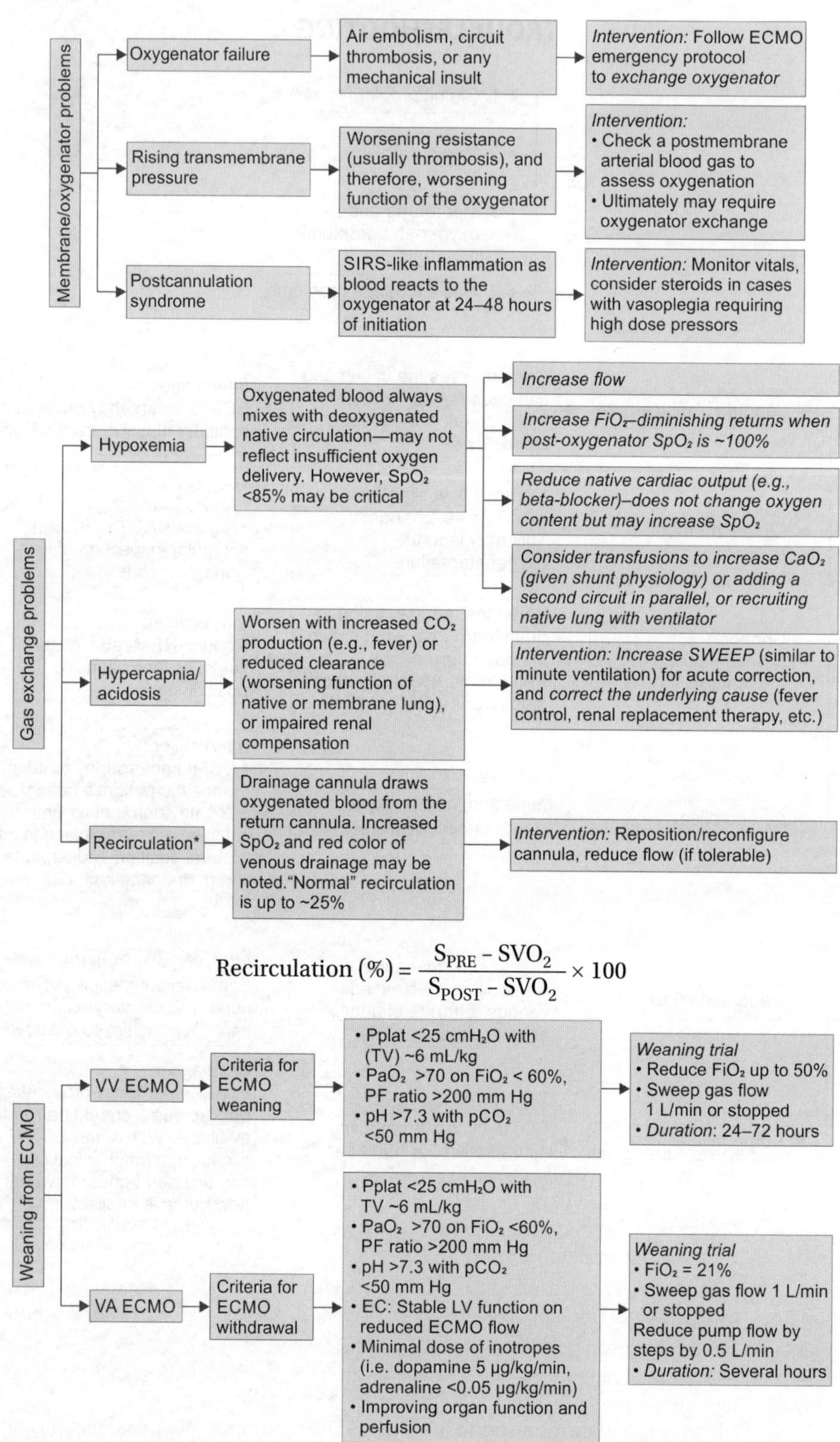

$$\text{Recirculation (\%)} = \frac{S_{PRE} - SVO_2}{S_{POST} - SVO_2} \times 100$$

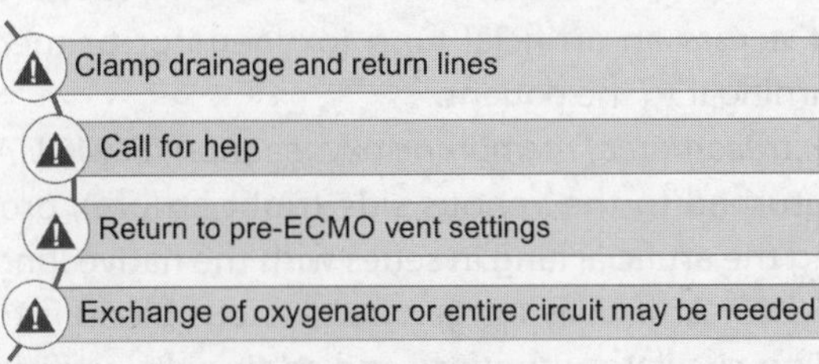

TABLE 1: Systemic monitoring on ECMO.

Neurological	• Monitor pupil size and equality as well as pupillary response to light (rule out cerebral bleed/intraventricular hemorrhage) • Monitor anterior fontanel for size and fullness • Cranial ultrasonography • Watch for any signs of seizure, electroencephalogram (EEG) monitoring if indicated • Cerebral function monitoring (CFM), near-infrared spectroscopy (NIRS) if available
Cardio-vascular	• Continuous cardiac monitoring • Assessment of electrocardiogram (ECG) for rhythm • Echocardiogram (ECHO) during weaning • Capillary refill time, peripheral and central pulses • Look for signs of edema
Respiratory	• Monitor pulse oximetry • Look for air entry and breathing sounds • Chest X-ray/lung ultrasound • Consider early tracheostomy if prolonged ECMO is predicted
Renal	• Monitor strict input output balance • Hemofiltration or hemodialysis may be added to ECMO circuit if renal failure does not improve
Abdomen	• Gastrointestinal bleed • Watch for necrotizing enterocolitis
Infection	• Complete blood count (CBC) with differential count, C-reactive protein (CRP) and surveillance cultures • Asses for signs of incisional and/or central access site infection • Antibiotics and fungal prophylaxis as per protocol
Pain and sedation	• Provide analgesia and sedation as appropriate to promote comfort and minimize stress (morphine/fentanyl, benzodiazepines) as per unit protocol • Avoid excessive movement which may result in cannula dislodgement or bleeding at the cannula site • Minimize use of muscle relaxants to assess neurological status and promote spontaneous respiratory effort
Family education	• Assess family's level of education, readiness to learn and provide information as appropriate • Utilize resources for support including social work, psychiatry, and chaplaincy as appropriate
Integument and immobility	• Gentle change in position every 2 hours as tolerated • Utilize pressure reducing surfaces as indicated (i.e., gel pads under pressure points) and monitor for pressure ulcers • Utilize appropriate resources to manage cannula and circuit during patient position

> ### Key Points to Remember
>
> - ECMO provides prolonged pulmonary and/or circulatory support by removing venous blood, pumping it across an artificial lung (oxygenator or membrane lung) for gas exchange, and returning it to the patient.
> - *Veno-venous (VV) extracorporeal membrane oxygenation (ECMO):* Artificially oxygenated venous blood is returned to the venous side (right atrium), providing no circulatory support, and adding the artificial lung in series with the native lung.
> - *Veno-arterial (VA) ECMO:* Artificially oxygenated venous blood is returned to the arterial side (aorta), providing circulatory support, and adding the artificial lung in parallel with the native lung.

■ FURTHER READING

1. Erdil T, Lemme F, Konetzka A, Cavigelli-Brunner A, Niesse O, Dave H, et al. Extracorporeal membrane oxygenation support in pediatrics. Ann Cardiothorac Surg. 2019;8(1):109.
2. Mufti HN, Rabie AA, Elhazmi AM, Bahaudden HA, Rajab MA, Al Enezi IS, et al. The Saudi Critical Care Society extracorporeal life support chapter guidance on utilization of veno-venous extracorporeal membrane oxygenation in adults with acute respiratory distress syndrome and special considerations in the era of coronavirus disease 2019. Saudi Med J. 2021;42(6):589-610.
3. Upadhyay G, Rao S, Joshi V, Joshi P. Pediatric cardiac ECMO: a review. J Pediatr Crit Care. 2017;4(2):54.

Management of Sepsis

Pratima Anand, Manisha Garg, Srishti Goel

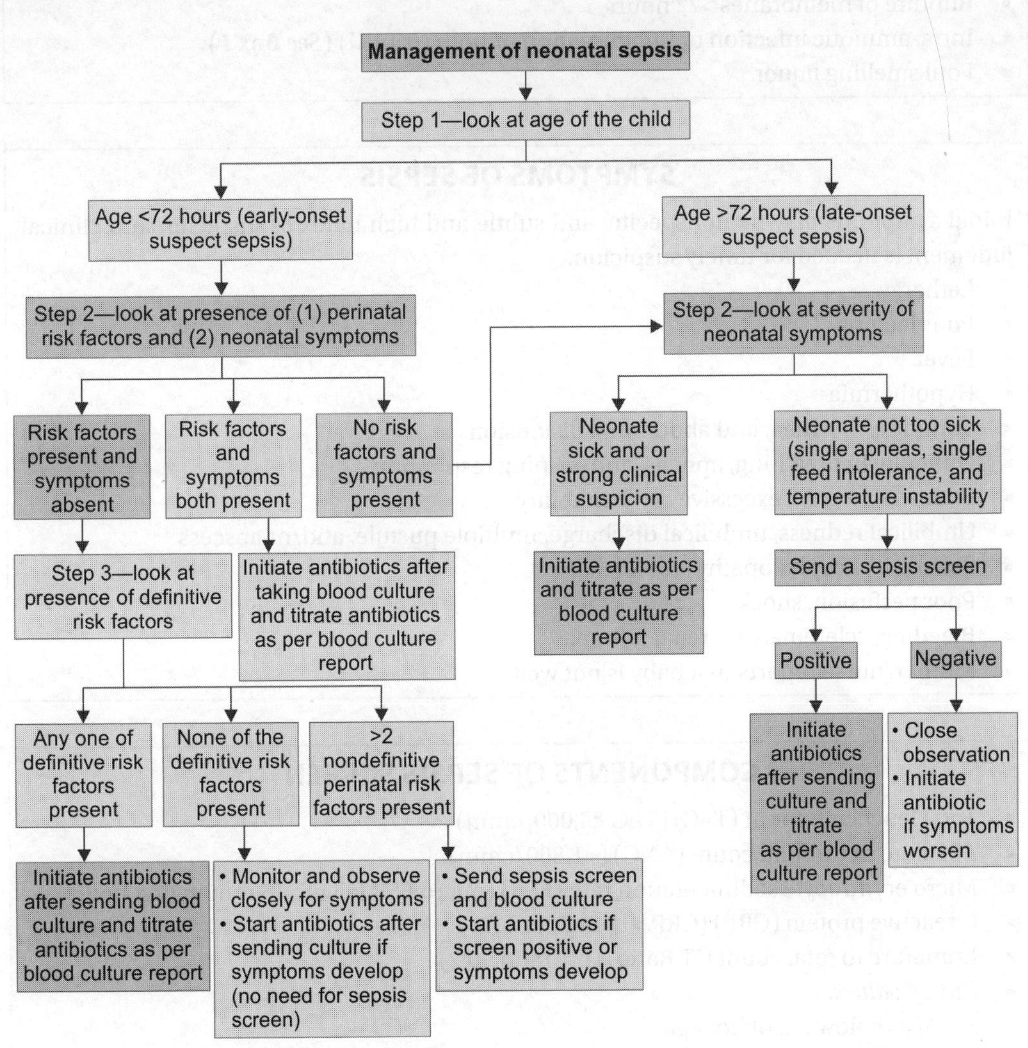

PERINATAL RISK FACTORS

- Rupture of membranes >24 hours
- Spontaneous preterm labor
- Presence of maternal fever >38°C
- Prolonged labor (duration of first and second stage labor >24 hours)
- Single unclean per vaginal examinations or >3 clean per vaginal examinations
- Perinatal asphyxia.

DEFINITIVE RISK FACTORS

- Rupture of membranes >72 hours
- Intra-amniotic infection or inflammation or both (triple I) (*See* **Box 1**)
- Foul smelling liquor.

SYMPTOMS OF SEPSIS

Initial symptoms may be nonspecific and subtle and high index of suspicion and clinical judgment is needed for timely suspicion.

- Lethargy
- Poor feeding
- Fever
- Hypothermia
- Vomiting, diarrhea, and abdominal distension
- Difficulty in breathing, apneas, and gasping respiration
- Poor weight gain, excessive cry/irritability
- Umbilical redness, umbilical discharge, multiple pustule, and/or abscess
- Seizures, encephalopathy
- Poor perfusion, shock
- Bleeding, sclerema, and renal failure.
- Mother/nurse reports that baby is not well

COMPONENTS OF SEPSIS SCREEN

- Total leucocyte count (TLC) (TLC <5,000/cmm)
- Absolute neutrophil count (ANC) (<1,800/cmm)
- Micro erythrocyte sedimentation rate (ESR) (micro ESR fall of >15 mm in first hour)
- C reactive protein (CRP) (CRP >10 mg per L)
- Immature to total count (IT Ratio) (I/T ratio >0.2)
- *Cut off values:*
  - ANC below cut off for age

Any two of the above constitute a positive sepsis screen.

Remember:
- Negative sepsis screen helps in ruling out sepsis; however, positive screen is not confirmatory of sepsis.
- There is no role of serial CRP in titrating the treatment of neonatal sepsis.

MANAGEMENT OF NEONATAL SEPSIS

Supportive Management

- Maintenance of temperature, airway, breathing and circulation
- Euglycemia
- Administration of vitamin K if not already administered.

Definitive Management

Initiation of appropriate antibiotics.

INDICATIONS OF INITIATING ANTIBIOTICS

- *First 72 hours of life:* Presence of definitive risk factors in the mother but asymptomatic neonate
- *First 72 hours of life:* Presence of more than two risk factors and symptomatic neonate
- *More than 72 hours of life:* Strong clinical suspicion of sepsis based on signs and symptoms, sick neonate
- *More than 72 hours of life:* Doubtful clinical symptoms and signs (single episode of fever/ single apnea/single feed intolerance episode) and well-baby: start if investigations are suggestive of sepsis.

CHOICE OF THE FIRST-LINE ANTIBIOTIC

- Do not start antibiotics without indication.
- Always send a blood culture before starting antibiotics.
- It is not possible to recommend a single antibiotic policy for use in all newborn units.
- It should be based on local culture and sensitivity data and profile of organisms for last 6-12 months. If not available, use data from nearby units or NNPD.
- Individual antibiotics and rational combinations of antibiotics must be evaluated for the percentage of organisms that they cover. The simplest and cheapest rational combination of antibiotics must be selected for each line.
- *First line:* Must cover approximately 75–80% of isolates
- *Second line:* Must cover approximately 90–95% of isolates
- *Third line:* Must cover approximately 95–100% of isolates

- Initial combination should cover both gram-negative and gram-positive organisms. One should use the lowest generation antibiotic combination which would cover about 70% of organisms. This is to ensure you have something to fall back on.
- Avoid cephalosporins as first-line antibiotics—proven harm (high risk of ELBS organisms, increased *Candida* infections, NEC, and mortality)—units who do not use have shown multiple benefits.
- Have a written unit/departmental/institutional antibiotic policy and practice antibiotic stewardship, i.e., have a written policy, write the reasons for starting the antibiotics, review the plan for antibiotics at 48 hours and again at 5 days based on culture reports and clinical course, have an exit plan, do not use reserve drugs without consultation.
- Antibiotic stewardship is the way forward to reducing the use of multiple antibiotics and resistance.

TITRATION OF ANTIBIOTICS

- Review the response of the antibiotics at 48 hours and clinical condition of the baby.
- If signs of sepsis disappeared and baby clinically improving, keep under observation and look for blood culture-sensitivity report.
- If signs of sepsis improving but still present, continue antibiotics and look for blood and CSF report.
- If signs of sepsis worsened or red signs appeared, upgrade antibiotics as per C&S report.
- Antibiotics need 48–72 hours to show effects, till that time aggressive supportive treatment should be the focus.
- When going from second-line to third-line antibiotics, give 72–96 hours at least for the effects to be seen.
- Empirical upgradation must be done if the expected clinical improvement with the ongoing line of antibiotics does not occur.
- Before changing, look for alternative reasons for sickness, diagnosis, and metabolic complications. Check whether dose is correct, dilution is correct, drug is not beyond shelf life and some drugs work better as infusions over few hours.
- Always take a repeat culture before changing.
- If the culture shows that the organism is sensitive to a lower generation antibiotic, in general one should downgrade.
- Believe a negative blood culture report and stop antibiotics if baby has recovered.
- Main utility of both CRP and procalcitonin is to rule-out sepsis. A positive test may also be due to several noninfective conditions. Therefore, a positive CRP or procalcitonin should be interpreted carefully giving due weightage to clinical course of the baby.

DURATION OF ANTIBIOTICS

- Blood culture positive sepsis (blood culture positive for growth of pathogenic organism)—14 days
- Meningitis (CSF culture positive of meningitis diagnosed based on CSF cellularity or biochemical parameters)—21 days
- Clinical sepsis—neonate symptomatic and clinician attributed the symptoms due to sepsis, but blood culture is negative for growth of any organism—5 days.

NO ROLE OF PROPHYLACTIC ANTIBIOTICS

- Extremely low birth weight/very low birth weight (ELBW/VLBW)
- Babies born by cesarean
- Twin of symptomatic baby
- Baby on IV fluids
- For colonization of—ET tube or elsewhere
- Meconium-stained liquor (MSL)
- Before or after exchange/partial transfusion.

No benefits—rather harmful. Increased mortality, increased necrotizing enterocolitis (NEC), increased fungal infections and late onset sepsis.

◼ MANAGEMENT OF FUNGAL SEPSIS

Risk factors.				
Immunity	*Medications facilitating fungal growth**	*Medications that suppress immune defense*	*Diseases*	*NICU practices*
• Extreme prematurity: Under developed immune system • Immune suppression • Neutropenia	• Cephalosporins* • Carbapenems* • Postnatal steroids*	• Histamine receptor antagonists* • Proton pump inhibitors (PPIs)* • Postnatal steroids*	• NEC • Prior BSI • Spontaneous intestinal perforation (SIP)/ focal bowel perforation • GI malformations • Hyperglycemia	• Prolonged use of antibiotics >5 days* • Multiple antibiotic usage* • Lack of enteral feeds* • Use of intralipid >7 days* • Indweller central venous catheter (CVC)* • Mechanical ventilation*

*Modifiable risk factors

Clinical Presentation

Nonspecific and variable course ranging from localized skin infection to disseminated end organ involvement.

Signs and symptoms	Common laboratory parameters
• *Mucocutaneous:* Oral thrush, diaper dermatitis • *Respiratory:* Frequent apnea, respiratory distress, pneumonia, increased oxygen requirement, and need for assisted ventilation • *Central nervous system:* Lethargy, hypotonia, meningitis, ventriculitis, and cerebral abscess	• Thrombocytopenia • Immature to total neutrophil ratio >0.2 • Increased CRP

Signs and symptoms	Common laboratory parameters
• *Gastrointestinal symptoms:* Feed intolerance, abdominal distension, blood in stools, peritonitis, and SIP (spontaneous intestinal perforation) • *Renal:* UTI and renal abscess • *Cardiac:* Hypotension, endocarditis, and thrombi • *Eye:* Endophthalmitis and chorioretinitis • *Bones and joints:* Septic arthritis and osteomyelitis	• Elevated WBC >20,000/cumm^3 • Hyperglycemia • Metabolic acidosis • Neutropenia <1,500/cumm^3

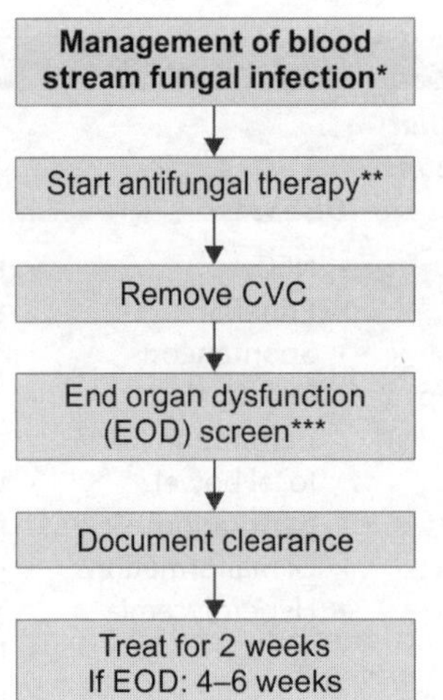

*Isolation of *Candida* species in blood culture

**Amphotericin B @ 1 mg/kg/day IV is initial DOC > fluconazole 12 mg/kg IV or PO Monitor for hypokalemia, renal tubular dysfunction, bone marrow toxicity

***Perform EOD screen at presentation and after 5–7 days of start of therapy. Involves:
• *Eye examination:* Retinitis/endophthalmitis
• Renal USG for fungal ball
• ECHO
• Cranial USG/CT/MRI

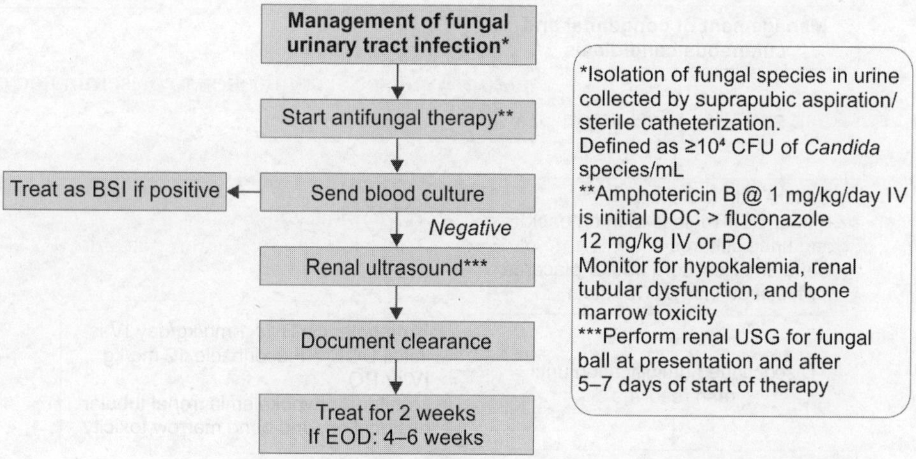

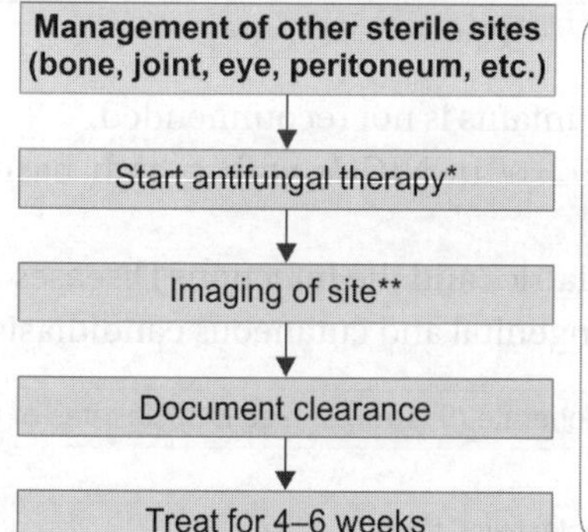

Management of fungal urinary tract infection*
Start antifungal therapy**
Send blood culture
Treat as BSI if positive
Negative
Renal ultrasound***
Document clearance
Treat for 2 weeks
If EOD: 4–6 weeks
*Isolation of fungal species in urine collected by suprapubic aspiration/ sterile catheterization.
Defined as ≥10⁴ CFU of *Candida* species/mL
**Amphotericin B @ 1 mg/kg/day IV is initial DOC > fluconazole 12 mg/kg IV or PO
Monitor for hypokalemia, renal tubular dysfunction, and bone marrow toxicity
***Perform renal USG for fungal ball at presentation and after 5–7 days of start of therapy

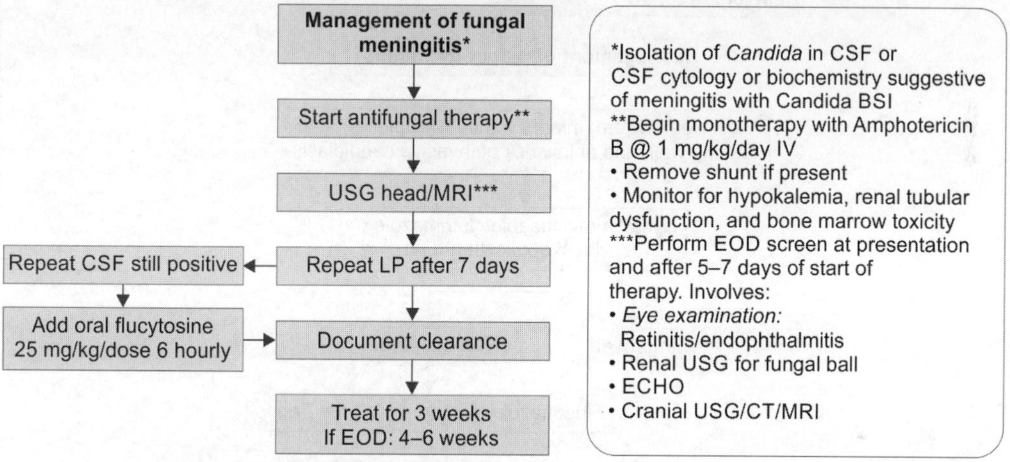

Management of fungal meningitis*
Start antifungal therapy**
USG head/MRI***
Repeat LP after 7 days
Repeat CSF still positive
Add oral flucytosine 25 mg/kg/dose 6 hourly
Document clearance
Treat for 3 weeks
If EOD: 4–6 weeks
*Isolation of *Candida* in CSF or CSF cytology or biochemistry suggestive of meningitis with Candida BSI
**Begin monotherapy with Amphotericin B @ 1 mg/kg/day IV
• Remove shunt if present
• Monitor for hypokalemia, renal tubular dysfunction, and bone marrow toxicity
***Perform EOD screen at presentation and after 5–7 days of start of therapy. Involves:
• *Eye examination:* Retinitis/endophthalmitis
• Renal USG for fungal ball
• ECHO
• Cranial USG/CT/MRI

Management of other sterile sites (bone, joint, eye, peritoneum, etc.)
Start antifungal therapy*
Imaging of site**
Document clearance
Treat for 4–6 weeks
* Amphotericin B @ 1 mg/kg/day IV is initial DOC > fluconazole 12 mg/kg IV or PO
Monitor for hypokalemia, renal tubular dysfunction, and bone marrow toxicity
** Perform EOD screen at presentation and after 5–7 days of start of therapy Involves:
• *Eye examination:* Retinitis/ endophthalmitis
• Renal USG for fungal ball
• ECHO
• Cranial USG/CT/MRI

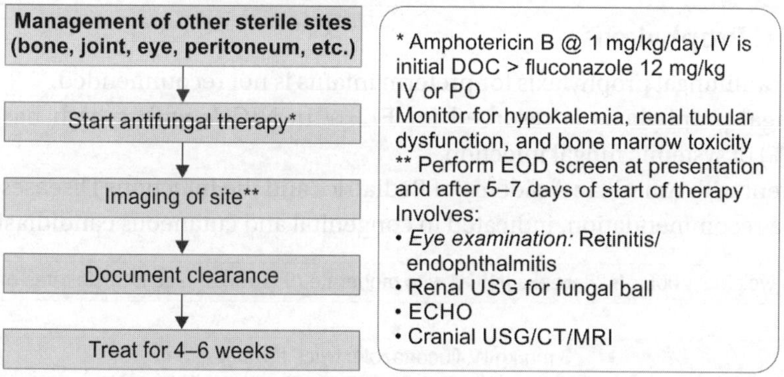

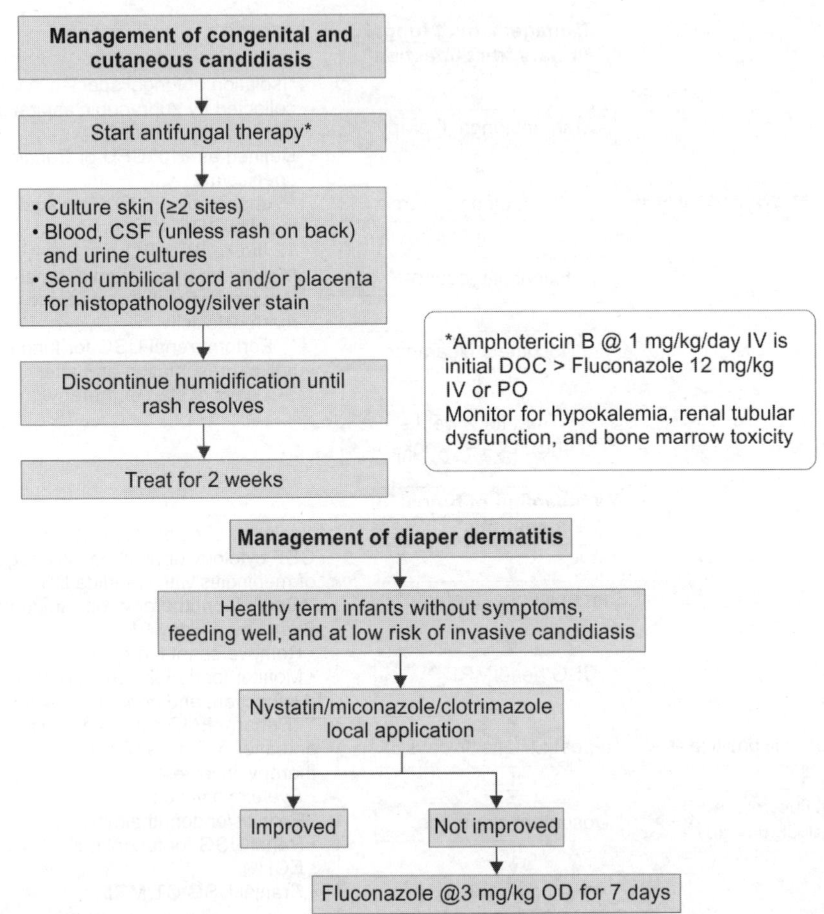

Antifungal Prophylaxis

- Routine antifungal prophylaxis for preterm infants is not recommended.
- Antifungal prophylaxis is reserved for ELBW in NICUs with a high baseline rate (>5–10%) of systemic fungal infection.
- Consistent with American Academy of Pediatrics and the Infectious Diseases Society of America recommendation, indicated in congenital and cutaneous candidiasis.

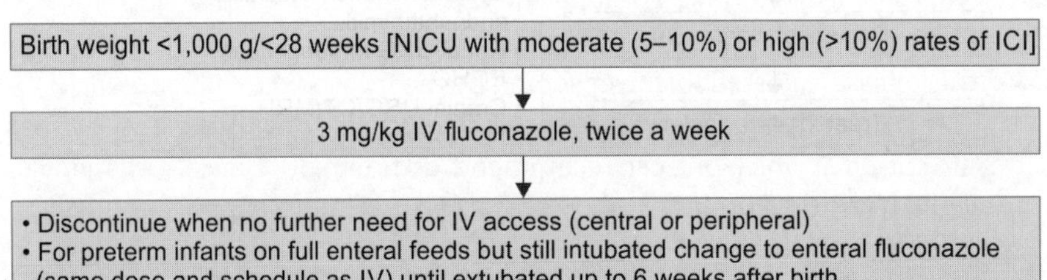

Key Points to Remember

Definition of Intra-amniotic Infection or Inflammation or Both (Triple I)

- *Maternal fever:* Maternal axillary temperature >38°C (100.4° F) on any one occasion.
- *Suspected triple I:* Fever without a clear source plus any of baseline fetal tachycardia (>160 BPM for >10 min)
- Maternal total leukocyte count (TLC) >15,000/cmm in absence of corticosteroids
- Definite purulent fluid from cervical os
- *Confirmed triple I:* All the above plus laboratory findings such as
  - Positive amniotic fluid gram stain/culture
  - Histopathological evidence of infection or inflammation or both in placenta.
- Early initiation and rapid advancement of enteral feeds.
- Minimize use and duration of IV alimentation.
- Rational use (dose, duration, type, and mode) of antibiotics.
- Removal of indwelling catheters when no longer required (within 7–10 days).
- Avoid usage of PPIs, H$_2$ antagonists, third-generation cephalosporins.

Management of Fungal Sepsis

- Invasive fungal infections encompass infections largely caused by *Candida* species (*C. albicans* > *C. parapsilosis* > *C. glabrata*) and with a small portion caused by *Aspergillus*, *Zygomycetes, Malassezia, and Trichosporon.*
- Invasive *Candida* infections (ICI) in neonates include congenital cutaneous candidiasis (CCC) and late-onset cutaneous candidiasis, bloodstream infections (BSIs), urinary tract infections (UTIs), meningitis, peritonitis, and infection of other sterile sites (bone and joint infections).
- *Incidence:* Inversely proportional to birth weight and gestational age 1–4% in VLBW and 2–8% in ELBW and 20% in <26 weeks/ <750 g neonates.
- *Definition of meningitis:*
  - *Culture positive meningitis:* Cerebrospinal fluid (CSF) culture is positive for growth of any organism.
  - Diagnosis of meningitis based on CSF cellularity and biochemical parameters:
    - *Preterm infants:* Treat if CSF WBC count ≥10 or glucose <24 or protein >170. Do not treat if "CSF WBC count <25 and glucose ≥25 and protein <170". For in-between results, clinical judgment will have to be used, keeping in mind clinical features (seizures, degree of altered sensorium, and fullness of fontanels) and prematurity (the lower the gestation, lower should be the threshold for diagnosis).
    - *Term infants:* Treat if CSF WBC count >8 or glucose <20 or protein >120. There is no safe cut-off at which one can recommend "do not treat". Clinical judgment as above would have to be used.

- *Lumbar puncture:*
  - It should be performed in all neonates with suspected late-onset sepsis prior to initiation of antibiotics.
  - In early-onset sepsis, lumbar puncture should be done in all symptomatic neonates suspected of sepsis, possible exceptions being (1) asymptomatic neonates where suspicion is due to maternal risk factors (LP in these cases also must be done if blood culture turns positive later) and (2) preterm neonates with respiratory symptoms attributed to surfactant deficiency/respiratory distress syndrome (RDS).

Best practices to prevent neonatal infections:

- Hand washing or alcohol-based hand rub should be practiced for hand hygiene
- Asepsis should be maintained during the delivery
- Early diagnosis and management of maternal infections
- Early and exclusive breastfeeding
- No prelacteal feeds
- Clean and dry cord
- Avoid overcrowding of NICUs
- Aseptic non-touch technique (ANTT) should be followed during all invasive procedures
- Neonatal units should implement central line insertion care bundle and ventilator associated pneumonia (VAP) prevention bundle
- Regular educational activities about prevention of healthcare associated infections should be conducted for healthcare professionals

■ FURTHER READING

1. Facility Based Newborn Care, Training Module for Doctors and Nurses, MoHFW, GoI; 2022.
2. Indian Council of Medical Research New Delhi. (2005). National Neonatal Perinatal Database Network: report for 2002–2003. [online] Available from https://www.newbornwhocc.org/pdf/nnpd_report_2002-03.PDF [Last accessed September, 2022].
3. Investigators of the Delhi Neonatal Infection Study (DeNIS) collaboration. Characterisation and antimicrobial resistance of sepsis pathogens in neonates born in tertiary care centres in Delhi, India: a cohort study. Lancet Glob Health. 2016;4(10):e752-60.
4. Sundaram V, Kumar P, Dutta S, Mukhopadhyay K, Ray P, Gautam V, et al. Blood culture confirmed bacterial sepsis in neonates in a North Indian tertiary care center: changes over the last decade. Jpn J Infect Dis. 2009;62:46-50.

Antibiotic Stewardship

Somosri Ray

DEFINITION

Antimicrobial stewardship (AMS) in simple term is defined as "the right antibiotic, for the right indication (right diagnosis), on the right patient, at the right time, with the right dose and route, causing the least harm to the patient and population".

GOAL

- Optimize clinical outcome
- Minimize adverse consequences of antimicrobial use (adverse drug reaction/toxicity of antimicrobials, drug resistance, necrotizing enterocolitis, and fungal infection)
- Reduction of healthcare cost
- Maintenance of quality of care.

PRINCIPLES

Remember the mnemonic of MINDME.
- M—Microbiology guides therapy
- I—Indication should be evidence based
- N—Narrowest spectrum required
- D—Dose should be appropriate
- M—Minimize duration of therapy
- E—Ensure monotherapy in most cases.

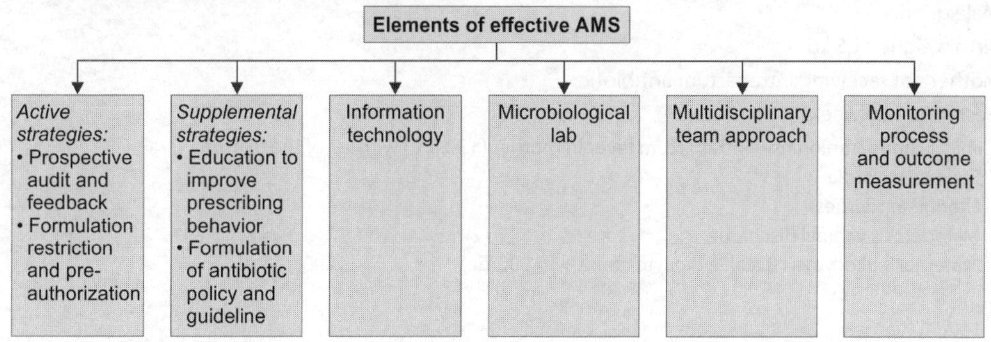

Q1: When to initiate empirical antibiotic in a neonate?

When sepsis is a possibility and patient is very sick with (red flag signs):
- Shock
- Sclerema
- Disseminated intravascular coagulation (DIC)
- Respiratory distress requiring intubation/Silverman score >6

When main differential diagnosis is sepsis (yellow flag signs):
- New-onset respiratory distress
- Worsened respiratory distress in case of primary diagnosis of transient tachypnea of newborn/meconium, aspiration, etc.
- Unexplained encephalopathy/lethargy/floppiness/refusal to feed
- Seizures
- Recurrent apnea
- Abdominal distension, bilious aspirate
- Unexplained bleeding diathesis
- Symptomatic neonate with positive sepsis screen
- Fever
- Diarrhea
- Heart rate (HR) >160 bpm persisting for 1 hour despite normal temperature

Asymptomatic neonates with risk of early-onset sepsis (EOS):
- High perinatal scores* (≥7) (for <35 weekers) (*see* **Table 1**)
  OR
- Presence of foul smelling liquor in any delivery
  OR
- Presence of any three of the following risk factors or two risk factors with positive sepsis screen in any neonate:
  - Low birth weight (<2,500 g) or prematurity
  - Febrile illness in mother with evidence of bacterial infection within 2 weeks prior to delivery
  - Rupture membrane ≥18 hours
  - Single unclean or >3 sterile vaginal examination during labor
  - Perinatal asphyxia (Apgar score <4 at 1 minute)
  - Prolonged labor (sum of first and second stage of labor >24 hours)
- Prolonged labor ≥24 hours

*Perinatal score—babies born <35 weeks, asymptomatic till 2 hours of life assessed for risk of EOS and evaluated using a score called perinatal score.
Score 0–6—observe for signs and symptoms of sepsis till 72 hours of birth
Score ≥7—send blood culture and start empirical intravenous antibiotics

TABLE 1: Perinatal score assessment.

Risk factor	*Score*
Intrapartum per vaginal examination ≥3	6
Clinical chorioamnionitis*	6
Male gender	3
Birth weight ≤1.5 kg	3
Mother not receiving intrapartum antibiotic	2
Gestation <30 weeks	2

*Clinical chorioamnionitis—intrapartum fever in mother (>37.8°C) with ≥2 of the features
- Fetal tachycardia
- Uterine tenderness
- Malodorous vaginal discharge
- Maternal leukocytosis (total leukocyte count >15,000/dL)

Q2: When not to initiate empirical antibiotic in a neonate?

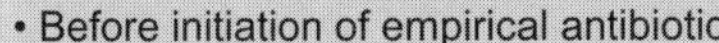

In situations where the signs and symptoms are subtle along with an alternative explanation and treating team feels the need for laboratory evidence to initiate antibiotics:
- Newborn with feed intolerance [may be due to absent/reversed end-diastolic flow in maternal Doppler (AEDF/REDF)/top feed/polycythemia]
- Preterm/small for gestational age (SGA) having hypoglycemia in first 72 hours
- Meconium aspiration syndrome (MAS) with persistent respiratory distress/oxygen requirement
- Fresh onset respiratory distress on D2-3 with oxygen requirement in preterm with clinical and echocardiographic features of patent ductus arteriosus (PDA)

Q3: When to send blood culture in a neonate?

- Before initiation of empirical antibiotic
- Before upgradation of antibiotic, nonresponsive to lower line antibiotic
- At least 1 mL of blood to be taken inside culture bottle
- Rapid blood culture method example, BACTEC is preferred method
- Culture bottle should be put for incubation within 1 hour of sample drawn

Q4: What should be choice of empirical antibiotic in neonate?

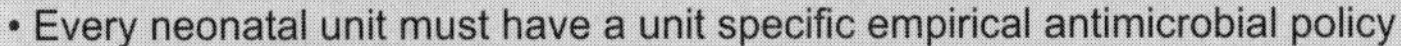

- Every neonatal unit must have a unit specific empirical antimicrobial policy
- Local antibiogram (list of antibiotics sensitive to kill the commonly isolated organisms) guides to form the policy: (Using 3–6 months @ last 30–40 culture reports)
  - First line should be able to cover roughly 75% of bacteria
  - The second line should be able to cover 95%
  - Third line should be able to cover 100% of organisms
- If ≥2 antibiotics/combinations qualify from antibiogram:
  - Choose the widest possible coverage
  - Choose with minimal side effects
  - Choose the cheapest
- The policy should be periodically reviewed and updated at an interval 1 year at least

Q5: How to prescribe antibiotic in neonate?

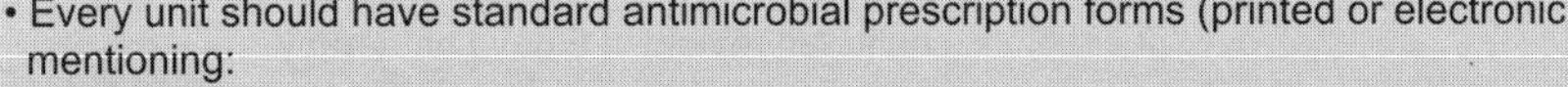

- Every unit should have standard antimicrobial prescription forms (printed or electronic) mentioning:
  - Indication
  - Dose
  - Dilution
  - Duration
  - Route

Q6: How fast to administer antibiotic once decision of antibiotic initiation taken?

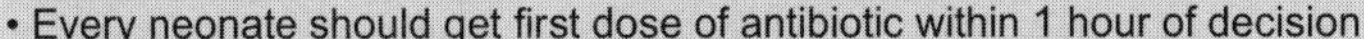

- Every neonate should get first dose of antibiotic within 1 hour of decision
- First dose preferably not to be given before drawing blood culture

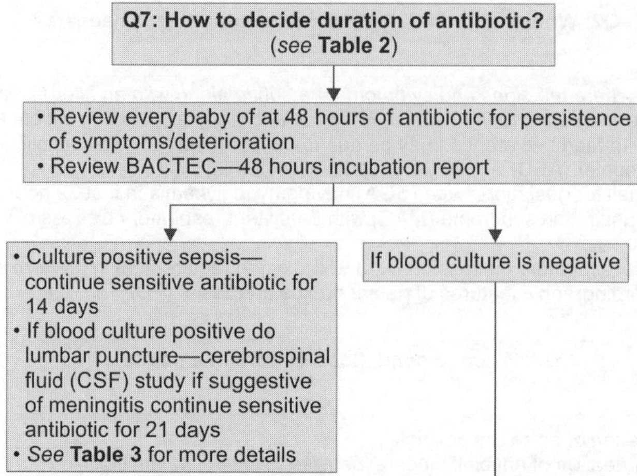

Clinical parameters	Baby receiving antibiotic	
	Alternative explanation other than sepsis present	*Alternative explanation other than sepsis absent*
Asymptomatic within 48 hours	Stop antibiotics	Stop antibiotics
Partially improves within 48 hours	Stop antibiotics	Follow clinically and stop whenever asymptomatic till 4–5 days
Baby condition static in first 48 hours	Stop antibiotics	Do C-reactive protein (CRP)/procalcitonin, stop antibiotics if twice CRP/procalcitonin is negative
Baby deteriorates within 48 hours	Don't escalate but If baby develops sclerema/shock/DIC, escalate to next line antibiotic after consultant review	
Baby deteriorates after 48 hours	Repeat blood culture, sepsis screen and upgrade antibiotic If alternative explanation other than sepsis is strong, serial septic screen is negative may stop antibiotic	Repeat blood culture, sepsis screen and upgrade antibiotic, assess baby along with laboratory reports at 48 hours and day 5 of antibiotic for continuation or further upgradation of antibiotic
Clinical parameters	**Baby receiving antibiotic**	
	If antibiotic continued review at 5 days of therapy	
If baby is well from last 48 hours, blood culture sterile and CSF are normal	Stop antibiotic	Stop antibiotic
If static	Stop antibiotic	Do CRP/procalcitonin, stop antibiotics if twice CRP/procalcitonin is negative
If deteriorates	Repeat blood culture, sepsis screen and upgrade antibiotic If alternative explanation other than sepsis is strong, serial septic screen is negative may stop antibiotic	Repeat blood culture, sepsis screen and upgrade antibiotic, assess baby along with laboratory reports for continuation or further upgradation of antibiotic
Blood culture negative meningitis	Continue same antibiotic 21 days provided asymptomatic	

TABLE 2: Duration of antibiotic in following situations.

Scenarios of proven sepsis	Duration in days
Blood culture positive sepsis	14
Blood culture negative and sepsis screen positive sepsis	5–7
Meningitis	21
Blood culture negative but chest X-ray suggestive pneumonia	5–7
Urinary tract infection (urine culture positive)	14
Urinary tract infection (urine culture negative)	10
Non-*Staphylococcus aureus* isolation without meningitis/deep seated infection in rapidly asymptomatic neonate	Shorter than 14 days with consultant review
Ventriculitis	42
Deep-seated infections	42
Bone infection	42–56

TABLE 3: Trouble shooting in blood culture positive sepsis situations.

Practical scenario	Possible explanation	How to tackle?
Empirical antibiotic reported sensitive but neonate has worsened on it	In vivo resistance	Start alternate sensitive antibiotic with narrowest spectrum
Empirical antibiotic reported resistant but neonate is improved	In vivo sensitivity	May continue same after consultant review
Empirical antibiotic reported resistant while isolated organism *Pseudomonas/Klebsiella/* Methicillin-resistant *Staphylococcus aureus/* deep-seated infection/meningitis	In vitro resistance	Must not continue with same antibiotic. Change to sensitive one with narrowest spectrum
If no antibiotic reported sensitive but one or more reported as "moderately sensitive"	–	Change to moderate sensitive antibiotic with highest permissible dose

Q8: If blood culture facility is not there how to take decision of duration of antibiotics, started as empirical therapy?

- A negative CRP (<12 mg/L) or procalcitonin (<1.1 ng/mL) at 48 hours after starting antibiotics, can help in early stopping of antibiotics
- If baby still symptomatic at 48 hours and alternative explanation other than sepsis is not there serial negative CRP/procalcitonin after 48 hours can help in early stopping of antibiotics
- During first 72 hours of life, CRP/procalcitonin may remain high due to physiological surge hence falling trend of serial values more assuring than absolute number
- CRP/procalcitonin can be high in various noninfective conditions, hence judgment regarding clinical course is mandatory

Q9: If *Pseudomonas aeruginosa/Acinetobacter baumannii* get isolated in BACTEC blood culture—do these require combination of sensitive antibiotics after getting culture sensitivity report?

Monotherapy is preferred than combination antimicrobial therapy for treatment of culture-positive systemic sepsis

Q10: How does culture sensitivity report guide choice of antibiotic?

- Down-gradation (de-escalation) of antibiotic is mandatory if the isolated organism is found to be sensitive to lower generation of antibiotic
- Selection of antibiotic preferably not to be based on the lowest minimum inhibitory concentration (MIC value) of antibiotics

Q11: Is there any process to monitor antimicrobial therapy of a neonate?

- Every unit should have a team of neonatologist, microbiologist, pharmacologist, pharmacist, and nurse to monitor the process of antimicrobial therapy
- This team should audit the following:
  - Selection
  - Indication
  - Duration
  - Dose
  - Route
  - Followed by feedback to SNCU/NICU staff

Q12: Can we switch to oral therapy from parenteral therapy after certain days?

In preterm and sick term hospitalized neonates completion of antibiotic course is preferred by parenteral route only rather than switching to oral therapy following short course of parenteral antibiotic

Q13: *Is there any role of prophylactic antibiotic specially in following situations to prevent sepsis?*
- Neonates with indwelling central arterial/venous catheters
- Neonates on invasive ventilation
- Neonates getting total parenteral nutrition
- Prematurity
- Noninfectious morbidities (e.g., MAS)

Systemic antibiotic should not be used if clinical symptoms, signs of sepsis not there

Key Points to Remember

- Do not start antibiotics without indication.
- Clinical features in neonates are nonspecific.
- Look for alternative reasons for sickness to avoid unnecessary use of antibiotics.
- Believe a negative blood culture report and stop antibiotics if baby has recovered.
- Every unit should have antibiotic stewardship protocol.
- Cochrane meta-analysis showed increased compliance to antibiotic policy and guideline along with reduction in antibiotic days following implementation of AMS in healthcare practices.
- No risk of increased sepsis or mortality in preterm neonates was observed in a recent systematic review on AMS while they achieved to reduce initiation of antibiotics in low-risk infants, reduction in duration of antibiotics.

■ FURTHER READING

1. Antibiotic_Stewardship_in_neonatal_care-NNFI_CPG_Dec2021.
2. Barlam TF, Cosgrove SE, Abbo LM, MacDougall C, Schuetz AN, Septimus EJ, et al. Implementing an Antibiotic Stewardship Program: Guidelines by the Infectious Diseases Society of America and the Society for Healthcare Epidemiology of America. Clin Infect Dis. 2016;62(10):e51-77.
3. Davey P, Marwick CA, Scott CL, Charani E, McNeil K, Brown E, et al. Interventions to improve antibiotic prescribing practices for hospital inpatients. Cochrane Database Syst Rev. 2017;2:CD003543.
4. Dutta S, Reddy R, Sheikh S, Kalra J, Ray P, Narang A. Intrapartum antibiotics and risk factors for early onset sepsis. Arch Dis Child Fetal Neonatal Ed. 2010;95(2):F99-103.
5. Rajar P, Saugstad OD, Berild D, Dutta A, Greisen G, Lausten-Thomsen U, et al. Antibiotic stewardship in premature infants: A systematic review. Neonatology. 2020;117(6):673-86.

Chapter 54

Management of Neonatal COVID-19

Swati Manerkar, Kalathingal Thaslima Aboobacker

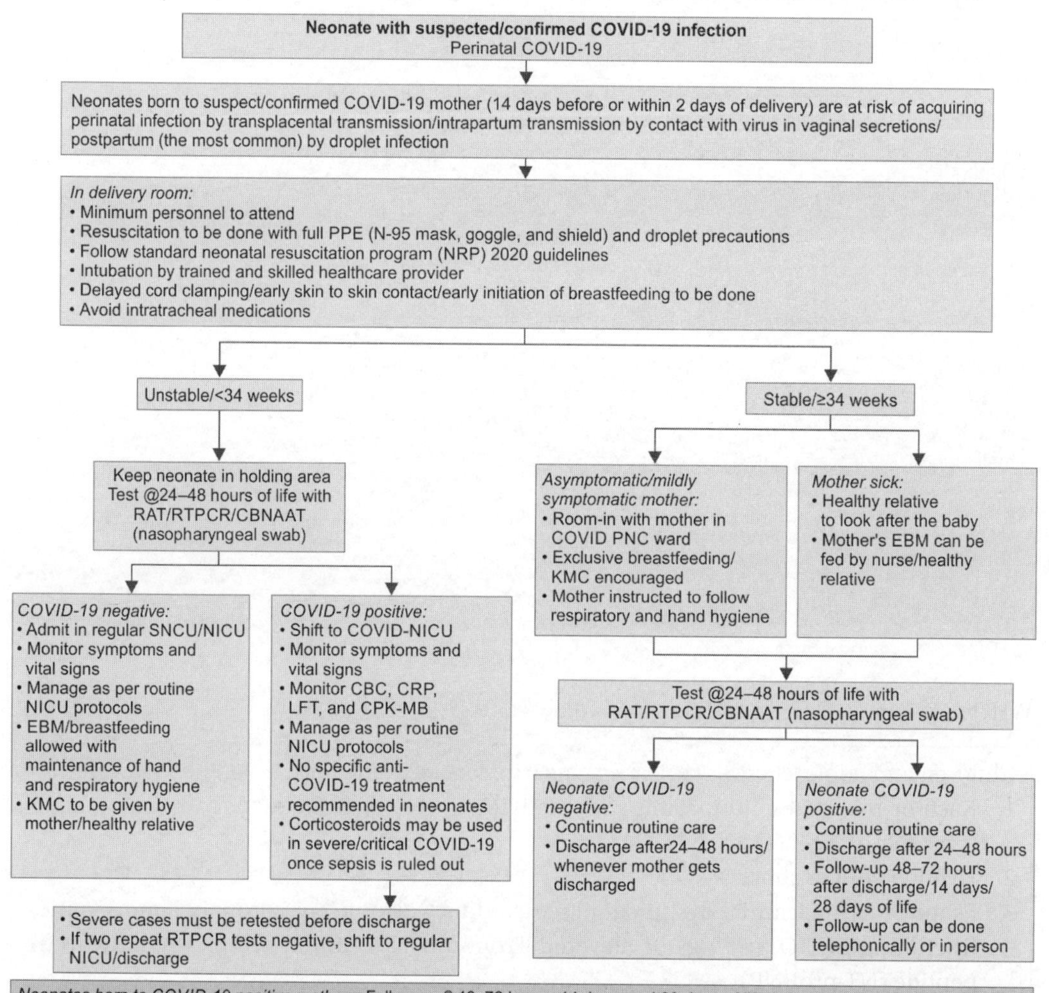

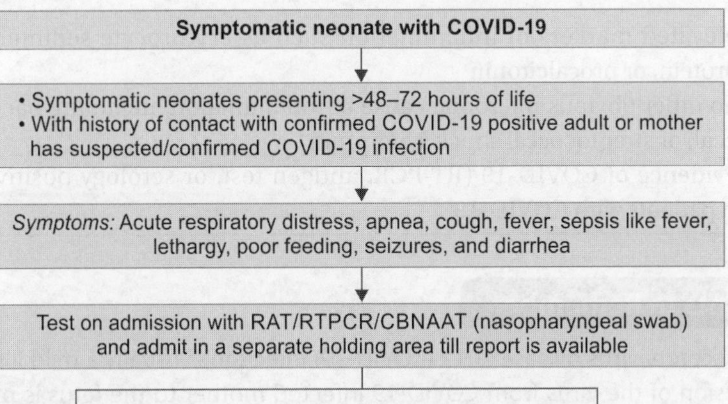

WHO definition of MIS in children and adolescents (0–19 years):

Children and adolescents 0–19 years of age with fever ≥3 days and *two* of the following:

1. Rash or bilateral nonpurulent conjunctivitis or mucocutaneous inflammation signs (oral, hands, or feet)
2. Hypotension or shock
3. Features of myocardial dysfunction, pericarditis, valvulitis, or coronary abnormalities [including ECHO findings or elevated Troponin/N-terminal pro b-type natriuretic peptide (NT-proBNP)]
4. Evidence of coagulopathy [by prothrombin time (PT), partial thromboplastin time (PTT), and elevated d-dimers)
5. Acute gastrointestinal problems (diarrhea, vomiting, or abdominal pain)

> AND—elevated markers of inflammation such as erythrocyte sedimentation rate, C-reactive protein, or procalcitonin
>
> AND—no other obvious microbial cause of inflammation, including bacterial sepsis, staphylococcal, or streptococcal shock syndromes
>
> AND—evidence of COVID-19 (RT-PCR, antigen test, or serology positive), or likely contact with patients with COVID-19

Key Points to Remember

- Neonatal coronavirus disease 2019 (COVID-19) infection is usually a mild illness. Vertical transmission of the virus from COVID-19 infected mother to the fetus is probable, but extremely rare.
- Most reported cases are in neonates are a result of horizontal transmission by droplets and aerosols. Incubation period is 5–14 days.

■ FURTHER READING

1. Groβ R, Conzelmann C, Müller JA, Stenger S, Steinhart K, Kirchhoff F, et al. Detection of SARS-CoV-2 in human breastmilk. Lancet. 2020;395(10239):1757-8.
2. NNF, IAP FOGSI. (2021). Perinatal-Neonatal Management of COVID-19. Clinical practice guidelines, Version 3.0. [online] Available from https://www.fogsi.org/wp-content/uploads/gcpr/perinatal-neonatal-management-of-covid-19.pdf [Last accessed September, 2022].
3. Vardhelli V, Pandita A, Pillai A, Badatya SK. Perinatal COVID-19: review of current evidence and practical approach towards prevention and management. Eur J Pediatr. 2021;180(4):1009-31.

Management of Neonates Born to Mothers with Tuberculosis, HIV, Varicella, and Hepatitis B

Tapas Bandyopadhyay, Rashi Gupta

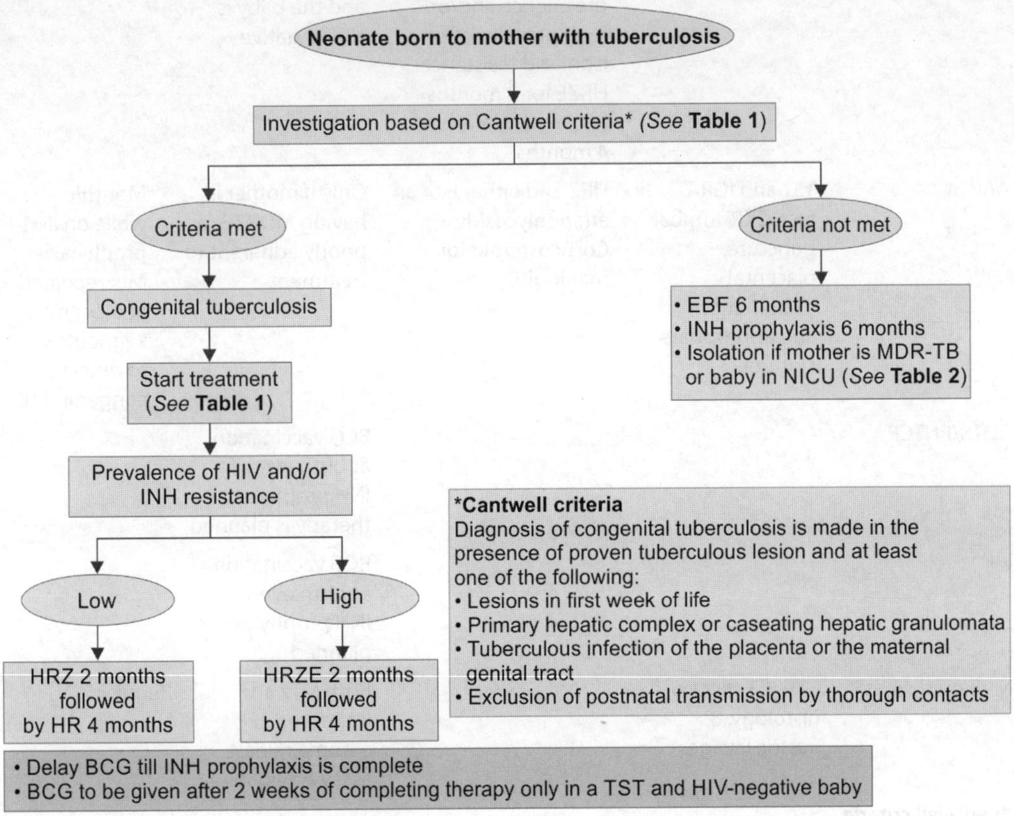

Neonate born to mother with tuberculosis

↓

Investigation based on Cantwell criteria* *(See **Table 1**)*

Criteria met

↓

Congenital tuberculosis

↓

Start treatment
*(See **Table 1**)*

↓

Prevalence of HIV and/or
INH resistance

Low → HRZ 2 months
followed
by HR 4 months

High → HRZE 2 months
followed
by HR 4 months

Criteria not met

- EBF 6 months
- INH prophylaxis 6 months
- Isolation if mother is MDR-TB
  or baby in NICU *(See **Table 2**)*

***Cantwell criteria**
Diagnosis of congenital tuberculosis is made in the presence of proven tuberculous lesion and at least one of the following:
- Lesions in first week of life
- Primary hepatic complex or caseating hepatic granulomata
- Tuberculous infection of the placenta or the maternal genital tract
- Exclusion of postnatal transmission by thorough contacts

- Delay BCG till INH prophylaxis is complete
- BCG to be given after 2 weeks of completing therapy only in a TST and HIV-negative baby

TABLE 1: Diagnosis, treatment, BCG vaccination, and follow-up management plan for congenital tuberculosis (TB).

Recommendation body	Criteria for diagnosis of congenital TB	Treatment recommendations for congenital TB	Timing of BCG vaccination	Follow-up management
WHO	Cantwell criteria*	• Areas with low HIV prevalence and/or low prevalence of isoniazid resistance: HRZ for 2 months followed by HR for 4 months • Areas with high HIV prevalence and/or high prevalence of isoniazid resistance: HRZE for 2 months followed by HR for 4 months	Delay until INH therapy is completed. BCG after 2 weeks of completing therapy only if TST remains negative and the baby is HIV-negative	Every 2 months till the treatment is complete
AAP	TST and IGRA test, CXR, lumbar puncture, placental examination, and appropriate cultures	• HRZ and either E or an aminoglycoside • Corticosteroid for meningitis	Only if mother is having MDR TB, or poorly adherent to treatment	• Monthly while on INH prophylaxis • Mtx repeated at 6, 9, and 12 months to detect congenital TB
DOTS/RNTCP	–	–	BCG vaccination at birth even if INH prophylaxis therapy is planned	–
IAP	–	–	BCG vaccination at birth even if INH prophylaxis is planned	–
NICE guidelines	CXR, CT thorax, histology, 3 gastric lavages	–	Both MTx and interferon-gamma release assay is negative	Regular

***Cantwell criteria**

Diagnosis of congenital tuberculosis is made in the presence of proven tuberculous lesion and at least one of the following:
• Lesions in first week of life
• Primary hepatic complex or caseating hepatic granulomata
• Tuberculous infection of the placenta or the maternal genital tract
• Exclusion of postnatal transmission by thorough contacts.

TABLE 2: Prevention of transmission of tubercular infection to the neonate from the mother.

Recommendation body	Breastfeeding recommendations	Role of isolation of mother-baby dyad	Prophylaxis for the neonate
WHO	Continue	Only if mother has MDR-TB or baby is managed in NICU (give expressed breast milk)	INH prophylaxis continued for 6 months
AAP	Only if the mother is on ATT	Only if mother is MDR-TB, noncompliant to therapy and before starting ATT	• INH for 3–4 months followed by Mtx test – *MTx negative:* Stop INH – *Mtx positive:* Search for congenital TB. If positive treat as congenital TB, if negative give INH for 9 months
DOTS/RNTCP	Breastfeeding	MDR TB or mother having active disease and noncompliant to treatment	• INH prophylaxis should be started after ruling out congenital TB and continued for 6 months • Chemoprophylaxis in MDR contacts is not recommended
IAP	Continue	Mother is sick, nonadherent to therapy or has MDR-TB	INH prophylaxis should be started after ruling out congenital TB and continued for 6 months
NICE	Continue	Mother and baby should not be separated	• INH + pyridoxine for exclusively breastfed babies for 6 weeks • MTx at 6 weeks – *Positive:* Reassess for active TB; if negative, continue isoniazid for 6 months – *Negative:* Reassess for active TB and consider an interferon-gamma release assay: - *Negative:* Stop INH - *Positive:* Reassess for active TB; if negative, continue isoniazid for 6 months

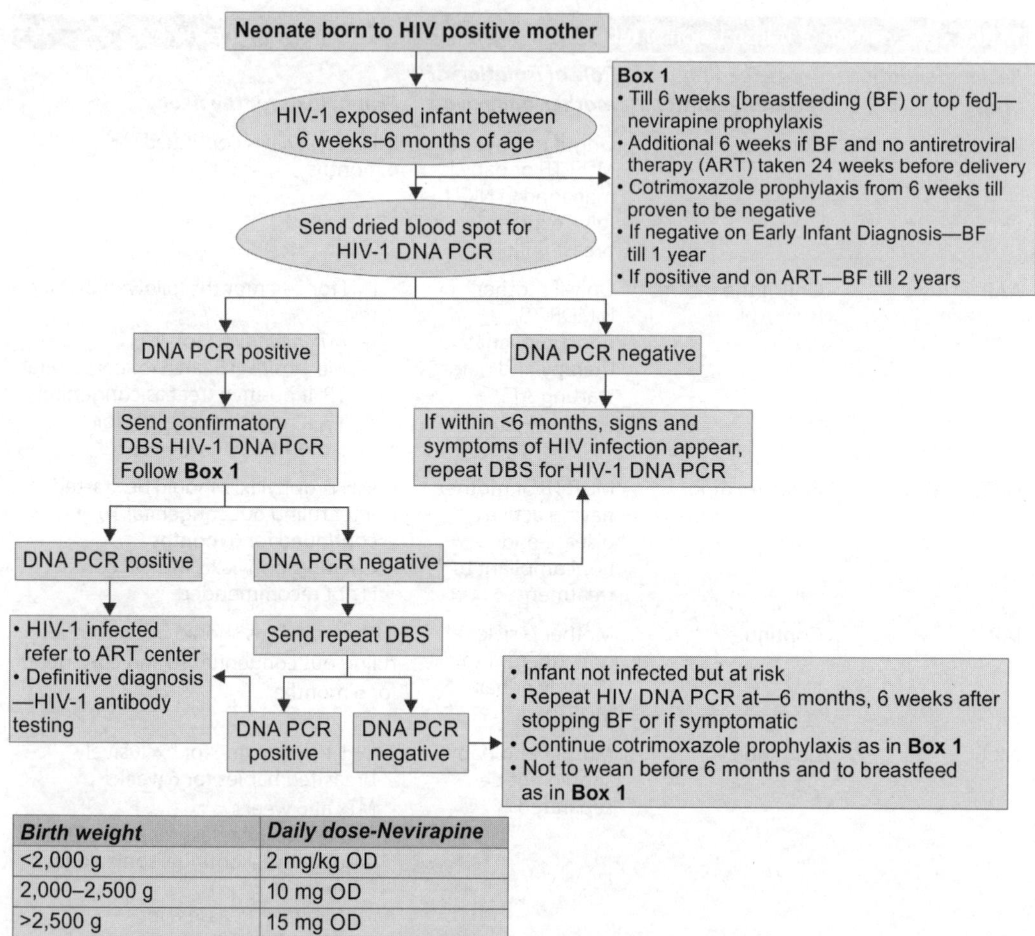

Birth weight	Daily dose-Nevirapine
<2,000 g	2 mg/kg OD
2,000–2,500 g	10 mg OD
>2,500 g	15 mg OD

Presumptive diagnosis of severe HIV disease

Infant's HIV-1 antibody test is reactive

and

Diagnosis of any AIDS-indicator conditions(s) can be made

Or

Presence of ≥ 2 of the following:

Oral thrush	Creamy white to yellow small plaques on red or normally colored mucosa which can be scraped off, or red patches on tongue, palate or lining of mouth, usually painful or tender
Severe pneumonia	Cough or difficult breathing with either chest in-drawing, stridor or any of the IMCI general danger signs; i.e., lethargic or unconscious, not able to drink or breast-feed, vomiting, and presence or history of convulsions during current illness; responding to antibiotics
Severe sepsis	Fever or hypothermia along with any severe sign such as tachypnea, chest in-drawing, bulging fontanelle, lethargy, reduced movement, not feeding or sucking breast milk, convulsions, etc

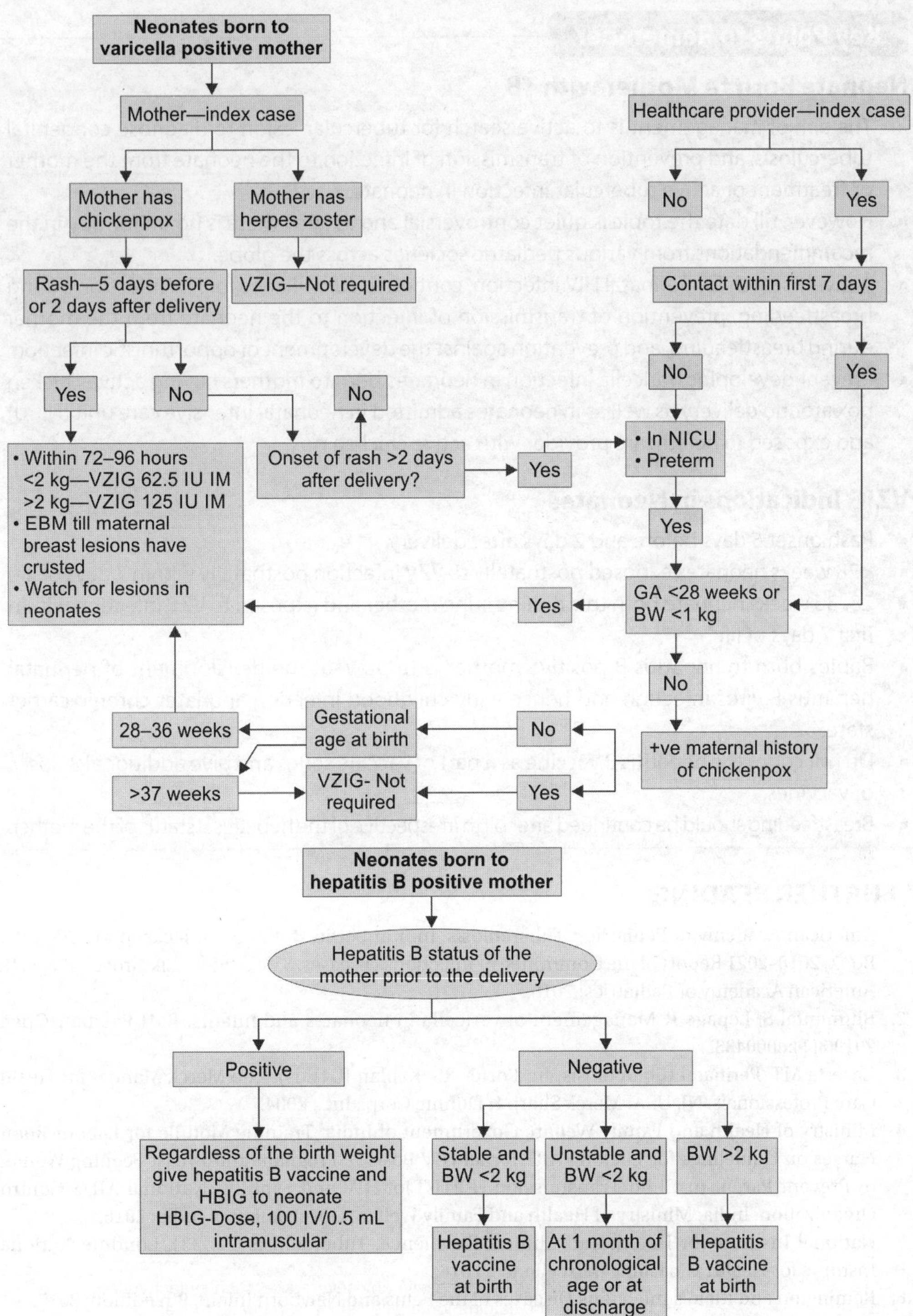
Neonates born to varicella positive mother
Mother—index case
Healthcare provider—index case
Mother has chickenpox
Mother has herpes zoster
No
Yes
Rash—5 days before or 2 days after delivery
VZIG—Not required
Contact within first 7 days
Yes
No
No
No
Yes
• In NICU
• Preterm
• Within 72–96 hours
  <2 kg—VZIG 62.5 IU IM
  >2 kg—VZIG 125 IU IM
• EBM till maternal breast lesions have crusted
• Watch for lesions in neonates
Onset of rash >2 days after delivery?
Yes
Yes
GA <28 weeks or BW <1 kg
Yes
No
28–36 weeks
Gestational age at birth
No
+ve maternal history of chickenpox
>37 weeks
VZIG- Not required
Yes
Neonates born to hepatitis B positive mother
Hepatitis B status of the mother prior to the delivery
Positive
Negative
Regardless of the birth weight give hepatitis B vaccine and HBIG to neonate HBIG-Dose, 100 IV/0.5 mL intramuscular
Stable and BW <2 kg
Unstable and BW <2 kg
BW >2 kg
Hepatitis B vaccine at birth
At 1 month of chronological age or at discharge
Hepatitis B vaccine at birth

> ## Key Points to Remember
>
> ### Neonate Born to Mother with TB
>
> - The aim of management is to active search for tubercular lesion to diagnose congenital tuberculosis, and prevention of transmission of infection to the neonate from the mother or treatment of active tubercular infection in neonate.
> - However, till date the topic is quiet controversial and as such there is no uniformity in the recommendations from various pediatric societies across the globe.
> - Actively search for perinatal HIV infection, continued surveillance for HIV infection during breastfeeding, prevention of transmission of infection to the neonate from the mother during breastfeeding, and prevention against the development of opportunistic infection.
> - Prevent developing varicella infection in neonates born to mothers having active chicken pox around delivery as well as in neonates admitted in neonatal intensive care unit (NICU) and exposed to healthcare provider with active chicken pox.
>
> ### VZIG Indications in Neonates
>
> - Rash onset 5 days before and 2 days after delivery
> - <28 weeks neonates exposed postnatally to VZV infection postnatally within 7 days of life
> - 28–36 weeks neonate born to a nonimmune mother and exposed to VZV infection within first 7 days of life.
> - Babies born to hepatitis B positive mother is to prevent the development of perinatal hepatitis B virus infection and hence early childhood infection and later chronic carrier state.
> - Do not count the hepatitis B vaccine as a part of vaccine series and give additional 3 doses of vaccines.
> - Breastfeeding should be continued after birth irrespective of the hepatitis B status of the mother.

◼ FURTHER READING

1. American Academy of Pediatrics. Tuberculosis. In: Kimberlin D, Brady M, Jackson M (Eds). Red Book: 2018–2021 Report of the Committee of Infectious Diseases, 31st edition. Elk Grove Village, IL: American Academy of Pediatrics; 2018.
2. Blumental S, Lepage P. Management of varicella in neonates and infants. BMJ Paediatr Open. 2019;3(1):e000433.
3. Caserta MT. Perinatal tuberculosis. In: Porter RS, Kaplan JL (Eds). The Merck Manual for Health Care Professionals. NJ, USA: Merck Sharp & Dohme Corp., Inc.; 2004.
4. Ministry of Health and Family Welfare Government of India. Training Module for Labour Room Nurses on Guidelines for Lifelong ART for all HIV Positive Pregnant and Breast Feeding Women to Prevent Parent-to-Child Transmission (PPTCT)of HIV and Syphilis. National AIDS Control Organization. India: Ministry of Health and Family Welfare Government of India; 2016.
5. National Institute for Health and Clinical Excellence. Tuberculosis (NG33). London: National Institute for Health and Clinical Excellence; 2016.
6. Remington and Klein's Infectious Diseases of the Fetus and Newborn Infant, 8th edition; 2015.
7. World Health Organization. Guidance for National Tuberculosis Programmes on the Management of Tuberculosis in Children, 2nd edition. Geneva: World Health Organization; 2014.

Chapter

56

Management of Congenital Infection

Vikram Bedi

■ 56.1 CONGENITAL TOXOPLASMOSIS

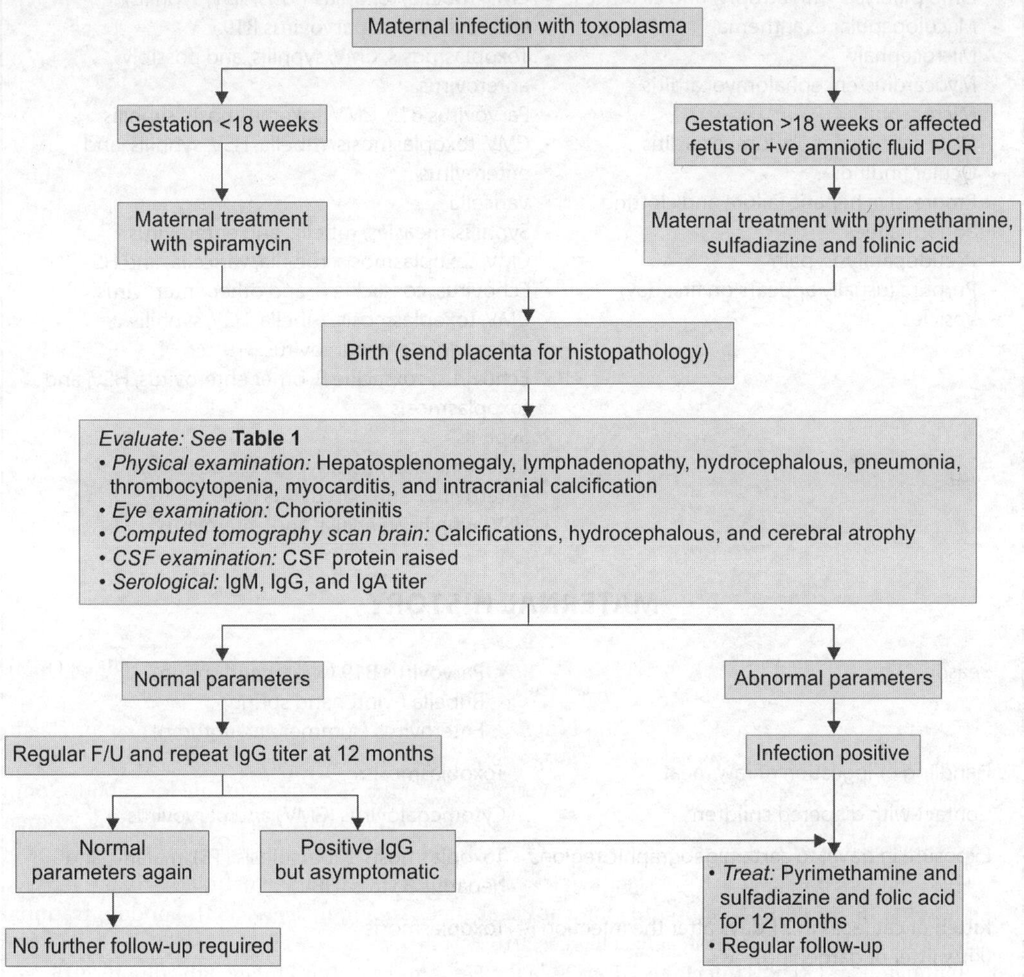

CLINICAL POINTERS SUGGESTIVE OF CONGENITAL INFECTION

Finding(s)	*Possible congenital infections*
• Intrauterine growth retardation	• Rubella, cytomegalovirus (CMV), and toxoplasmosis
• Anemia with hydrops	• Parvovirus B19, syphilis, CMV, toxoplasmosis
• Bone lesions	• Syphilis, rubella
• Cerebral calcification	• Toxoplasmosis (widely distributed)
• Congenital heart disease	• CMV and herpes simplex virus (HSV) (usually periventricular)
• Hearing loss (commonly progressive)	• Parvovirus B19, rubella, human immunodeficiency virus (HIV)
• Hepatosplenomegaly	• Lymphocytic choriomeningitis virus
• Hydrocephalus	• Rubella
• Hydrops, ascites, pleural effusions	• Rubella, CMV, toxoplasmosis, and syphilis
• Jaundice with or without thrombocytopenia	• CMV, rubella, toxoplasmosis, HSV, syphilis, enterovirus, and parvovirus B19
• Limb paralysis with atrophy and cicatrices	• Toxoplasmosis, CMV, syphilis, and possibly enterovirus
• Maculopapular exanthema	• Parvovirus B19, CMV, toxoplasmosis, syphilis
• Microcephaly	• CMV, toxoplasmosis, rubella, HSV, syphilis, and enterovirus
• Myocarditis/encephalomyocarditis	• Varicella
• Microcephaly	• Syphilis, measles, rubella, and enterovirus
• Myocarditis/encephalomyocarditis	• CMV, toxoplasmosis, rubella, varicella, and HSV
• Ocular findings	• Echovirus, coxsackie B, and other enterovirus
• Progressive hepatic failure and clotting abnormalities	• CMV, toxoplasmosis, rubella, HSV, syphilis, enterovirus, and parvovirus B19
• Pseudoparalysis, pain	• Echovirus, coxsackie B, other enterovirus, HSV, and toxoplasmosis
• Purpura (usually appears on first day)	• Syphilis
• Vesicles	• CMV, toxoplasmosis, syphilis, rubella, HSV, enterovirus, and parvovirus B19
	• HSV, syphilis, varicella, and enterovirus

MATERNAL HISTORY

Season	• Parvovirus B19 (winter and spring) • Rubella (winter and spring) • Enterovirus (summer and autumn)
Handling or ingestion of raw meat	Toxoplasmosis
Contact with diapered children	Cytomegalovirus (CMV) and parvovirus
Exposure in travel to certain geographic regions	Toxoplasmosis, tuberculosis (TB), malaria, and hepatitis B virus (HBV)
Kitten or cat feces in 21 days after the infection (kitty litter or gardening)	Toxoplasmosis

Number of sexual partners, sex industry worker, and illicit drug use	Syphilis, HSV, HBV, hepatitis C virus, and human immunodeficiency virus (HIV)
Rash	Syphilis, rubella, parvovirus B19, and enterovirus
Arthritis	Parvovirus B19 and rubella
Mononucleosis-like fatigue, lymphadenopathy	CMV, toxoplasmosis, and HIV

- In the absence of suggestive maternal laboratory results, suspect congenital infections in neonates with:

• Hydrops fetalis	• Microcephaly	• Seizures
• Cataract	• Hearing loss	• Congenital heart disease (CHD)
• Hepatosplenomegaly	• Jaundice	• Rash
• Thrombocytopenia	• Intrauterine growth restriction (IUGR)	

- Majority clinically inapparent ("asymptomatic") at birth.

INVESTIGATION

Specimen	Tests	Interpretation
Urine	Viral culture or detection* (CMV, HSV, and rubella)	• Urine for CMV must be obtained at younger than age 2–3 weeks • If positive, diagnostic for infection
Throat swab	Viral detection* (CMV, HSV, rubella, and enteroviruses)	If positive, diagnostic for infection
Blood	Viral detection* (CMV, parvovirus B19)	If positive, diagnostic for infection
Neonatal serum (single specimen)	Rubella-specific IgM	If positive, test is diagnostic, although determination of status at 10–12 months of age is confirmatory
Sequential neonatal, infant sera over 6–12 months	IgG antibody for etiological agents of concern	Passive maternal antibody in uninfected infant disappears at • 4–9 months of age for CMV (unless peri- or postnatally transmitted) eight months for *Toxoplasma gondii*; and • 6 months VDRL/rapid plasma reagent and 12–15 months treponemal test (e.g., fluorescent treponemal antibody absorbed with nonpallidum treponemes)
		Positive specific antibody at 8–12 months suggests congenital toxoplasmosis parvovirus B19, rubella or varicella zoster virus infection

Contd...

Contd...

Specimen	Tests	Interpretation
Single maternal serum at delivery	Toxo-specific IgM (or toxoplasmosis-specific)	If IgM-specific antibody is positive, reference laboratory testing of maternal and infant sera is recommended
Serology of both mother and infant	IgG antibody for etiological agents of concern	• Negative maternal serology rules out source of infection • Serial infant serology identifies passive maternal antibody (titers fall) and active infection (titers remain the same or rise over months)
Cerebrospinal fluid culture, detection	Detection* CMV, enteroviruses, HSV, toxoplasmosis (reference laboratory), parvovirus B19 Rubella-specific IgM antibody VDRL	If positive, usually diagnostic for that infection
Skin lesions culture, detection	If vesiculated at birth: detection* of herpes, enteroviruses, varicella zoster virus and dark-field for *Treponema pallidum* (syphilis)	If positive, diagnostic for infection
Nasopharyngeal secretions	Dark-field for *T pallidum* (syphilis)	If positive, diagnostic for infection
Stool culture	Enteroviruses	If positive, diagnostic for infection
Placenta	Pathology	Variable

*Detection refers to culture or polymerase chain reaction testing.

Key Points to Remember

- Transmission—ingestion of cysts from cats

Trimester of maternal acquisition	Incidence of transmission (%)	Relative severity of disease
I	17	Severe
II	25	Intermediate severity
III	65	Milder or asymptomatic

- *Clinical manifestation:* Most neonates with congenital toxoplasmosis are asymptomatic.

Abnormal spinal fluid	Hepatomegaly	Mental retardation
Anemia	Hydrocephalus[#] (20%)	Microcephaly
Chorioretinitis[#] (86%)	Intracranial calcifications[#] (37%)	Spasticity and palsies
Convulsions	Jaundice	Splenomegaly
Deafness	Learning disabilities	Thrombocytopenia
Fever	Lymphadenopathy	Visual impairment
Growth retardation	Maculopapular rash	

[#]Sign in the classic triad suggesting the presence of congenital toxoplasmosis.

TABLE 1: Evaluation of the newborn/infant	
Test	*Comment*
Clinical evaluations	
Physical examination	Fever, jaundice, hepatosplenomegaly, and lymphadenopathy
Eye examination	Chorioretinitis may be the only manifestation
Auditory brainstem response	Routine newborn hearing screening is performed
Lumbar puncture	
CSF glucose, protein, and cell count	• CSF abnormalities may be the only manifestation (Pleocytosis) • CSF protein >1 g/dL in severely affected infants • Lower in mild or subclinical disease
Toxoplasma-specific PCR	When strong suspicion for congenital toxoplasma infection; can establish the diagnosis
Neuroimaging	Intracranial calcifications or hydrocephalus
Serology (performed in conjunction with maternal serology)	
Toxoplasma-specific IgG	Does not differentiate maternal from infant infection
Toxoplasma-specific IgM (ELISA)	• Indicative of congenital infection if not contaminated with maternal blood • Negative IgM does not exclude congenital toxoplasmosis
Toxoplasma-specific IgA (ELISA)	• Especially useful if IgG and IgM assays are indeterminate • Indicative of congenital infection if not contaminated with maternal blood
Blood tests (primarily performed before initiating treatment in confirmed or suspected cases)	
CBC with differential and platelet count	Anemia and thrombocytopenia are common in symptomatic infants
Evaluation for G6PD deficiency (before initiation of treatment)	Treatment with sulfadiazine may cause hemolysis in G6PD-deficient children
Liver function tests	Primarily for baseline studies before initiating treatment; both direct and cholestatic jaundice may occur in infected infants

- *Follow-up:* Neurological and ophthalmologic examination every 3 monthly till 2 years of age, thereafter 3 yearly till adolescence.

■ 56.2 CONGENITAL CYTOMEGALOVIRUS (CMV) INFECTION

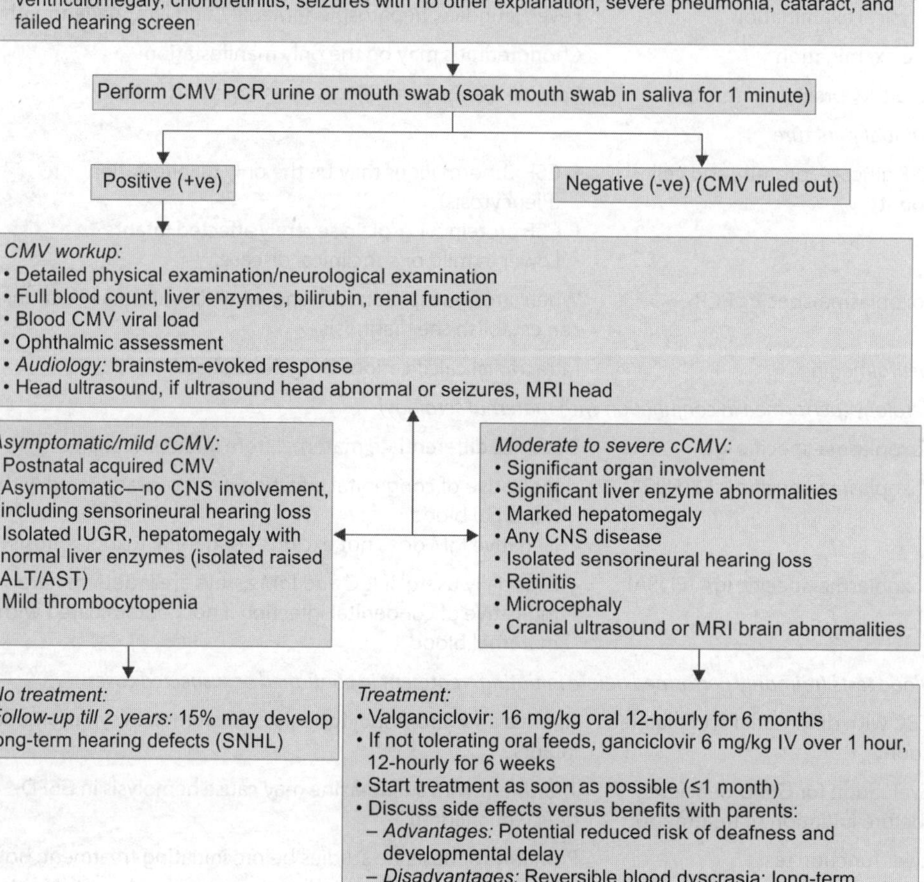

Key Points to Remember

- In utero transmission of CMV can occur during primary maternal infection, reactivation, or reinfection of seropositive mothers.

Maternal CMV serology (IgG and IgM) and viral loads		
IgG negative	IgM negative	Unlikely to be CMV infection
IgG positive	IgM negative	Past maternal infection
IgG positive	IgM positive	Check CMV IgG avidity (if low likely to be maternal CMV infection within last 3–4 months)

- *Antenatal ultrasound:* Intrauterine growth restriction, intracranial ventriculomegaly/ calcification, microcephaly, ascites, hydrops fetalis, pleural or pericardial effusions, oligo- or polyhydramnios, hepatomegaly, abdominal calcification, pseudomeconium ileus, and thickened placenta.
- Follow-up:
  - *Ganciclovir IV:* Perform CBC (neutropenia), LFT (transaminitis), U&E at least twice weekly
  - *Valganciclovir oral:* CBC, LFT, U&E weekly for first 4 weeks, then monthly until completion
  - CMV viral load on antiviral therapy
  - *Audiology:* 3 monthly for first year, then 6 monthly for 3 years, then annually until aged
  - 6 years for both asymptomatic and symptomatic congenitally infected babies
  - *Pediatric infectious diseases specialist:* As soon as possible in first month, then annually until aged 2 years
  - *Ophthalmology:* At least annually until aged 5 years if symptomatic/signs at birth
  - *Neurodevelopmental assessment:* Aged 1 year, if delayed development discusses MRI brain with radiology

■ 56.3 CONGENITAL RUBELLA

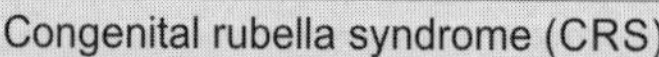

• Review of maternal history to confirm documentation of rubella immunity • Complete physical examination assessing for stigmata consistent with the syndrome (*See* **Table 2**) • Complete blood count • Liver enzymes and bilirubin (total and direct) • Lumbar puncture • Cardiac evaluation—some experts suggest echocardiography for all infants in whom CRS is suspected, whereas others suggest cardiology consultation and echocardiography based upon clinical examination findings • Radiographs of long bones • Ophthalmologic evaluation • Audiologic evaluation • Neuroimaging (e.g., ultrasonography and computed tomography) • Rubella serology

Congenital rubella syndrome (CRS)

Clinical case definition

An illness, usually manifesting in infancy, resulting from rubella infection in utero and characterized by clinical findings from the following categories:
- *Category A:* Cataracts/congenital glaucoma, congenital heart disease (most commonly, patent ductus arteriosus, or peripheral pulmonary artery stenosis), hearing impairment, and pigmentary retinopathy
- *Category B:* Purpura, hepatosplenomegaly, jaundice, microcephaly, developmental delay, meningoencephalitis, and radiolucent bone disease

Laboratory criteria (any one of the following)

- Demonstration of rubella-specific IgM
- Infant rubella antibody level (IgG) that persists at a higher level and for a longer time than expected from passive transfer of maternal antibody (i.e., rubella titer that does not drop at the expected rate of a twofold dilution per month)*
- Isolation of rubella
- PCR positive for rubella virus

Classification	Criteria
Suspected	An infant that does not meet the criteria for a probable or confirmed case but has one of more of the above clinical findings (category A or B)

Probable¶	• An infant without an alternative etiology that does not have laboratory confirmation of rubella infection but has either:
	  – At least two clinical findings from category A above
	  – One finding from category A and one or more from category B above

Confirmed	• An infant with at least one of the above clinical findings that is clinically consistent with CRS (category A or B), and • Laboratory evidence of congenital rubella infection, as demonstrated by any of the above laboratory criteria
Infection only△	An infant without any clinical symptoms or signs but with laboratory evidence of infection, as demonstrated by any of the above laboratory criteria

*Infants with symptoms consistent with CRS who test negative soon after birth should be retested at age 1 month. Approximately 20% of infected infants tested for rubella IgM may not have detectable titers before age 1 month

¶In probable cases, either or both of the eye-related findings (cataracts and congenital glaucoma) count as a single complication

△If any compatible signs or symptoms (e.g., hearing impairment) are identified later, the case is reclassified as confirmed

MANAGEMENT

Supportive care and surveillance are the cornerstones of management for congenital rubella infection.

- *No role for antiviral therapy:* The clinical course of congenital rubella syndrome (CRS) is not altered by treatment with antiviral or biological agents, nor are there any agents that have any long-term effect on the duration of viral shedding.
- *Management of complications:* Most infants with CRS have multiple medical problems and require multidisciplinary management. At the time of diagnosis, a comprehensive evaluation should be performed to determine the extent of disease severity.

The medical problems that may occur in CRS are generally managed in the same manner as in patients without CRI:

- Hearing loss—may require hearing aids and early intervention program.
- Eye disease—cataracts, retinopathy, infantile glaucoma, and other eye complications—pediatric eye care specialist.
- Central nervous system (CNS) manifestations—CNS disease may manifest as meningoencephalitis (abnormal neurologic findings, seizures). Initial supportive care measures may CNS stabilization and treatment of seizures.
- After infancy, CNS manifestations may include intellectual disability, autism, and cerebral palsy, which may require referral to developmental specialist, speech, language, occupational, and/or physical therapy.
- Congenital heart disease—patent ductus arteriosus and pulmonary stenosis are most common.
- *Endocrine abnormalities:* The late-onset endocrine abnormalities (e.g., diabetes and thyroid dysfunction) should be managed by an endocrinologist.
- *Neonatal thrombocytopenia:* Thrombocytopenia is generally mild to moderate and transient. Although purpura and petechiae may be severe, clinically significant bleeding is uncommon.
- Neonatal respiratory distress—neonates with respiratory distress should be managed with oxygen or ventilatory support as necessary.
- Neonatal hyperbilirubinemia—hyperbilirubinemia in CRS is typically conjugated and rarely severe; it generally does not require any specific therapy.

TABLE 2: Clinical pointers suggestive of rubella infection.

Clinical manifestation	Frequency	Typical time of onset	Course
Hearing impairment	60%	Early infancy	Permanent
Heart defect	45%		
Patent ductus arteriosus	20%	Early infancy	Permanent
Peripheral pulmonic stenosis	12%	Early infancy	Permanent
Microcephaly	27%	Neonatal	Permanent
Cataracts	25%	Early infancy	Permanent
Low birth weight (<2,500 g)	23%	Neonatal	Poor weight gain may persist
Hepatosplenomegaly	19%	Neonatal	Transient
Purpura	17%	Neonatal	Transient
Intellectual disability (mental retardation)	13%	Variable	Permanent
Meningoencephalitis	10%	Neonatal	Transient
Radiolucent bone lesions	7%	Neonatal	Transient
Retinopathy	5%	Early infancy	Permanent
Late-onset manifestations			
Hearing loss			Permanent
Intellectual disability			Permanent
Diabetes mellitus			Permanent
Thyroid dysfunction			Permanent
Progressive panencephalitis			Permanent

Other findings include petechiae and purpura ("blueberry muffin lesions"), thrombocytopenia, hemolytic anemia, hepatosplenomegaly, jaundice, hepatitis, diarrhea, interstitial pneumonia, myocarditis, radiolucent bone lesions (in the long bones), and lymphadenopathy.

Key Points to Remember

Congenital Rubella

- *Transmission:* Often from primary maternal rubella with a rash:
  - >80% during the first 12 weeks of pregnancy
  - 54% at 13–14 weeks
  - 25% at the end of the second trimester
- *Defects:*
  - <11th week—CHD and deafness
  - 13–16 weeks—deafness
  - >16 weeks—rare

■ 55.4 NEONATE BORN TO A MOTHER WITH HERPES GENITAL LESIONS

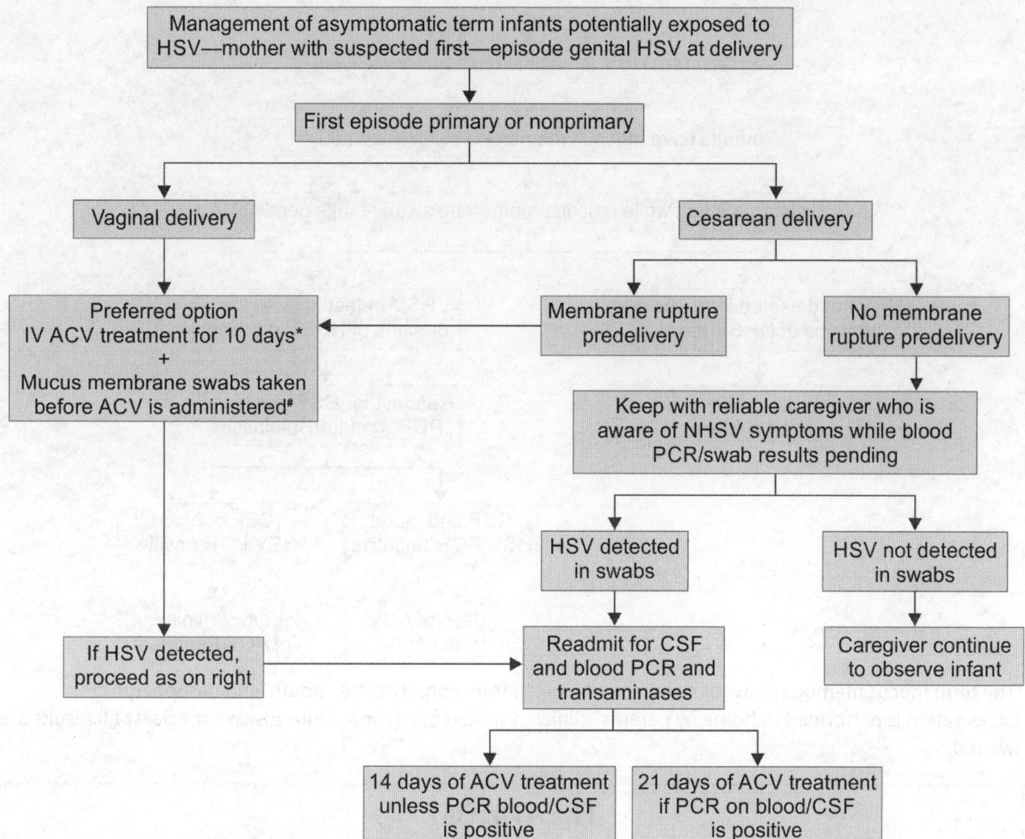

*If type-specific serology is available and shows that the mother has recurrent HSV and all the swabs obtained from the infant are negative, acyclovir can be stopped and the infant discharged for close observation at home.
#The term mucus membrane swabs denotes swabs taken from conjunctivae, mouth and nasopharynx. In addition to mucous membrane swabs, some experts recommend blood for PCR. Consider CSF cell count, chemistries, and PCR when mucous membrane swabs are taken.

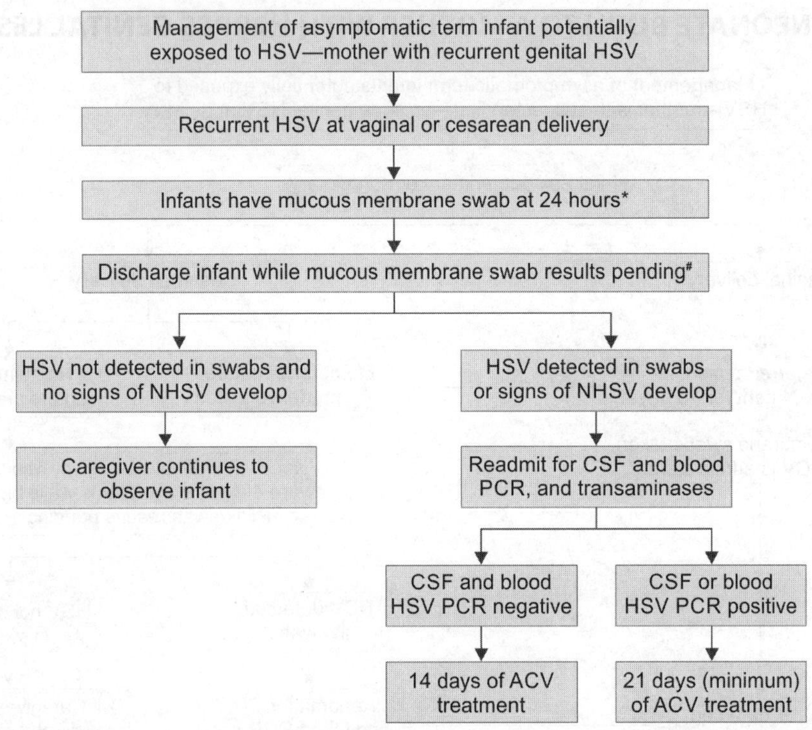

*The term mucus membrane swabs denote swabs taken from conjunctivae, mouth, and nasopharynx.
#Observation is performed at home by parents. Clinician should talk to infectious disease specialist till results are awaited.

TREATMENT

Primary HSV (Genital herpes ≤6 weeks before vaginal delivery):
- Swab infant's nasopharynx, conjunctiva, mouth, and rectum in viral transport medium for HSV PCR
- Check infant's ALT and send blood for HSV PCR
- Start acyclovir 20 mg/kg IVI (over 1 hour) 8-hourly
- If ALT abnormal/other signs of infection send CSF for HSV PCR
- Recommend breastfeeding unless herpetic lesions around nipple treatment.

Duration acyclovir IV:
- If neonatal HSV PCR negative, stop acyclovir
- If active infection ruled out, stop acyclovir
- If skin, eye or mouth lesions, lumbar puncture
- if CSF HSV negative and ALT normal, acyclovir IV for 10 days
- If ALT raised and CSF negative, acyclovir IV for 14 days
- If CSF HSV positive, repeat LP at 14 days and if negative stop at 21 days
- If any confirmed HSV disease: give suppressive therapy with acyclovir 300 mg/m^2 oral 8-hourly for 6 months.

Key Points to Remember

- Types:
  - Herpes simplex virus (HSV) type 1: 25%
  - Herpes simplex virus (HSV) type 2: 75%
- Transmission:
  - Intrauterine 5%
  - Perinatal 85–90%
  - Postnatal 5–10%

Maternal genital HSV cases may be classified as follows:

- *Newly acquired:* First-episode primary infection (mother has no serum antibodies to HSV-1 and 2 at onset)
  - First-episode nonprimary infection (mother has a new infection with one HSV type in the presence of antibodies to the other type)
- *Recurrent* (mother has preexisting antibodies to the HSV type that is isolated from the genital tract).
- Classification of neonate herpes:
  - *Disseminated HSV (22%):* Most severe form (50% mortality), pneumonitis, fulminant hepatitis, encephalitis, disseminated intravascular coagulation (DIC), and respiratory failure
  - *Localized CNS HSV (28%):* Lethargy, seizures, temperature instability, hypotonia, and encephalitis
  - *Skin, eye and mucous membrane (SEM) infection (50%):* Clustering of vesicles on skin (usually appears on 6–9th day), eye pain, keratoconjunctivitis, and orophageal ulceration.

FURTHER READING

1. Arvin AM, Whitley RJ. Herpes simplex virus infections. In: Remington JS, Klein JO (Eds). Infectious Diseases of the Fetus and Newborn. 7th edition. Philadelphia: WB Saunders; 2006.
2. Cherry J, Demmler-Harrison GJ, Kaplan SL, Hotez P. Rubella virus. In: Feigin and Cherry's Textbook of Pediatric Infectious Diseases, 8th edition. Philadelphia: Elsevier; 2018. p.1601.
3. Johnson KE. (2012). Overview of TORCH infections. [online] Available from https://www.uptodate.com/contents/overview-of-torch-infections [Last accessed September, 2022].
4. Plotkin SA, Reef SE, Cooper LZ, Alford Jr CA. Rubella. In: Remington, JS, Klein, JO, Wilson, CB, et al (Eds). Infectious Diseases of the Fetus and Newborn Infant, 7th edition. Philadelphia: Elsevier Saunders; 2011. p. 861.
5. Remington and Klein's Infectious Diseases of the Fetus and Newborn Infant, 8th edition; 2015.

Chapter 57

Management of Feeding in Low Birth Weight Neonate

Srishti Goel

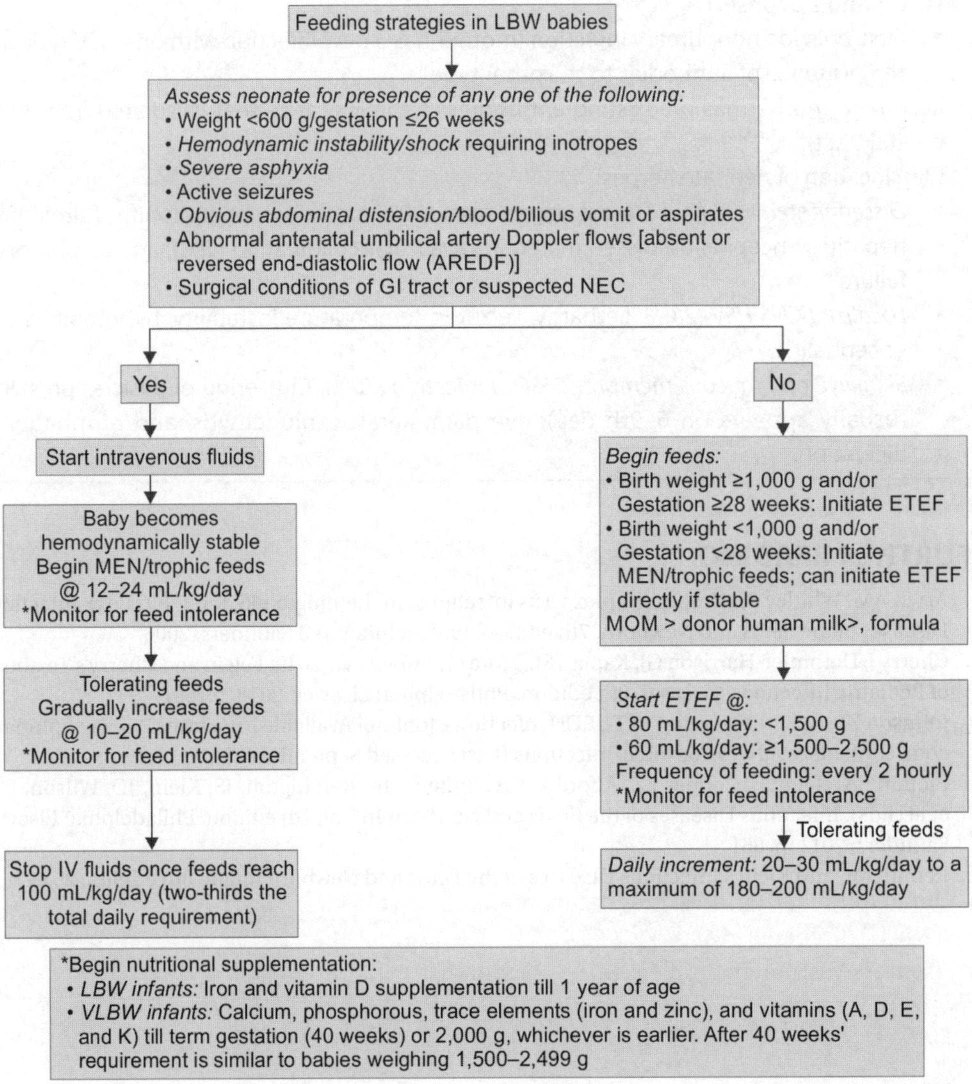

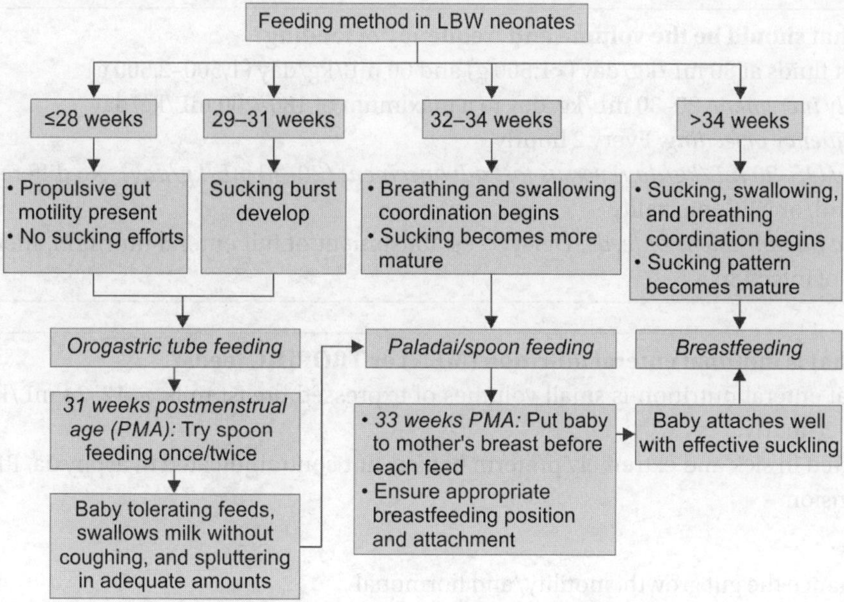

Q1. When to start feeds?

Enteral feeding should be initiated *as early as possible* in all babies:

- *Early versus delayed introduction of feeds:* No difference in feed intolerance and/or necrotizing enterocolitis (NEC)
- *Delayed initiation:* Intestinal villous atrophy, longer time to achieve full feeds, poor growth, delay in regaining birth weight, prolonged duration of hospital stay, and complications of IV alimentation (sepsis and cholestasis)
- Presence of RD, need for ventilation, moderate asphyxia, patent ductus arteriosus, and extreme prematurity are not contraindication to feeding.
- *Contraindication to feed initiation:* Presence of hemodynamic instability requiring vasopressor support, and suspected GI surgical anomalies.

Q2. Which milk to give?

Mothers own milk (MOM) is the best option. Results in dose specific reduction in risk and severity of

- Necrotizing enterocolitis
- Late-onset sepsis
- Retinopathy of prematurity
- Rehospitalization after neonatal intensive care unit (NICU) discharge
- Neurodevelopment problems at 18–22 months.

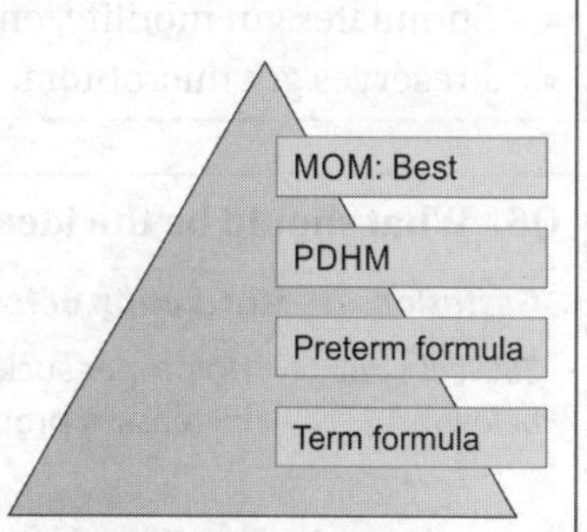

Q3. What should be the volume and frequency of feeding?

- Start fluids at 80 mL/kg/day (<1,500 g) and 60 mL/kg/day (1,500–2,500 g)
- *Daily increment:* 20–30 mL/kg/day to a maximum of 180–200 mL/kg/day
- *Frequency of feeding:* Every 2 hourly
- *Slow (15–20 mL/kg/day) versus fast advancement (30–40 mL/kg/day):* No difference in FI and/or NEC, mortality
- *Slow advancement of feeds:* Delayed establishment of full enteral nutrition, increased risk of infection.

Q4. What is minimal enteral nutrition (MEN) or TROPHIC feeds?

Minimal enteral nutrition is small volumes of expressed breast milk @ 12–24 mL/kg/day every 1–3 hourly

Started in sick and extremely preterm babies; not contraindicated in asphyxia, RD, and hypotension.

Benefits:
- Enhance the gut growth, motility, and hormonal
- Less feed intolerance
- Reduction in days required for attaining full feeds; fewer days on parenteral nutrition
- Improved weight gain and decreased hospital stay.

Q5. What is role of early total enteral feeding (ETEF) in very low birth weight (VLBW) babies?

Early total enteral feeding (ETEF) is an effective intervention to improve outcomes in VLBW neonates in resource limited settings.

Benefits:
- Avoid prolong intravenous access and its related complications
- Improved postnatal growth
- Gut maturation and reduced intestinal permeability
- Stimulates gut motility, enzyme production, and GI hormone release
- Preserves gut microbiota.

Q6. What should be the ideal mode of feeding?

Gestation	Maturation of feeding skills	Initial feeding method
28 weeks and below	• No proper sucking efforts • Increasing propulsive motility of gut	• Initiate *tropic feeds/MEN* • Initiate ETEF if clinically stable • Hike the feeds after monitoring for feed intolerance
29–31 weeks	• Sucking bursts develop • No suck/swallow and breathing coordination	*Orogastric (OG) tube feeding*

| 32–34 weeks | • Slightly mature sucking pattern
• Breathing and swallowing coordination develops | *Spoon/paladai feeds* |
| >34 weeks | • Mature sucking pattern
• Sucking/swallow and breathing coordination develops | *Breastfeeding* |

Q7. What nutritional supplements should be given in LBW and VLBW infants?

Low birth weight, especially preterm needs supplements to meet their high demands.

Nutritional supplementation in LBW infants:

- Require iron and vitamin D supplementation till 1 year of age.

Nutritional Supplementation in VLBW infants:

- Feeds should be supplemented for protein, energy, calcium, phosphorous, trace elements (iron and zinc) and vitamins (A, D, E, and K) till term gestation (40 weeks) or 2,000 g, whichever is earlier.
- After 40 weeks requirement is similar to those with birth weight 1,500–2,499 g.

Methods of supplementation:

- Giving individual nutrients
- Fortification with preterm formula/human milk fortifier (HMF)

Nutrients	Dose	When to start	Till
Vitamin D	400 IU/day	Feeds at 100 mL/kg/day	1 year of age
Iron	3 mg/kg/day	2–4 weeks	1 year of age
Vitamin D	400 IU/day (ELBW: 800–100 IU)	Feeds at 100 mL/kg	1 year of age
Calcium and phosphorus	140–160 mL/kg/day and 60 mg/kg/day (2:1 ratio) (Syrup ostocalcium 8–10 mL/kg/day)	Feeds at 100 mL/kg	40 weeks PMA or 2 kg whichever is later
Zinc, vitamin A, B6	Multivitamin drops (Visyneral Z 1 mL OD)	Feeds at 100 mL/kg	40 weeks PMA or 2 kg whichever is later
Iron	2–3 mg/kg/day	2 weeks	1 year of age

Fortification of breast milk:

- Supplementation with multicomponent HMF improves short-term increase in weight, length, and head circumference (HC).
- It reduces hospital stay, total parenteral nutrition (TPN) days with no effect on biological activity of human milk.
- Started when neonate is on 100 mL/kg/day enteral feeds with EBM @ 0.4 g per 10 mL and continued till weight of 2 kg or PMA 40 weeks, whichever is later.
- Provide optimal calories, protein, and micronutrients except zinc which needs to be added separately.

Q8. What are the good NICU practices to promote optimal feeding?

- *Family participatory care:* Involvement of mothers in the care of their babies
- Promoting and supporting kangaroo mother care (KMC)
- Oropharyngeal therapy with MOM in all preterm <32 weeks soon after birth (sick as well as healthy) @ 0.2 mL q 2 hourly has immunomodulatory effects and decreases NEC/late-onset sepsis
- Non-nutritive sucking on empty breast as soon as baby is clinically stable.

Q9. How to monitor growth in LBW infants?

- All LBW infants should be weighed daily till the time of discharge from the hospital. Both term and preterm LBW infants tend to lose weight (about and 15% respectively) in the first 7–14 days of life.
- Birth weight is regained by 10–14 days. Thereafter, the weight gain should be at least 15–20 g/kg/day till a weight of 2–2.5 kg is reached. After this, a gain of 20–30 g/day is considered appropriate.

Q10. How to initiate feeds neonates with absence or reversal of end-diastolic flow (AREDF) in umbilical artery Doppler?

- Preterm neonates born to mothers with AREDF in umbilical artery Doppler (6% of all high-risk pregnancy) are at an increased risk of *feed intolerance* (FI and NEC) leading to undue delay in initiation and advancement of enteral feeding resulting in prolonging the time to reach full enteral feeds as well the duration of hospital stay.
- *Feeding in AREDF:* What does the current evidence suggest?
  - *Early (6–48 hours) versus delayed initiation of enteral feeds:* No difference in incidence of FI and/or NEC. Delayed feed initiation group: Increased time to reach full feeds
  - *Slow (10–20 mL/kg/day) versus rapid (20–40 mL/kg/day):* No difference in FI and/or NEC

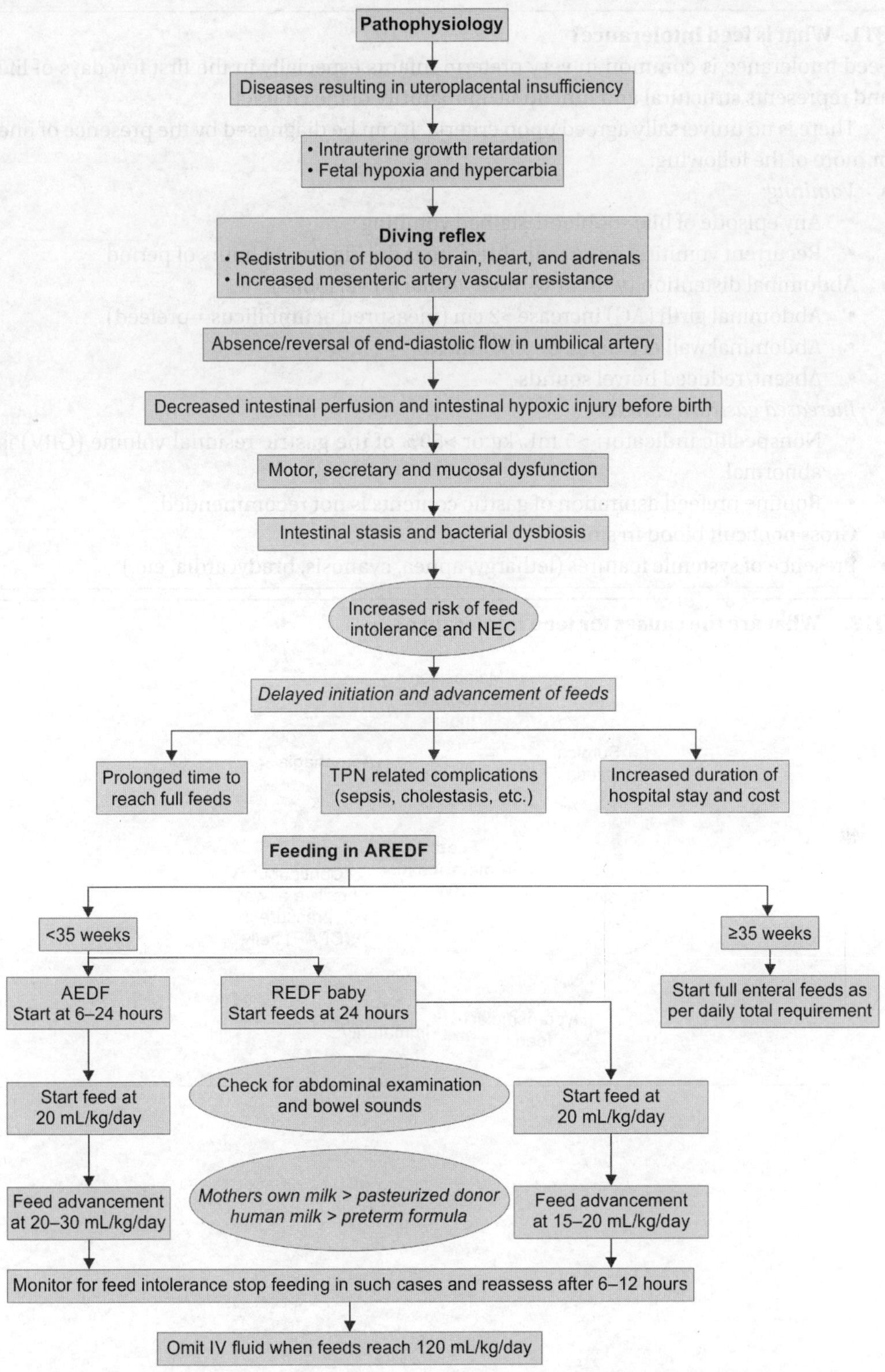

Pathophysiology
Diseases resulting in uteroplacental insufficiency
• Intrauterine growth retardation
• Fetal hypoxia and hypercarbia
Diving reflex
• Redistribution of blood to brain, heart, and adrenals
• Increased mesenteric artery vascular resistance
Absence/reversal of end-diastolic flow in umbilical artery
Decreased intestinal perfusion and intestinal hypoxic injury before birth
Motor, secretary and mucosal dysfunction
Intestinal stasis and bacterial dysbiosis
Increased risk of feed intolerance and NEC
Delayed initiation and advancement of feeds
Prolonged time to reach full feeds
TPN related complications (sepsis, cholestasis, etc.)
Increased duration of hospital stay and cost
Feeding in AREDF
<35 weeks
≥35 weeks
AEDF
Start at 6–24 hours
REDF baby
Start feeds at 24 hours
Start full enteral feeds as per daily total requirement
Start feed at 20 mL/kg/day
Check for abdominal examination and bowel sounds
Start feed at 20 mL/kg/day
Feed advancement at 20–30 mL/kg/day
Mothers own milk > pasteurized donor human milk > preterm formula
Feed advancement at 15–20 mL/kg/day
Monitor for feed intolerance stop feeding in such cases and reassess after 6–12 hours
Omit IV fluid when feeds reach 120 mL/kg/day

Q11. What is feed intolerance?

Feed intolerance is common in very preterm infants especially in the first few days of life and represents structural and functional immaturity of the GI tract.

There is no universally agreed upon criteria. It can be diagnosed by the presence of one or more of the following:

- *Vomiting:*
  - Any episode of bile- or blood-stained vomiting
  - Recurrent vomiting more than three times during any 24 hours of period
- Abdominal distention (with or without visible bowel loops):
  - Abdominal girth (AG) increase >2 cm (measured at umbilicus—prefeed)
  - Abdominal wall erythema or tenderness
  - Absent/reduced bowel sounds
- *Increased gastric residuals:*
  - Nonspecific indicator; >5 mL/kg or >50% of the gastric residual volume (GRV) is abnormal
  - Routine prefeed aspiration of gastric contents is not recommended.
- Gross or occult blood in stools
- Presence of systemic features (lethargy, apnea, cyanosis, bradycardia, etc.)

Q12.   What are the causes for feed intolerance?

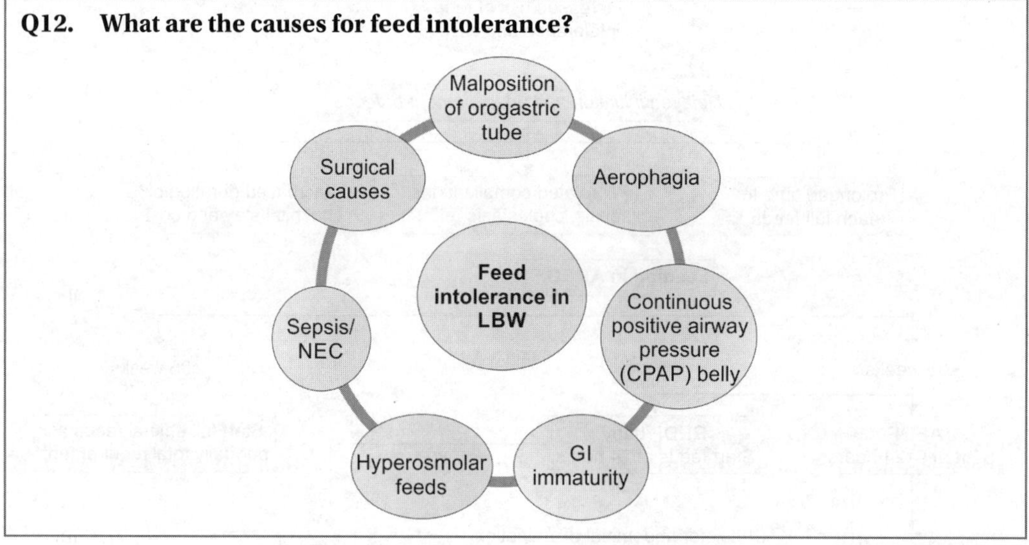

Q13. How to manage neonates with feed intolerance?

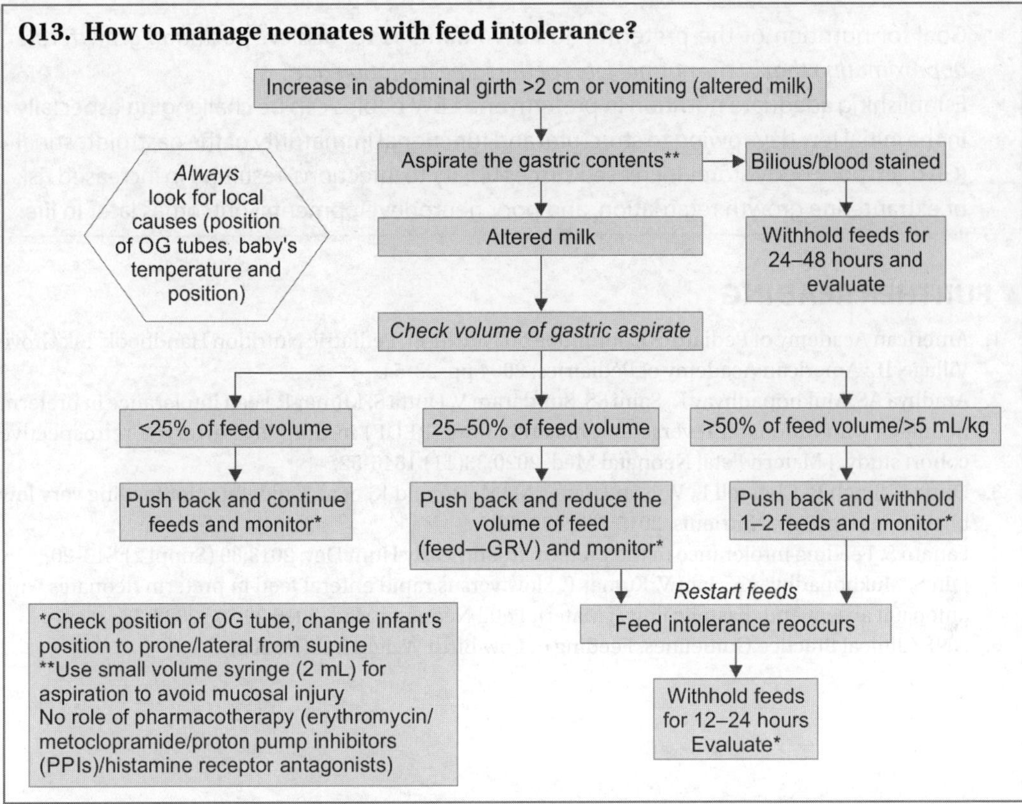

Key Points to Remember

- Skilled professional support should be provided to all the lactating mothers.
- Metoclopramide should not be used to enhance the breast milk. Interventions like breast massage, breast warming, and relaxation techniques should be used to enhance breast milk supply in mothers whose preterm infants are admitted in the NICU.
- Nonnutritive sucking (NNS) should be encouraged in preterm VLBW neonates admitted in neonatal unit.
- Peer support should be provided to the mothers to help in initiating and sustaining breastfeeding.
- Preferred mode of feeding <32 weeks—OG tube, 32–34 weeks—katori spoon/paladai, ≥35 weeks—breastfeeding.
- *Frequency of feeding:* Every 2 hourly if <32 weeks PMA/<1,500 g and every 3 hourly if ≥32 weeks/weight ≥1,500 g
- India accounts >40% of the global burden of low birth weight (LBW) babies with 7.5 million babies (or 30% of the country's total annual live births) being born with a birth weight <2,500 g.

- Goal for nutrition of the preterm and LBW infants is to *"achieve postnatal growth rate approximating that of the normal fetus of the same gestation age".*
- Establishing adequate nutrition in preterm and LBW babies can be challenging especially in the initial few days owing to structural and functional immaturity of the gastrointestinal (GI) tract, poor body stores increased susceptibility to infections, resulting in increased risk of extrauterine growth retardation, and poor neurodevelopmental outcomes later in life.

FURTHER READING

1. American Academy of Pediatrics Committee on Nutrition. Pediatric Nutrition Handbook. Elk Grove Village, IL: American Academy of Pediatrics; 2004 pp. 23-54.
2. Aradhya AS, Mukhopadhyay K, Saini SS, Sundaram V, Dutta S, Kumar P. Feed intolerance in preterm neonates with antenatal reverse end diastolic flow (REDF) in umbilical artery: a retrospective cohort study. J Matern Fetal Neonatal Med. 2020;33(11):1846-52.
3. Dutta S, Singh B, Chessell L, Wilson J, Janes M, McDonald K, et al. Guidelines for feeding very low birth weight infants. Nutrients. 2015;7(1):423-42.
4. Fanaro S. Feeding intolerance in the preterm infant. Early Hum Dev. 2013;89 (Suppl 2):S13-20.
5. Jain S, Mukhopadhyay K, Jain V, Kumar P. Slow versus rapid enteral feed in preterm neonates with antenatal absent end diastolic flow. J Matern Fetal Neonatal Med. 2016;29(17):2828-33.
6. NNF Clinical Practice Guidelines. Feeding of Low Birth Weight babies; 2020.

Total Parenteral Nutrition

Chinmay Chetan

■ COMPONENTS

1. Energy

- *Recommended energy supply:*
  - First day in preterm infants—at least 45–55 kcal/kg/day
  - After initial weight loss, energy should be given to target weight gain of 17–20 g/kg/day
  - 90–120 kcal/kg/day of calories are required by VLBW babies—to match intrauterine accretion rates and adequate weight gain.
- Energy requirement when given by enteral route—10–20% higher than when given by parenteral route
- Energy supplied is calculated from carbohydrate, proteins, and lipids by Atwater factor. Energy supplied by:
  - 1 g protein—4 kcal/g
  - 1 g carbohydrates—4 kcal/g
  - 1 g lipid—9 kcal/g.

2. Protein

- Adequate protein intake—required for accretion of lean body mass and anabolism
- Inadequate calorie supply with adequate protein also leads to protein catabolism to energy, so wastage of the protein being given.
- For utilization of amino acids in accretion—ensure adequate calorie intake of 30–40 kcal/g amino acids.
- Day 2 onward ensure nonprotein energy intake of >65 kcal/kg/day for effective utilization of amino acids for anabolism.
- *CNR (nonprotein calorie nitrogen ratio):*
  - Formula = Total nonprotein calorie/Total nitrogen
  - 1 g nitrogen = 6.25 g of proteins
  - Target—150–250 kcal/g of nitrogen

Protein intake (G/kg/day).		
Preterm infant	Day 1 1.5–2.5	Day 2 onwards 2.5–3.5
Term infant	1.5–3.0	

- *Commonly available amino acid preparation:*
  - 10% aminoven
    - Total amino acids—100 g/L
    - Ph—5.5–6.0
    - Osmolarity—800-900 mOsm/L

3. Carbohydrates

- In TPN, carbohydrate is provided by dextrose.
- Maintain blood sugar level between 60 mg/dL and 145 mg/dL
- Recommended dextrose supply is given in **Table 2**.

Dextrose supply in mg/kg/min (g/kg/day).					
			Day 2 onward		
	Day 1		**Target**	**Minimum**	**Maximum**
Preterm infant	4–8 (5.8–11.5)	Increase gradually over 2–3 days (keeping sugar in normal range)	8–10 (11.5–14.4)	4 (5.8)	12 (17.3)
Term infant	2.5–5 (3.6–7.2)		5–10 (7.2–14.4)	2.5 (3.6)	12 (17.3)

Note: To convert from mg/kg/min to g/kg/day—multiply by 1.44

- If baby become sick, e.g., in infection, shock—then the carbohydrate can be given according to day 1 requirement, to be guided by blood sugar levels. Higher sugar intake during the acute illness does not prevent protein catabolism.

4. Lipids

- *Provides:*
  - Energy
    - 25–50% of nonprotein calories by lipids are recommended.
  - Essential fatty acids
  - Helps in delivery of lipid soluble vitamins A, D, E, and K
- *Types of lipids available:*
  - Pure soybean oil based
  - Medium chain triglycerides (MCT) based
  - Newer lipids with fish oil (FO), e.g., SMOF 20%
    - 30% soyabean oil (SO), 30% MCT, 25% olive oil (OO), and 15% FO
    - Osmolality—380 mOsm/kg H_2O

- Benefits of mixed (SO/OO/MCT/FO)-based lipids compared to only SO-based lipid preparation:
  - Higher docosahexaenoic acid (DHA)
  - Lesser adverse immunological effect—lesser sepsis rates
  - Decreased rates of cholestasis and TPN associated liver dysfunction
  - Lesser oxidative stress
  - Decreased phytosterol load
- Gradual increase of lipids—improves fat tolerance:
  - Start with 1–1.5 g/kg/day—increase gradually by 0.5–1 g/kg/day
  - Maximum dose (both term/preterm) 4 g/kg/day
- Should always be given by light protected tubing or covered with opaque material.
- *Complications of lipids*:
  - Increased chances of sepsis (nonconclusively proven)
  - *Excess lipids may lead to:*
    - Bilirubin displacement from albumin binding sites by free fatty acids (FFAs)—jaundice and kernicterus
    - Stored in adipose tissue and may increase the risk of fat overload syndrome.
    - Plasma triglyceride (TG) concentration may rise and may cause adverse effects including reticuloendothelial system overload.
  - *Photo peroxidation:* If not covered by light protected tubing then may lead to peroxidation—causing free radical injury in infants.
- *Monitoring:*
  - *Plasma TG levels:*
    - To be done within approximately 1–2 days after initiation or adjustment of lipid infusion. Thereafter, weekly to monthly depending on the stability and history of the patient.
    - Reduction of dosages of lipids—to be considered if serum TG exceeds 265 mL/dL
  - *Liver enzymes and direct bilirubin levels:* 2 weeks after initiation of PN and weekly/monthly thereafter
- *Recommended lipid supply:* To prevent essential fatty acid deficiency, a minimum of 0.5 g/kg/day of an SO lipids and 1 g/kg/day of SMOF lipids should be provided.

5. Electrolytes

	Preterm	*Term*
Sodium (mmol/kg/day)	• First week of life 0–3 • Later 2–5	• First week of life 0–2 • Later 2–3
Potassium (mmol/kg/day)	• First week of life 0–3 • Later 1–3	• First week of life 0–3 • Later 1–3
Chloride (mmol/kg/day)	• First week of life 0–3 • Later 2–5	• First week of life 0–3 • Later 2–3

Note: Electrolytes should be added to the maintenance fluid after 2–3 days of life.

6. Micronutrients and Trace Elements

Minerals	Preterm	Term	When to give
Calcium	• During first few days 40–80 mg/kg/day • Growing preterm 60–150 mg/kg/day	30–60 mg/kg/day	To be given in all babies on TPN
Phosphate	• During first few days 30–60 mg/kg/ day • Growing preterm 50–100 mg/kg/day	20–40 mg/kg/day	To be given in all babies on TPN
Magnesium	• During first few days 2.5–5.0 mg/kg/day • Growing preterm 5.0–7.5 mg/kg/day	2.5–5.0 mg/kg/day	To be given in all babies on TPN
Zinc	400–500 µg/kg/day	250 µg/kg/day	• To be given in all babies on TPN • Maximum 5 mg/day
Copper	40 µg/kg/day	20 µg/kg/day	• To be given in all TPN • Maximum 0.5 mg/day
Iron	200–250 µg/kg/day	50–100 µg/kg/day	• Only if prolonged TPN • Maximum 5 mg/day
Manganese	No >1 µg/kg/day		• Only if prolonged TPN • Maximum 50 µg/day
Selenium	7 µg/kg/day	2–3 µg/kg/day	• To be given in all TPN • Maximum of 100 µg/day
Chromium	0.2 µg/kg per day		• Supplementation is unnecessary since Cr contaminates PN • Maximum 5 µg/day

For example, of trace element preparation is available in Indian market—Otski, Igrace, and Celecel.

7. Vitamins

Vitamin	Function	Dose in term	Dose in preterm
Vitamin A	• Vision • Epithelial cell function and differentiation • Immune function • Growth	2,300 IU/day	700–1,500 IU/kg/day
Vitamin D	• Regulation of calcium and phosphate • Bone accretion • Immune function	400 IU/day	800–1,000 IU/day

Contd...

Contd...

Vitamin	Function	Dose in term	Dose in preterm
Vitamin E	Antioxidant	≤11 mg/day	2.8–3.5 mg/kg/day
Vitamin K	• Coagulation factors • Anticoagulation factors	10 µg/kg/day	10 µg/kg/day
Vitamin C	Cofactor for many enzymes and a strong antioxidant	15–25 mg/kg/day	15–25 mg/kg/day
Thiamine (Vitamin B_1)	Involved in carbohydrate and lipid metabolism	0.35–0.50 mg/kg/day	0.35–0.50 mg/kg/day
Riboflavin (Vitamin B_2)	Energy metabolism	0.15–0.2 mg/kg/day	0.15–0.2 mg/kg/day
Pyridoxine (Vitamin B_6)	• As a cofactor in glucose, amino acid metabolism • Immune function	0.15–0.2 mg/kg/day	0.15–0.2 mg/kg/day
Cobalamin (Vitamin B_{12})	Involved in DNA nucleotides formation	0.3 µg/kg/day	0.3 µg/kg/day
Niacin	• Energy metabolism • DNA synthesis	4–6.8 mg/kg/day	4–6.8 mg/kg/day
Pantothenic acid	Synthesis of coenzyme A and therefore essential for fatty acid metabolism	2.5 mg/kg/day	2.5 mg/kg/day
Biotin		5–8 µg/kg/day	5–8 µg/kg/day

Lipid soluble vitamins especially vitamin A and vitamin B_2—photo degraded. Therefore, all vitamin preparations should ideally be mixed with lipid preparation—and given by photo-protected tubings.

8. Fluids

Total fluid rate is started at 60–80 mL/kg/day. Increased by 15–20 mL/kg/day depending on the adequate weight loss/gain. Increased to a maximum of 150–160 mL/kg/day. It can be increased further depending on the intravascular status of the neonate.

■ CALCULATION OF TOTAL PARENTERAL NUTRITION

TPN Chart			
Name: X			*Weight:* 1.2 kg
DOL: 3rd day			*TFI:* 120 mL/kg/day
	Target	*Total requirement*	*Fluid amount for one day*
Feeding	Nil		
Protein	3 g/kg/day	3.6 g/day	36 mL aminoven (10% aminoven)
Lipids	3 g/kg/day	3.6 g/day	18 mL of SMOF (20% SMOF)
3% saline	3 mEq/kg/day	3.6 mEq/day	7.2 mL of 3% saline (1 mL of 3% saline has 0.5 mEq of sodium)
KCL	2 mEq/kg/day	2.4 mEq/day	1.2 mL of KCL (1 mL of KCL has 2 mEq of potassium)
MVI*	0.2 mL/kg/day	0.25 mL/day	0.25 of MVI
Calcium gluconate	6 mL/kg/day	7.2 mL/day	7.2 mL/day of 10% calcium gluconate
$MgSO_4$	5 mg/kg/day	6 mg/day	0.1 mL (50% $MgSO_4$–500 mg $MgSo_4$/1 mL—equivalent to 50 mg elemental mg/1 mL)
OTSKI (trace element)	0.2 mL/kg/day	0.25 mL/day	0.25 mL
Total			70.2 mL

*Amount to be taken depending on which preparation being used. To be calculated depending on the constituent dose of the vitamins

$$\text{Total fluid intake—}120 \ mL/kg/day = 144 \ \text{mL}$$
$$\text{Carbohydrate—}10 \ mg/kg/min = 14.4 \ \text{g/kg/day} = 17.3 \ \text{g/day}$$
$$\text{Fluid left for carbohydrate} = 144 \ \text{mL} - 70.1 \ \text{mL} = 74 \ \text{mL}$$

For achieving 17.3 g in 74 mL fluid

- *Assuming:*
  - x mL of 10% Dx and y mL of 25% Dx
    - $x + y = 74$ mL
    - $10/100 \ x + 25/100 \ y = 17.3$
  - So, 8 mL of 10% Dx and 66 mL of 25% Dx per day
- Therefore, final order

Mix (Solution 1):

- 36 mL of 10% aminoven
- 7.2 mL of 3% NaCl
- 1.2 mL KCL
- 7.2 mL of 10% calcium gluconate
- 0.1 mL of 50% $MgSO_4$

- 0.25 mL of OTSKI
- 8 mL of 10% Dx
- 66 mL of 25% Dx
- (Total—126 mL)
- To be given at 126 mL/24 h – 5.25 mL/h

And (solution 2):

- 18 mL of 20% SMOF
- 0.25 mL MVI
- To be given at 18.25/24 h – 0.76 mL/h
- Lipid and MVI are light sensitive – so should be given by light protective assembly [syringe/PMO line to be covered by aluminum foil/opaque paper]

Solution 1 and 2 should be given by separate line and tubings, but can be mixed at the end via a Y connector and given by same long line/peripheral cannula.

Total Calories (kcal/kg/day): Protein (3 g/kg/day × 4 kcal/g = 12 kcal/kg/day) + lipid (3 g/kg/day × 9 kcal/g = 27 kcal/kg/day) + carb (14.4 g/kg/day × 4 kcal/g = 57.6 kcal/kg/day) = 96.6 kcal/kg/day

Total energy per gram of amino acid: 96.6 kcal/kg/day / 3 g/kg/day = *32.2 kcal/g of proteins* (Target = 30–40 kcal/g)

Nonprotein calorie = 57.6 + 27 = 84.6 kcal/kg/day (Target > 65 kcal/kg/day)

CNR (Nonprotein – calorie nitrogen ratio): – (27 + 57.6 / 3) × 6.25 = 176.25 kcal/g of nitrogen (Target: 150–250 kcal/g of nitrogen)

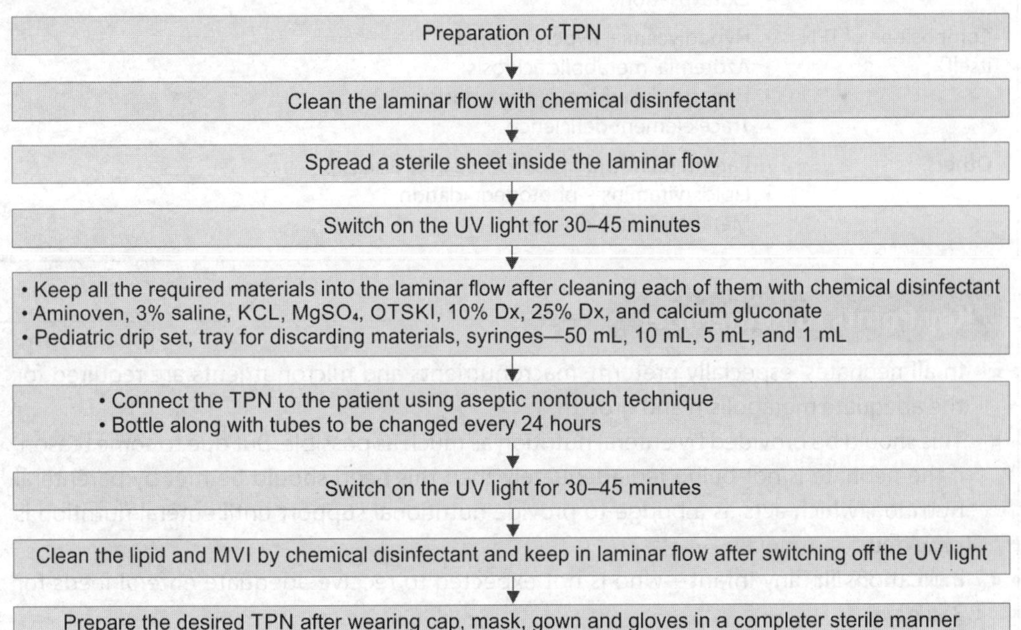

Monitoring

Frequency	Sample
Multiple times in a day	Blood sugar (in the beginning)
Daily	• Blood sugars (after few days—when sugars and GIR stabilized), Urine sugar • Weight
Twice a week	Sodium*, potassium*, and chloride
Weekly	• Calcium*, phosphorous, magnesium, blood gases, CBC, LFTs, creatinine, and blood urea nitrogen • Head circumference and length
As required	• Triglycerides 1–2 days after initiation or adjustment of lipid infusion. Thereafter, weekly to monthly depending on the stability and history of the patient • Trace element levels

*Initially may be sent every 1–2 days till stabilized.

Frequency may be increased/decreased individualized on patients' requirement

Complications

Central venous catheter related	• Infection • *Mechanical complication:* Leakage, blockage, dislodgement, and migration • Extravasation
Composition of TPN itself	• Hypoglycemia, hyperglycemia • Azotemia, metabolic acidosis • Hypertriglyceridemia, cholestasis • Trace element deficiency
Others	• Parenteral nutrition associated liver disease • Lipids/vitamins—photodegradation • Metabolic bone disease

Key Points to Remember

- In all neonates, especially preterm, macronutrients and micronutrients are required for the adequate metabolism and growth.
- This should be provided by enteral nutrition as much as possible. But due to some reason, if the neonate is not being fed adequately then this need should be met by parenteral nutrition, which acts as a bridge to provide nutritional support until enteral nutrition is provided.
- Indications (In any infant—who is not expected to receive adequate enteral feeds for 3–5 days)
  - Extremely preterm infants

- Necrotizing enterocolitis
- Septic ileus
- Infants with surgical abdomen, e.g., intestinal atresia, perforation, and tracheoesophageal fistula
- Short bowel syndrome
- Infant too sick to receive enteral nutrition, e.g., shock requiring high dose inotropes and pressors

- In such infants, it should be started as soon as possible.
- If aggressive total parenteral nutrition (TPN) is not provided, it leads to extrauterine growth retardation (EUGR) and its associated problems such as infections, prolonged requirement of respiratory support, prolonged hospital stay, signs of micronutrient, and vitamin deficiency.
- Preterm infants, who required TPN, should be started soon after birth on the first day itself.
- Extrauterine growth retardation itself leads poor neurodevelopmental outcome. To prevent such complications, it is essential to start TPN if indication arises.
- If possible, parenteral nutrition should be given by central line.
- Umbilical venous catheter or peripherally inserted central catheter (PICC) line can be used as central line in neonates.
- Till securing the central line, parenteral nutrition can be started with peripheral line, but central line should then be secured as soon as possible.
- For short-term TPN, peripheral line can be used if osmolality is kept below 900 mOsm/L.
- Dextrose concentration of >12.5% should not be given by peripheral line in view of high osmolarity and acidic pH, which can irritate the vein and cause thrombophlebitis.
- Central line used for parenteral nutrition should not be used for any other purpose, if possible. It should be handled as less frequently as possible to prevent infection.

When to Discontinue TPN?

When baby reaches feeds of at least 50–70 mL/kg/day then parenteral nutrition can be started to wean off. It can be stopped if the neonates reach 100–120 mL/kg/day of feeds.

■ FURTHER READING

1. Gleason CA, Juul SE. Avery's Diseases of the Newborn e-book. Philadelphia: Elsevier Health Sciences; 2017.
2. Hartman C, Shamir R, Simchowitz V, Lohner S, Cai W, Decsi T, et al. ESPGHAN guidelines on Pediatric Parenteral Nutrition. Clin Nutr. 2018;37(6 Pt B):2418-29.
3. NICE. (2020). National Institute for Health and Care Excellence. Neonatal parenteral nutrition. [online] Available from https://www.nice.org.uk/guidance/ng154 [Last accessed September, 2022].

Management of Donor Human Milk

Malvika Haldwani, Avadhesh Ahuja

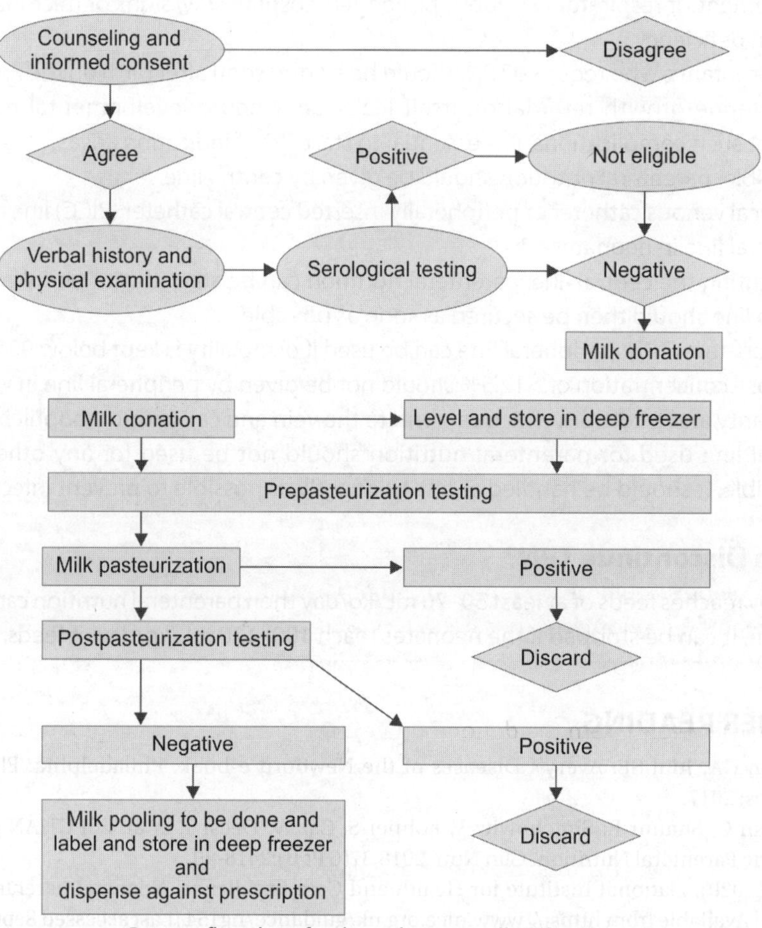

Process flowchart for donor human milk utilization.

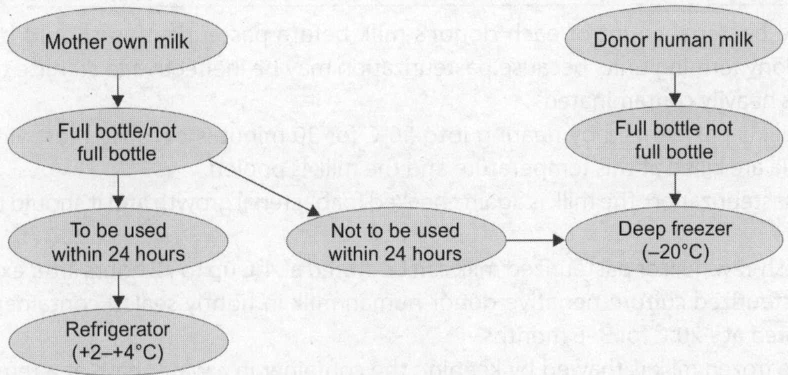

Process flowchart for prepasteurization storage of donor human milk (DHM).

Key Points to Remember

- Human breast milk banks provide service for screening, collecting, processing, storing, and distributing donated human milk.
- Banked or pooled human milk is regarded as "the next best option" for feeding the babies, if biological mother is unable to breastfeed or breastfeeding is contraindicated.
- Indications for the use of donor human milk
  - Decreased or absent supply of breast milk (inadequate lactation)
  - Abandoned babies, adopted child, or orphaned babies
  - Sick neonates transferred to neonatal intensive care unit (NICU) without mother
  - Infant at health risk from breast milk of the biological mother
- Screening
  - A detailed medical history of the donor is taken to exclude infectious diseases which can be transmitted through breast milk.
  - Her blood should be screened for human immunodeficiency virus-1 (HIV-1) and 2, human T-lymphotropic virus (HTLV), cytomegalovirus (CMV), hepatitis B virus (HBV), HCV, and syphilis.
- Consent
  - A consent form from the donor mother is required that her infant will not suffer and there are no financials involved in it.
- Collection
  - Strict aseptic precautions should be taken while collecting the milk.
  - The milk can be expressed either manually or with the help of a manual or an electric pump.
  - The milk is pooled from 4 to 6 donors after pasteurization and best collected in the stainless steel containers because leukocytes and macrophages may stick to the surface of glass container while polyethylene bags are associated with the decrease in the IgA content of the milk.

- The bacterial count of each donor's milk before pasteurization should be <1,000 colony forming units because pasteurization may be ineffective to sterilize the milk if it is heavily contaminated.
- The milk is pasteurized by heating it to 56°C for 30 minutes because most viruses and bacteria are killed at this temperature and the milk is pooled.
- After pasteurization, the milk is again checked for bacterial growth and it should be sterile.
- Storage
  - Fresh-raw milk or pasteurized milk can be stored at 4°C up to 72 hours after expression.
  - Pasteurized culture-negative donor human milk in tightly sealed containers can be stored at −20°C for 3–6 months.
  - The frozen milk is thawed by keeping the container in a water bath at a temperature not exceeding 37°C or under running lukewarm water, thawing at high temperatures result in reduction of IgA content of milk.
  - Breast milk, under all circumstances, should be handled using aseptic techniques and at all times.
- Impact of donor human milk on vulnerable infants
  - *Sepsis:* Risk is reduced for late onset-sepsis in vulnerable, low birth-weight infants during the neonatal period.
  - *Necrotizing enterocolitis (NEC):* Human milk feeding whether mothers own milk or donor human milk reduces the chances of developing NEC.
  - *Feeding intolerance:* Preterm infants fed with unfortified donor human milk have fewer vomits, less gastric stasis, and reduced diarrhea compared with the formula milk.
  - Reduced length of NICU stay
  - Cost saving
  - *Neurodevelopmental outcomes and long-term outcomes:* Lesser rates of metabolic syndromes, increased white matter and brain volume and significantly greater scores for mental, motor, and behavior settings.
  - Under NHM, lactation management centers are being established in the country at three level to provide lactation support to the mothers.
    - **Comprehensive Lactation Management Centre (CLMC):** Established at tertiary/regional health facility.
    - **Lactation Management Unit (LMU):** Established at a secondary level health facility—district hospital with SNCU.
    - **Lactation Support Unit (LSU):** Established at the sub-district hospital/CHC/PHC with delivery points.

■ FURTHER READING

1. Arslanoglu S, Moro GE, Bellu R, Turoli D, De NG, Tonetto P, et al. Presence of human milk bank is associated with elevated rate of exclusive breastfeeding in VLBW infants. J Perinat Med. 2013;41:129-31.
2. Bharadva K, Tiwari S, Mishra S, Mukhopadhyay K, et al. Infant and Young Child Feeding Chapter, Indian Academy of Pediatrics, Human Milk Banking Guidelines. Indian Pediatr. 2014;51(6):469-74.
3. Mantri N, Goel AD, Joshi NK, Bhardwaj P, Gautam V, Gupta MK. Challenges in implementation of mother milk banks in Rajasthan: a situational analysis. J Mother Child. 2022;25(2):86-94.

Chapter 60

Management of Extrauterine Growth Retardation

Anita Singh

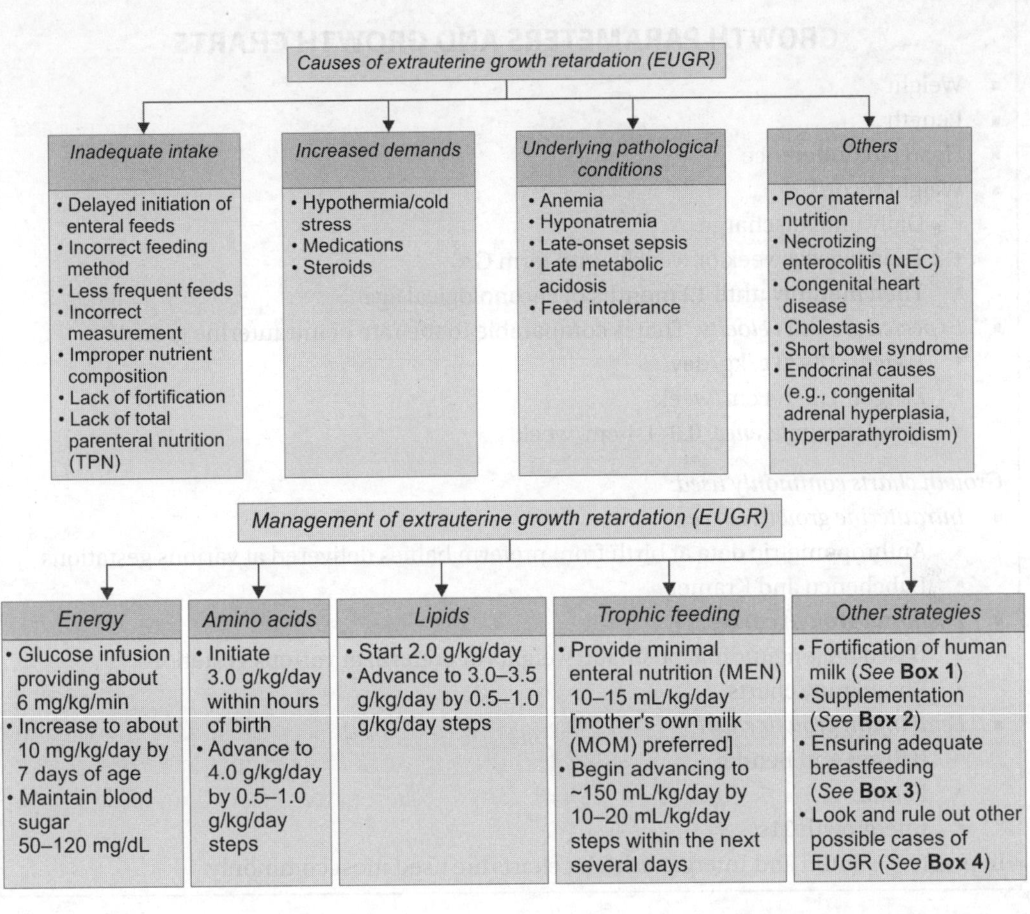

EXPECTED NUTRITIONAL AND GROWTH PARAMETERS

The *American Academy of Pediatrics Committee on Nutrition* recommends the nutritional goals of preterm infants is to "provide nutrient that permits the postnatal growth rate and the composition of weight gain to approximate that of a normal fetus of the same PMA and to maintain normal concentrations of blood and tissue nutrients."

- *For ELBW and VLBW infants:*
  - Enteral intake of 125–130 kcal/kg/day or parenteral intake of 100–110 kcal/kg/day
  - 3.5–4 g/kg/day of protein
  - The recommended dietary allowance (RDA) of all nutrients is given in **Table 1**.

GROWTH PARAMETERS AND GROWTH CHARTS

- Weight
- Length
- Head circumference
- Weight record
  - Daily until discharge
  - Then twice a week or weekly until term GA
  - Then monthly until 12 months of chronological age
- *Expected growth velocity:* That is comparable to the rate of intrauterine growth.
  - *Weight:* 18–20 g/kg/day
  - *Length:* 1.1–1.4 cm/week
  - *Head circumference:* 0.9–1.1 cm/week.

Growth charts commonly used:
- *Intrauterine growth curves:*
  - Anthropometric data at birth from preterm babies delivered at various gestations
  - Lubchenco and Kramer
- *Postnatal growth curves:*
  - Based on longitudinal postnatal weights of preterm at various gestations
  - Ehrenkranz charts
- *Fetal infant growth chart:*
  - Babson and Benda
  - Fenton
  - Intergrowth 21st

In practice, Fenton and Intergrowth 21st charts are used most commonly.

PREVENTION AND MANAGEMENT

- *Early aggressive nutrition:*
  - To reduce the cumulative caloric and protein deficits in acute stage to a minimal degree
  - Early parenteral and enteral nutrition
  - Monitoring for feed intolerance
  - Not withholding feeds for gastric residuals without signs of NEC.

- *Enteral nutrition:*
  - Starting trophic feeding within 1–2 days of birth in small volume as possible
  - *Type of milk feed:* Mother's own milk should be the first choice followed by pasteurized donor human milk.
  - Formula should only be considered if first two options are unavailable.

BOX 1: Fortification of human milk.

- Unsupplemented mature human milk is not enough to meet the requirement of protein to support the growth and lean body mass accretion of very preterm infants.
- The concentrations of calcium and phosphorus in human milk are also significantly below that to match levels of in utero accretion.
- *Indications:*
  - ≤34 weeks of gestation
  - ≤1,500 g BW
  - On TPN >2 weeks
  - >1,500 g with suboptimal growth
  - >1,500 g with limited ability to tolerate increased volume.
- *How to use:*
  - Human milk fortifier (HMF) is started once baby has reached 100 mL/kg/day of feeds.
  - Fortification should be continued till the infant reaches 2–2.5 kg or 40 weeks postmenstrual age whichever comes later, however, it may be continued till 9–12 months.
- *Types of fortifiers:*
  - Monocomponent (protein only, carbohydrate only, and fat only) or multicomponent
  - Powder or liquid form
  - From animal milk or human milk source (pasteurized human donor milk).
- *Method of fortification:*
  - *Standard fortification:* The composition of human milk is assumed and fortifier is added as per manufacturer's recommendation.
  - *Individualized fortification:* Protein and energy content of human milk are measured and fortifier is added as per results.
- Currently four different HMF brands are available in our country. The details of the fortifiers are given below.

Composition of HMFs available in India.

Nutrient	Lactodex (per g)	HIJAM (per g)	Prenan (per g)	Neolacta (per g)
Calories (kcal)	3.37	3.5	4	3.5
Carbohydrate (g)	0.49	0.49	0.68	1.8
Protein (g)	0.27	0.25	0.3	0.12
Fat (g)	0.04	0.25	0.1	0.02
Calcium (mg)	15.8	25	16	2.51
Phosphorus (mg)	7.9	12.5	9	1.77
Iron (mg)	0.3	0.36	0.36	0.00
Vitamin D (IU)	133	100	24	-
Osmolarity	393	<400	366	<400
			Partially hydrolyzed whey protein with EFA	

BOX 2: Supplements.

- *Calcium, phosphorus, and vitamin D:*
  - Recommended dietary allowances as per European Society of Pediatric Gastroenterology, Hepatology, and Nutrition (ESPGHAN)
  - *Calcium:* 120–140 mg/kg/day
  - *Phosphorus:* 60–90 mg/kg/day
  - *Vitamin D:* 800–1,000 IU/day
  - *Optimal Ca:* P ratio in enteral feeds: 1.5–2.0 (mg/mg).
- *Iron:*
  - Recommended dietary allowance as per ESPGHAN: 2–3 mg/kg/day
  - Start at 2–6 weeks of age (2 weeks in VLBW)
  - To be continued after discharge (till 6–12 months of age)
  - Increased requirement during rHuEPO therapy (up to 6–8 mg/kg/day)
  - Routine monitoring of iron indices, especially Hb and ferritin
- *Multivitamin drops:* Multivitamin drops are supplemented as 1 mL/day.

BOX 3: Facilitation and ensuring adequate feed.

- Positioning and technique of breastfeed are explained below. Make sure that baby is properly clothed.
- Assessing adequacy of paladai/cup feeds
  - Swallows milk without coughing or spluttering
  - Accepts required amount

For all feeding modes, baby should have adequate weight gain and should pass urine 6–8 times in 24 hours.

Postdischarge Nutrition
- Infants discharged with a subnormal weight for postconceptional age should be continued on fortified human milk.
- If breast milk is not available then the babies should be fed on special postdischarge formula with high contents of protein, minerals, and trace elements.

BOX 4: Look and rule out other possible cases of EUGR.

- *Avoid hypothermia/cold stress:* The preterm and very low birth weight babies should be adequately clothed to prevent cold stress.
- *Correct anemia:* If a baby is having weight gain of <10 g/day for 4 days on 100 kcal/kg/day with Hct of <31%, the packed cell transfusion is recommended.
- *Correct hyponatremia:* Preterm neonates may continue to lose sodium till 34–36 weeks postmenstrual age because of tubular dysfunction. Thereby babies should be screened for hyponatremia and correction should be done accordingly by sodium supplementation.
- *Metabolic acidosis:* Preterm babies often have nonanion gap metabolic acidosis because of tubular dysfunction related to prematurity. This is a frequently encountered cause of suboptimal weight gain. In such cases, oral sodium bicarbonate supplementation by 1–2 mEq/kg/day helps.
- *Look for occult infection:* The sepsis and urinary tract infection are one of the important causes of poor weight gain. Babies with suboptimal weight gain should be thoroughly screened for sepsis and treated.
- *Judicious use of drugs:* Diuretics, caffeine, and steroids are commonly used medication which interferes with weight gain. These drugs should be judiciously used and stopped proactively once no longer needed.
- *Increase volume:* Conventional total feed maximum volume at full feeds is usually 150–180 mL/kg/day in preterm very low birth weight babies. It can be increased to 200 mL/kg/day in babies if weight gain is lesser despite adequate calories and if it is tolerated well.
- *Kangaroo mother care:* Kangaroo mother care is a low cost intervention that can improve weight gain in preterm and low birth weight babies.

TABLE 1: Recommended intake of macro and micronutrients expressed per mg/kg/day and per 100 kcal unless otherwise denoted.

Maximum–Minimum	Per/kg/day	Per/100 kcal
Fluid, mL	135–200	
Energy, kcal	110–135	
Protein, g <1 kg body weight	4.0–4.5	3.6–4.1
Protein, g 1–1.8 kg body weight	3.5–4.0	3.2–3.6
Lipids, g (of which MCT <80%)	4.8–6.6	4.4–6.0
Linoleic acid, mg*	385–1540	350–1400
A Linoleic acid, mg	>55 (0.9% of fatty acid)	>50
DHA, mg	12–30	11–27
AA, mg†	18–42	16–39
Carbohydrate, g	11.6–13.2	10.5–12
Sodium, mg	69–115	63–105
Potassium, mg	66–132	60–120
Chloride, mg	105–177	95–161
Calcium salt, mg	120–140	110–130
Phosphate, mg	60–90	55–80
Magnesium, mg	8–15	7.5–13.6
Iron, mg	2–3	1.8–2.7
Zinc, mg‡	1.1–2.0	1.0–1.8
Copper, µg	100–132	90–120
Selenium, µg	5–10	4.5–9
Manganese, µg	≤27.5	6.3–35
Fluoride, µg	1.5–60	1.4–55
Iodine, µg	11–55	10–50
Chromium, ng	30–1,230	27–1,120
Molybdenum, µg	0.3–5	0.27–4.5
Thiamin, µg	140–300	125–275
Riboflavin, µg	200–400	180–365
Niacin, µg	380–5,500	345–5,000
Pantothenic acid, µg	0.33–2.1	0.3–1.9
Pyridoxine, µg	45–300	41–273
Cobalamin, µg	0.1–0.77	0.08–0.7
Folic acid, µg	35–100	32–90
L-ascorbic acid, mg	11–46	10–42
Biotin, µg	1.7–16.5	1.5–15
Vitamin A, µg RE, 1 µg ~3.33 IU	400–1,000	360–740
Vitamin D, IU/day	800–1,000	
Vitamin E, mg (a-tocopherol equivalents)	2.2–11	2–10

Contd...

Contd...

Maximum–Minimum	Per/kg/day	Per/100 kcal
Vitamin K$_1$, µg	4.4–28	4–25
Nucleotides, mg		≤5
Choline, mg	8–55	7–50
Inositol, mg	4.4–53	4–48

Calculation of the range of nutrients expressed per 100 kcal is based on a minimum energy intake of 110 kcal/kg.

*The linoleic acid to a-linolenic acid ratio is in the range of 5–15:1 (wt/wt).

†The ratio of AA to DHA should be in the range of 1.0–2.0–1 (wt/wt), and eicosapentaenoic acid (20:5n-3) supply should not exceed 30% of DHA supply.

‡The zinc to copper molar ratio in infant formulae should not exceed 20.

Key Points to Remember

- EUGR is defined if weight, height, and head circumference <10th percentile at discharge or 36 weeks postmenstrual age.
  - *Cross-sectional definition* (weight at a given t-time <10th centile) or
  - *Longitudinal definition* (weight loss between birth and a given t-time >1SD)
- Extrauterine growth retardation (EUGR) is commonly seen in preterm/extremely low birth weight (ELBW) and very low birth weight (VLBW) infants.
- The incidence of EUGR in VLBW infants is strikingly high, reaching 43–97%.
- "97% VLBW are <10th centile at 36 weeks postmenstrual age (PMA)" (Ehrenkranz et al.).
- Early growth faltering is associated with an increased risk of chronic diseases in later life.

OSCE/Checklist 1: Steps of formula milk preparation.

S. No.	Performance steps	Yes	No
1.	Washed hands properly before formula preparation		
2.	Identified the need of formula feed (should be only used when mother's own milk or donor human milk is not available)		
3.	Chosen the appropriate formula type as per term/preterm or low birth weight condition		
4.	Sterilized the container/bottle in which formula has to be prepared		
5.	Used pre-boiled lukewarm water for formula preparation		
6.	Measured the correct amount of water as per need (generally 30 mL for 1 scoop) in a sterile syringe (ideally every time) and pour in the container/bottle		
7.	Added the required scoop of milk powder		
8.	Taken the milk powder in scoop properly as leveled (should neither heaped nor under filled)		
9.	Mixes it properly by spoon. There should not be any lump		
10.	Chosen cup/paladai for feeding (not bottle)		
11	Consumed the prepared formula as early as possible or within an hour		
	Total score (maximum score: 11)		

OSCE/Checklist 2: Steps of adding human milk fortifier (HMF).			
S. No.	Performance steps	Yes	No
1.	Washed hands properly		
2.	Arranged for preparation on a clean firm surface		
3.	Ensured hygienic collection of expressed breast milk (EBM)		
4.	Ensured addition of fortifier just before giving feed to the baby		
5.	Wore sterile gloves for addition of HMF		
6.	Kept sterile paper of gloves handy on which human milk fortifier powder can be placed to cut if needed		
7.	Identified the correct amount of milk in which one sachet needs to be added as per manufacturer's recommendation (Generally one sachet of HMF is added to 25 mL of EBM, however in extremely low birth weight baby it may needs to be given in lesser amount. In such cases the content of HMF sachet needs to be divided)		
8.	Properly levels up the HMF sachet content to distribute the content equally before cutting it (when it is needed in smaller amount of milk) *For 12 mL EBM feed it can be cut in two equal half by sterile blade*		
9.	Put the sachet on sterile surface for cutting (sterile surface of gloves paper can be used)		
10.	Cut the sachet with sterile blade		
11.	Mix the content of one half cut sachet in measured amount of EBM by spoon so that no lumps are left.		
12.	Fed the prepared EBM with fortifier to the baby either by gavage, paladai, or cup (bottle should not be used)		
	Total score (maximum score: 12)		

■ FURTHER READING

1. Agostoni C, Buonocore G, Carnielli VP. Enteral nutrient supply for preterm infants: commentary from the European Society for Paediatric Gastroenterology, Hepatology and Nutrition Committee on Nutrition. J Pediatr Gastroenterol Nutr. 2010;50(1):85-91.
2. Fenton TR, Cormack B, Goldberg D, Nasser R, Alshaikh B, Eliasziw M, et al. "Extrauterine growth restriction" and "postnatal growth failure" are misnomers for preterm infants. J Perinatol. 2020;40(5):704-14.
3. Kler N, Thakur A, Modi M, Kaur A, Garg P, Soni A, et al. Human milk fortification in India. Nestle Nutr Inst Workshop Ser. 2015;81:145-51.
4. Prince A, Groh-Wargo S. Nutrition management for the promotion of growth in very low birth weight premature infants. Nutr Clin Pract. 2013;28(6):659-68.

Management of the Newborn: In Postnatal Ward

Ravi Sachan

CARE IN THE POSTNATAL WARD

- *Maintenance of temperature:*
  - Maintain room temperature in all weathers. Avoid air draughts by closing windows, doors, and switching off fans and air-conditioners.
  - Practice rooming-in 24 × 7. Start Kangaroo mother care (KMC) as early as possible for eligible neonate.
  - Promote exclusive breastfeeding.
  - Advice the mother to keep the baby clean and dry at all times. Remove wet diaper/clothes as early as possible.
  - Ensure that the baby is kept warm. During winter, prewarm the linen, and clothes of the baby before dressing. Cover the baby adequately using cap socks and mittens.
  - During summer, dress the baby in loose cotton clothes. Exposure of the baby to direct sunlight during the hot summer months can lead to serious hyperthermia.
  - Educate mother regarding identification of hypothermia using touch method.
- *Assessment of tone, cry, and activity:*
  - During the first few days of life, babies sleep throughout the day and they are awake, noisy, and troublesome during the night.
  - Babies cry when they are hungry or in discomfort. Discomfort may be due to the unpleasant sensation of a full bladder before passing urine, painful evacuation of hard stools, or soiling by urine and stools.
  - An experienced mother or nurse can usually distinguish between the cry used as a signal for food and the cry of discomfort.
  - Persistent crying needs examination and evaluation.
- *Breastfeeding:*
  - Ensure that the baby is exclusively breastfed, every 2–3 hours cue-based feeding during day and night or on demand.
  - During each feed, one breast should be completely emptied before the baby is put to the other breast.
  - Educate the mother about the benefits of giving breast milk to the baby and the mother should be counseled that there is no need for additional water.
  - An adequately fed baby passes urine at least six to eight times in a day.
  - Regular and optimal feeding will avoid any excessive weight loss.

- *Passage of urine/meconium:*
  - Any baby who has not passed meconium for 24 hours after birth or urine within 48 hours needs to be evaluated.
  - *Transitional stools* (day 3–4 of life) are often semi-loose and greenish-yellow with increased frequency and settle within 24–48 hours, need no treatment. Reassure mother if baby continues to feed well.
  - *Stools*: Breastfed babies pass frequent golden yellow, sticky, semi loose stools, and often while being fed or soon after a feed. This is due to exaggerated gastrocolic reflex, which may persist for a couple of weeks. These infants, however, generally continue to gain weight satisfactorily.
- *Assessment of jaundice:*
  - All the infants must be examined in daylight for the development and severity of jaundice, twice a day for first few days of life.
  - Transcutaneous bilirubinometer (TcB) should be used to screen the assessment of jaundice.
- *Weight record:* Most healthy term babies lose weight during the first 2–3 days of life and regain birth weight by the end of first week; averaging 20–30 g/day; whereas a preterm takes 10–14 days of age to regain birth weight.
  - Any weight loss >5% in a 24-hour period is abnormal. However, preterm may loss 2–3% daily up to maximum 10–15%
- *Possetting/vomiting:*
  - Many normal babies regurgitate or spit out some amount of milk soon after feeds. This is often due to faulty technique of feeding and aerophagy. Counsel all mothers regarding feeding and burping.
  - If the vomiting is persistent, projectile, or bile stained or is associated with abdominal distension baby need to be evaluated further.
  - *Detection of birth defect:* The baby should be thoroughly examined at birth from head-to-toe and the finding should be recorded in neonatal record sheet.
  - Birth defect should be detect and reported as per RBSK operational guidelines.
- *Look for physiological conditions*: Counsel the mother and manage accordingly (*See* **Table 1**).
- *Ask mother's concern*, if any.

DISCHARGE AND FOLLOW-UP

- *Maintenance of body temperature*: Explain about prevention and recognition of hypothermia.
- Ensure successful establishment and adequacy of breastfeeding before discharge.
- *Skin care/bathing:*
  - Ask mother to take special precautions during bathing. Bathing should be delayed until the cord falls off by itself.
  - Sponge bath with cotton dipped in lukewarm water is preferred.
  - Daily baths may be avoided during the winter months and the baby can be sponged in a warm room to prevent hypothermia and to keep the baby clean.

- • Cleaning the perineal area after changing the diaper helps to prevent diaper rashes.
- • Educate the mother about how to provide KMC to keep the baby warm.
- ▪ *Care of the umbilical cord:*
  - • Let the umbilical cord get dry in the air. Make sure the diaper is taped below the cord.
  - • Application of any antiseptic solution is not recommended.
  - • Watch for bleeding and for presence of anyle purulent discharge from the cord.
  - • The cord usually falls after 4–10 days.
- ▪ *Care of the eyes:*
  - • Routine application of antiseptic ointment/drops for prevention of ophthalmia neonatorum is not recommended.
  - • If purulent discharge and eyes are sticky, use sterile cotton swabs dipped in lukewarm sterile water for cleaning. Wipe the eyes from inner canthus to outer using separate swabs for each stroke.
  - • Some neonates may develop persistent epiphora (watering) due to blockage of nasolacrimal duct by epithelial debris.
  - • The mother should be advised to massage the nasolacrimal duct area (by massaging the either side of the nose adjacent to the medial canthus) five to eight times daily, each time before she feeds the baby.
- ▪ *Immunization:*
  - • Birth immunization Bacillus Calmette–Guérin (BCG) vaccine, zero dose of oral polio vaccine and Hepatitis B vaccine as per Universal Immunization Program (UIP) schedule and document it in the mother and child protection (MCP) card.
  - • Newborn screening (NBS) blood test/DBS should be done before discharge.
  - • The mother should be informed about the date of the next visit.
- ▪ *Nutrition supplements:* Required for all low birth weight (LBW) baby and should be started before discharge.
- ▪ *Traditional practices:*
  - • Mother may continue with a variety of beneficial traditional practices such as oil massage or inconsequential practice such as putting black mark on forehead.
  - • However, she should be discouraged to follow harmful traditional practices such as applying kajal/surma in eyes as it may transmit infections, cause injury or even cause lead poisoning.
- ▪ *Explain the danger signs:* When to return to the facility?
  - • Not feeding well, undue lethargy
  - • Sudden rise or fall in body temperature
  - • Respiratory difficulty, not breathing or bluish discoloration of the body
  - • Sudden abnormal movement of the body
  - • Appearance of jaundice within 24 hours of age (If discharge early) or yellowing of palms and soles
  - • Excessive crying
  - • Drooling of saliva or choking during feeding
  - • Persistent vomiting
  - • Bleeding from any site

TABLE 1: Common neonatal physiological developmental conditions.

	Description	Action
Breast hyperplasia (Mastitis neonatorum)	Engorgement of breasts in-term babies of both sexes on the third or fourth day and may last for days or even weeks due to persistence of maternal hormones	Local massage, fomentation and expression of milk should not be done as it may lead to infection
Vaginal bleeding	Seen in female babies about 3–4 days after birth because of withdrawal of maternal hormones. The bleeding is mild and lasts for 2–4 days	Additional vitamin K is unnecessary
Mucoid vaginal secretions	Most female babies have thin, grayish, mucoid, and vaginal secretions	Should not be mistaken for purulent discharge
Tongue tie	A fibrous frenulum with a notch at the tip of the tongue	Does not interfere with sucking or later speech development
Nonretractable prepuce	Normally nonretractable in all male newborn babies, should not be diagnosed as phimosis. The urethral opening is often pinpoint and is visualized with difficulty	Mother should be advised against forcibly retracting the foreskin
Hymenal tags	Seen at the margin of hymen in two-thirds of female babies	
Umbilical hernia	Manifest after the age of 2 weeks or later	Most of these disappear spontaneously by one or two years of age
Peeling skin	Dry skin with peeling and exaggerated transverse sole creases are seen in all post-term and some term babies	Consider application of coconut oil
Milia	Yellow-white spots on the nose or face due to retention of sebum, are present in practically all babies	Disappear spontaneously
Erythema neonatorum	An erythematous rash of unknown cause with a central pallor appearing on the second or third day in-term neonates, which begins on the face and spreads down to the trunk and extremities in about 24 hours. This should be differentiated from pustules, which need treatment	It disappears spontaneously after 2–3 days without any specific treatment
Stork bites (Salmon patches or nevus simplex)	These are discrete, pinkish-gray, sparse, capillary hemangiomata commonly seen at the nape of neck, upper eyelids, forehead and root of the nose, which invariably	Disappears after a few months
Mongolian blues pots	In babies of Asiatic origin, irregular blue areas of skin pigmentation are often present over the sacral area and buttocks, though extremities and rest of the trunk may also be affected	These spots disappear by the age of 6 months

Contd...

Contd...

	Description	*Action*
Subconjunctival hemorrhage	Semilunar arcs of subconjunctival hemorrhage are a common finding in normal babies	The blood gets reabsorbed after a few days without leaving any pigmentation
Epstein pearls	These are white spots, usually one on either side of the median raphe of the hard palate. Similar lesions may be seen on the prepuce	They are of no significance
Sucking callosities	The presence of these button like, cornified plaques over the center of upper lip	Has no significance

Key Points to Remember

- The immediate postnatal period, i.e., first 48 hours after birth when the mother and baby are in the hospital is critical to their health and survival.
- Postnatal care during the first 2 days of birth in facilities provides an opportunity for preventive care practices and routine assessments to identify and manage common conditions in the baby.
- All babies delivered at the health facility should be monitored in the postnatal ward and provided:
  - Routine care and support for feeding difficulties.
  - Appropriate treatment for danger signs and prompt referral if required.
  - Examine a baby for life-threatening congenital malformations and appropriate management.
  - Recognize minor physical peculiarities or developmental variations.
  - Provide advice at discharge including recognition of danger signs.

OSCE/Checklist: Discharge from postnatal ward			
S. No.	*Performance steps*	*Yes*	*No*
1.	Checks newborn and mother is free from any illness and mother is confident to take care of her infant at home		
2.	Newborn has been immunized		
3.	Assessed the adequacy of breastfeeding		
4.	Estimated normal weight loss/gain pattern		
5.	Explain the danger signs clearly and check by reinforcement		
6.	Mother oriented with the use of discharge card/MCP card		
7.	Next follow-up visit has been explained and scheduled		
Signature of the doctor/nurses		*Signature of parents*	

■ FURTHER READING

1. Facility based newborn care, training module for doctors and nurses. MoHFW, GoI; 2022.

Breastfeeding

Malvika Haldwani

Signs of successful breastfeeding.

Signs of good positioning	Signs of good attachment	Signs of good effective suckling	Signs of successful lactation
• Baby's body is well supported • The head, neck and the body of the baby are kept in same plane • Baby's body turned towards the mother • Baby's abdomen touching the mother's abdomen	• The baby's mouth is wide open • The baby's chin touches the breast • The baby's lower lip is everted • Majority of areola inside the baby's mouth	• Baby suckles slowly and pauses in between to swallow (suck, suck, suck, and swallow) • Baby's cheeks are full and not hollow or retracting during sucking	• Newborns will normally pass urine 4–6 times/day • Adequate weight (15–20 g/day) gain would be seen in neonates • Baby sleep after feeding

Advantages of breastfeeding.

To mother	To baby	To society
• Enhances emotional bonding between mother and baby • Can act as lactational amenorrhea • Faster maternal recovery (involution of uterus) • Weight loss is faster • Less postpartum depression • Lower risk for maternal cancers (ovarian and breast)	• Optimum nutrition for growth and development • Easily available • Easily digestible • Lower risk of overweight/obesity in later life • Improved cognition and motor development • Fewer infections including diarrhea, respiratory illness and allergies • Less ear infections, skin conditions, sudden infant death syndrome (SIDS), etc.	• Decrease the overall cost of care • Decreases the duration of hospital stay • Promotes family planning • More economical than artificial feeding • Decrease the re-hospitalization rate and therefore ↓ NMR and IMR

Types of breast milk.

Type	Colostrum	Transition milk	Mature milk
Secretion	• As early as second trimester and during first week of delivery • Thick, sticky, and yellowish in color	• During first 2 weeks (starting from 2nd to 5th day) • Breastfeeding becomes fuller and warmer, color changes to bluish-white	After transition milk secretion the breast starts to secrete mature milk comprising of foremilk and hindmilk
Contents	• Anti-infective proteins and white cells • Vitamin A and vitamin K • Growth factors	• Higher levels of fat (medium chain fatty acids) • Increase lactose low levels of sodium and chloride • Decreasing levels of lactoferrin and IgA antibody and increasing lysozymes • Concentrations of minerals, zinc, copper and manganese decreases	• *Foremilk*—thin Milk (More water, low levels of fats, high lactose, sugar, proteins, vitamins, minerals) • *Hindmilk*—thicker more whiter (Less water, more fats)
Functions	• Protective and provides immunity against diseases • Prevents jaundice (purgative effect) • Helps in digestion and prevents allergies	• Increase in quantity to meet the demands of baby • Bacteria killing enzyme property increases	• Foremilk-satisfies thirst of the baby • Hindmilk-supplies energy and improve growth of baby

■ REFLEXES IN BREASTFEEDING

Reflexes in mother.

Prolactin reflex (anterior pituitary gland)	Oxytocin reflex (posterior pituitary gland)
Baby suckles on the breast	As baby suckles
Sensory stimulus provided through nerve endings in nipple and areola	Induce secretion of oxytocin from posterior pituitary gland
Responsible for milk production	Responsible for milk ejection
	Requires 2–3 minutes of suckling of this response

Reflexes in the baby.

Rooting reflex	Sucking reflex	Swallowing reflex
When something touches lips, baby opens mouth put tongue down and forward	When something touches palate, baby sucks	When mouth fills with milk, baby swallows

■ FACTORS DETERMINING THE OXYTOCIN PRODUCTION

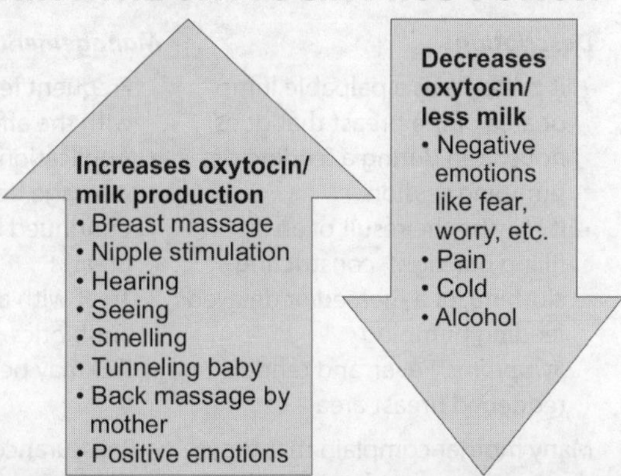

Pathological problems of breastfeeding and management.

Condition	Description	Management
Inverted/flat nipple	Should be diagnosed in the antenatal period	• Teach mother to roll out nipple between thumb and five fingers several times a day • Explain syringe method to be done by the mother • Mothers need additional support to feed their babies
Sore, tender nipples	Caused by incorrect attachment to the breast	• Explain correct positioning and attachment • Apply hind expressed breast milk after each feed and nipple should be aired • No other cream should be applied • If fungal infection is suspected, treat with antifungal medication
Traumatized, painful nipples (includes bleeding, blisters, and Crains)	Possible caused—includes ineffective, poor latch on to breast, improper suckling technique, removing infant from breast without first breaking suction and underlying nipple condition on infection (i.e., eczema, bacterial, fungal infection)	• Assessment of infant position and latch on technique with corrective measures • Diagnose any underlying nipple conditions and prescribe appropriate treatment • In case of severely traumatized nipples, temporary cessation of breastfeeding may be indicated to allow for healing. Instruct the mother to maintain lactation with mechanical/hand expression until direct breastfeeding is resumed
Engorgement	Severe form of increased breast fullness that usually presents on day 3 to day 5 postpartum signaling the onset of milk production. It may be caused by independent breast stimulation resulting in swollen, hard breasts that are warm to touch	• Start early and frequent feed to prevent engorgement • Application of local warm, packs to be applied • Gentle massage of breast during feeding and/or milk expressions • Mild analgesic (paracetamol) for pain relief

Contd...

Contd...

Condition	Description	Management
Breast abscess/ mastitis	• It presents as a palpable lump or area of the breast that does not soften during a feeding or pumping session • It may be the result of an ill—filling bra, tight, constricting clothing, or a messed or delayed feeding pumping • *Symptoms:* Fever, and tender, reddened breast area	• Frequent feeding/pumpings begging with the affected breast • Application of mist heat and breast massage before and during feeding • Continued breastfeeding on unaffected breasts • Treat with appropriate analgesic and antibiotics • I&D may be indicated
Reduced milk supply/ not enough milk	Many mother complain that they do not have enough milk	• Reassurance to the mother • If baby passing urine 6–8 times/day, sleeping 2–3 hours after each feed and gaining weight adequately

---

TEN STEPS TO SUCCESSFUL BREASTFEEDING

1. Written policy regarding breastfeeding.
2. Training of healthcare staff in skills in implementing this policy.
3. Inform all mothers about benefits and management of BF.
4. Help mother to initiate BF within half an hour of delivery.
5. Show mothers, how to breastfeeding and maintain location.
6. Teach mothers to only exclusive BF for 6 months and no food, drinks for 6 months.
7. Promote rooming in within 24 hours of delivery.
8. Encourage BF on demand.
9. Not to give artificial pacifiers and teats.
10. Foster establishment of BF support groups and refer mother to them on discharge from hospitals, clinics.

Key Points to Remember

- Breastfeed at least 8–10 times/day including night feeds or cue-based feeding
- Feeding cues how to recognize baby is ready to feed:
  - Fully opened eyes
  - Widely opens mouth
  - Increased alertness
  - Tongue sucking
  - Hand movements to mouth and sucking hands
- Empty one breast completely then offer another breast.
- Counsel the mother about balanced diet, adequate rest, and avoid stress.
- Exclusive breastfeeding (EBF) is most important and effective tool to decrease infant mortality rate and under-5 mortality rates.
- *Exclusive breastfeeding:* Only breastfeeding till 6 months and medication (if indicated).

Checklist: Breastfeeding counseling			
S. No.	*Performance steps*	*Yes*	*No*
1.	Washed hands		
2.	Explain mother regarding the importance of breastfeeding to mother and baby		
3.	Provide comfortable position to mother		
4.	*Ensure correct position:* • Baby's body is well supported • Keep baby's head in line with body and well supported • Entire body of the baby faces the mother • Baby's abdomen touches mother's abdomen		
5.	*Explain and ensure good attachment:* • Baby's mouth is widely open • Chin touching the breast • Lower lip turned outwards • Majority of areola inside the baby's mouth		
6.	Make sure that baby is sucking properly		
	Total score		

■ FURTHER READING

1. Facility based newborn care, training module for doctors and nurses. MoHFW, GoI; 2022.

Management of Hypothermia

Tanushree Joshi Bahuguna

Grading and management of hypothermia
(Axillary temperature <36.5°C)

↓

- Immediate stabilization of the baby check vital parameters heart rate (HR), respiratory rate (RR), blood pressure (BP), oxygen saturation (SpO_2), and capillary refill time (CRT)
- Remove the cause of hypothermia (wet clothes, cold environment)

Mild hypothermia (36.4–36.0°C)

- Warm room 26–28°C
  – Skin-to-skin contact [Kangaroo mother care (KMC)]
- Cover the baby well
- Continue breastfeeding
- Monitor for apnea and hypoglycemia
- Monitor axillary temperature every 1/2 hour till reaches 36°C, then hourly for next 4 hours
- If hypothermia persists even after 1 hour of supervised KMC, treat as moderate hypothermia

Moderate hypothermia (32–35.9°C)

- Warm under radiant warmer
- KMC (if warmer not available)
- Monitor temperature every 15–30 minutes
- Blood sugar monitoring, if <45 mg/dL manage hypoglycemia
- Follow all steps of mild hypothermia

Severe hypothermia (<32°C)

- Admit the baby. Place under radiant warmer
- Injection vitamin K, if not given or active bleeding
- Provide nasal oxygen, if saturation <90% IV fluid NS@10 mL/kg, if perfusion is poor
- Manage hypoglycemia
- Reassess temperature every 15–30 minutes
- Supportive care

Prevention of hypothermia—maintenance of warm chain

Delivery room (DR)	Postnatal wards	Warm chain during transport
• Radiant warmer is must in neonatal care corner • Area should be air draught free • All DRs should have room thermometer • Maintain DR temperature >25°C • Switch on radiant warmer 20–30 minutes before delivery • Radiant warmer should be in manual mode with heater output being 100% • Prewarm two to three sterile towels by keeping them under radiant warmer for 20 minutes • Practice early skin-to-skin contact for stable neonates for 1 hour or at least till first breastfeeding • Dry newborn immediately after birth • Remove wet linen immediately • Weighing and checking temperature should be done after breastfeeding	• Cover neonate adequately • Practice rooming-in 24 × 7 • Avoid air draughts by closing windows, doors, and switching off fans and air conditioners • Start KMC as early as possible for eligible neonate • Promote exclusive breastfeeding • Delay bath till after discharge • Remove wet diaper/clothes as early as possible • Educate mother regarding identification of hypothermia using touch method	• *Without external heat source:* – A fully wrapped neonate with cap can be transported in an adult's arms in a closed vehicle – Neonate can be transported in skin-to-skin contact – Ensure that the neonate is in upright position and covered snuggly with the person's clothes and a blanket • *With external heat source:* – A thermal mattress or a transport incubator – Indigenous insulated boxes can be used in resource-limited settings – No neonate should be placed naked in a trolley or bed without an external heat source

Key Points to Remember

Why Newborns Prone to Develop Hypothermia?

- Larger surface area.
- Decreased thermal inulation due to lack of subcutaneous fat (LBW neonates).
- Reduced amount of brain fat (LBW neonates).
- Lack of shivering.
- Prevention of hypothermia is essential component of neonatal care.
- Neonatal hypothermia is important cause of neonatal mortality as it predisposes to hypoglycemia, acidosis, apnea, bleeding diathesis, pulmonary hemorrhage, respiratory failure, and shock.
- Rule out underlying cause, such as sepsis, hypoglycemia, shock, seizure, and treat accordingly.

Mechanism of Heat Loss in Newborns

- *Evaporation:* Amniotic fluid from skin
- *Conduction:* Contact with cold objects like tray
- *Convection:* Cold air currents
- *Radiation:* To colder nearby surfaces and objects like walls

Methods of Recording Temperature

- *Touch method*—back of the hand is used to touch and assess the skin temperature of the abdomen and feet of the baby. Abdominal temperature represents the core temperature **(*See* Annexure 1)**.
- *Thermometer*—digital thermometer should be placed against the roof of the axilla parallel to the side of the chest to measure the temperature **(*See* Annexure 1)**.
- *Thermistor probe*—in the radiant warmer is attached to the upper right abdomen to measure the temperature **(*See* Annexure 1)**.

Hypothermia in Preterm Babies

- In preterm and low birth weight (PT and LBW) neonates, the signs and symptoms of hypothermia may be subtle and nonspecific.
- Preterm babies have higher risk of hypothermia and increased risk of complication.
- Additional measures thermal mattress during neonatal transport and polyethylene plastic bag or wrap during neonatal resuscitation are required for maintaining temperature of preterm babies.

■ FURTHER READING

1. Facility based newborn care, training module for doctors and nurses. MoHFW, GoI; 2022.
2. Weiner GM, Zaichkin J, Kattwinkel J, American Heart Association Editors. Textbook of Neonatal Resuscitation, 8th edition. United States: American Academy of Pediatrics; 2021.
3. WHO. (1997). Thermal protection of newborn: a practical guide. [online] Available from https://apps.who.int/iris/handle/10665/63986 [Last accessed September, 2022]

Kangaroo Mother Care

Mahendra Jain

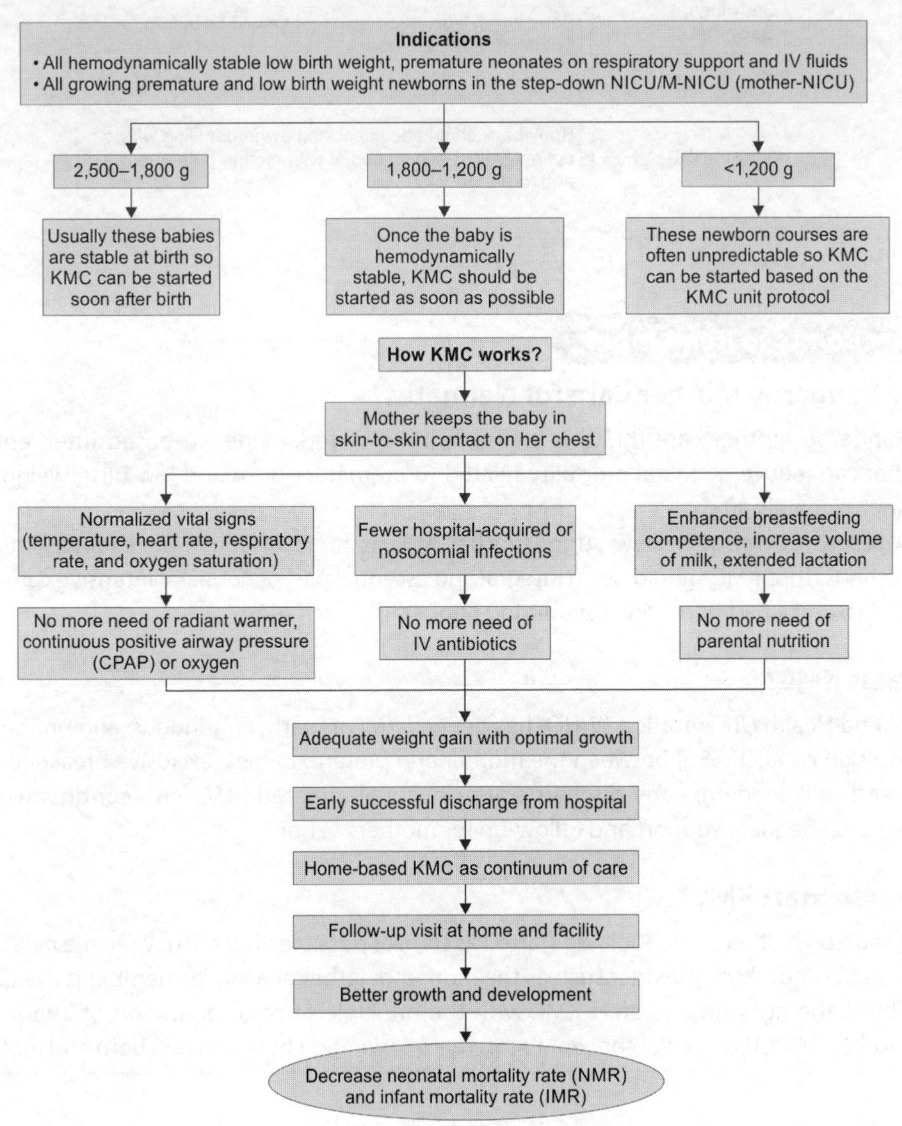

■ KMC POSITION

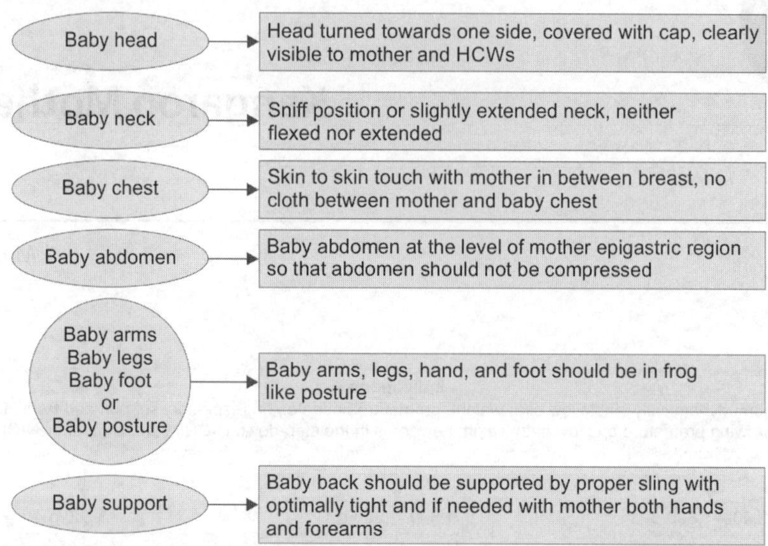

Key Points to Remember

Why Kangaroo Mother Care for Neonates?

- Kangaroo mother care (KMC) is a simple, time-tested, evidence-based intervention that can reduce neonatal mortality related to premature birth and low birth weight by approximately 40%.
- A recent Cochrane review suggests that KMC is more effective in resource-limited settings. Thus KMC should be an integral and essential part of neonatal intensive care unit (NICU) and a part of routine care during neonatal resuscitation.

What is KMC?

The World Health Organization (WHO) has defined KMC as early, continuous, and prolonged skin-to-skin contact (SSC) between the mother and preterm babies; exclusive breastfeeding or breast milk feeding; early discharge after hospital-initiated KMC with continuation at home; and adequate support and follow-up for mothers at home.

When to Start KMC?

- Kangaroo mother care should be started as soon as possible after birth when the newborn is stable and a KMC provider such as the mother or father or a family member is available.
- This is the right time to start KMC with the principle of zero separation of infant and mother. MNICU is a novel concept to start zero separation between newborn and mother.

Who can Provide?

- Mother who is willing, free of illness and maintain a good hygiene
- Alternative KMC provider (AKP)—father OR any relatives who is ready to spend quality time for KMC.

The mother is the best KMC provider because KMC also improves the amount of breast milk (nonpharmacological interventions to improve lactation) and also leads to successful breastfeeding.

How to Provide?

- Have a written KMC policy that is routinely communicated to staff and parents.
- Establish a KMC audit system that ensures availability of manpower, goods and materials, space for KMC, and documents for KMC.
- Ensure that staff has sufficient knowledge, competence, and skills to initiate, guide, and support KMC.
- Discuss the advantage, importance, detail procedure of KMC with mother or other alternate KMC provider.
- Facilitate immediate and uninterrupted SSC and support mothers to initiate KMC as soon as possible once newly born baby hemodynamically stable.
- Educate mother about breastfeeding and monitor respiration.

Where can be Given?

Kangaroo mother care can be given at NICU, SNCU, PNC during transport and at home.

What Supplies are Needed to Provide?

- *Kangaroo mother care chair:* Recliner bed for KMC provider (back adjustable and comfortable for back support)
- Water absorbable nappies or diapers, cap, socks, and front open dresses for baby
- Mother can wear whatever she finds comfortable or front open gowns, shirts, or blouse, and sari.
- Chart that includes duration of KMC, vital, feeding, urine/stool frequency.
- During KMC, the mother can be seated/sleep in a semilying position, the baby should be held vertically up, in between the breast, vital (HR and SpO_2) monitoring is very important.
- During KMC, the mother can do her routine work, e.g., walking, sitting, eating, or sleeping, etc.

How Much Time can be Deliver?

- KMC should be provided as long as possible, duration should be 1 hour.
- KMC may be continued till the baby find it comfortable.
- When baby in KMC wriggles, pulls limb out or cries, KMC may be discontinued.
- KMC duration defined as short (4 hours), extended (5–8 hours), long (9–12 hours), and continuous (more than 12 hours).

OSCE/Checklist: For KMC		
*Name of the participants:*____		
Performance steps	*Yes*	*No*
Place: ☐ NICU ☐ SDNICU ☐ LR ☐ MNICU ☐ PNC ☐ Home		
Infrastructure		
Institute has a written KMC policy		
KMC policy routinely communicated to nursing staff		
Institute has set up KMC audit system, which ensures availability of work force, material, and space for KMC		
Health care provider (HCP) has adequate knowledge, capability, and skills to initiate guide and support the KMC		
KMC process		
HCP has introduced themselves and built rapport with mother/KMC provider		
HCP discussed KMC benefits, importance, with mother or AKP (alternative care provider)		
HCP counsel the mother and take her consent for initiating KMC		
The mother is confident, comfortable, and fit to provide KMC		
Ensure the privacy for the mother		
Ensure mother is sitting or reclining comfortably		
HCP has placed the baby in proper KMC position with napkin, socks and cap on		
Baby prone on mother's chest in an upright position (Frog like) between the breast		
Turns baby's head to one side to ensure airway is open		
Support baby's bottom using appropriate sling or binder		
Cover mother and baby with blanket or shawl		
Appreciates the mother during KMC and encourage breast feeding every 2 hours		
Noted down the start time of KMC and monitoring vitals (HR, RR, temperature, and SpO_2) and danger signs during KMC		
Documented the duration of KMC per session and per day		
HCP responded to the queries/concerns of the parents regarding KMC after the KMC session		
Is the KMC interrupted due to a maternal in the neonatal cause? Document details of incident.		
Hand hygiene and asepsis maintained during KMC		
Time of starting the KMC and end of KMC with duration		
Growth monitoring, i.e., weight, head circumference, and length has been done and plotted in the growth chart		
Advised after discharge from hospital and during neonatal transport		
Mother advised follow-up visit		

FURTHER READING

1. KMC Manual, KMC foundation of India.
2. MOHFW, GOI. (2014). Kangaroo Mother Care and Optimal feeding in low birth weight infants, operational guidelines. [online] Available from https://www.nhm.gov.in/images/pdf/programmes/child-health/guidelines/Operational_Guidelines-KMC_&_Optimal_feeding_of_Low_Birth_Weight_Infants.pdf [Last accessed September, 2022].
3. WHO. (2003). Kangaroo mother care: a practical guide. [online] Available from https://apps.who.int/iris/handle/10665/42587 [Last accessed September, 2019].

Chapter 65

Supportive Management on Ventilator

Sonia Thomas

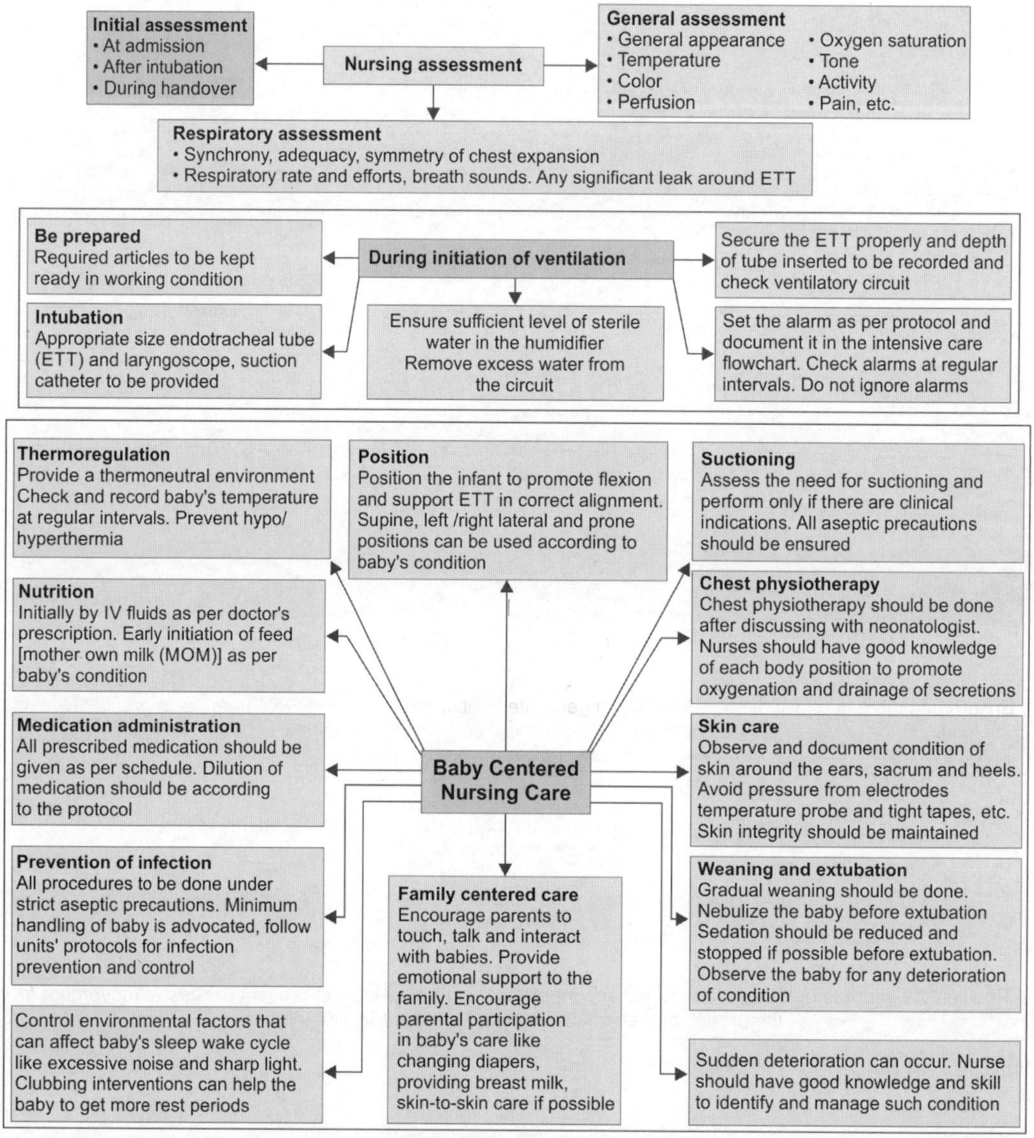

Nursing assessment

Initial assessment
- At admission
- After intubation
- During handover

General assessment
- General appearance
- Temperature
- Color
- Perfusion
- Oxygen saturation
- Tone
- Activity
- Pain, etc.

Respiratory assessment
- Synchrony, adequacy, symmetry of chest expansion
- Respiratory rate and efforts, breath sounds. Any significant leak around ETT

During initiation of ventilation

Be prepared
Required articles to be kept ready in working condition

Intubation
Appropriate size endotracheal tube (ETT) and laryngoscope, suction catheter to be provided

Ensure sufficient level of sterile water in the humidifier
Remove excess water from the circuit

Secure the ETT properly and depth of tube inserted to be recorded and check ventilatory circuit

Set the alarm as per protocol and document it in the intensive care flowchart. Check alarms at regular intervals. Do not ignore alarms

Baby Centered Nursing Care

Thermoregulation
Provide a thermoneutral environment Check and record baby's temperature at regular intervals. Prevent hypo/hyperthermia

Nutrition
Initially by IV fluids as per doctor's prescription. Early initiation of feed [mother own milk (MOM)] as per baby's condition

Medication administration
All prescribed medication should be given as per schedule. Dilution of medication should be according to the protocol

Prevention of infection
All procedures to be done under strict aseptic precautions. Minimum handling of baby is advocated, follow units' protocols for infection prevention and control

Control environmental factors that can affect baby's sleep wake cycle like excessive noise and sharp light. Clubbing interventions can help the baby to get more rest periods

Position
Position the infant to promote flexion and support ETT in correct alignment. Supine, left /right lateral and prone positions can be used according to baby's condition

Family centered care
Encourage parents to touch, talk and interact with babies. Provide emotional support to the family. Encourage parental participation in baby's care like changing diapers, providing breast milk, skin-to-skin care if possible

Suctioning
Assess the need for suctioning and perform only if there are clinical indications. All aseptic precautions should be ensured

Chest physiotherapy
Chest physiotherapy should be done after discussing with neonatologist. Nurses should have good knowledge of each body position to promote oxygenation and drainage of secretions

Skin care
Observe and document condition of skin around the ears, sacrum and heels. Avoid pressure from electrodes temperature probe and tight tapes, etc. Skin integrity should be maintained

Weaning and extubation
Gradual weaning should be done. Nebulize the baby before extubation Sedation should be reduced and stopped if possible before extubation. Observe the baby for any deterioration of condition

Sudden deterioration can occur. Nurse should have good knowledge and skill to identify and manage such condition

Supportive Management on CPAP

Jubilant James

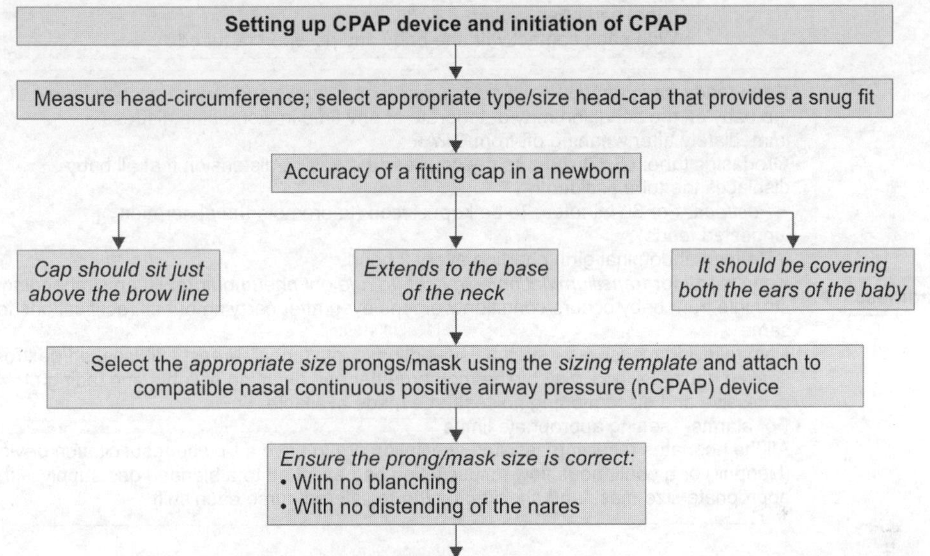

■ NURSING MANAGEMENT

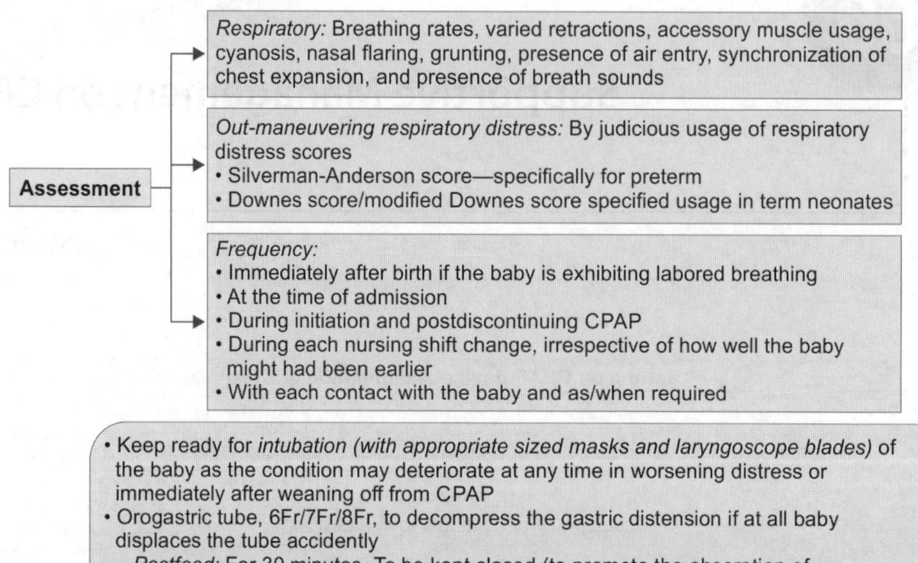

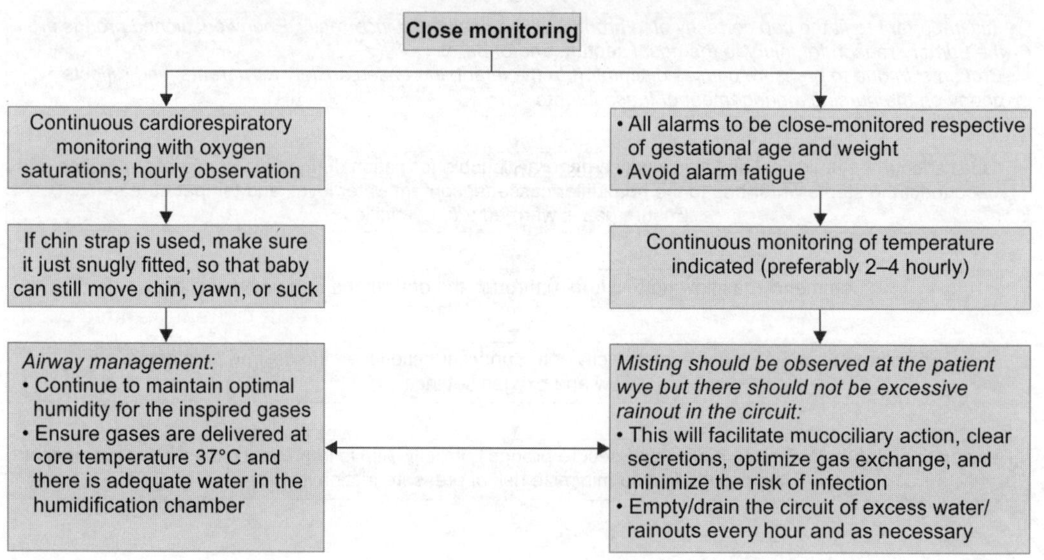

■ NEED-BASED CARE

S. No.	Needs-led assessment	Care frequency	Handling/management
1.	*Airway suction*	• Not routine based • Is performed on a needs basis • *Indications for suction may include:* increasing frequency and severity of apnea, slowing of response to tactile stimulation and increasing oropharyngeal secretions	• The nurse should always optimize work of breathing (confirm patency of nasal prongs), humidification, infant position, the thermal environment, and enteral feeding techniques • If suction is required the color, consistency, and quantity of secretions should be documented
2.	*Positioning of the neonate*	Every 2–4 hourly • To facilitate comfort and optimize the respiratory effort • Different positions to be considered and used intermittently to promote upper airway stability, reduce work of breathing, facilitate physiological flexion of the trunk and limbs, prevent posture and movement problems and encourage midline orientation of the hands to face	• Use of the prone, supine, and lateral body stance • Document preferred and best tolerated position
3.	*Skin-integrity*	• To minimize pressure/friction injury to the nasal septum and nares • Nasal septal injury—3 stages: – *Stage 1: Erythema* nonblanching, on an otherwise intact skin – *Stage 2:* Superficial ulcer or erosion, with partial thickness skin loss – *Stage 3:* Necrosis with full thickness skin loss • Cue-based nursing care generally 2–4th hourly	• Limit excessive movement of prongs/mask/nasal tubing's and of the baby too • Maintain good alignment of prongs • Avoid excessive moisture from frequent rainouts in the CPAP circuit • Frequently check the CPAP tubing and remove excess water • *DO NOT* use any lubricants except for a few drops of saline if necessary for initial prong placement • Dry the nares and prongs/mask as needed • Ensure the cap remains fitted over the glabella to anchor prongs/mask effectively • Do not tolerate cap that slide back over the forehead

Contd...

Contd...

S. No.	Needs-led assessment	Care frequency	Handling/management
			• *Avoid* poorly fitting prongs/masks that pinch, blanch or distend the nares, tight security straps causing excessive pressure on cheeks or orbital edema • *Prevent twisting* or tension on the nCPAP circuit, this will cause incorrect positioning of the prongs or mask • Routine pressure releases *every 2 hourly* • *Gently massaging* the nares to assess the blanching
4.	*Eye-care*	Upon each handling/2 hourly	• Check for puffiness of eyes • Choose appropriate sized hats and prongs • Keep a watch on fluid volume excess • Maintain the continuity in position change
5.	*Euthermia/ normothermia*	• Every 2–4th hourly • This prevents the neonate from suspected sepsis or cold stress (if baby is hypo/hyperthermic) • Promotes and enhances the neonate to grow in an environment as close to in-utero environment magnifying the spurts in development of major core-body and organ functions	• Provide euthermia by keeping the neonate/infant in radiant warmer/incubator/transport incubator • Achieve optimal humidification of inspired gases
6.	*Capillary filling time (CFT)*	Every 4th hourly/at least once per shift	• Over mid-sternum • *Normal:* <3 seconds • *Prolonged:* ≥3 seconds
7.	*Parental involvement*	• The parents should be kept informed and involved in all aspects of their infant's management • Encourage questions and opportunities to interact with their infant	• Once the infant can tolerate some handling the parents should be encouraged to participate in their routine care • Methods commonly used to comfort and contain infants in the neonatal intensive care unit (NICU) should be demonstrated and discussed with parents

Contd...

Contd...

S. No.	Needs-led assessment	Care frequency	Handling/management
			• Frequent skin-to-skin contact should be encouraged especially when the infant is having on off CPAP so the parents can see more of their baby and less of the ICU equipment
8.	*If skin integrity is lost/ deteriorates with resultant break*	Every hour for the first initial 4 hours progressing to 2 hours	• Hydrocolloid adhesive used to be removed • Nares should be assessed by senior nurse/nurse-in-charge as well as the doctors on duty • Commence an individualized neonate care plan and discuss management with parents • If tolerated; wean-off from CPAP • CPAP for postextubation distress is often for not so significant duration for infants between the gestations 35–40 weeks • Start cycling off from CPAP, once FiO_2 is at the lowest, peep is 5 cmH_2O • Documentation of the wound, appearance, color and care undertaken • Pressure release hourly

9.	• *Prevention of complications:*
	  – Pneumothorax
	  – Retinopathy of prematurity
	  – CPAP belly
		• Every 2 hourly
		• Every hour and as needed
		
		• 30 minutes postfeed
			• Check for air-leaks/pressure leaks
			• Maintain closed circuit functioning of CPAP
			• Ensure judicious usage of oxygen therapy
			• Keep OG feeding tube open

Pressure leak:
- Position the neonate adequately so that the chin is closed
- Apply chin-strip, only snug-fitting, not to leave in-situ for longer periods of time (review periodically)

Air leak:
- Maintain closed-circuit system for delivery of CPAP without any breakage in continuity
- Check the disconnection/loosening of heating wires

Bubble-loss:
- Adequate sized hat/cap with appropriate sized mask/prongs
- Increase oxygen flow rate to reach desired bubbling of water

CPAP belly:
- Inserting orogastric (OG) feeding tube (bridge of nose-earlobe-midway between xiphisternum and umbilicus)
- Post OG tube feeding, keep the feeding tube closed for half an hour
- Remaining periods—OG tube to be kept open always

Increased work of breathing:
- Good positioning of baby
- Decent alignment of gas/pressure inlet tubing as well as nasal tubings
- Ensure delivery of humidified gas at core body temperature

Troubleshooting

Nasal septum erythema/skin breakdown:
- Minimize using over-sized/under-sized nasal mask or prongs and hat as well
- Use neobond (hydrocolloid dressing)/cannula ide (different sizes available according to birth weight of the baby) over columella before inserting prongs or nasal mask
- Use Tegaderm's (size 1610) white adhesive part across the bridge of the nose/the area surrounding upon which nasal mask will be put on for a minimum of two to three layers
- Provide pressure-release every 2 hourly and provide cycling alternating between mask and prongs

Periorbital edema/facial edema:
- With changing head-circumference immediately after birth (due to varying birth process), head-cap should be judiciously chosen appropriately
- Retaining nasal—tubing's with optimal length to allow defined baby movement. The head tie and the prong ties should not be too tight
- Have a check on neonate's fluid consumption per day to verify for fluid-retention or any underlying cardiac disease

Frequent apnea/desaturations:
- Optimizing optimal FiO_2 requirement to reach target SpO_2 levels
- Clear frequent build-up of airway secretions by wiping—off or suctioning (mouth/nares)
- Instilling nasal saline drops into each nares as required

Checklist for initiating CPAP.

- Connect circuit to the blender and turn on gas flow
- Confirm the circuit is correctly setup and the 1 liter bag of sterile water to fill the water chamber
- Set the required level of nCPAP by inserting the rod under the water to desired pressure, occlude end and ensure system is bubbling
- Ensure the invasive or ventilator mode is used, the temperature display should read 37.0°C + 0.20°C and measures the temperature delivered at the patient wye
- The nCPAP device should be connected lo the blended gas supply and oxygen concentration titrated with the infant's SpO_2%
- Choose the appropriate cap size (17–22, 22–25, 25–29, and 29–36 cm)
- Connect the correct size nasal extension tubing—50 mm for premature infants, 70 mm for larger infants
- Measure width of the infant's nares and septum using the reference guide and select an appropriate set of prongs/mask
- Connect prongs/nasal mask to the circuit
- Position the prongs gently in the nares/mask over the nose and secure with the lateral tapes to the cap
- The prongs should rest gently inside the nares, with the tapes securing the prongs flat to the philtrum—avoid excessive pressure on cheeks and septum
- The prongs should rest approximately 2–3 mm from the nares and should NOT be in contact with the columella (end of septum)
- Very premature infants may need to alternate between prongs and mask to reduce pressure to the nares/septum
- Four sizes available—XS (extrasmall), S (small), M (medium), and L (large)

Supportive Management of a Newborn During the Procedure

Athira Thilakan

67.1 CARE OF THE BABY UNDERGOING EXCHANGE TRANSFUSION

Prerequisites

1. Keep donor blood ready (<3 days old)
2. Blood should be cross-matched against mother's blood
3. Fresh heparinized blood/blood preserved with acid-citrate dextrose is preferred
4. In Rh incompatibility, transfusions are to be performed with Rh negative group 'O' blood. Volume to be transfused is 160–180 mL/kg
5. Keep ready for intubation In case of any cardiopulmonary compromise

NURSING MANAGEMENT

Before Procedure

- Priming the parents about the procedure and obtaining their consent.
- Collect the blood product from blood bank, check the details of the baby and the blood group of the component along with collection date and expiry.
- Bring down the temperature of the blood unit to room-temperature/blood-warmer machine can be used for the same in case of emergency.
- Baby should be kept NPO at least 4–6 hours prior the commencement of the procedure with intravenous fluid administration for fluid-volume maintenance.
- If baby appears to be hemodynamically labile, unstable or critical—carry out the intubation by assisting the neonatologist prior to performing double volume exchange transfusion (DVET).
- Perform baseline sampling of arterial blood gas (ABG), random blood sugar (RBS), Sr. calcium, Sr. potassium, and Hb before the start of the procedure.

During the Procedure

- Expose and immobilize the baby on the cross-splint.
- Procedure to be carried out in the incubator/radiant-warmer depending upon patient's allotted place in the manual mode with 100% heater output (heater output can be decreased as well according to the person's comfort who is performing the procedure).
- Assist in appropriate surgical asepsis and open the dressing pack.

- Assist in cleaning of umbilical stump, maintenance of umbilical venous or arterial lines, helping in fixation of position of the catheters.
- Pour 100 mL normal saline into sterile bowl and add 0.1 mL of heparin (5,000 IU) into it.
- Ensure heat source is available throughout the procedure.
- Hemodynamic monitoring of the baby's vital statistics (especially heart rate, saturations, respiratory rate, and BP monitoring) throughout the procedure.
- The physician removes the calculated amount of blood and replaces it with the exact same amount of fresh blood until the entire calculated volume is exchanged.
- Conduct the same set of blood sampling for baby once DVET crosses half phase.

After the Procedure

- Once the procedure ends, wrap the ends of the central lines with a sterile hub cover and start on with infusion fluids for patency/else remove the lines and stop bleeding.
- Check the baby's response to the procedure, if the baby is having no untoward reaction stabilize the baby and start on the phototherapy and continue it.
- Document the start time, duration, completion time, amount, and type of blood exchanged, no. of cycles done, condition of baby during and after procedure, any drugs if at all given during the procedure and samples sent to the lab.
- Postprocedural lab values of hemoglobin, calcium, potassium, bilirubin, and blood sugar to be conducted.

67.2 CARE OF BABY UNDERGOING PHOTOTHERAPY

- Care should be aimed at attaining optimal body temperature between 36.5 and 37.5°C.
- Expose as much of the skin surface as possible to the close proximity of the phototherapy light.
- Nurse the neonate naked apart from application of eye shield (eye protector) and diaper.
- The phototherapy unit should be directly above the skin surface and can be kept as close as 18–25 cm. Care should be taken to place the plastic cover or cling wrap to cover the bulb lights or illuminating surfaces of the phototherapy unit, if in case there is a danger of breakage of lights.
- Ensure safe removal of eye protectors every 4–6 hourly for eye care. Document for any changes and observe for any discharge, redness, swelling, or damage.
- To keep a close watch and check on adequacy of hydration (urine output) and nutrition (weight gain). Daily fluid requirements should be reviewed, individualized and titrated for gestational and postnatal age.
- Assess general skin color while recording and monitoring vital statistics.
- Breastfeeds may be limited to 20 minutes only to minimize the time out time of the phototherapy units.
- Normal hand hygiene measures to be followed while caring for a baby undergoing phototherapy regimen.

67.3 CARE OF BABY UNDERGOING SURFACTANT THERAPY

Storage and Handling

- Surfactant is stored in a refrigerator at +2 to +8°C.
- Vial should be slowly warmed to room temperature.
- While taking the medication from the vial, it should be turned upside down in order to obtain a uniform suspension.
- Unopened, unused vials of surfactant suspension that have warmed to room temperature can be returned to refrigerator within 24 hours for future use.
- Protect from light
- Do not warm to room temperature and return to refrigerator more than once.
- **Before the procedure:**
  - Continuous cardiovascular monitoring to be maintained throughout the procedure.
  - Keep ready at and for intubation, bag and mask ventilation and suction equipment.
  - Requires two-personnel at least to perform.
  - *Record baseline observations:* Heart rate, respiratory rate, and oxygen saturations; if required a blood-gas analysis.
  - Ensure and confirm correct position of the endotracheal tube via chest X-ray prior to administering surfactant.
  - Ensure patency of endotracheal tube prior to procedure; perform suction as necessary prior to procedure.
  - Perform in-out procedure of surfactant administration if baby does not require ventilation postsurfactant administration. InSurE technique widely followed.
- **During the procedure:**
  - On clean surface, gather and prepare for equipment.
  - Perform proper hand wash.
  - Ensure bed is flat and neonate is placed supine.
  - Open and assist for supplies and maintaining surgical asepsis throughout the procedure.
  - Before administering surfactant, disconnect endotracheal tube from ventilator and administer in 2–4 aliquots or bolus as quickly as the neonate tolerates.
  - Surfactant can occlude the endotracheal tube and it may be necessary to cease administration until the tube is cleared and chest wall movement resumes.
  - *Ventilator settings:* [FiO_2/pressure delivered] may be increased temporarily.
  - Vitals stats monitoring to be carried out throughout the procedure and recorded along with the procedure tolerance.
  - Clean surface, empty the clutter and area; again perform hand-hygiene.
- **After the procedural considerations:**
  - Marked improvements are noted within few moments of surfactant administration. Hence, FiO_2 requirement needs to be optimized to avoid hyperoxygenation and peak inspiratory pressures needs to be titrated.
  - At high ventilator rates (>40 bpm) regurgitation of surfactant may occur, ET tube may be held straight for few minutes postadministration of surfactant and ventilator rates can be brought down.

- Blood-gas analysis 1 hour postsurfactant therapy may be preferred and close monitoring of vitals post–SRT administration; every 15 minutes for first 30 minutes note changes in nonpulmonary hemodynamics (especially in extreme prematures).
- After surfactant is instilled into the airway, *do not* suction airways for at least after 1 hour, unless any signs of significant airway obstruction occurs.

67.4 CARE OF BABY UNDERGOING THERAPEUTIC HYPOTHERMIA

- Commence therapeutic hypothermia therapy within 1–6 hours of birth itself and maintain rectal temperature between 33 and 34°C for a duration of 72 hours.
- If necessary, ensure intubation is carried out prior.
- Avoid hyperthermia to prevent degenerating effects to the brain of the baby, whereas; head-cooling delivers a neuroprotective coating to the brain of the baby.
- Nurse the infant in a diaper with radiant warmer kept off.
- Record baseline observations before commencing the head-cooling therapy such as heart rate, respiratory rate, temperature, oxygen saturations, and blood-pressure. There will be usually changes in heart rate and respiratory rate on lower side. Keep a close watch for the same.
- Watch for hypovolemia and arrhythmias.
- Insert rectal probe not more than 5 cm into the anus and tape the probe to the upper thigh.
- Monitor skin temperature regularly.
- Gain access to central lines such as umbilical venous catheters and umbilical arterial catheters to maintain capillary filling as perfusion mostly diminishes during cooling therapy.
- Neonates are at greater risk for electrolyte imbalances, they need frequent monitoring and sampling and tracing of the serum levels of electrolytes. Carry out the correction based on laboratory values.
- Sodium and magnesium levels to be kept at upper limits of normal range for neuroprotective effects.
- Intravenous sedation (preferably fentanyl) to be initiated to decrease the basal metabolic rate which in-turn increases the effectiveness of cooling therapy. Gradual tapering-off should be considered at 48–72 hours.
- Neonates should be watch for any change in hemodynamics and closely watched for any occurrence of seizure activity.
- Check pupils, evaluate level of consciousness and for signs of raised intracranial pressure (ICP).
- Start with aEEG monitoring for evaluation of seizure occurrence. As they peak within first 48 hours.
- Frequent position change and evaluation of skin integrity to be carried out for color change, any breakdown, perfusion and signs of subcutaneous fat necrosis (induration erythematous nodules and plaques over bony prominences such as arms, chest, back, thighs, and buttocks.

- Head-end to be kept elevated.
- Place urinary catheter in-situ as urinary retention will be noted.
- Document the date and time of starting head-cooling therapy, baby's tolerance to the procedure.
- Encourage family-centered care and involve infant–parent bonding by providing space for touching the baby and letting them know that their baby will be cold throughout the procedure.

67.5 CARE OF BABY WITH COLOSTOMY

- Colostomy pouch to be applied to collect gas and stool.
- Pouch is to be sealed tightly against the baby's skin.
- Do not apply any wet soaks or wet the pouch as it may cause the leakages and causes the seal to loosen.
- If pouch seal is not maintained appropriately then skin redness and irritation usually occur, hence; usually it requires the mandate to change the pouch.
- Always keep the extrasupplies of pouch, stoma powder, and adhesives ready.
- Empty the pouch when it is one-third full (almost half) filled with stool/gas.
- Change the pouch three to four times a week.
- Always check the stoma and the site surrounding for redness, breakage, necrosis, and swelling.
- Do not use baby-wipes on the skin around the stoma.
- Clean the stoma site aseptically with normal saline with sterile gauze pieces.
- Loosen the clothing around the stoma site and avoid any tightening.
- Check for any foul smell from the stoma site and for any new occurrence of any grade of fever. Antibiotics will be started.
- For redness/irritation, apply stoma powder after cleaning and drying the area.

Stoma Appearances and Their Interpretation

- *Red stoma/dark pink stoma:* Adequate blood supply/healthy
- *Pale pink stoma:* Diminished Hb/poor perfusion
- *Dark red/purplish stoma:* Bruising
- *Gray to black stoma:* Ischemia and potential necrosis (immediate surgical review required)

Developmentally Supportive Care

Sonia Thomas

Nursing Management

Healing environment
- Nurse baby in thermoneutral environment
- Provide soothing environment for babies (minimize lights, sound)
- Protect sleep by nesting, kangaroo mother care (KMC), cluster care
- Restrict number of visitors, allow parents
- Practice good empathetic care giving behavior

Light
- Rate of 100–600 lux is recommended
- Turn-off unnecessary light and dim lights at night
- Cover the bassinet for preterm infants
- Eyes should be covered when using examination light and phototherapy

Cue-based care and clustering of care
- Use appropriate strategy like timeout or modification of care
- Clustering of activities encourages a minimum handling approach

Noxious stimuli
- Minimize baby's exposure to noxious stimuli such as strong fragrances

Family-centered care
- Involvement of families in care giving activities (visitor to care provider)
- Educating and empowering
- Emotional support during critical care

Noise
- Noise level should not exceed 40–45 db
- Avoid unnecessary talking at bedside
- Reduce volume of monitor noises
- Close incubator portholes/cabinet gently
- Avoid writing or putting bottles and equipment directly on the incubator
- Remove water bubbling in oxygen and ventilator tubing

Touch
- Minimal handling
- Talk to baby before touching
- Allow handling the baby by mother, KMC

Stimulation
- *Tactile:* Position, nesting, swaddling, facilitated tuck, and massage
- *Auditory:* Music therapy, allow mothers to sing or talk in soft voice
- Provide skin to skin contact
- *Vestibular stimulation:* Gently roll the baby side-to-side
- Keep gauze or cotton soaked in mother's milk to stimulate olfactory system

Stressful or painful procedure
- Minimize painful procedures
- Use comforting techniques like NNS, swaddle or gently hold the baby, using containment technique, breastfeeding the baby at the time of injection if appropriate oral sucrose can be given

End-of-Life Care

Purvi Patel

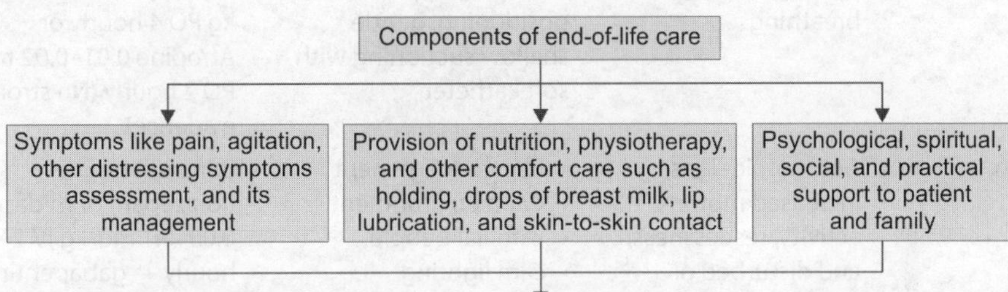

Symptom and management.

Symptoms	Assessment tool	Nonpharmacological intervention	Pharmacological intervention

Pain: Types of pain
• Nociceptive
• Somatic
• Visceral
• Neuropathic
	• Behavioral indicators of infant pain (BIIP)
	• Premature infant pain profile (PIPP)
	• COMFORTneo Scale
	• CRIES (cry, requirement for more oxygen, increased vital signs, expressions, and sleeplessness)
	• NPASS (neonatal pain, agitation, and sedation scale)
		• Less noxious stimuli—less vitals monitoring
		• Breastfeeding
		• Swaddling
		• Skin-to-skin care/kangaroo care
		• Non-nutritive sucking with or without oral sucrose
			• Mild pain—acetaminophen 6–8 mg/kg IV 8 hourly
			• *Moderate:*
			  – Morphine 0.15–0.5 mg/kg PO/sublingual 2–4 hourly
			  – Fentanyl 0.5–2 mcg/kg IN/IV 2 hourly
			• *Severe pain:*
			  – Morphine IV infusion 0.01–0.05 mg/kg/h IV continuous
			  – Hydromorphone IV infusion + - Ketamine IV infusion

Respiratory distress	• Tachypnea • Retractions • Grunting • Nasal flaring • Gasping	• Positioning modifications such as head end elevation and side-lying or prone position • Air movement of fan towards patient • Skin-to-skin contact • Fluid restriction • Gentle suction • Oxygen for comfort if appropriate	• Morphine 0.15–0.5 mg/kg PO/sublingual 2–4 hourly or • Fentanyl IN/IV 0.5–2 µg/kg IN/IV 2 hourly If not improving • Fentanyl 1–4 µg/kg/h IV continuous + lorazepam 0.05–0.1 mg/kg PO/IV 4–6 hourly

Contd...

Contd...

Symptoms	Assessment tool	Nonpharmacological intervention	Pharmacological intervention
			For refractory dyspnea • Morphine infusion 0.01–0.05 mg/kg/h IV continuous or • Hydromorphone infusion+-dexmedetomidine infusion 0.5–1 µg/kg IV/IN 2 hourly
Excessive secretions	Pooling of secretions leading to noisy breathing	Fluid restriction, side-lying or prone positioning, gentle shallow suctioning with soft catheter	If not improving • Glycopyrrolate 0.04–0.1 mg/kg PO 4 hourly or • Atropine 0.01–0.02 mg/kg PO 2 hourly (No strong evidence)
Agitation	Autonomic signs, increased motor activity, restlessness, and disturbed or disrupted sleep	• Pain management • Calm environment • Familial people • Dim lighting • Familial music and toys • Massage therapy • Swaddling • Skin-to-skin contact	• Benzodiazepines (lorazepam or midazolam 0.05–0.1 mg/kg IV 2–4 hourly +- gabapentin PO 5–15 mg PO every 8 hourly If not improving • Dexmedetomidine 0.5–1 µg/kg IV/IN 2 hourly or • Ketamine 0.5–1 mg/kg PO/IV 2–4 hourly • Morphine 0.05–0.2 mg/kg IV/IM 2–4 hourly
Seizure		No role	Anticonvulsant like Phenobarbital 5 mg/kg every 24 hours PO/PR
Constipation-Opioid induced most likely			• Liquid glycerine • Methylnaltrexone—opioid antagonist
Skin care	Dusky erythema, mottling, or cool surfaces	Prevention of excessive pressure, friction, moisture, and immobilization	Topical emollients
Eye care	Incomplete eye closure—signs of exposure keratopathy	Complete eye closure	Artificial tear drops
Mouth care	Mouth xerostomia	Moist sterile water swabs	Topical petroleum jelly
Nutrition	• Decision regarding giving artificial hydration and nutrition or	Lactation consultant to assist mothers who want to breastfeed their infant or donate breast milk at the end of life	

Contd...

Contd...

Symptoms	Assessment tool	Nonpharmacological intervention	Pharmacological intervention
	• Natural hydration and nutrition should be based on risk versus benefit ratio and should be clearly communicated with parents		
Familial existential distress	Assess parental preferences for memory making activities	Preparing the family for what to expect during the dying process via healthy discussion and effective communication	

CODE KRISHNA: AN EXPERIENCE

In our institute, we practice named "Code Krishna" as an attempt to dignify the event of death and respect cultural convictions of community at the Shree Krishna Hospital, Karamsad, for every death taking place in the hospital since 2016.

Process

- Treating team paying its respects to the departed soul and empathizing with the bereaved family.
- *Visible component:* Treating team members assembling at the bedside of the deceased, team and bereaved relatives offering floral tributes to the deceased, and reciting a prayer according to the family's religious faith followed by a few minutes of meditative silence.
- *Invisible component:* Respectful body language for the deceased, sharing bereaved family's grief, and creating a silent environment.

  We believe and have experienced too that seeking and fulfilling culture-specific wishes help to create healing moments in the story of each dying person, besides reducing emotional trauma and achieving closure.

Key Points to Remember

End-of-life (EOL) care in neonates is one aspect of palliative care of a newborn who has advanced, progressive, and incurable illness such as extreme prematurity, complex congenital anomalies, genetic abnormalities, or other lethal conditions, till their final outcome to support a peaceful, dignified death for the newborn and support to the family till the last phase of life and into bereavement.

Ethical principles followed while taking EOL decisions:
- Autonomy—patient/parents or a legal guardian has the right to decide about the treatment.

- Beneficence—act in the best interest of the patient.
- Nonmaleficence—do not harm.
- Justice—fair patient management using health resources optimally.

In cases of resuscitation of newborn, the autonomy of newborn and to take decision in life-threatening emergency situations are both exceptions of general rules of ethics. There are no legal guidelines in our country regarding withdrawal of care or EOL decisions.

End-of-Life Care Pathway

- Treating doctor's subjective and objective assessment of the medical futility. Consensus among palliative team members.
- Honest, accurate, and early disclosure of the prognosis to the family.
- Discussion and communication of all modalities of EOL care with the family—it can be provided in home-like environment in a location in or near the neonatal intensive care unit (NICU).
- Shared decision-making—consensus through open and repeated discussions.
- Transparency and accountability through accurate documentation.
- Ensure consistency among caregivers
- Implementing the process of withholding or withdrawing life support—communicate effectively with parents regarding further consequences and respect their preferences for any rituals or memory making activities along with continuation of supportive care including nutrition.
- Effective and compassionate palliative care with proper assessment of symptoms and its management and allow active participation of parents in comfort care along with appropriate support to the family.
- After death, ensure cessation of breastfeeding and genetic counseling and/or autopsy if cause of death is suspected to affect again in next pregnancy.
- Bereavement care support, palliative care after an infant's death should be continued by keeping the follow-up of parents or connect them with identified community services.
- Review of care process—facilitated debriefing by team.

■ FURTHER READING

1. Mishra S, Mukhopadhyay K, Tiwari S, Bangal R, Yadav BS, Sachdeva A, et al. End-of-life care: consensus statement by Indian Academy of Pediatrics. Indian Pediatr. 2017;54(10):851-9.
2. Vaishnav B, Nimbalkar S, Desai S, Vaishnav S. Code Krishna: an innovative practice respecting death, dying and beyond. Indian J Med Ethics. 2017;2(4):289-92.

Infection Prevention Practices: Nursing Perspective

Jubilant James

PRINCIPLES OF INFECTION PREVENTION PRACTICES

- Directly/in immediate contact with the baby—use soap and water only.
- Away from baby—alcohol/aldehyde/hypochlorite-based solutions to be used.
  - Alcohol-based solutions to be avoided on transparent surfaces.
  - High-potent disinfectants to be used for terminal cleaning.
  - To guide and supervise housekeeping personnel.
  - Ensure appropriate use of PPE and dilution.
    - Progression to be made from least moist area to the most soiled (e.g., metallic part of bassinet to be cleaned first followed by wheels).
    - Before redipping, mop 120 square feet
    - Solution to be changed—once cleaning surface area of 240 square feet is reached.
    - Rinse-off any solutions used prior to current cleaning/mopping.
  - Atmosphere to be kept free from dust.
  - All holes and crevices should be sealed.
  - Ambient temperature to be maintained between 25 and 28°C.
  - Overcrowding to be prevented.
  - Every person entering the unit should perform hand-hygiene.
  - Number of handling by any professional cadre (doctors/nurses/any unit therapist) should be reduced.

Equipment decontamination.

S. No.	Items	Decontamination procedures	Frequency
1.	*Thermometers, tape measures, stethoscope, monitor-probes (SpO_2 and temperature), torches, BP cuffs*	• Surface disinfect with *70% isopropyl alcohol* impregnated wipes (in between patients as well) • Infected O_2 hood-disinfect with *2% Bacillocid*	Daily and after each use
2.	*Oxygen hoods, multichannel monitors, and ventilator screen*	• Dry dusting, clean using a moist wipe (soap and water) • If infected—with Bacillocid 2%	Daily
3.	*Ventilator's air filter*	Clean with moist wipe and dust off	Daily

Contd...

Contd...

S. No.	Items	Decontamination procedures	Frequency
4.	*Incubators/radiant warmers/transport incubators*	• If occupied by baby—with soap and water • For terminal cleaning—with 2% Bacillocid *Always dismantle the parts which can be removed and clean*	Daily
5.	*Bassinet/baby cot*	Wipe with 2% Bacillocid	Daily and after each use
6.	*Weighing machine*	Wipe with Bacillol	Daily and after each use
7.	*Resuscitation and accessories*	• Dismantle, wash with soap and rinse under running water, clean dry and immerse in *2% CIDEX* for 6–8 hours. After that rinse-off with distilled water. Once dried, ready for use OR • Clean with soap and water after dismantling and send for ETO (ethylene oxide)	Daily and after each patient contact/usage
8.	*Laryngoscope*	• Wipe with spirit • Once in a week/infected patient—soak in CIDEX for 30 minutes	After each use/else daily
9.	*Ventilator tubings and continuous positive airway pressure (CPAP) tubings*	If clean, can be sent for ETO	• Not to be changed weekly • Only to be changed if visibly soiled/any breakage in the tubes
10.	*Nebulizer tubings (ventilator attached)*	• Dismantle the parts and wash under running water • Send for ETO OR • After washing, dry it and immerse in CIDEX for 30 minutes	After each use
11.	*CPAP body, ventilator body, nitric oxide machine*	Clean with Bacillol spray, use soap and water for monitor screens	Daily
12.	*Incubator humidifiers*	• Primary cleaning with soap solution and after dried, send for ETO • Humidifier water to be changed at least every 8 hours	Daily when in use

Contd...

Contd...

S. No.	Items	Decontamination procedures	Frequency
13.	Suction bottles and O$_2$ humidifiers	• Noninfected—clean with soap and water • If infected add 1% hypochlorite solution—30 minutes clean	Daily
14.	• Linens (baby sheets, baby frocks, draw sheets, towels, and hand towels), procedure sets • Glass bottles/articles, steel swab containers, and Cheatle forceps	Clean with soap and water and send for autoclaving	• After each and every use • Daily
15.	Syringe pump, infusion pump, and I/V stand	Wipe with Bacillol	Daily
16.	Phototherapy units, Biliblanket	Wipe with Bacillol	Daily
17.	Head-cooling machines (e.g., Techotherm, Blanketrol)	Wipe with Bacillol	Daily
18.	Feeding utensils (small bowls, paladai, spoons, and small trays)	Wash with soap and water and roll-boil for 15–20 minutes	After each use
19.	USG probe (any size), transilluminator	• Wipe with 70% isopropyl alcohol • If infected—wipe with 1% hypochlorite solution	Daily and after each use
20.	Ultrasound Machines	Wipe with Bacillol	Daily
21.	Sponge Bowls	Primary wash and send to CSSD for autoclaving	Daily
22.	Breast-pumps	• Specifically individualized use for each patient (one per person) • Wash with soap and water and then sterilize the accessories by boiling it for 15–20 minutes	After each use
23.	Breast-pump machine	Wipe with Bacillol	Daily

Environmental cleaning.

S. No.	Area/surface	Decontamination procedures	Frequency
1.	Walls	Wipe with 2% Bacillocid	Once in each shift
2.	Nursing station/counter	Wipe with 2% Bacillocid	Once in each shift
3.	Chairs/KMC chairs/feeding chairs/tables/trolleys	Wipe with 2% Bacillocid	Once in each shift and after every use
4.	Door-handle, bedrails/control panels, call-buttons, room inner door-knob	Wipe with 2% Bacillocid	Daily
5.	Sink	Soap and water	Daily
6.	Biomedical waste bins	Soap and water	Once in each shift

Contd...

Contd...

S. No.	Area/surface	Decontamination procedures	Frequency
7.	*Buckets*	With soap and water	Empty during each shift
8.	*Refrigerator*	Defrost, clean with wet mop using soap and water	Weekly
9.	*Floors (with A/C switched off)*	• Wet mop with 200 mL of Bacillocid in 10 L of water • Wet mop with 50 mL of Bacillocid in 10 L of water	• Once (8 AM) • Once (2 PM, 8 PM and 2 AM) and in between if/as required
10.	*Telephone*	Wipe with 2% Bacillocid	Daily
11.	*Feeding pillows/normal pillows*	• Send to laundry for washing followed by autoclaving • Contaminated pillows must be discarded. Torn pillow covers must be replaced before pillow is reused • If contaminated with body-fluid, the blood spill management protocol of the respective hospital should be followed	• Daily • Should not be used if cover is damaged
12.	*A/C*	Surface and filters to be washed with soap and water	• Surface to be cleaned on daily basis • Filters to be cleaned on weekly basis
13.	*Windows*	Clean with soap and water	Daily
14.	*Curtains (if any)*	• Cleaning depends on the material used • If plastic panes are used—clean with soap and water	Daily
15.	*Duster cloth*	Washed with soap and water and dried	• After each use • To be discarded if torn or visibly very dirty
16.	*Locker tops, medicine lockers*	Damp dust with solution and allow it to dry	Daily
17.	*Flooring mopping*	• *Item:* Three-bucket trolley and one clean mop with handle and one mechanized squeezer • *Disinfectant:* 2% Bacillocid 20 mL in 1,000 mL • Make disinfectant solution in two buckets as cleaning solution and plain water, in the third bucket as rinsing solution	Once in each shift

Contd...

Contd...

S. No.	Area/surface	Decontamination procedures	Frequency

		• Use clean and dry mop. Wet mops are rich source of contamination
		  – I-bucket *empty* for rinsing
		  – II-bucket normal concentration—plain water
		  – III-bucket double the concentration—disinfectant solution
		• **Process**
		  – Step 1—dip mop in plain water and squeeze generously, mechanical wringer can also be used
		  – Step 2—dip mop in disinfectant solution and sweep
		  – Step 3—squeeze in the bucket kept for dirty water
		  – Step 4—dip in the plain water
		  – Step 5—dip in disinfectant solution then sweep again
		  – *Do not dry mop or sweep* the newborn care unit as this causes dust, debris, and microorganisms to become airborne and contaminate clean surfaces	

Functional Echocardiography

Kunal P Ahya

ESSENTIAL MORPHOLOGY—SEGMENTAL ANALYSIS AND ANATOMIC CORRELATES

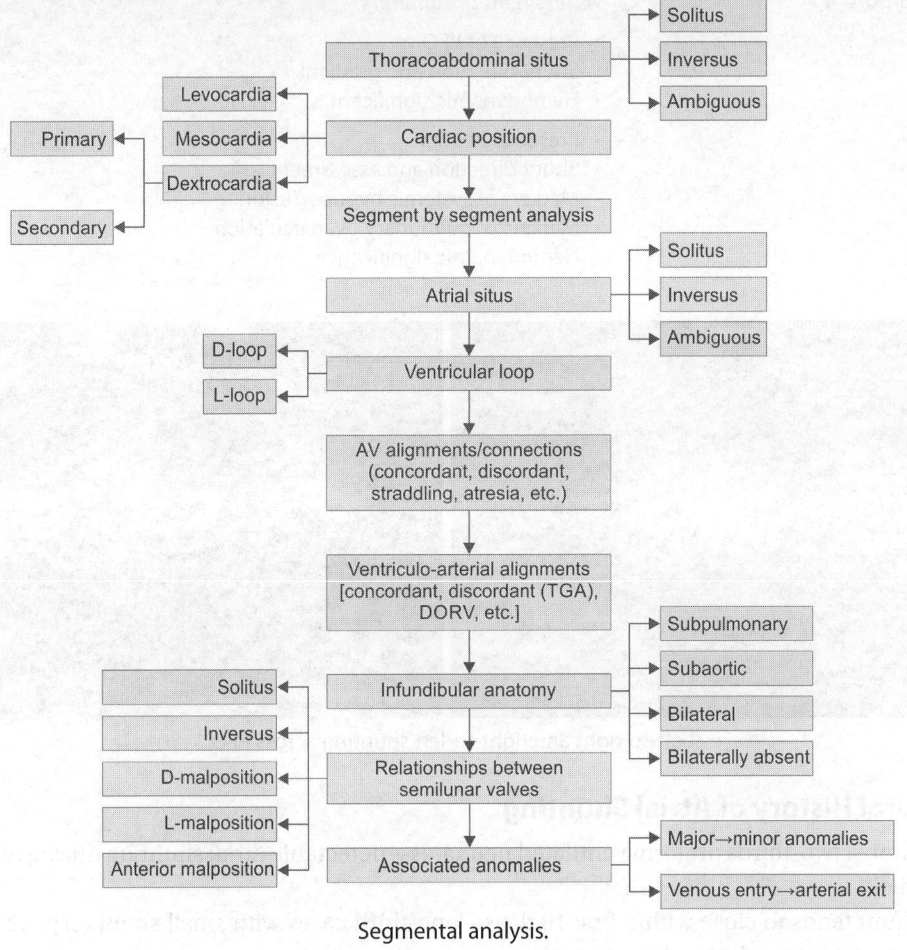

Segmental analysis.

INDICATIONS

Hemodynamics of shunt:
- Patent foramen ovale/atrial septal defect (PFO/ASD)
- Patent ductus arteriosus (PDA)

- Suspected persistent pulmonary hypertension (PPHN)
- Assessment of hemodynamics in neonatal shock
- Perinatal asphyxia
- Neonatal sepsis
- Suspected pericardial effusion
- Central line assessment

■ NEONATAL FUNCTIONAL ECHOCARDIOGRAPHY (FECHO): SHUNTS

Condition	Assessment parameters
PFO	• Presence of PFO • Shunt direction and gradient • Hemodynamic significant
PDA	• Presence of PDA • Shunt direction and assessment • Markers of systemic hypoperfusion • Markers of pulmonary overcirculation • Hemodynamic significance

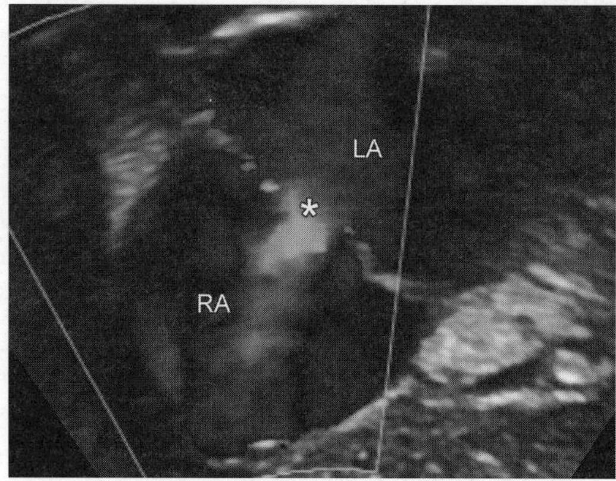

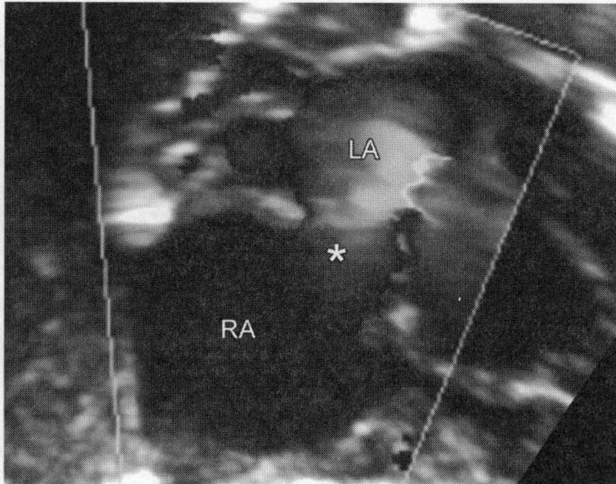

Left-to-right and right-to-left shunting across PFO.

Natural History of Atrial Shunting

- Almost two-thirds preterm ventilated neonates—detectable atrial shunting during the first week.
- Shunt tends to close within first 10 days—one-third cases with small shunt (size <3 mm), detectable even beyond first month.

- The foramen ovale is functionally closed by the 3rd month of life followed by anatomical closure by the age of 1 year.
- Babies with larger PFOs and those in whom PFO remained open for longer time had a significantly higher incidence of chronic lung disease.
- Pulmonary overcirculation caused by PFO—considered very significant—no direct treatment available to treat it.
- Pure right-to-left atrial shunts are uncommon, but need to rule out critical congenital heart disease (CCHD).

■ HEMODYNAMIC ASSESSMENT OF DUCTAL SHUNTING

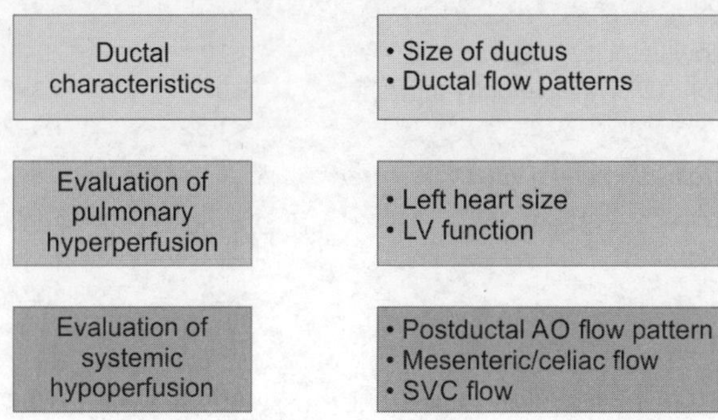

Parameter	View	Mode
Duct characteristics		
• Duct visualization/diameter	• Ductal view	• Color Doppler
• Duct direction	• Ductal view	• Pulse Doppler
Pulmonary over circulation		
• Main pulmonary artery (MPA) flow	• Short axis view	• Pulse Doppler
• Left pulmonary artery (LPA) flow	• Short axis view	• Pulse Doppler
• Pulmonary vein Doppler	• Apical view	• Pulse Doppler
• Left atrium (LA): Ascending aorta (AO)	• PLAX view/short axis	• M Mode
• Left ventricular end-diastolic diameter (LVEDD): AO	• PLAX view/short axis	• M Mode
• E:A ratio	• Apical view	• Pulse Doppler
• Isovolumic relaxation time (IVRT)	• Apical view	• Pulse Doppler
• Left ventricular outflow tract (LVOT)	• Apical/PLAX	• Pulse Doppler
Systemic hypoperfusion		
• DA flow	• Arch view	• Pulse Doppler
• Anterior cerebral artery (ACA) flow	• Midline sagittal	• Pulse Doppler
• Superior mesenteric artery (SMA)	• Subcostal view	• Pulse Doppler
• Renal artery (RA)	• Abdominal RA View	• Pulse Doppler

■ MARKERS OF PULMONARY HYPERPERFUSION

Overview of Echocardiographic Indices of Transductal Shunt Volume

Echocardiographic indices of shunt volume	*Small*	*Moderate*	*Large*
Characteristics of the PDA			
• Absolute diameter (mm)	<1.5	1.5–2.0	≥2.0
• PDA:LPA diameter ratio	<0.5	0.5–1.0	≥1.0
• PDA diameter indexed to body weight (mm/kg)	-	-	≥1.4
• Transductal peak systolic velocity (m/s)	>2.0	1.5–2.0	<2.0
• Transductal systolic-to-diastolic velocity gradient	<2.0	2.0–4.0	>4.0
Pulmonary hypertension			
• End-diastolic blood flow velocity in LPA (cm/s)	<20	20–50	>50
• Pulmonary vein diastolic (D)-wave velocity (cm/s)	<0.3	0.3–0.5	>0.5
• LA:Ao ratio	<1.5	1.5–2.0	>2.0
Left ventricular end-diastolic diameter (LVEDD) (Z-score)			
• LVO (mL/kg/min)	<200	200–300	>300
• Mitral valve E:A ratio	<1	1	>1
• LV:IVRT (ms)	>40	30–40	<30
Systemic hypoperfusion			
Diastolic blood flow pattern in systemic arteries (DAo, MCA, PCA, CT, SMA, and RA)	Antegrade	Absent	Retrograde
Qp:Qs ratio			
LVO:superior vena cava flow (SVCf) ratio	-	-	≥4.0

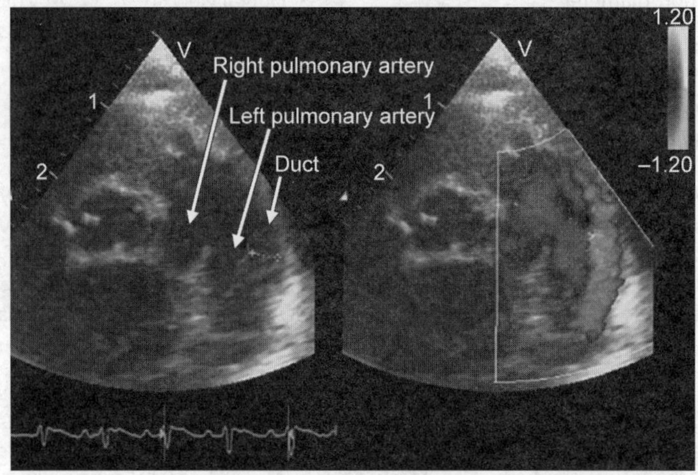

PDA—three leg view.

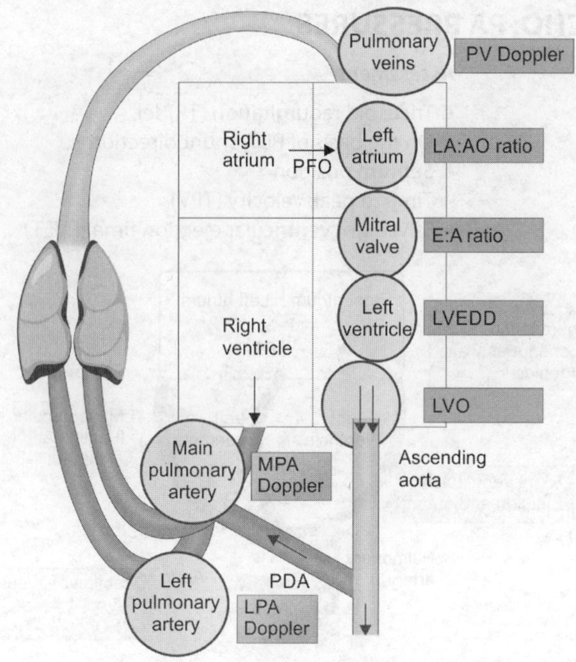

Overview of echocardiographic indices of transductal shunt volume.

ULTRASOUND PARAMETERS OF DUCTAL HEMODYNAMIC SIGNIFICANCE

Parameter	Hemodynamic significance		
	Mild	*Moderate*	*Severe*
PDA diameter			
• 2D diameter (mm)	<1.5	1.5–3	>3
• PDA to LPA ratio	<0.5	0.5–1	>1
PDA Doppler			
• Vmax (m/s)	>2.5	1.5–2.5	<1.5
• Systolic to diastolic velocity ratio	<2	2–4	>4
• LV chamber dilatation (Z score)	<+ 2.0	+2.0 – +3.0	>+3.0
Pulmonary overcirculation			
• LA to Ao ratio	<1.5	1.5–2.0	>2.0
• Mitral valve E to A ratio	<1	<1	>1
• IVRT (milliseconds)	>40	30–40	<30
• LPA Vmax diastole (m/s)	<0.3	0.3–0.5	>0.5
• LVO (mL/kg/min)	<200	200–300	>300
• PV D wave (m/s)	<0.35	0.35–0.45	>0.45
Systemic hypoperfusion			
• Abdominal Ao diastolic flow	• Forward	• Absent	• Reversed
• Celiac artery diastolic flow	• Forward	• Absent	• Reversed
• MCA diastolic flow	• Forward	• Forward	• Absent/Reversed

■ NEONATAL FECHO: PA PRESSURES

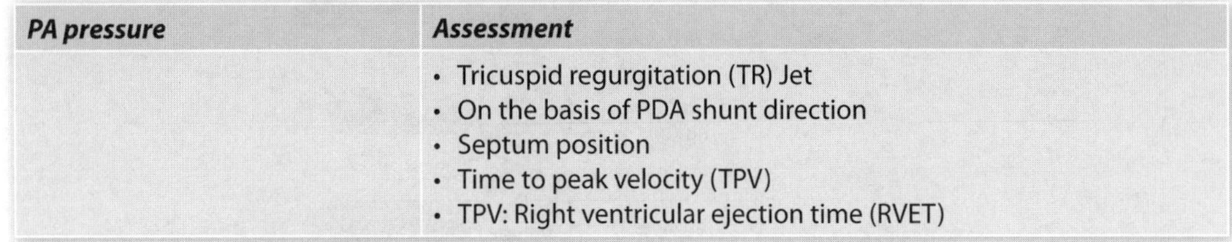

PA pressure	Assessment
	• Tricuspid regurgitation (TR) Jet • On the basis of PDA shunt direction • Septum position • Time to peak velocity (TPV) • TPV: Right ventricular ejection time (RVET)

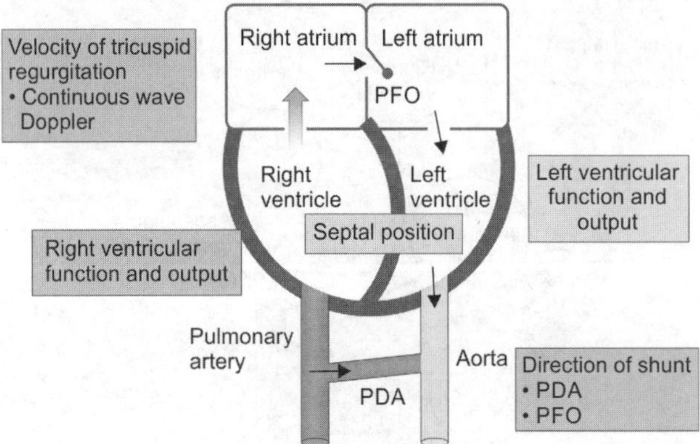

Echocardiographic assessment for high pulmonary vascular resistance.

■ STEPS OF PULMONARY ARTERIAL PRESSURE CALCULATIONS

- Apical four chamber/PLAX
- Color—TR jet
- CW application
- Measure—TR Jet velocity in m/s
- Velocity = Apply $4V^2$ (m/s)
- Right ventricular systolic pressure (RVSP) = $4V^2$ + RA pressure
- RA pressure = 5 mm Hg
- Hence RVSP = $4V^2$ + 5

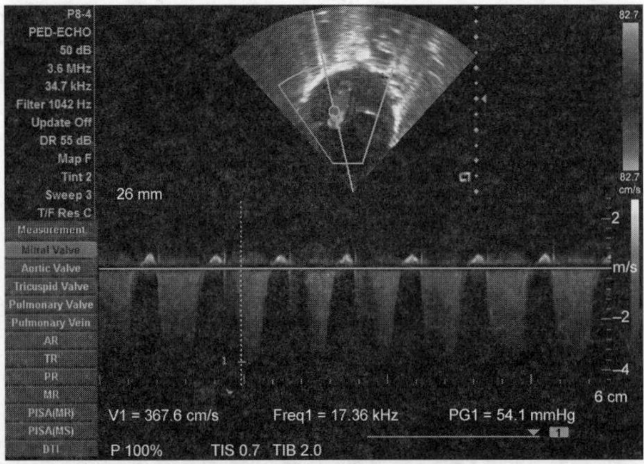

Calculation of pulmonary arterial pressure (PAP) in continuous wave Doppler mode from TR jet.

Pulmonary arterial pressure calculations on the basis of PDA.

PDA	PAP measurement
Left to right PDA	Systolic BP (invasive/noninvasive)—PG of left to right PDA (+ Doppler)
Right to left PDA	Systolic BP (Invasive/noninvasive) + PG of right to left PDA (Doppler)
Bidirectional (right-to-left component >30% of cardiac cycle)	Systolic BP (Invasive/noninvasive) + PG of right to left PDA (Doppler)

Pulmonary arterial pressure and persistent pulmonary hypertension.

PAP (TR jet/PDA direction)	PPHN
<35	Normal
35–45	Mild PPHN
45–60	Moderate PPHN
>60	Severe PPHN

Estimation of PAP on the basis of pulmonary artery acceleration time/TPV.

Pulmonary artery acceleration time (PAAT)/TPV	PAP
>100	Normal PAP
<90	Moderately raised PAP
<40	Significantly raised PAP

Estimation of PAP on the basis of TPV: RVET (PAAT: RVET).

TPV: RVET (PAAT: RVET)	PAP
>0.3	Normal PAP
0.3–0.2	Moderately raised PAP
<0.2	Significantly raised PAP

Estimation of RVP based on LV configuration.

Left ventricular configuration	Estimated RVP
O-shaped LV	<50% of LVP
D-shaped LV	50–100% of LVP
Crescent–shaped LV	>100% of LVP

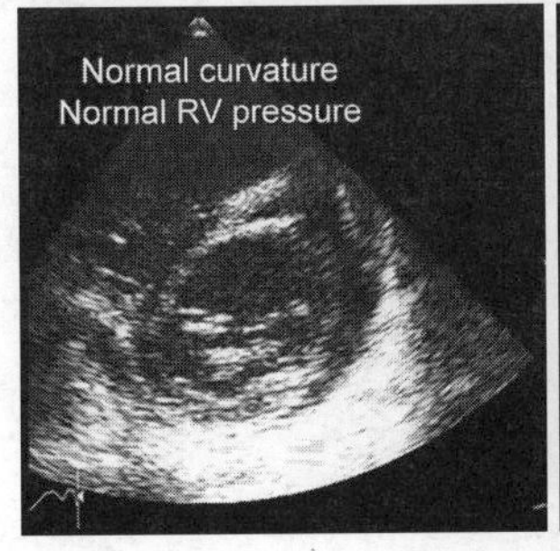

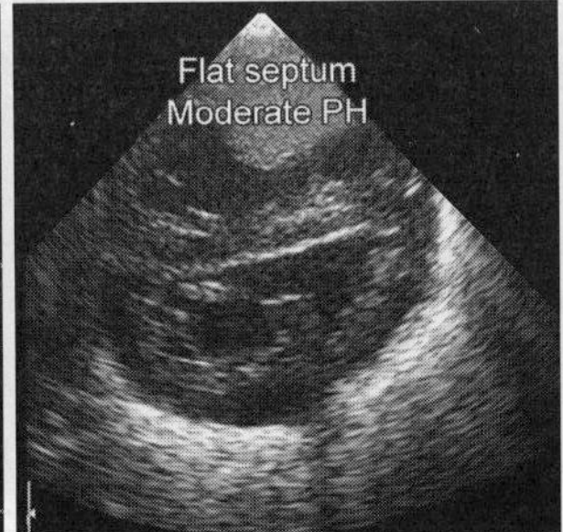

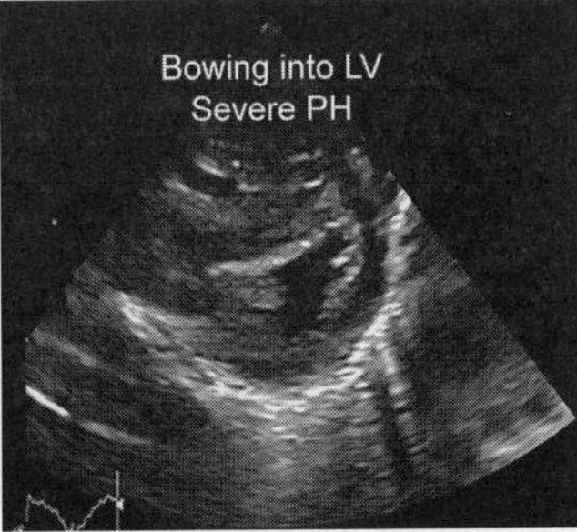

Position of intraventricular septum.

ECHO parameters in PPHN.

ECHO parameter	Assessment	View
RV hypertrophy and dilatation	Eyeball visual assessment	Apical four-chamber
Estimation of PAP	TR Jet	Apical four-chamber/PLAX
PDA shunt direction	Bidirectional or right to left	High parasternal ductal view
TPV (PAAT)	Time to peak velocity	Short-axis view
TPV: RVET (PAAT: RVET)	TPV versus right ventricular ejection time ratio	Short axis
IVS and LV shape	Visual inspection of septum	Parasternal short axis

Neonatal fECHO: ventricular function.

Ventricular function	Assessment
RV systolic function	• Tricuspid annular plane systolic excursion (TAPSE) • Fractional area change (FAC) • MPA
RV diastolic function	E:A ratio
LV systolic function	• Visual contractility • FS/EF • MPA
LV diastolic function	• E:A Ratio • Tissue Doppler • Pulmonary vein Doppler

Neonatal fECHO: cardiac and systemic blood flow.

Blood flow	Assessment
Cardiac blood flow	• RVOT • LVOT • SVC
Systemic blood flow	• ACA/MCA • SMA • RA

Cardiac blood flow.

Blood flow	Normal value (mL/kg/min)	Low output (mL/kg/min)	High output (mL/kg/min)
LVOT	150–300	<150	>300
RVOT	150–300	<150	>300
SVC flow	70–100	<50	>100

$$\text{Flow} = \frac{3.14 \ (\text{diameter cm})^2 \times \text{VTI (cm)} \times \text{HR}}{4 \times \text{Birth weight (kg)}}$$

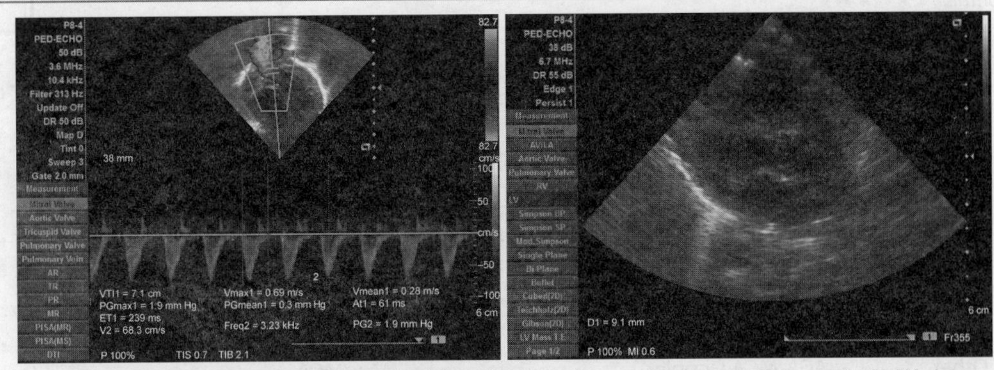

Aortic velocity time integral (VTI) in apical five-chamber view and aortic root diameter in PLAX view.

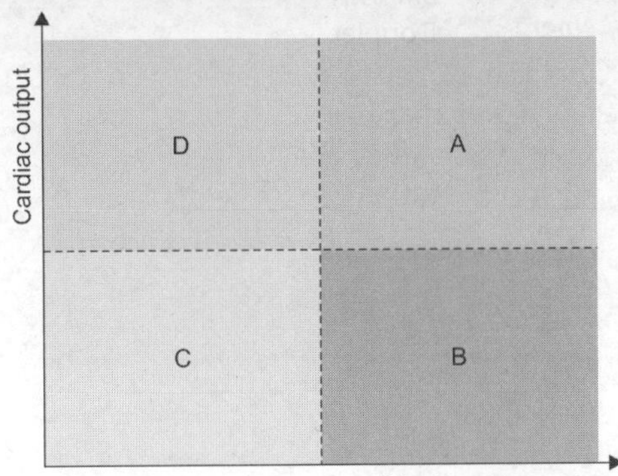

	Cardiac output	Blood pressure	Situation
A	Normal/high	Normal/high	Normal
B	Low	Normal/high	Compensated shock
C	Low	Low	Uncompensated shock
D	Normal/high	Low	Hyperdynamic circulation

ECHO assessment of shock: measurement of cardiac output and blood pressure.

Key Points to Remember

fECHO Assessment.

View	PDA	PPHN	Blood flow	V function
Subcostal		Atrial shunting	SVC VTI	
Apical 4/5 chamber	• LA/LV dilatation • Pulmonary vein D • E:A ratio • IVRT • LVOT—aortic VTI	• RA/RV dilatation • TR Jet—PASP measurement	LVOT—aortic VTI	• TAPSE • FAC • RV S/D • E:A of TV/MV • Pulmonary vein D • Tissue Doppler • Tei
PLAX	• LA:AO • LVEDD: AO • AO Diameter—LVOT	RV inflow—TR Jet measurement	• AO diameter • RV outflow for VTI and diameter • SVC diameter	• FS/EF • AO diameter

Contd...

Contd...

View	PDA	PPHN	Blood flow	V function
PSAX	• MPA Doppler • LPA Doppler • LA AO • LVEDD:AO	• TPV/PAAT • TPV:RVET • Septal deviation • LV shape	RV outflow for VTI and diameter	RV outflow for VTI and diameter
Ductal view	• Duct assessment • Direction and Doppler	• Duct assessment • Direction and Doppler		
Arch view	DA Doppler		DA Doppler	
Other	• ACA/MCA Doppler • SMA/RA Doppler		• ACA/MCA • SMA/RA Doppler	

Reporting

- Structure
- *Shunts:*
  - PFO
  - PDA
- PA pressures
- *RV and LV—ventricular functions:*
  - Systolic
  - Diastolic
- *Cardiac blood flow:*
  - RVOT
  - LVOT
  - SVC
- *Systemic blood flow:*
  - ACA/MCA
  - SMA
  - Renal

■ FURTHER READING

1. Suryawanshi P, Nagpal R, Ahya K. Atlas of neonatal functional echocardiography. Thane: Perfect prints; 2021.
2. Suryawanshi P, Sahni M, Parikh T. Point of care neonatal ultrasound; 2016.

Cranial Ultrasound

Rema S Nagpal

Indications for cranial ultrasound in neonates

- Routine screening in preterm neonates for germinal matrix hemorrhage-intraventricular hemorrhage (GMH-IVH), cerebellar bleeds
- Congenital malformations (e.g., holoprosencephaly)
- Acquired lesions—hypoxic-ischemic encephalopathy (HIE), hydrocephalus (postmeningitis/posthemorrhagic), and periventricular leukomalacia (PVL)
- Encephalopathic neonate including neonate with seizures
- Evaluation of intracranial bleeds
- Unexplained cardiac failure (to rule out AV malformations)
- Neonatal sepsis, meningitis, and congenital infections

Initial evaluation
- Intracranial bleeds—GMH-IVH, parenchymal hemorrhage, and subgaleal bleed
- Neonates with abnormal neurological signs
- Neonatal seizures
- Cerebral Doppler studies—assessment of Doppler flows in patent ductus arteriosus (PDA) suggestive of hemodynamic significance, resistive index in neonates with HIE

Ongoing/sequential imaging
- Posthemorrhagic or postinfective ventricular dilatation
- Evolution of white matter injury (PVL)
- Cranial infections—ventriculitis, brain abscess

WHICH BABIES SHOULD BE SCREENED (TABLE 1)

- Routine cranial ultrasound (CUS) of all neonates <32 weeks, or <1,500 g for GMH-IVH
- Neonates >32 weeks, >1,500 g, if there are risk factors such as asphyxia, abnormal neurological signs
- All ventilated neonates, term or preterm, to rule out intracranial hemorrhage.

Repeat imaging if Indicated:
- At 37–42 weeks, it may show PVL, ventriculomegaly (due to white matter injury, or posthemorrhagic dilatation), and structural anomalies.
- Neonate <32 weeks or birth weight <1,500 g
- Neonates with moderate to severe anomalies on CUS (≥grade 3 IVH, PHVD, or grade 3–4 PVL)
- Neonates with risk factors [mechanical ventilation, vasopressor use, necrotizing enterocolitis (NEC), and major surgery]

TABLE 1: Suggested CUS screening protocol for preterm neonates.		
<28 weeks or BW <1,000 g or 28–31 + 6 weeks and/or BW <1,500 g on life support	28–31 + 6 weeks or BW 1,000–1,500 g without life support	*32–34 weeks with risk factors:* Monochorionic twins, head circumference <3rd centile, ventilation and/or surfactant need, fetal distress, acidosis 5 minute APGAR score of <6, or hypotension
• 6 hours of age • Day 3 to 1 week • 4 weeks Term age equivalent (TAE) or discharge whichever occurs first	• Day 3 to 1 week • 4 weeks • TAE or discharge	Day 5 to 1 week and then as indicated
One week after any "new" sick event such as sepsis, hypotension, necrotizing enterocolitis (NEC), etc. In case of IVH other than GMH also, weekly scans are indicated CUS anytime in case of clinical suspicion of IVH		

WHICH ULTRASOUND WINDOWS ARE USED FOR THE PERFORMANCE OF CUS?

- *Standard CUS (Figs. 1 to 5):* Through anterior fontanel as the main acoustic window—in 6 standard coronal, and 5 mid and parasagittal planes—frontal horns, all ventricles
- Supplemental acoustic windows (**Figs. 6 and 7**):
  - Temporal Window—circle of Willis, mid brain
  - Mastoid Window—midbrain, posterior fossa, and cerebellum
  - Post Fontanel—occipital parenchyma, occipital horns, and posterior fossa

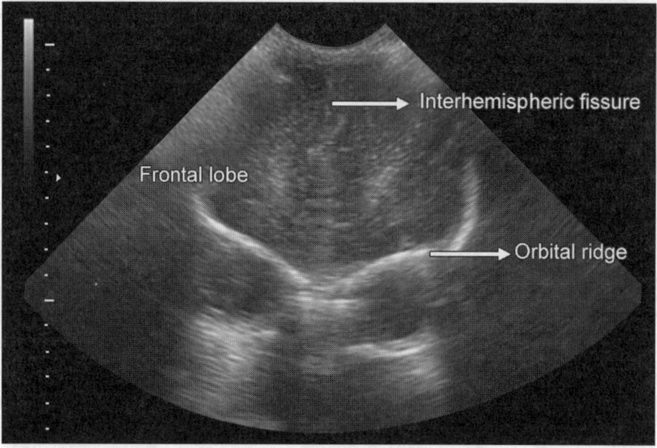

Fig.1: Coronal view through frontal lobe.

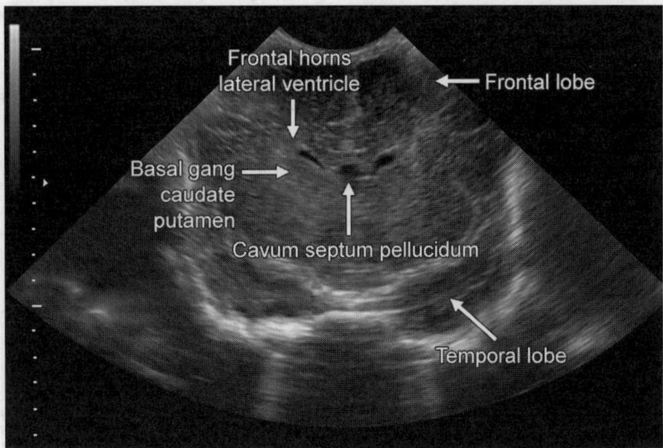

Fig. 2: Coronal view through frontal horns of lateral ventricle.

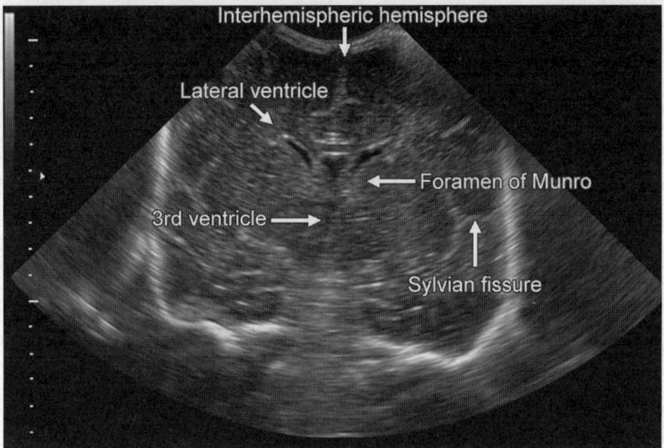

Fig. 3: Coronal view through foramen of Munro.

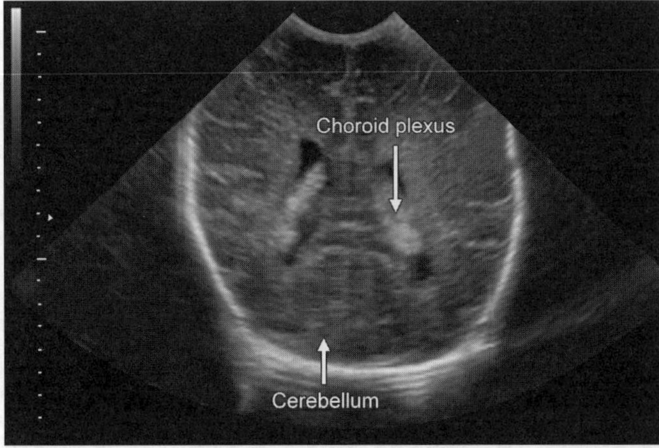

Fig. 4: Coronal view of Trigone.

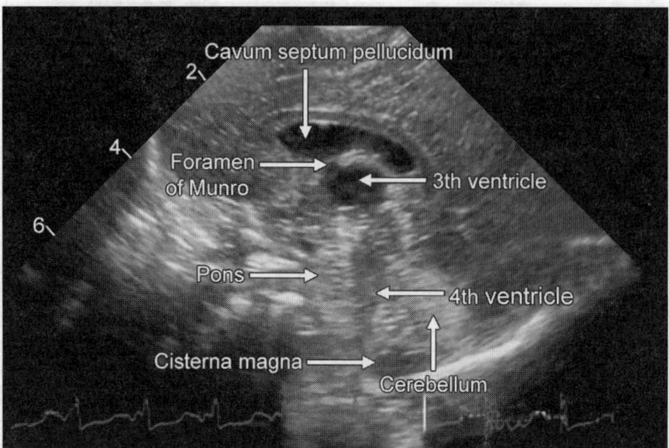

Fig. 5: Midline sagittal view.

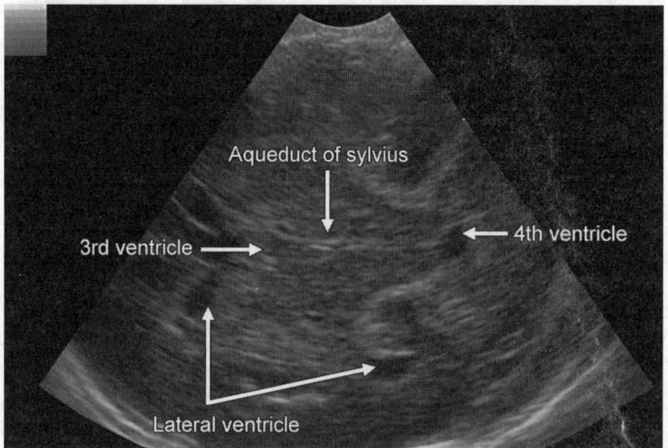

Fig. 6: Temporal view of midbrain.

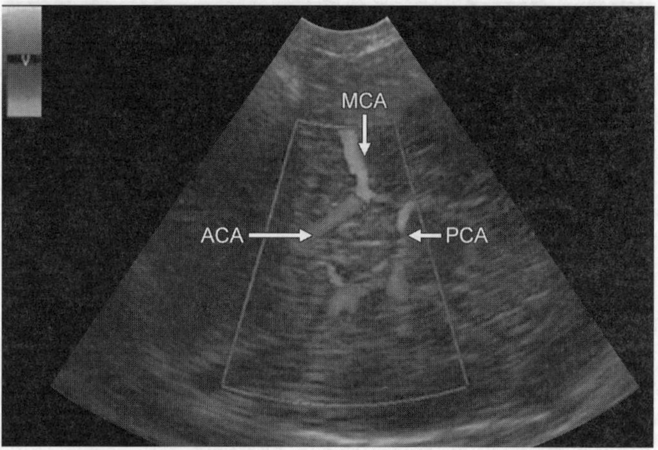

Fig. 7: Temporal window: reveals the circle of Willis.

GERMINAL MATRIX HEMORRHAGE-INTRAVENTRICULAR HEMORRHAGE

- *Incidence:* 20–25% amongst very low birth weight (VLBW) neonates. In >34 weeks gestation, severe IVH is seen in 0.2–4% neonates.
- *Germinal matrix (GM):* It forms the complete floor of the ventricular system in early gestation, progressively decreases with increase in gestational age, and involutes by 34–36 weeks gestation. The GM is never seen on CUS unless there is a bleed. Bleeds should be identified in 2 or more CUS views, and never in a single view. Acute hemorrhages are highly echogenic on CUS, and become less echogenic over 1–2 weeks. Absence of echogenicity on CUS is very unlikely to be an acute bleed.
- *Pathogenesis and risk factors for IVH:* Gestational age is the single independent risk factor. Contributing factors include fragility of GM, fluctuations in cerebral blood flow during hemodynamic instability, and limited cerebral autoregulation. Single-independent factor that decreases risk of GMH-IVH is antenatal corticosteroids.
- *Time of onset:* 50% by 24 hours; 90% by 72 hours. The maximum progress of lesion is between 3 and 5 days after initial diagnosis.
- *Classifications:* Volpe's (1989) **(Table 2)** classification and the Papile and Burstein Classification (1978) **(Table 3)** are currently used to grade IVH bleeds. Grades 1 and 2 are considered mild, while Grades 3 and 4 are considered severe IVH.

TABLE 2: Volpe classification for GMH-IVH (1989).	
Grade 1	Germinal matrix hemorrhage with no or minimal IVH (<10% of ventricular area on parasagittal view)
Grade 2	IVH (10–50% of ventricular area on parasagittal view)
Grade 3	IVH (>50% of ventricular area on parasagittal view; usually distends at least 1 lateral ventricle at the time of diagnosis)
Separate notation	Concomitant periventricular echo density (location and extent), referred to as "IPE" (intraparenchymal echo density), periventricular or parenchymal hemorrhagic infarction, or venous infarction

TABLE 3: Papile and Burstein classification for GMH-IVH (1978) (Figs. 9 to 11).	
Grade 1	A small hemorrhage, confined to the germinal matrix, and without effect on the adjacent parenchyma
Grade 2	Hemorrhage originating within the germinal matrix, where small amount of blood has leaked into the lateral ventricle, with no ventricular dilatation
Grade 3	Hemorrhage originating within the germinal matrix, where large amount of blood has leaked into the ventricular system, leading to acute ventricular dilatation
Grade 4	Larger hemorrhage into germinal matrix, along with evidence of venous infarction of the adjacent periventricular white matter (PHI)

This study was based on CT scans performed on neonates <1,500 g, a majority of whom had IVH. Grade 3 IVH must be differentiated from IVH with posthemorrhagic ventricular dilatation. The ventricular dilatation in Grade 3 IVH is acute and may be transient only.

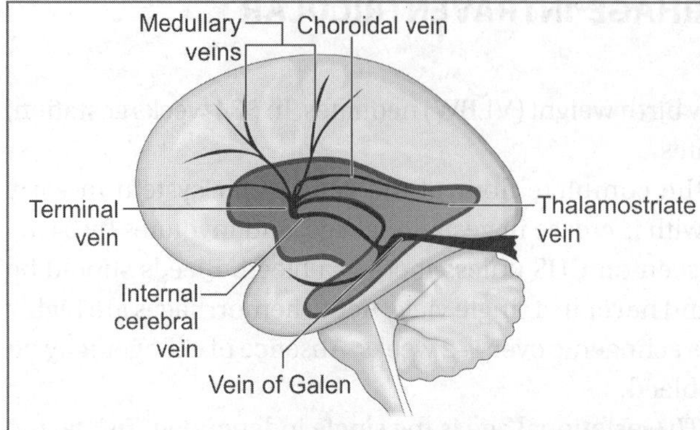

The medullary, choroidal and thalamostriate vein form the terminal vein. This vein courses through the GM to empty into the internal cerebral vein, but takes a sharp turn at this junction, making it prone to bleeds (*see* **Fig. 8**).

Large bleeds obstruct the terminal vein, and impair blood flow in the medullary vein, leading to a venous infarct called the periventricular hemorrhagic infarct.

Fig. 8: Venous drainage of galenic system and germinal matrix.

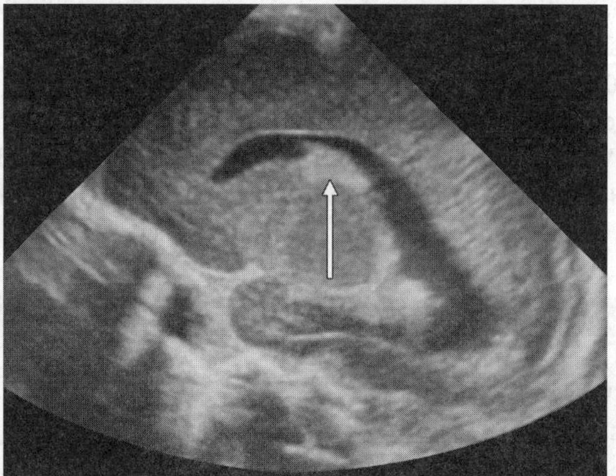

Fig. 9: Grade 1 IVH seen just anterior to the caudothalamic notch in the sagittal view (arrow).

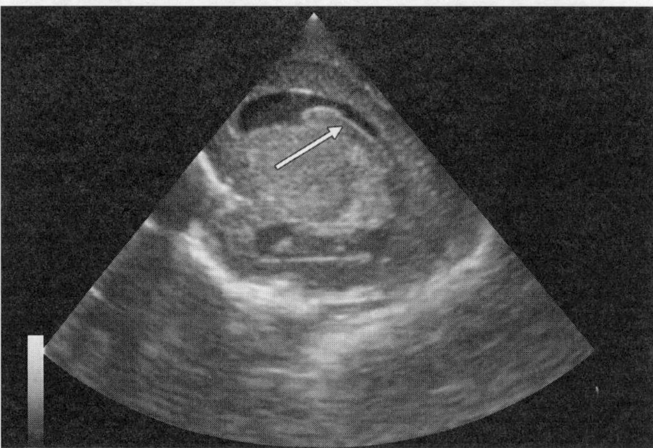

Fig. 10: Grade II IVH: IVH has drained into ventricular cavity, without dilatation. Choroid Plexus has the same echogenicity as the IVH.

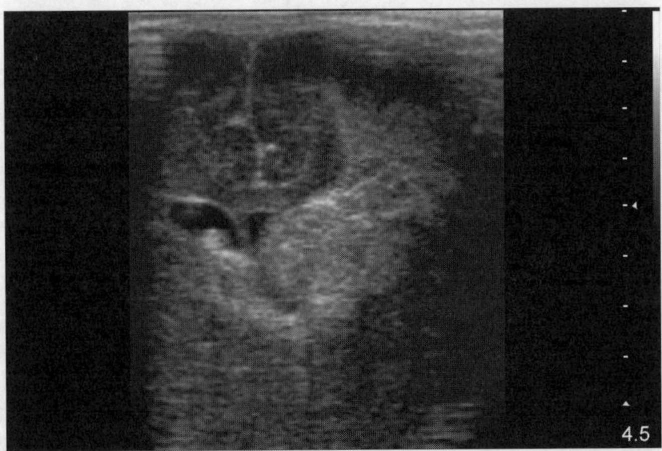

Fig.11: Periventricular hemorrhagic infarct (PVHI) seen in the coronal view is unilateral.

Prediction of abnormal neuromotor function by cranial ultrasound.		
Grade of GMH-IVH	*Pathological effect*	*Clinical impact on neonate*
Grade I-II IVH	• Microstructural impairment in periventricular and subcortical white matter • Relevant loss of glial precursor cells, leading to impaired myelination and cortical development	Robust data lacking
Grade III IVH	IVH triggers inflammation in adjacent white matter through activated microglia, passage of red blood cells and red blood cell degradation, resulting in perilesional tissue injury secondary to free radical release and the presence of free iron	Cerebral palsy 7–63%
Parenchymal hemorrhagic infarct (PHI)	• GMH-IVH leads to venous obstruction, resultant ischemia and secondary hemorrhagic infarct • Evolves into cavitation within periventricular white matter • Cavitation resulting from PHI is usually single, asymmetric and persistent	• CP and severe cognitive impairment • Bilateral PHI has high mortality • Redirection of care may be discussed
Grade I-II IVH	• Microstructural impairment in periventricular and subcortical white matter • Relevant loss of glial precursor cells, leading to impaired myelination and cortical development	Robust data lacking
Grade III IVH	IVH triggers inflammation in adjacent white matter through activated microglia, passage of red blood cells and red blood cell degradation, resulting in perilesional tissue injury secondary to free radical release and the presence of free iron	Cerebral palsy 7–63%

Contd...

Contd...

Grade of GMH-IVH	Pathological effect	Clinical Impact on neonate
Parenchymal hemorrhagic infarct (PHI)	• GMH-IVH leads to venous obstruction, resultant ischemia and secondary hemorrhagic infarct • Evolves into cavitation within periventricular white matter • Cavitation resulting from PHI is usually single, asymmetric and persistent	• CP and severe cognitive impairment • Bilateral PHI has high mortality • Redirection of care may be discussed
Posthemorrhagic ventricular dilatation (PHVD)	Obstruction of liquor pathways around cerebellum	• 25% of neonates with GMH-IVH develop progressive PVHD • 80% of progressive PVHD follow Grade III IVH • 40% resolve spontaneously • 15% resolve after nonsurgical treatment • 35% require surgical treatment • 10% die

Posthemorrhagic ventricular dilatation (Figs. 12 to 15).

The parameters considered and the actionable levels for PHVD are:
• Ventricular index: 4 mm >97th centile
• Anterior horn width >4 mm (>1 mm over 97th centile)
• Thalamo-occipital distance >26 mm (>1 mm over 97th centile)
• Third ventricular width >3 mm (>1 mm over 97th centile)

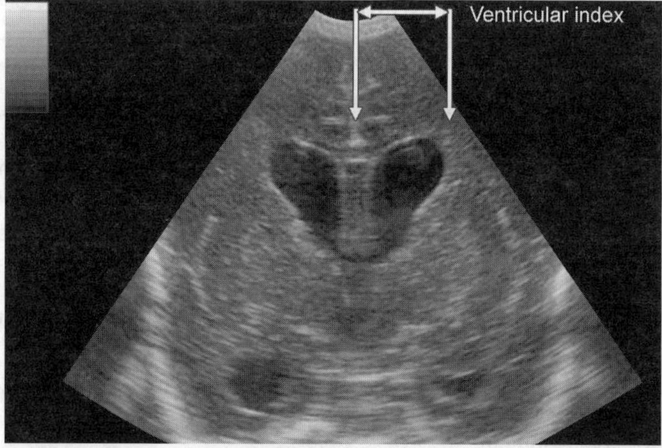

Fig.12: Posthemorrhagic ventricular dilatation of the lateral ventricles measured by ventricular index (VI).

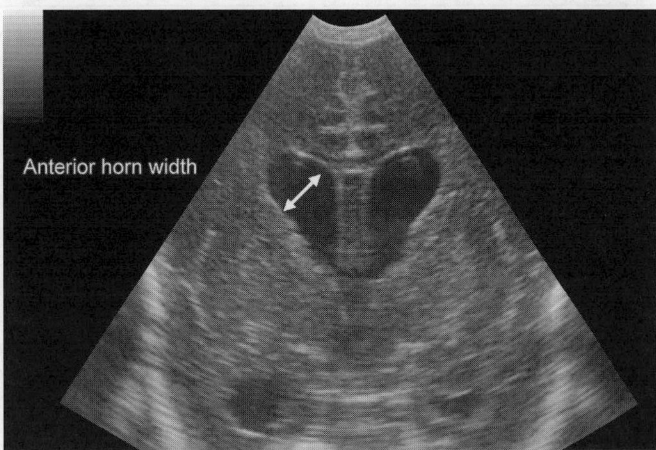

Fig. 13: PHVD with increased anterior horn width.

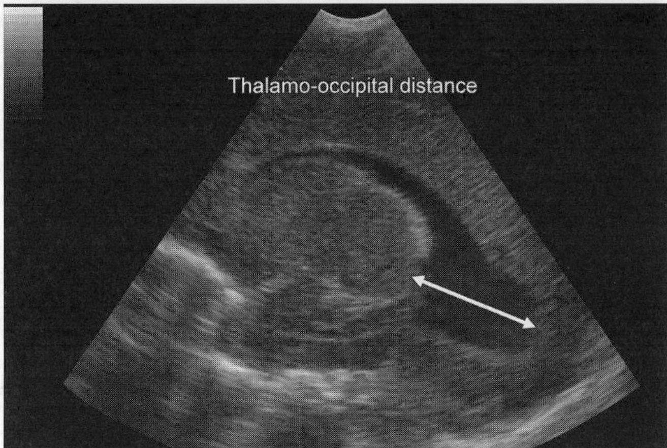

Fig.14: PVHD with increased thalamo-occipital distance.

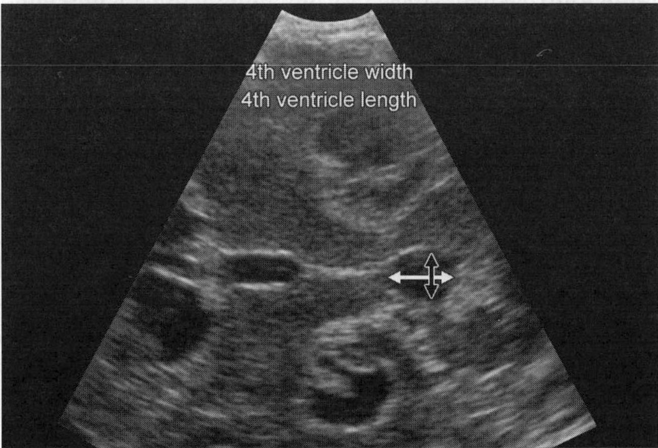

Fig. 15: Mastoid view reveals dilated 4th ventricle.

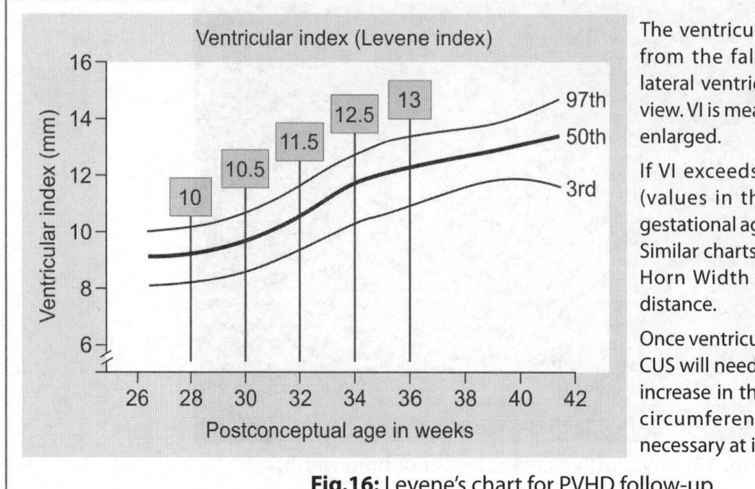

The ventricular index (VI) is the distance from the falx to the outermost part of lateral ventricle in the Foramen of Munro view. VI is measured if the ventricles appear enlarged.

If VI exceeds the 97th centile by 4 mm (values in the green boxes) at a given gestational age, an intervention is required. Similar charts are available for the Anterior Horn Width and the Thalamo-occipital distance.

Once ventricular dilatation is noted, weekly CUS will need to be performed, to note the increase in the size of the ventricles. Head circumference measurements are also necessary at increasing frequency.

Fig.16: Levene's chart for PVHD follow-up.
Source: Levene M. Archives of Disease in Childhood. 1981;56(12):9004-4.

- *Parenchymal hemorrhagic infarction (PHI):* Occurs in 15–20% VLBW with IVH.
- *Posthemorrhagic ventricular dilatation (PHVD):* Defined as ventricular enlargement >97th centile for gestational age. 30–50% neonates with severe IVH develop PHVD. This may be nonprogressive or progressive requiring intervention. PHVD is typically seen 7–14 days after IVH.
- *Levene's charts* were the first published reference curves for ventricular index (VI) measurements following IVH. *Davies* has produced reference charts for anterior horn width, thalamo-occipital distance, and third ventricular width.
- Cerebellar injury is seen in 10–20% preterm neonates <32–34 weeks gestation.

PERIVENTRICULAR LEUKOMALACIA

- Symmetrical nonhemorrhagic necrosis of white matter, dorsal, and lateral to the external angles of the lateral ventricles
- Focal necrosis (with subsequent cyst formation) and diffuse gliosis may be seen.
- Echo densities on the ultrasound may be transient (<7 days), or prolonged (>7 days).
- Extensive cysts may develop 2–3 weeks following insult, localized cysts may take 3–6 weeks to develop.
- Periventricular hemorrhagic infarct needs to be differentiated from PVL.

Grades of periventricular leukomalacia (Figs. 17 and 18).	
Grade I	Transient periventricular echo densities lasting >7 days (periventricular flare)
Grade II	Transient periventricular echo densities evolving into small localized frontoparietal cysts (localized cystic PVL)
Grade III	Periventricular echo densities evolving into extensive periventricular cystic lesions (extensive cystic PVL)
Grade IV	Densities extending into the deep white matter evolving into extensive cystic lesions

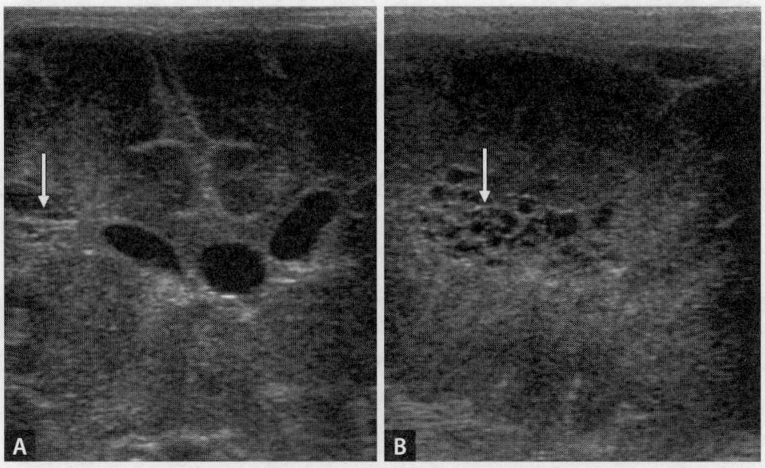

Figs. 17A and B: Localized cystic PVL (Grade II PVL)—cystic lesions seen in frontoparietal area in the coronal (A) and the parasagittal view (B).

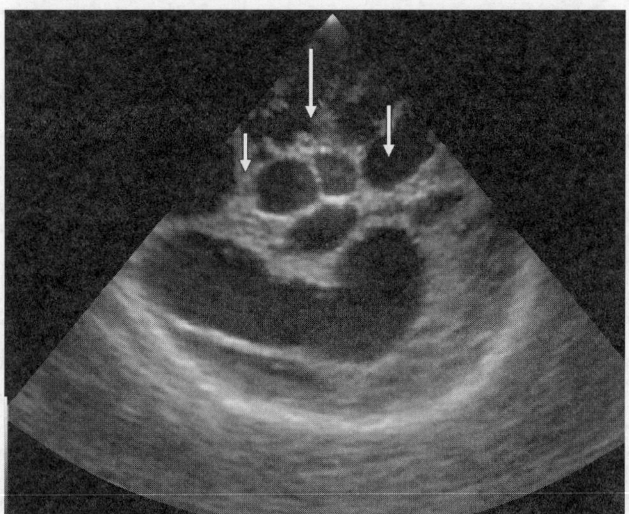

Fig. 18: Grade IV PVL with lesions extending deep into the white matter.

Differences between periventricular hemorrhagic infarction and cystic PVL.	
Periventricular hemorrhagic infarction	*Cystic PVL*
Usually, unilateral	Mainly bilateral
Associated ipsilateral large IVH	No/small IVH
Fan shaped echo density	Patchy appearance
Sharply delineated	Irregular border
Regular shape	Irregular shape
Signs of increased pressure	No signs of increased pressure
Almost half develop hemiplegia	Invariably develop CP

■ DOPPLER STUDIES

- The Doppler flows of the neonatal brain are used to assess the hemodynamics of the neonatal circulation and the perfusion of the brain. It determines the velocity of blood flow in the cerebral vasculature (anterior, middle, and posterior cerebral artery)

- *Resistive index of Pourcelot (RI)* $= \dfrac{\text{Peak systolic velocity} - \text{End-diastolic velocity}}{\text{Peak systolic velocity}}$

- *Normal value of RI* $-$ 0.75 $\pm$ 0.08

Resistive indices in various diseases (Figs. 19A to C).	
Disease	**Resistive index**
GMH-IVH	Increased
PVL	Increased
Hydrocephalous	Increased
PDA	Increased
Gram-negative sepsis	Increased
Asphyxia	• Decreased in the initial stages • Increased in the later stages
Vascular malformations	Decreased

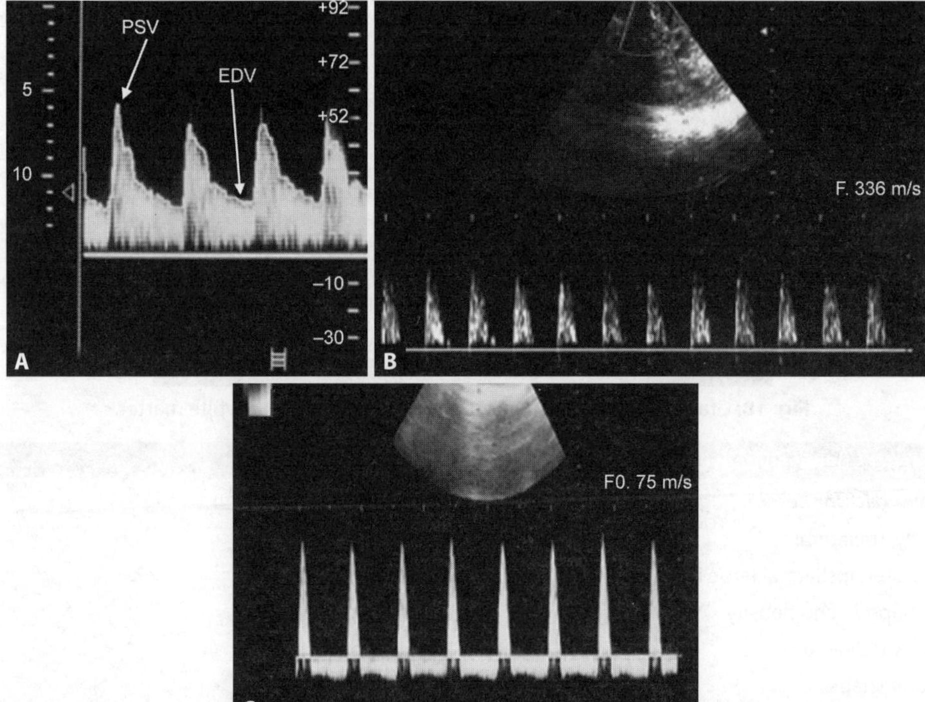

Figs. 19A to C: Doppler studies performed in the cranial US. (A) Normal RI; (B) Reveals absent diastolic flow; and (C) Reveals reversal of diastolic flow.

Key Points to Remember

Limitations of Cranial Ultrasonography

- Brain convexity may not be well visualized, small arterial infarcts and lesions in the water shed areas may be overlooked.
- Extracerebral hemorrhages on the cerebral hemisphere convexity may be difficult to detect (e.g., subdural, epidural, and subarachnoid hemorrhages).
- Hypoglycemic parenchymal injury to the occipital lobes may not be noted unless posterior fontanel CUS is performed.
- Myelination cannot be recognized on CUS.
- Diffuse white matter injury, seen in preterm neonates, may not be reliably detected on CUS.

■ FURTHER READING

1. Guillot M, Chau V, Lemyre B. Routine imaging of the preterm neonatal brain. Paediatr Child Health. 2020;25(4):249-62.
2. Lowe LH, Bailey Z. State-of-the-art cranial sonography: Part 1, Modern techniques and image interpretation. Am J Roentgenol. 2011;196:1028-33.
3. Lowe LH, Bailey Z. State-of-the-art cranial sonography: Part 2: Pitfalls and variants. Am J Roentgenol. 2011;196(5):1034-9.
4. Parodi A, Govaert P, Horsch S, Bravo MC, Ramenghi LA, Ramenghi LA, Agut T, et al. Cranial ultrasound findings in preterm germinal matrix haemorrhage, sequelae and outcome. Pediatric Research. 2020;87:13-24.
5. Rath C, Suryawanshi P. Point of care neonatal ultrasound-head, lung, gut and line localization. Indian Pediatr. 2016;53:889-99.

Chapter 73

Chest Radiographs

Sarvani Sattiraju, Shriyan Ashvij

OBJECTIVES

- Schematically read and describe a neonatal chest X-ray.
- Identify the typical radiologic features of common conditions.
- Understand the variations and overlap.
- Identify the complications of a disease.

NEONATAL CHEST X-RAY—HOW IS IT DIFFERENT?

- Almost always anteroposterior (AP) view.
- Diaphragm is up to 6 ribs anteriorly and 8 ribs posteriorly.
- Ribs are more horizontal.
- Normal cardiothoracic (CT) ratio is up to 0.6.
- Air bronchogram can be present in retrocardiac areas.
- Thymus may be prominent.

WHAT DO YOU SEE?

Five radiographic densities in order of increasing brightness:

1. Air—black
2. Fat—dark gray
3. Fluid—gray
4. Bone—white
5. Metal—bright white

Interpretation

- Projection [AP vs. posterioranterior (PA) film]
- Exposure (hard vs. soft films)
- Rotation
- Bones and soft tissue
- *Lungs:* Expansion/parenchyma/cardiac and diaphragmatic margins
- *Cardiac:* CT ratio/pulmonary vascular markings/specific chamber enlargement
- Lines and tubes.

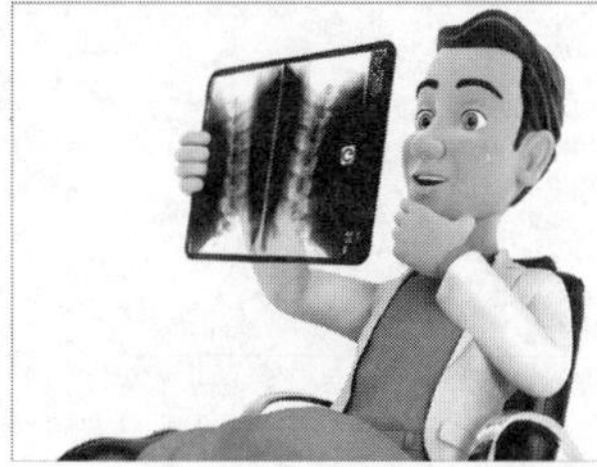

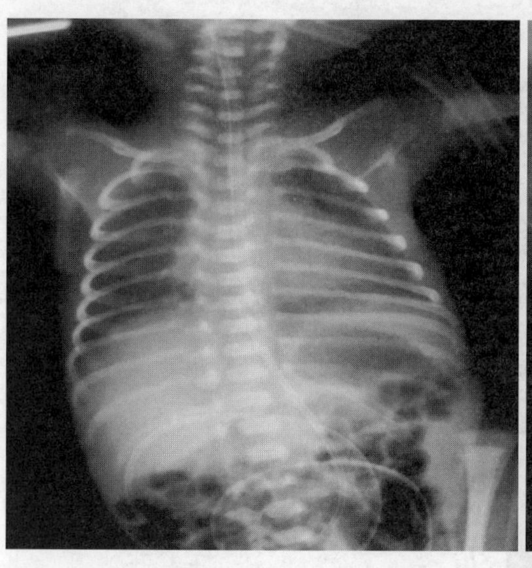 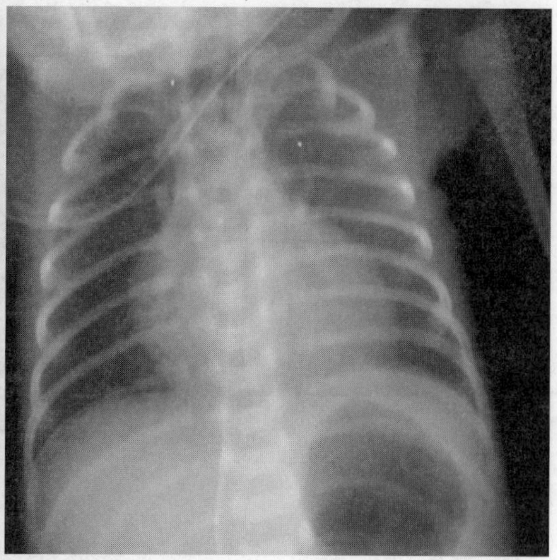

PA films	AP films
Scapulae lie posterolaterally, away from lung fields	• Scapulae overlap the lungs • Heart appears larger
Lamina more prominent	• Cervicothoracic vertebral end plates are more prominent • Ribs appear horizontally placed

Overexposure

- Darker the soft tissue, more the exposure
- Retrocardiac vertebrae easily seen, over exposed
- Long bones disappear, over exposed

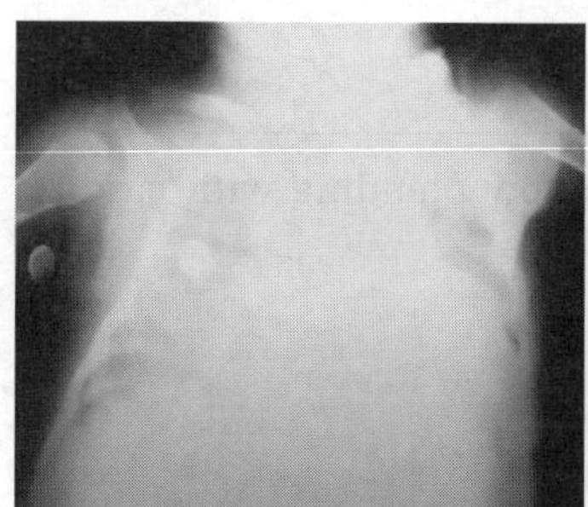 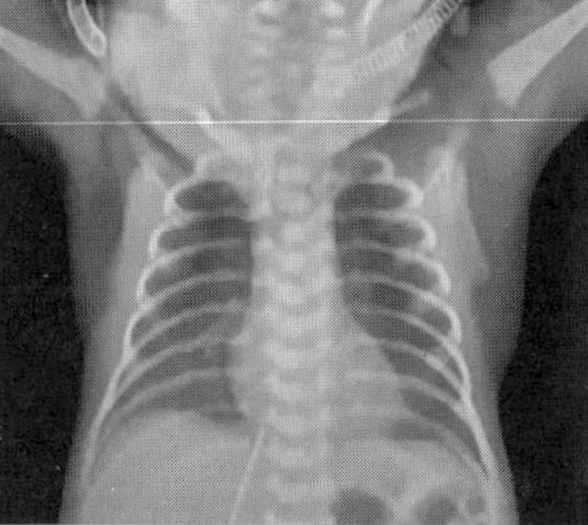 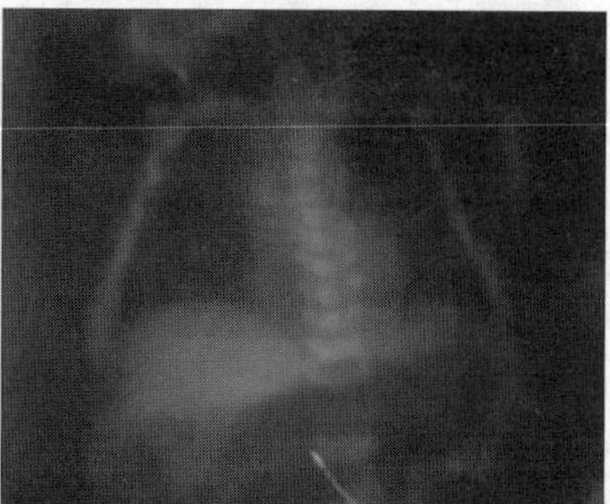

Rotation

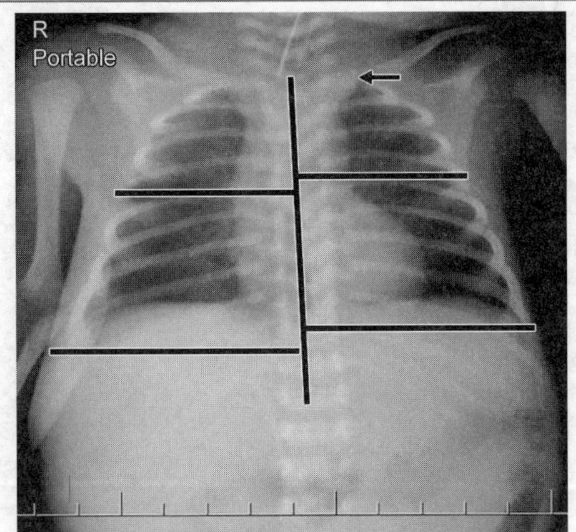

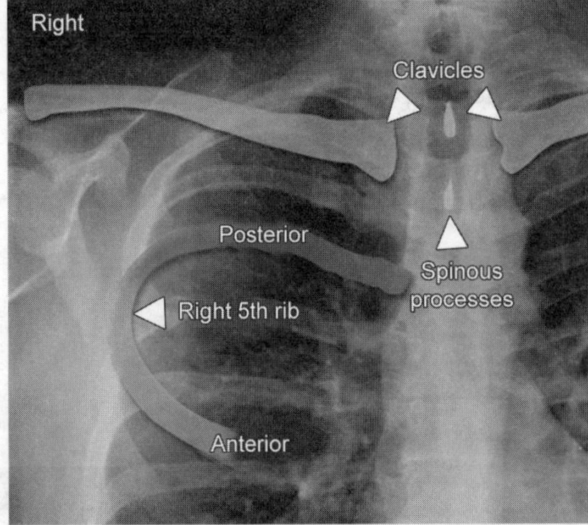

Rotated if:
- Distance of anterior ends of ribs from midline is unequal.
- Medial end of clavicles.

Normal thymus: Bilateral smooth superior mediastinal shadow blending with cardiac silhouette.

Normal thymus variants:
- Notch sign—prominent notch on inferior left border
- Sail sign—sail like border
- Wavy thymus sign—undulating border due to ribs indentation.

Schematic Reading

ABCDEF approach:

A—Airways

B—Bones and soft tissues

C—Cardiac size, shape, and position

D—Diaphragm
E—Extras (UAC, UVC, ET, and PICC)
F—Fundus bubble.

Respiratory Distress Syndrome

- Underaerated lungs
- Reticulogranularity
- Air bronchograms
- Diffuse granularity
- White out lungs

Mild respiratory distress syndrome (RDS)	• Normal to decreased aeration • Reticulogranularity
Moderate RDS	• Decreased aeration • Air bronchograms • Indistinct diaphragm and heart borders
Severe RDS	White out lung

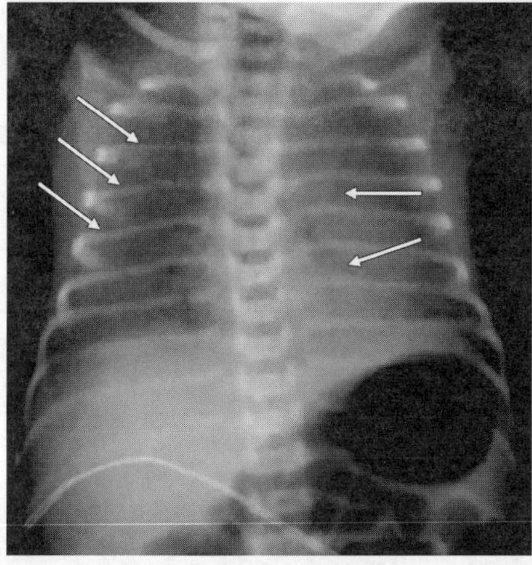
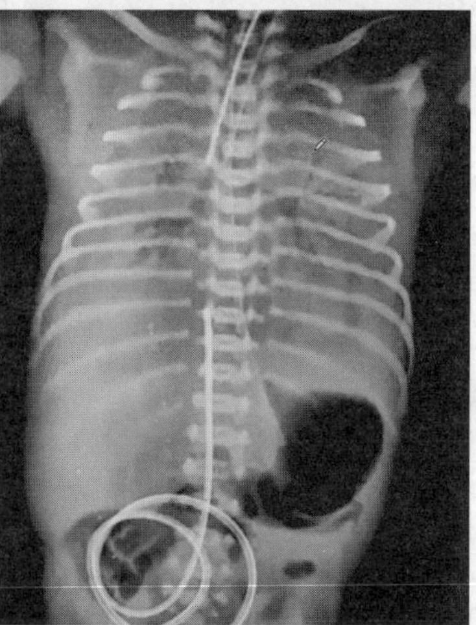

Transient Tachypnea of Newborn

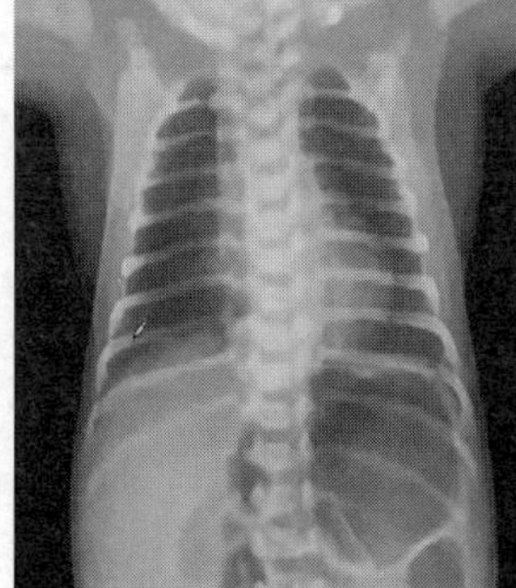
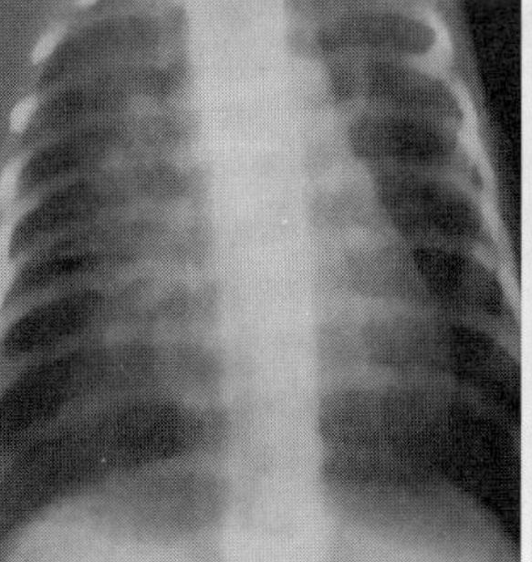
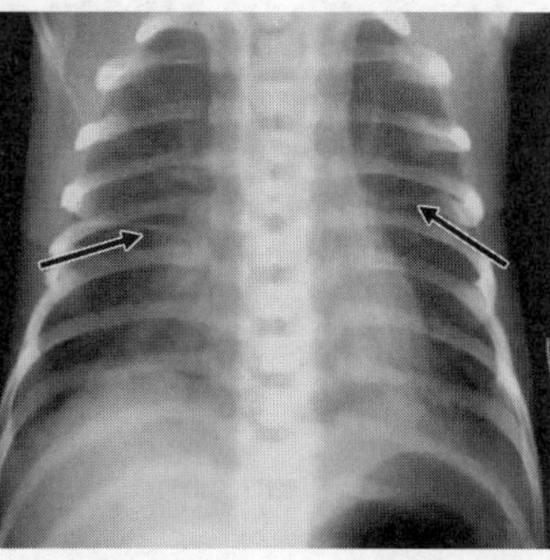

- Overaeration of lung fields
- Fluid filled horizontal fissures
- Small pleural effusions
- Lung volume good
- Streaky densities.

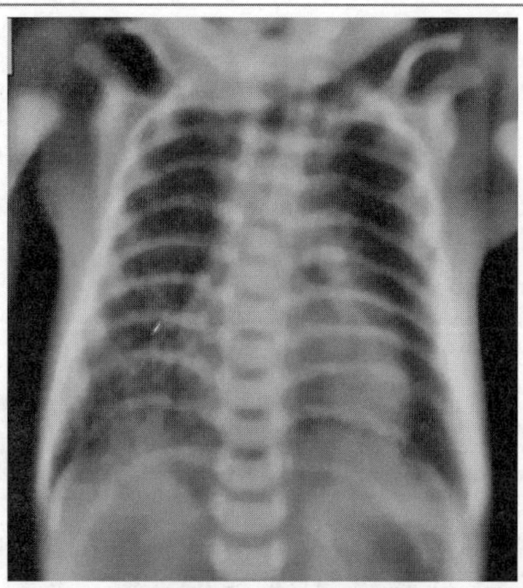

Meconium aspiration syndrome
- Hyperaeration
- Asymmetric
- Coarse nodular opacities
- Air leaks.

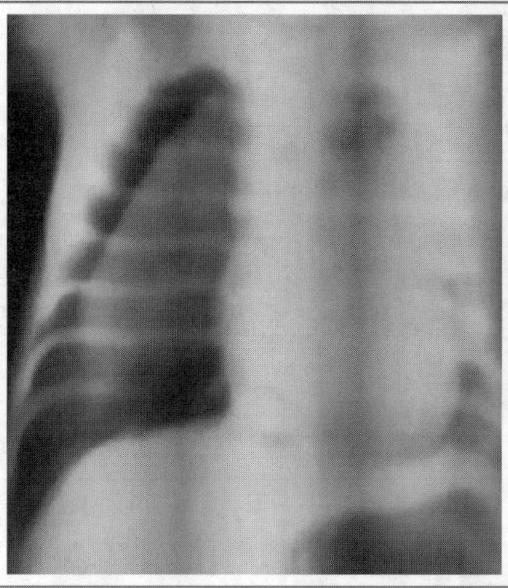

Pneumothorax
- Clear border of collapsed lung
- Absent lung markings
- Mediastinal shift
- Herniation into the contralateral side.

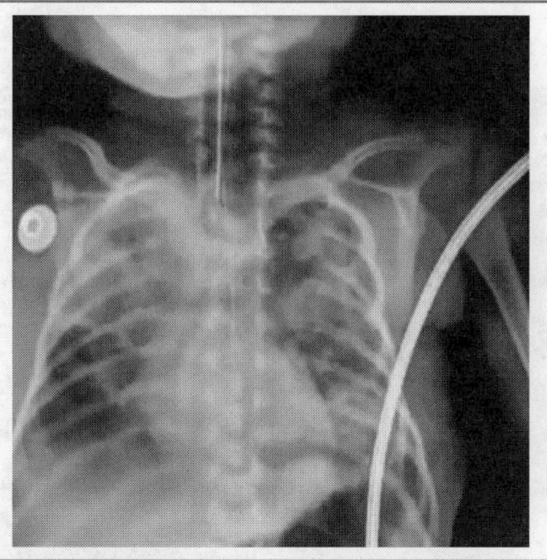

Pneumonia
- May range from reticulogranularity to lobar or segmental consolidation
- Air bronchograms may be seen
- Coarse granular patchy infiltrates with irregular areas of hyperinflation.

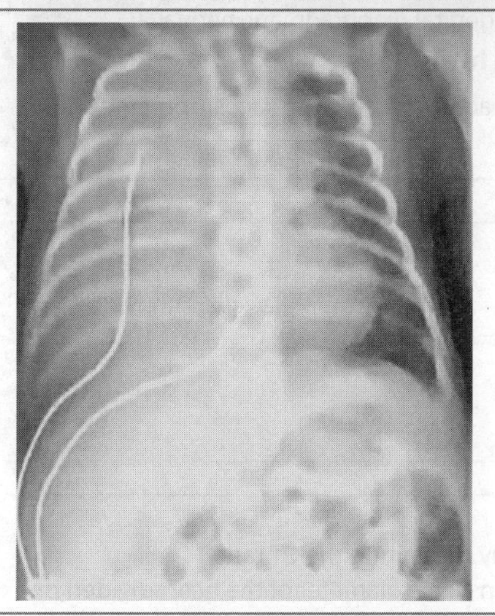

Pleural effusion
- Blunting of lateral costophrenic angles (erect film)
- Decreased transradiancy of the lung with preserved pulmonary vascular markings (supine film).

Bronchopulmonary Dysplasia

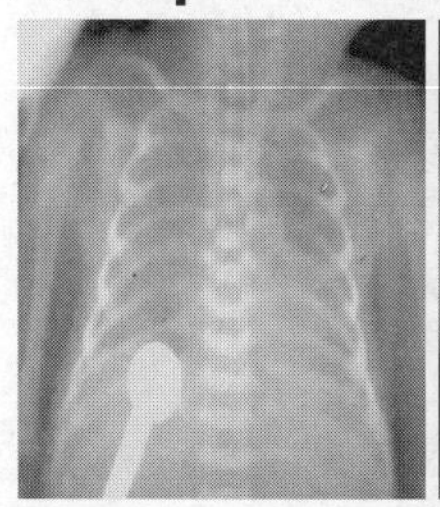
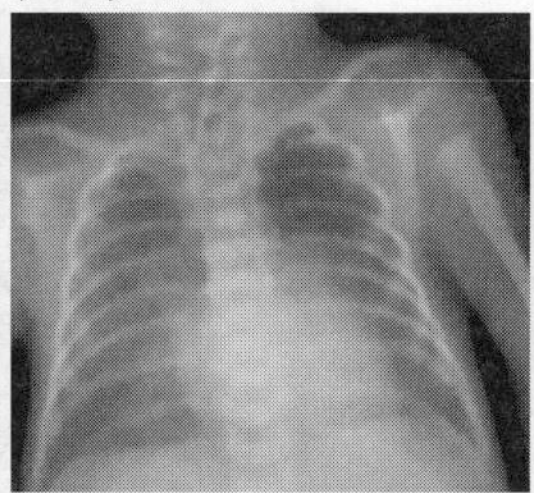
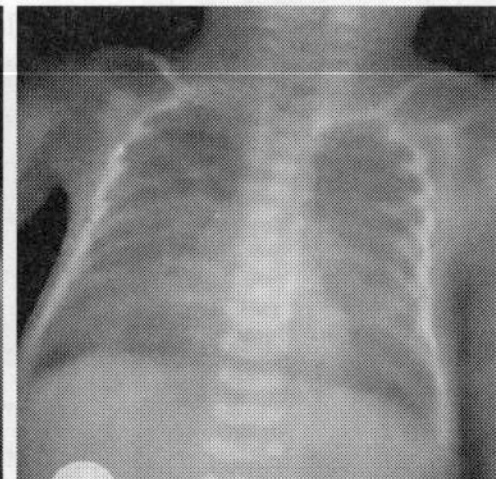
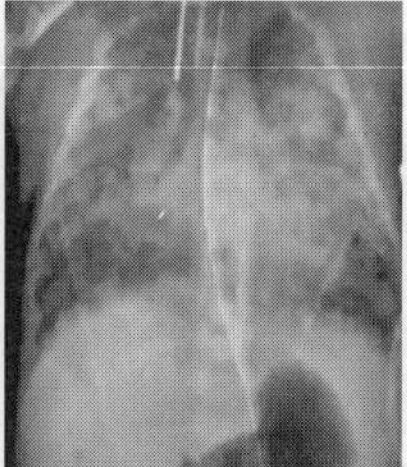

Stage 1	*Stage 2*	*Stage 3*	*Stage 4*
2–3 days	4–10 days	11–20 days	1 month
• Air bronchogram • Reticulogranularity	• Opacification • Coarse irregular densities	Small generalized radiolucent cysts	• Dense fibrotic strands • Generalized cystic areas • Hyperinflated lungs

Congenital Diaphragmatic Hernia

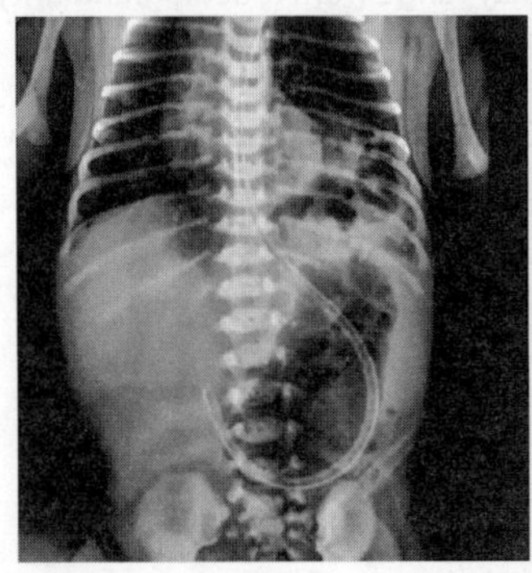 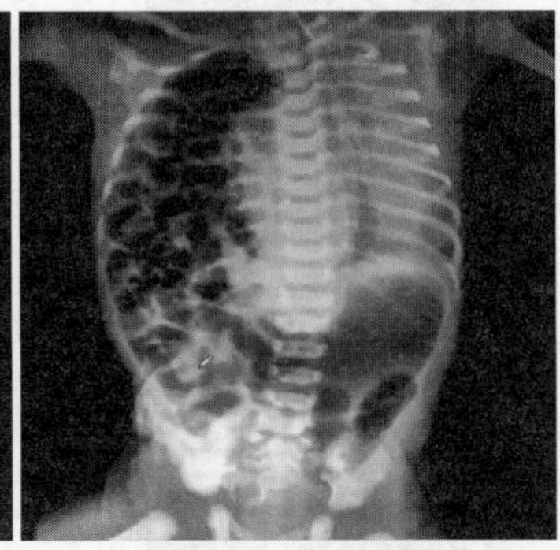

Left congenital diaphragmatic hernia	Right congenital diaphragmatic hernia
Bochdalek defects	Morgagni hernias
Well defined dome-shaped soft tissue opacity on left chest	Opacities adjacent to the right costophrenic angle

Interpretation of the Cardiac Shadow

- Cardiac size
- Pulmonary vasculature
- Cardiac situs
- Shape and size of chambers.

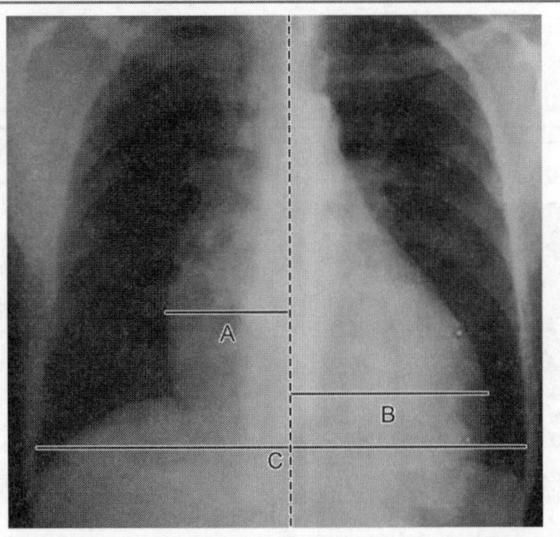

Cardiac size
- Assessed by measuring the CT ratio
- Largest transverse diameter of the heart divided by the maximum internal diameter of the chest
- Cardiothoracic ratio >0.6 suggests cardiomegaly in newborns.

Pulmonary Vasculature Pattern

- Normal vascularity
- Increased vascularity or plethora
- Decreased vascularity or oligemia

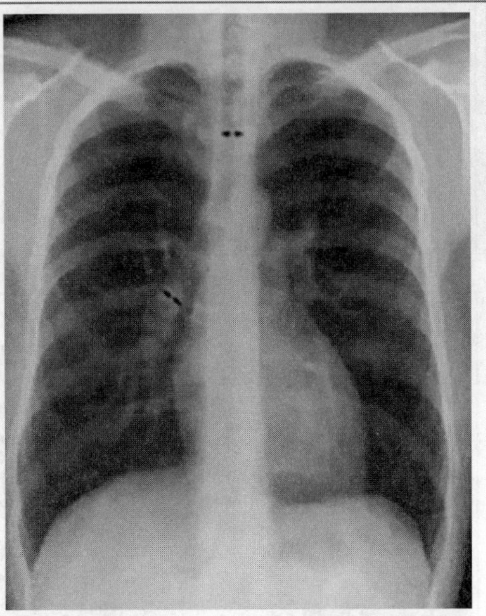

Normal vascularity
- Symmetric.
- Gradual tapering toward periphery.
- Diameter of right descending pulmonary artery is equal to that of trachea.
- In peripheral lung fields, the pulmonary vessels and accompanying bronchi are of equal size.

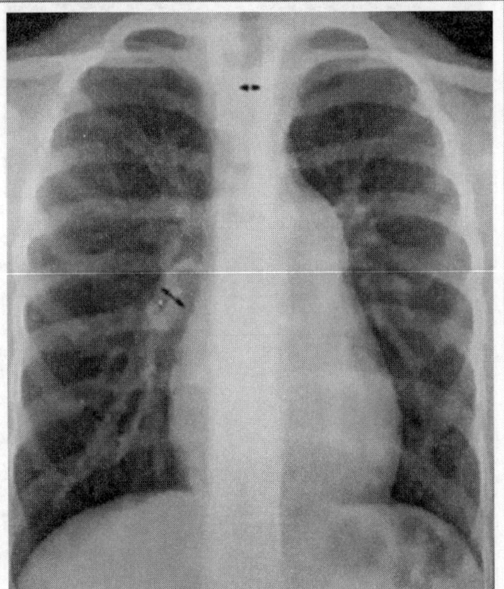

Plethora
- Uniformly enlarged vessels at hilum and within lung fields
- Dilated and tortuous vessels extending to lateral third of lung fields
- More than 3–5 end on views of vessels at hilum
- Diameter of right descending pulmonary artery more than trachea size
- Diameter of peripheral pulmonary artery more than adjacent bronchus.

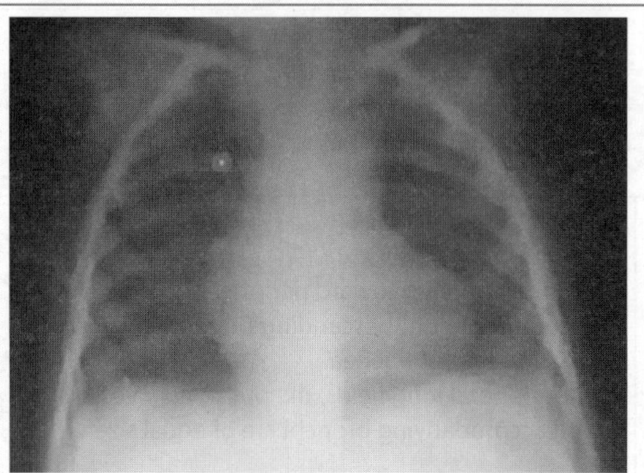

Oligemia
Small size of pulmonary vessels at hilum and lung fields.

Cardiac Situs

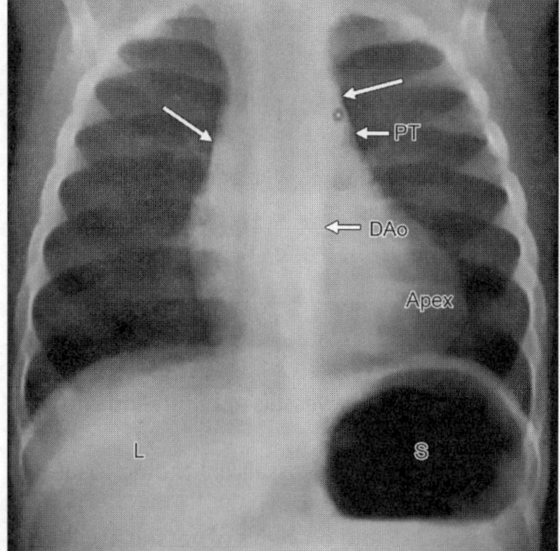

Situs solitus with levocardia

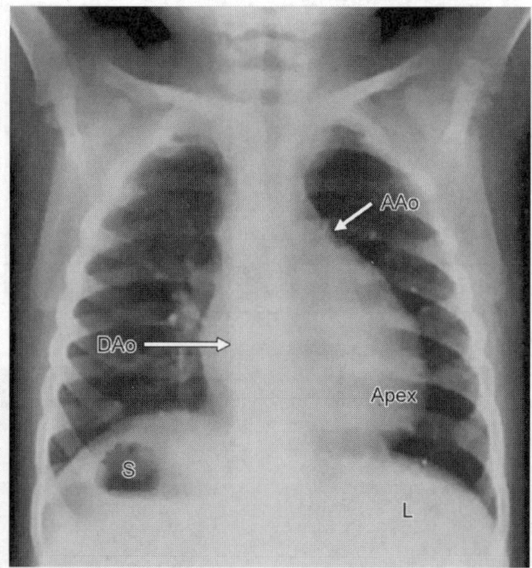

Situs inversus with levocardia

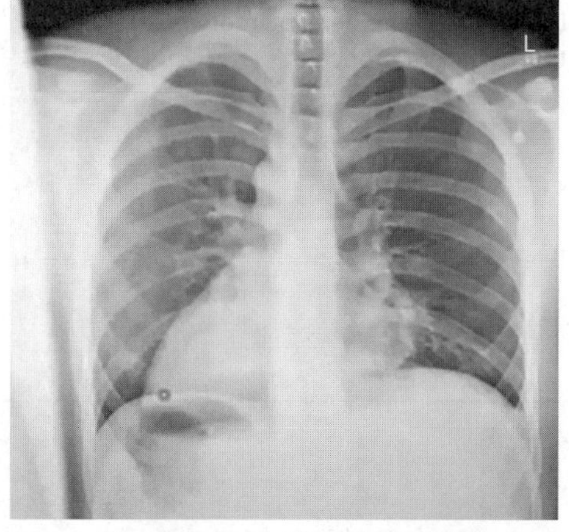

Situs inversus with dextrocardia

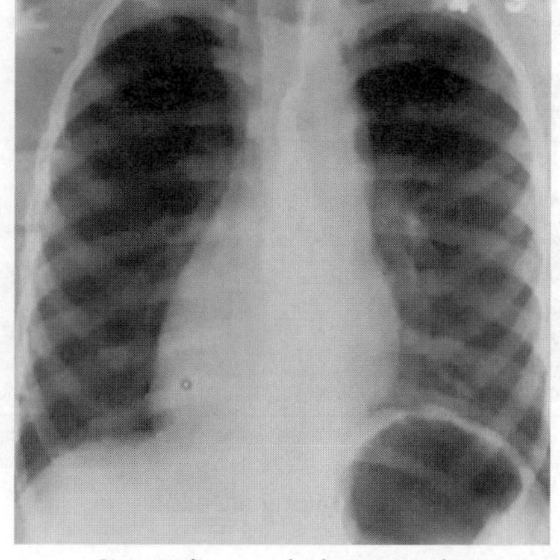

Situs solitus with dextrocardia

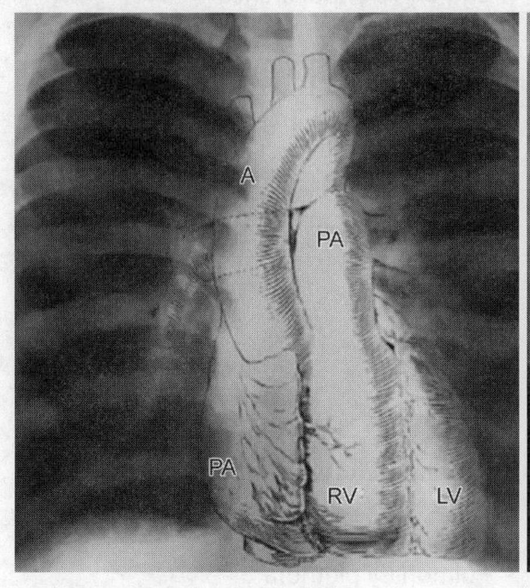

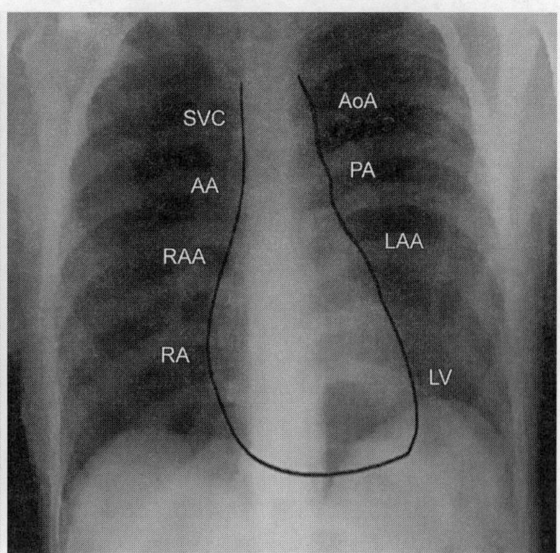

Shape and Size of Chambers

Right heart border	**Superior vena cava (SVC)** • Ascending aorta (AA) • Right atrial appendage (RAA) • Right atrium (RA)
Left heart border	• Aortic arch (AoA) • Main pulmonary artery (PA) • Left atrial appendage (LAA) • Left ventricle (LV)

■ SPECIFIC X-RAY FINDINGS IN FEW CONGENITAL HEART LESIONS

Specific heart lesion	*X-ray finding*
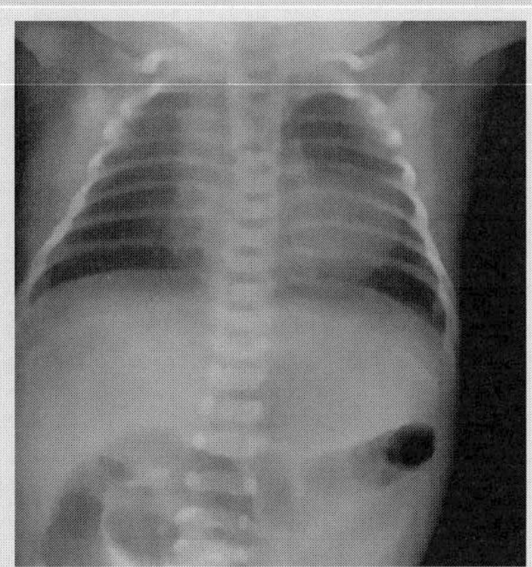 Tetralogy of Fallot	**Tetralogy of Fallot** • Cœur en sabot (boot shaped) heart • Pulmonary oligemia • RV hypertrophy • Small pedicle

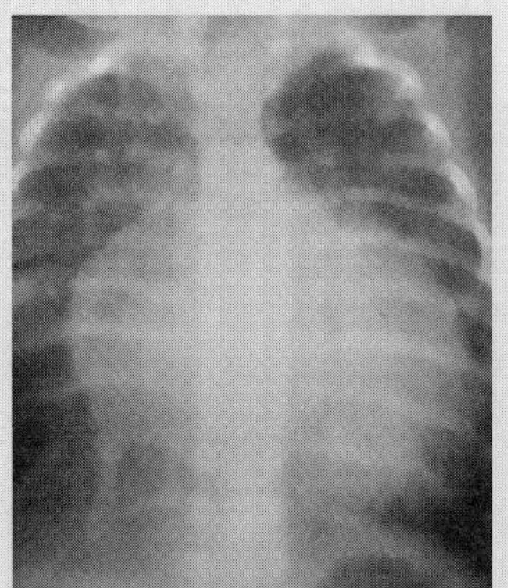

Transposition of great arteries

Transposition of great arteries
- Egg on side appearance
- Narrow pedicle
- Pulmonary plethora

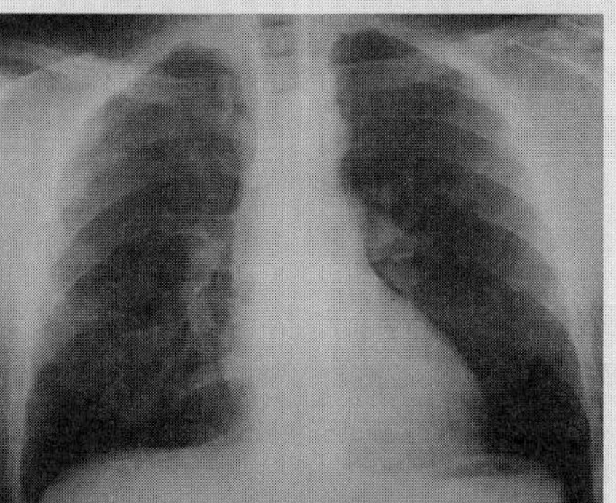

Coarctation of aorta

Total anomalous pulmonary venous connection (supracardiac)
- Snowman appearance
- Pulmonary plethora

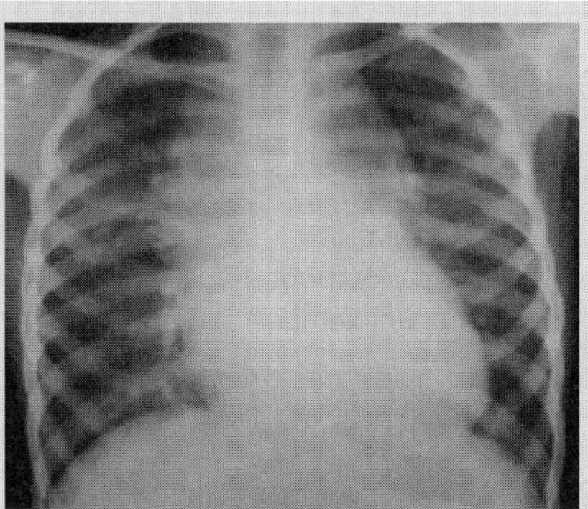

Total anomalous pulmonary venous connection (supracardiac)

Coarctation of aorta
- Reverse 3 sign
- Inferior rib border notching

Checklist for the Interpretation of the Chest X-ray (RIPES)			
1.	Rotation of film (R)	*Yes*	*No*
2.	Inspiratory versus expiratory film (I)		
3.	Projection—AP versus PA view (P)		
4.	Exposure of film (E)		
5.	Soft tissues/bones (S)		
6.	Lung expansion bilateral and parenchyma		
7.	Diaphragm		
8.	Cardiac size, shape, and position		
9.	Ribs		
10.	Extralines and tubes		

Management of Follow-up of a High-risk Neonate

Murugesan A

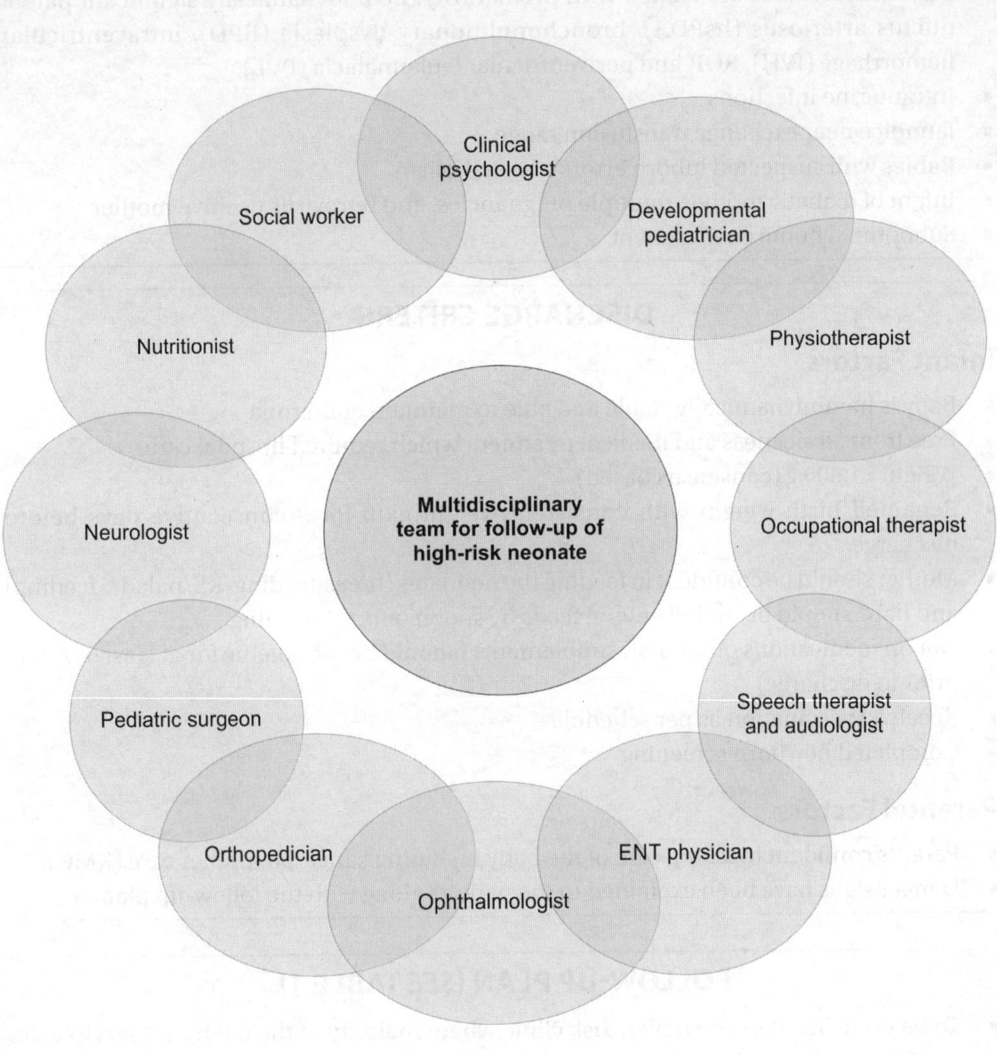

FOLLOW-UP OF A HIGH-RISK NEONATE

- Preterm <34 weeks, birth weight <1,800 g
- Severe IUGR (<3rd centile) and large for gestational age (LGA) (>97th centile)
- Major malformations
- Abnormal neurological examination at discharge
- *Turbulent NICU course:* Perinatal asphyxia [Apgar <3 at 5 minutes, Hypoxic ischemic encephalopathy (HIE) stage 2, or more], shock, sepsis, meningitis, mechanical ventilation for 24 hours or more, hypoglycemia, seizures, necrotizing enterocolitis (NEC), cholestasis, etc.
- Major morbidities associated with prematurity: hemodynamically significant patent ductus arteriosus (hsPDA), bronchopulmonary dysplasia (BPD), intraventricular hemorrhage (IVH), ROP, and periventricular leukomalacia (PVL)
- Intrauterine infections
- Jaundice near exchange transfusion range
- Babies with suspected inborn errors of metabolism
- Infant of diabetic mother, multiple pregnancies, and retrovirus positive mother
- Suboptimal home environment

DISCHARGE CRITERIA

Infant Factors

- Baby is hemodynamically stable and able to maintain euthermia
- Free from all sickness and medical treatment which required hospital care.
- Weight >1,500 g (consensus based)
- Regained birth weight with consistent weight gain for 3 consecutive days before discharge.
- Mother should be confident in feeding the neonates (breastfeeding/KS/paladai feeding) and baby should be on full enteral feeds by spoon or breastfeeding.
- Not on medications other than supplements (should be off caffeine for at least 5–7 days prior to discharge)
- Received vaccination as per schedule
- Completed newborn screening

Parental Factors

- Parents confident in taking care of the baby including kangaroo mother care (KMC).
- Danger signs have been explained to the parents along with the follow-up plan.

FOLLOW-UP PLAN (*SEE* TABLE 1)

- To be done in a dedicated high-risk clinic where majority of the follow-up services are available under single roof under the primary care of neonatologist/pediatrician.
- Should be done until a minimum of 2 years corrected age and ideally till 8 years of age.

- Use corrected age for assessing growth and development, and postnatal age for vaccination and establishing complementary feeding.
- High risk follow-up team

Follow-up schedule: 48 hours after discharge, 2 weeks after discharge, at 6, 10, and 14 weeks, 3, 6, 9, 12, 15, 18, and 24 months

TABLE 1: Follow-up plan

S. No.	Intervention	Frequency	Details
A	Anthropometry	Every visit	Intergrowth postnatal follow-up charts till 64 weeks postmenstrual age (PMA) followed by WHO charts after 64 weeks
B	Breastfeeding	Every visit	Address breastfeeding problems
C	Counseling	Every visit	• Hygiene • Feeding • KMC • Ongoing issues
D	Developmental screening and neuro-logical examination	Every visit	• Trivandrum developmental screening chart • DDST-II • BSID
E	Eye	• ROP screen as per RBSK • 4 weeks postnatal age (at 3 weeks if <28 weeks and/or <1,200 g) and repeat as required based on stage of ROP until 44 weeks PMA • Evaluation for fixation at 3 months and refractive errors and visual acuity at 9 months	Formal visual assessment at 9–12 months
F	Follow-up USG	At discharge/36 weeks PMA	To look for PVL and other abnormalities
G	Growth monitoring	Every visit	
H	Hearing	BERA at 34 weeks PMA	If normal, screen at 9 and 18–24 months, or if there is parental concern of hearing problems
I	Immunization	6, 10, 14 weeks, 9 months, 15–18 months, and 24 months	As per UIP
L	• Language/speech • Behavior at/after IQ testing	• 1, 2, and 3 years • 1 and 3 years	Any delay detected should prompt early intervention

> ## Key Points to Remember
>
> - Improvement in maternal and neonatal care has led to increased survival of babies at risk of long-term morbidities which include growth failure, ongoing medical illness, and long-term neurodevelopmental sequelae (motor, cognitive, and sensorineural impairment).
> - Comprehensive discharge and follow-up program are required for early detection and management of these morbidities.
> - Discharge planning should begin well in advance before the discharge. Caregivers should be explained about routine care of the baby at home.

OSCE/Checklist: Items in the discharge summary.

S.No.	Parameter	Details	Yes	No
1.	Morbidity	Details of important morbidities in chronological order, e.g., hyaline membrane disease (HMD), Sepsis, Asphyxia, meconium aspiration syndrome (MAS), etc.		
2.	Treatment during NICU stay	Oxygen, antibiotics, anticonvulsants, inotropes, prolonged tube feeding, etc.		
3.	Anthropometry	Weight, length, and occipital frontal circumference (OFC) at birth and discharge		
4.	Special consultation if any	For example, endocrine, genetics, pulmonologist, pediatric cardiologist pediatric surgeon, etc.		
5.	Neurological examination	Mention abnormality in tone, posture, reflexes, movements, orientation, and behavior		
6.	Retinopathy of prematurity (ROP) screening as per RBSK	Mention previous reports and date of next screen		
7.	Hearing screen	Results at time of discharge and date of next screen		
8.	Neuroimaging if required	USG, CT, and/or MRI: mention earlier reports along with date of next screen		
9.	Nutrition counseling	Along with quality, quantity, and the supplements		
10.	Counseling regarding temperature maintenance	(Including KMC) along with hand hygiene		
11.	Immunization	Mention date of next immunization visit		
12.	Explain danger signs	As per Integrated Management of Newborn and Childhood Illness (IMNCI)		
13.	Next follow-up	Date, time, and place		

■ FURTHER READING

1. Facility based newborn care: Training module for doctors and nurses. MoHFW, GoI; 2022.

Chapter 75

Growth Charts

Sidharth Nayyar

GROWTH AND GROWTH CHARTS

- *Growth* is defined as an increase in mass or size of the bodily tissues. Rapid growth occurs by five to six times between 24 through 40 weeks gestation and is influenced by maternal, placental, and fetal factors. Postnatal growth depends on genetic potential, internal, and external factors.
- A growth chart is graphic representation of growth of reference population for daily clinical use.
- It comprises growth representations by curves displaying the size of child at a certain age and his/her rate of growth over time.

Importance of Growth Monitoring

- It helps to locate any deviation of physical growth from the normal trajectory.
- It helps in the early identification of neonates at an increased risk of neurodevelopmental impairment.

History

- Count Philibert de Montbeillard, a French, developed first growth chart in the 18th century.
- Centiles were first used by Henry Bowditch in 1891.
- The first intrauterine growth chart to be widely used in neonates was the Lubchenco's chart which also classified newborn's size at birth.

Types

Growth references versus growth standards:

Growth references	Growth standards
• A statistically derived summary of anthropometry in a specific group of children taken as a reference, but their health status is not considered • Descriptive	• A statistically derived summary of anthropometry in a reference population whose health status is taken into consideration • Prescriptive represents a normal healthy growth pattern

Contd...

Contd...

Growth references	Growth standards

• Shows how the children actually grow rather than showing the ideal growth pattern
• Data is cross sectional
• Has a large sample size
• *Examples:*
  – Intrauterine growth charts
  – Postnatal growth charts
  – Fetal–infant growth charts
	• Shows how a child should ideally grow
	• Based on prospective and longitudinal monitoring of growth so difficult to acquire large sample size
	• *Examples:*
	  – WHO–Multicenter Growth Reference Study (MGRS) charts
	  – INTERGROWTH–21st

GROWTH REFERENCES

Intrauterine Growth Charts

- Data is derived from anthropometry of neonates at different gestational ages at birth
- Small sample size
- Cross-sectional and nongender specific
- Most importantly, a preterm baby is different from a fetus which might cause a bias in anthropometric measurements
- Examples are Lubchenco (1966), Usher and McLean (1969), Brenner (1976), Kramer (2001), etc.

Lubchenco Charts (1948–1961) (Fig. 1)

- Included a data of 4,700 newborns between 26 and 42 weeks gestation.
- This was a multicentric retrospective study which provided weight, length, and head circumference (HC).
- First described small-for-gestational-age/appropriate for gestational age/large for gestational age (SGA/AGA/LGA).

Benefits	Drawbacks
• Used ponderal index, a new parameter • Better accepted than previous models • Helps to identify unusual intrauterine growth patterns • Forms a basis for future research	• Intrauterine growth is depicted in terms of length, HC, weight, and weight-length ratio. These are an approximate depiction of the pattern of fetal growth with advancing gestational age • Data obtained from single country and of high altitude

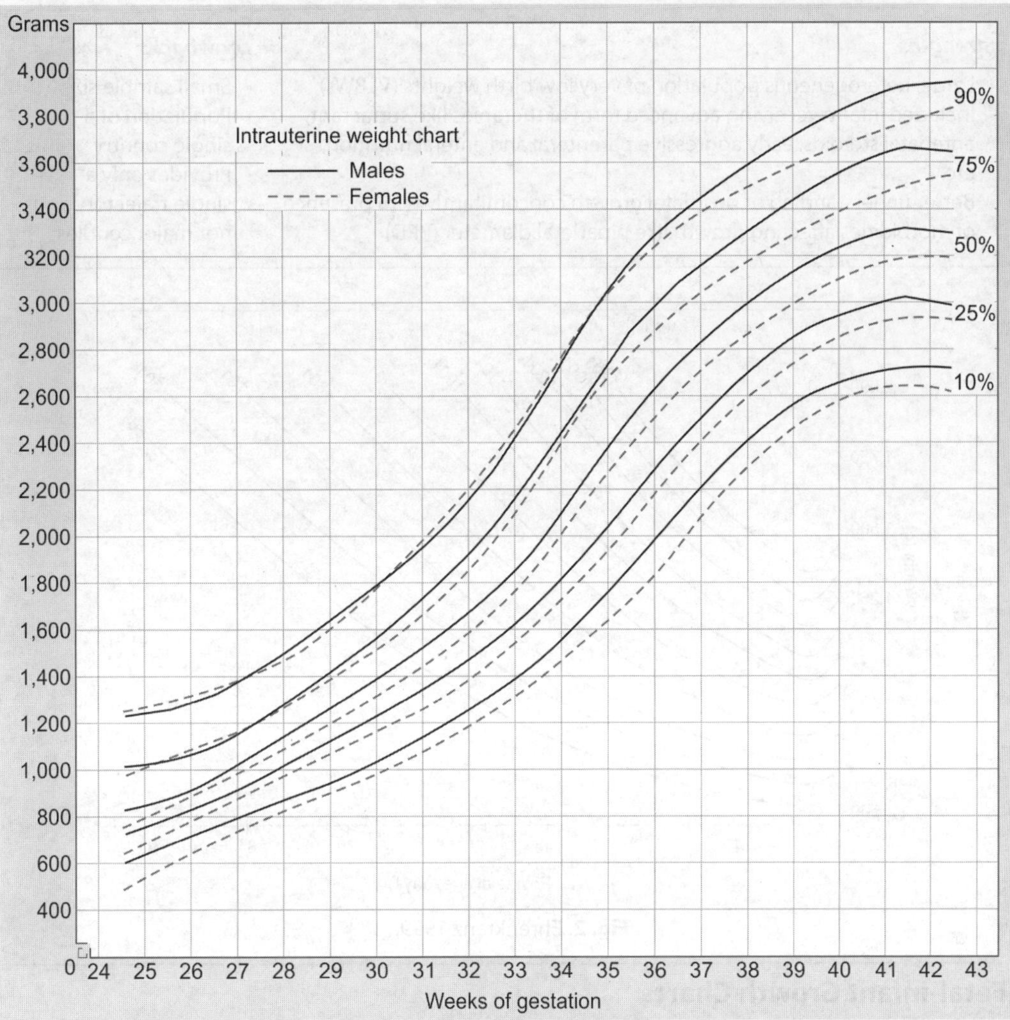

Fig. 1: Lubchenco charts.

Postnatal Growth Charts

- Longitudinal measurement parameters of infants are followed.
- Provides real world pattern of infant's postnatal growth (including postnatal weight loss).
- Examples include Dancis 1948, Wright 1993, and Ehrenkranz 1999.

Ehrenkranz 1999 (Fig. 2)

Multicentric prospective longitudinal Cohort study.

- 1,660 infants in 12 US centers with birth weight 500–1,500 g admitted ≤24 hours of age were included.
- Weight, length, HC, and mid-upper arm circumference (MUAC) were measured from birth onward till discharge or transfer or death till the age of 120 days, or a weight of 2 kg.

Strengths	Drawbacks
• Large, heterogeneous population of very low birth weights (VLBWs) • Included infants receiving advanced form of therapies like surfactant, antenatal steroids, early aggressive parenteral and enteral nutrition, etc. • Better understanding of postnatal growth concomitantly with presence of morbidities affecting growth like biparietal diameter (BPD)	• Small sample size • Population of a single country • Provides only a single trajectory and not major centiles

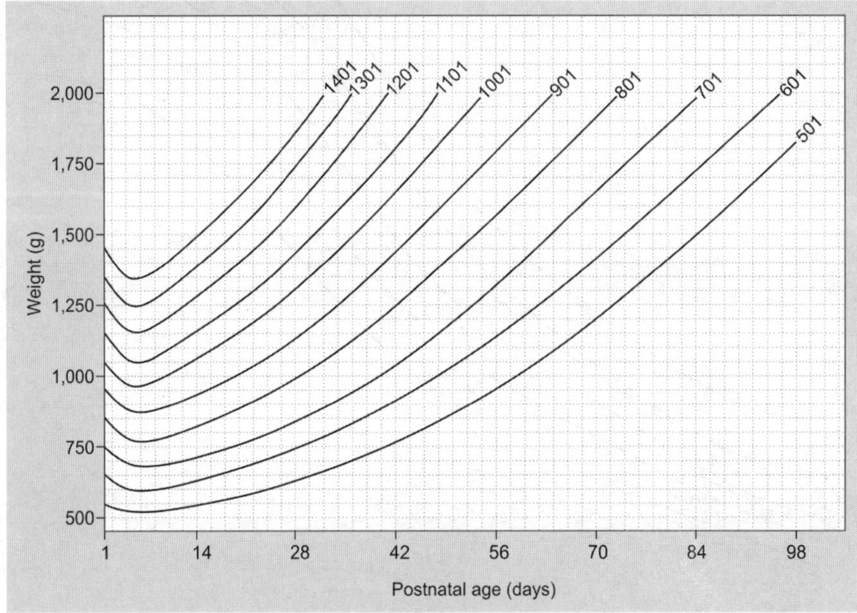

Fig. 2: Ehrenkranz 1999.

Fetal-infant Growth Charts

- Two reference data sets are merged to construct these charts. These include anthropometric *cross-sectional data* and *postnatal longitudinal data* of preterm infants at birth and term infants postnatally, respectively.
- Permits comparison of growth with fetus followed by term anthropometry standards.
- Advantage is assessment of catch up growth.
- Examples, Babson and Benda charts 1967, Fenton chart 2003 and 2013.

Babson and Benda Chart

Includes Mean ± SDs for weight at birth, length, and HC from 26 weeks to 1 year of postnatal age.

	Limitations:
• Data from mostly Caucasian infants from 1959 through 1966 • 39,743 infants from 27 to 44 weeks were included	• X axis starts at 26 weeks postmenstrual age (PMA) • Y axis depicts 500 g interval increments which make exact plotting tricky • Limited sample size

Fenton 2003 (Fig. 3)

Updated Babson–Benda charts which included gestational ages between 22 through 50 weeks PMA.

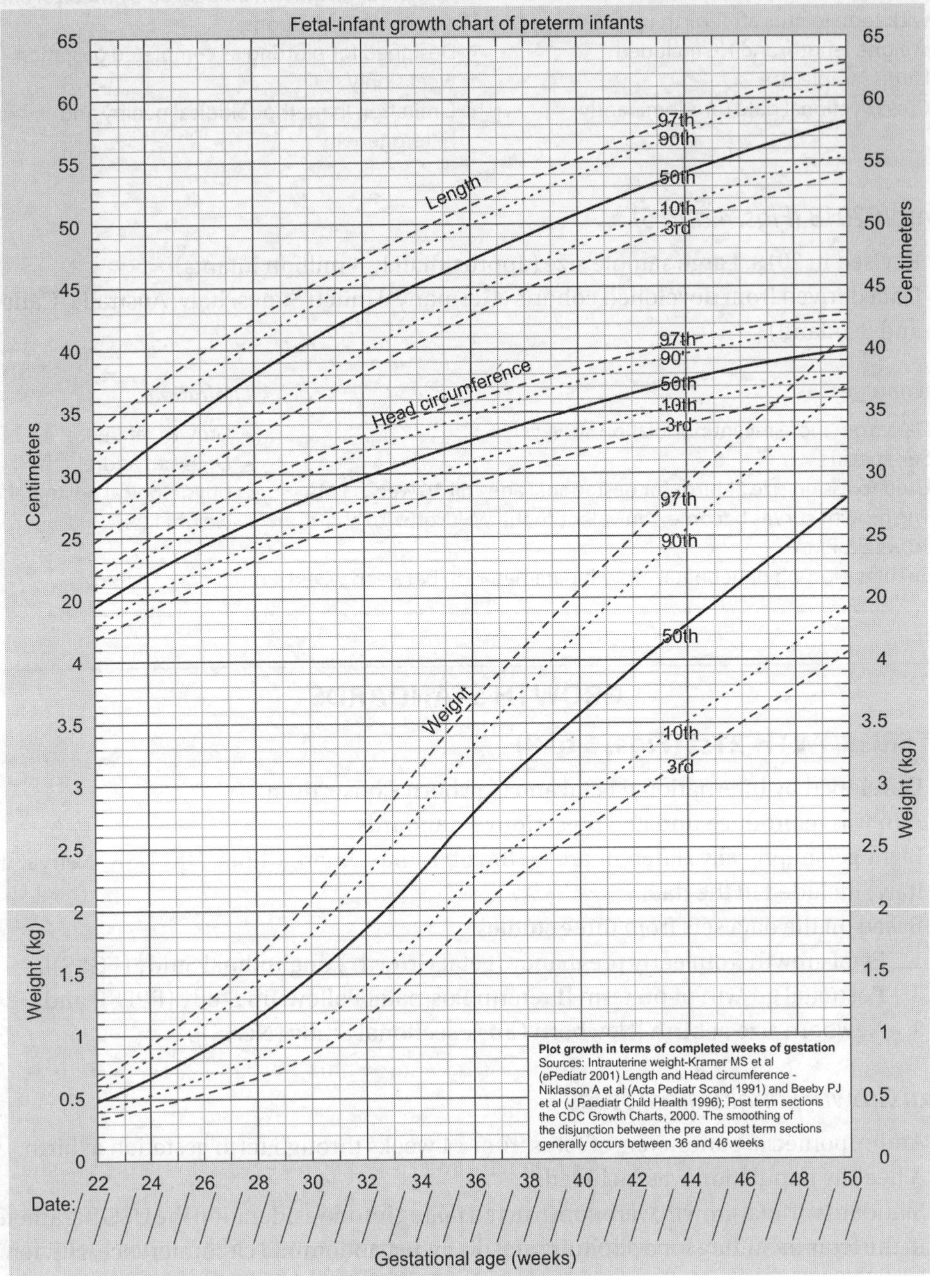

Fig. 3: Fenton 2003.

Advantages	Limitations
• Growth of a preterm infant is compared with that of fetus starting at 22 weeks PMA which is followed till 36 weeks PMA and then later with term infants after birth up to 50 weeks • Weight, length, and HC included • Large sample size • Cross-sectional data (predominantly)	• Not sex specific and change in weight pattern not represented • Longitudinal growth influenced by medical and nutritional conditions • Designed for plotting as completed gestation weeks only • Limitation in methodological quality and heterogeneity

Fenton 2013 (Figs. 4 and 5)

- Revised in 2013. Large sample size (approximately 4 million infants).
- Data derived from developed cohorts (Germany, United States, Italy, Australia, Canada, and Scotland).

Advantages	Limitations
• Data from more recent population surveys • Sex specific • Used to assign size at birth for gestational ages till 36 weeks PMA • The growth curves become equivalent to the WHO growth charts at 50 weeks PMA • Enables plotting of neonatal growth parameters in between weeks	• Growth reference • Does not address the physiological postnatal weight loss

GROWTH STANDARDS

INTERGROWTH 21st (Figs. 6 to 9)

- Developed by International Fetal and Newborn Consortium.
- Aim was to produce updated prescriptive standards.
- Eight geographically different areas (Brazil, India, Oman, China, UK, USA, Kenya, and Italy) included in the data.
- Based on the data sets from three studies.
  1. Fetal growth from early pregnancy [Fetal Growth Longitudinal Study (FGLS)],
  2. Postnatal growth of preterm [Preterm Postnatal Follow-up Study (PPFS)] and
  3. Newborn size at birth [Newborn Cross-sectional Study (NCSS)].

Fetal Growth Longitudinal Study

- Anthropometric parameters of fetus from 14 weeks through term gestation at birth.
- A healthy population was included.
- Standards of fetal growth were constructed taking into consideration the USG parameters in the fetus including for occipitofrontal diameter, abdominal circumference, HC, femur length, and biparietal diameter.
- Both LMP and USG were used to ascertain the gestation age.

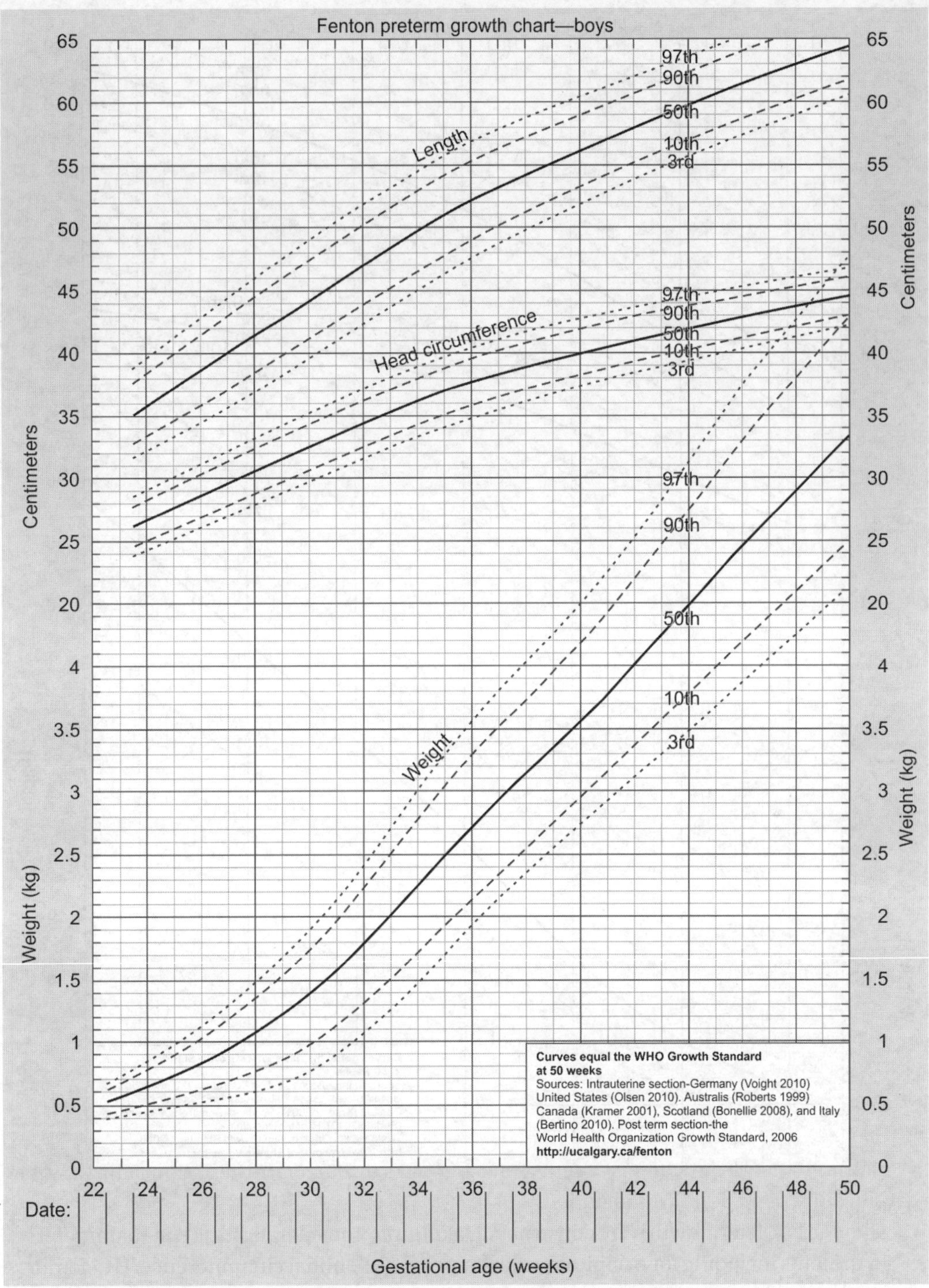

Fig. 4: Fenton 2013 boys.

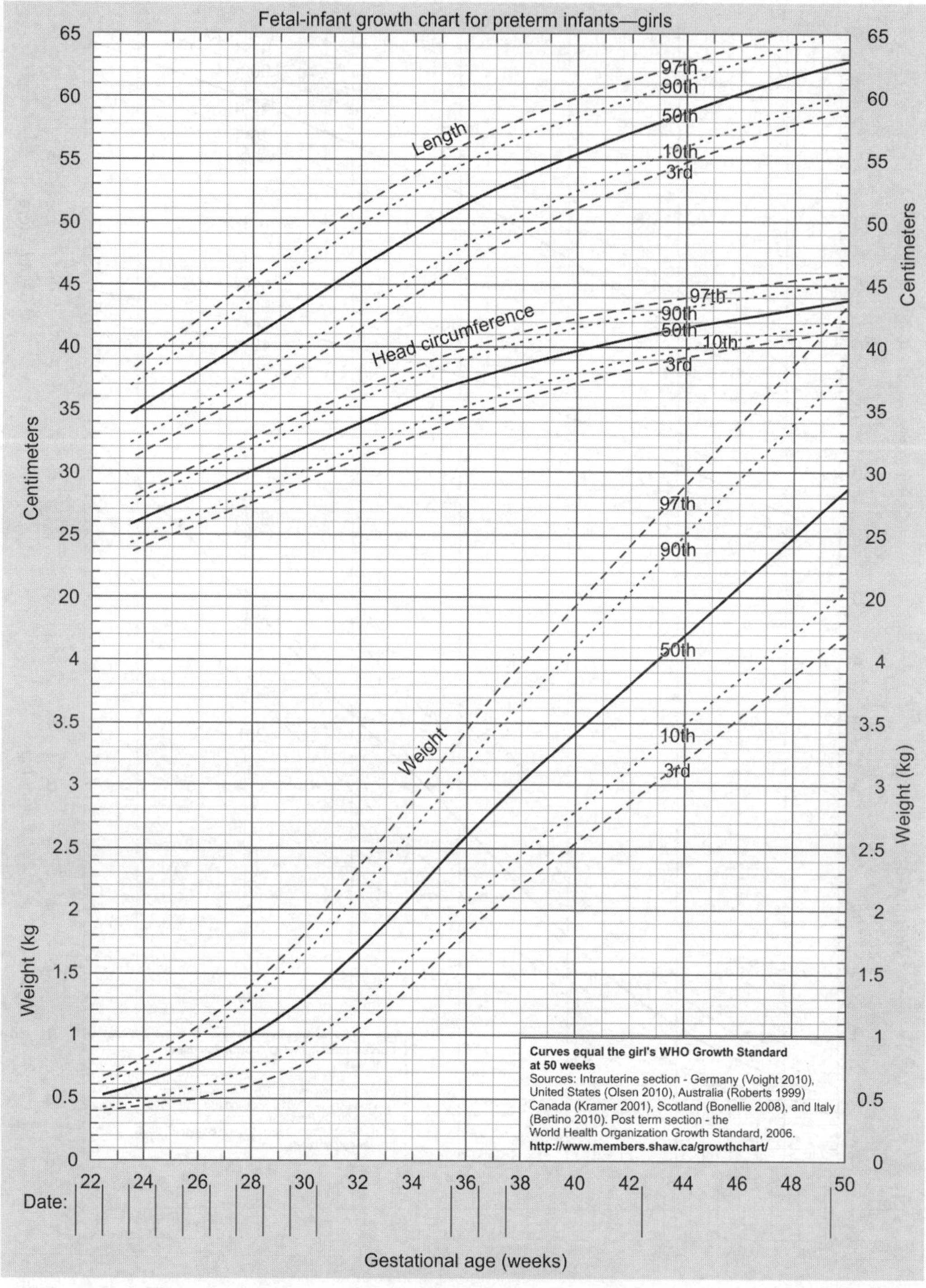

Fig. 5: Fenton 2013 girls.

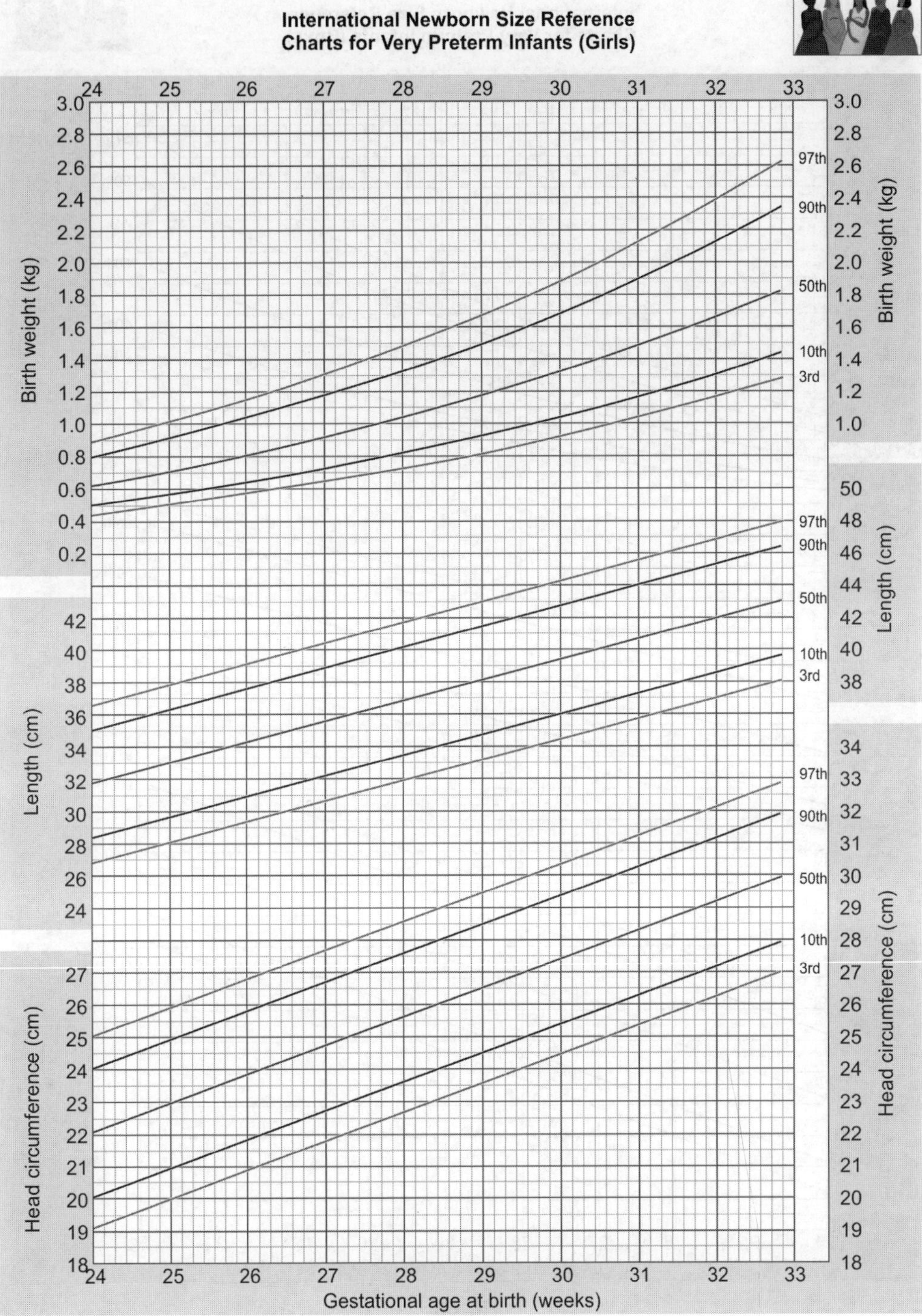

INTERGROWTH-21st
International Newborn Size Reference
Charts for Very Preterm Infants (Girls)
Birth weight (kg)
Birth weight (kg)
Length (cm)
Length (cm)
Head circumference (cm)
Head circumference (cm)
Gestational age at birth (weeks)
97th
90th
50th
10th
3rd

Fig. 6A

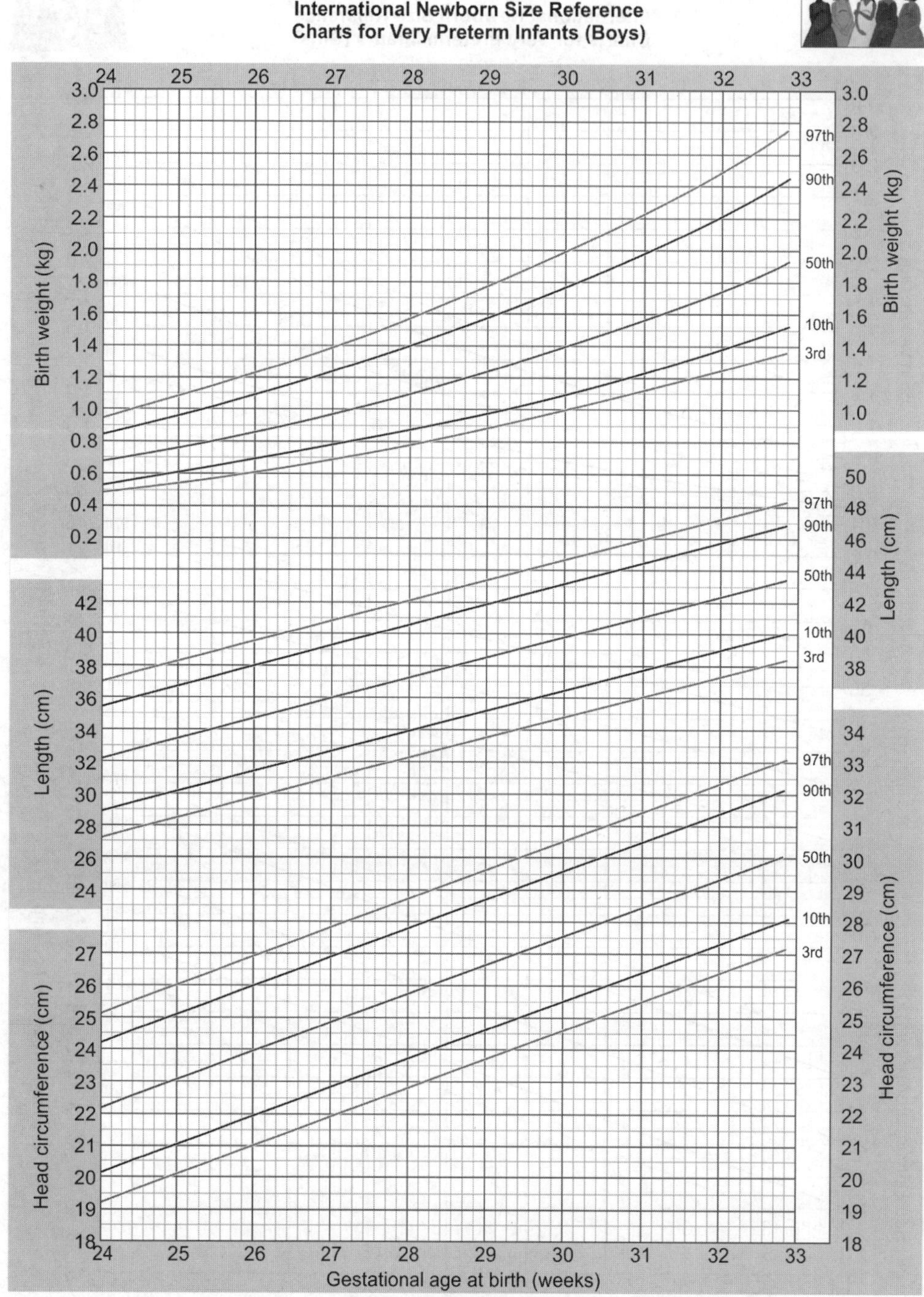

Fig. 6B

Figs. 6A and B: Growth references INTERGROWTH 21st for very preterm.

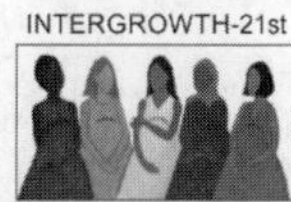

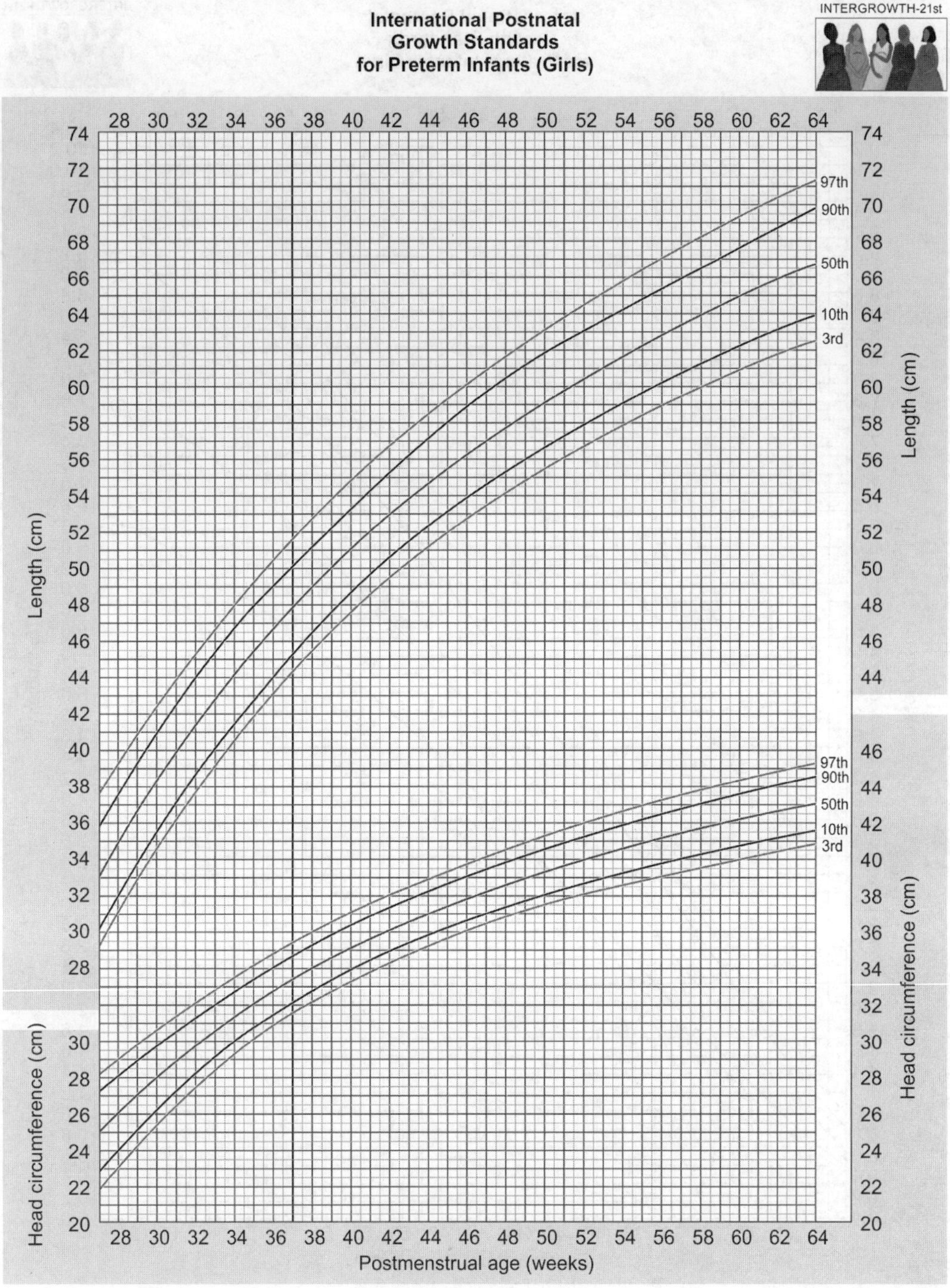
International Postnatal
Growth Standards
for Preterm Infants (Girls)
INTERGROWTH-21st
Length (cm)
Head circumference (cm)
Postmenstrual age (weeks)
97th
90th
50th
10th
3rd
97th
90th
50th
10th
3rd
28 30 32 34 36 38 40 42 44 46 48 50 52 54 56 58 60 62 64
74 72 70 68 66 64 62 60 58 56 54 52 50 48 46 44 42 40 38 36 34 32 30 28
46 44 42 40 38 36 34 32 30 28 26 24 22 20

Fig. 7A

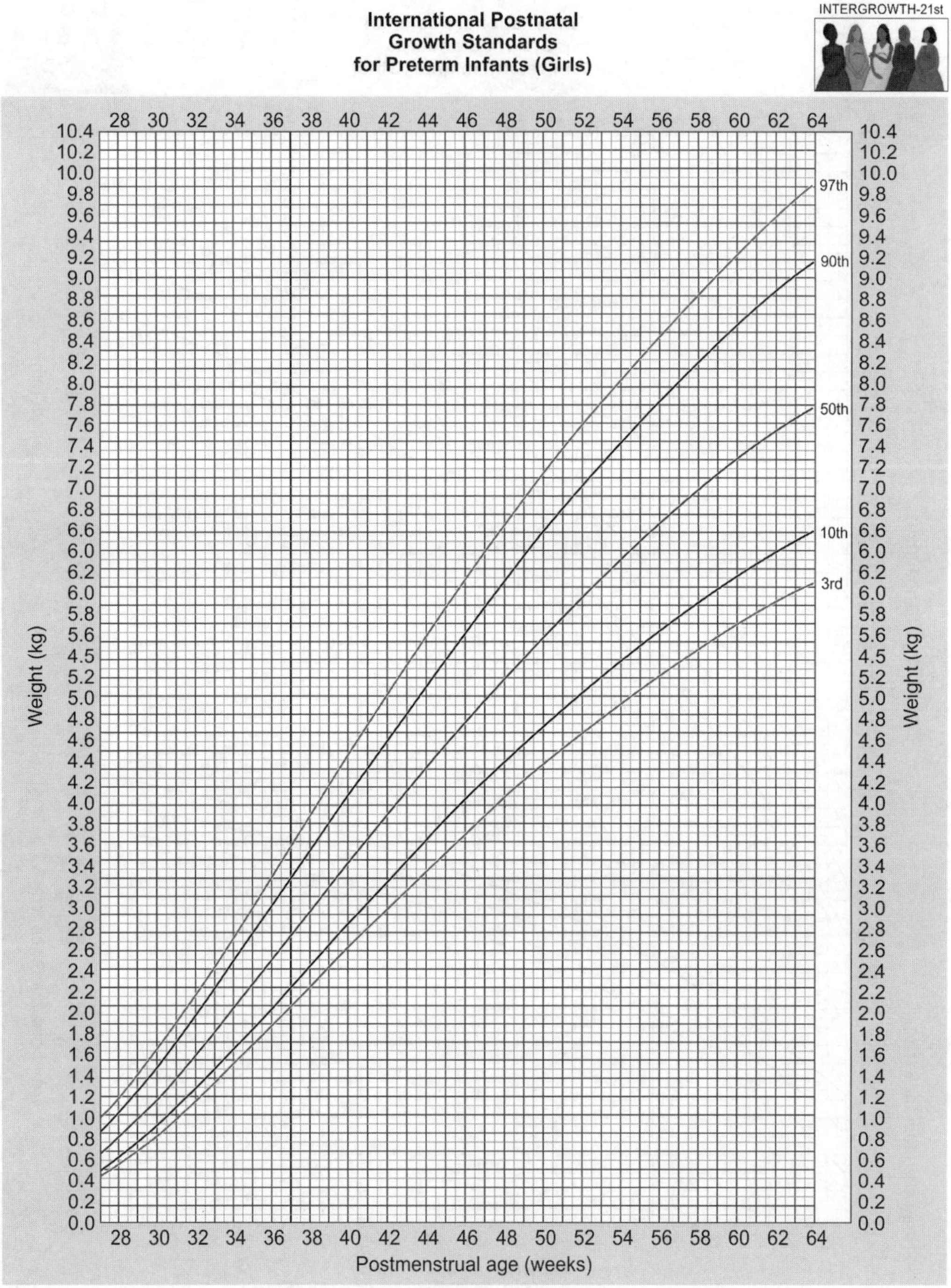

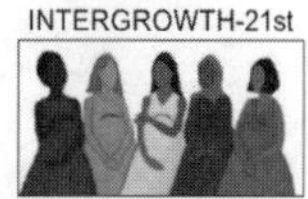

Fig. 7B

Figs. 7A and B: INTERGROWTH 21st postnatal growth standards for preterms (girls).

**International Postnatal
Growth Standards
for Preterm Infants (Boys)**

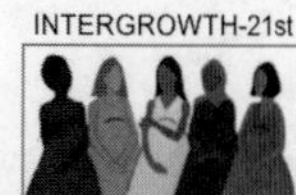

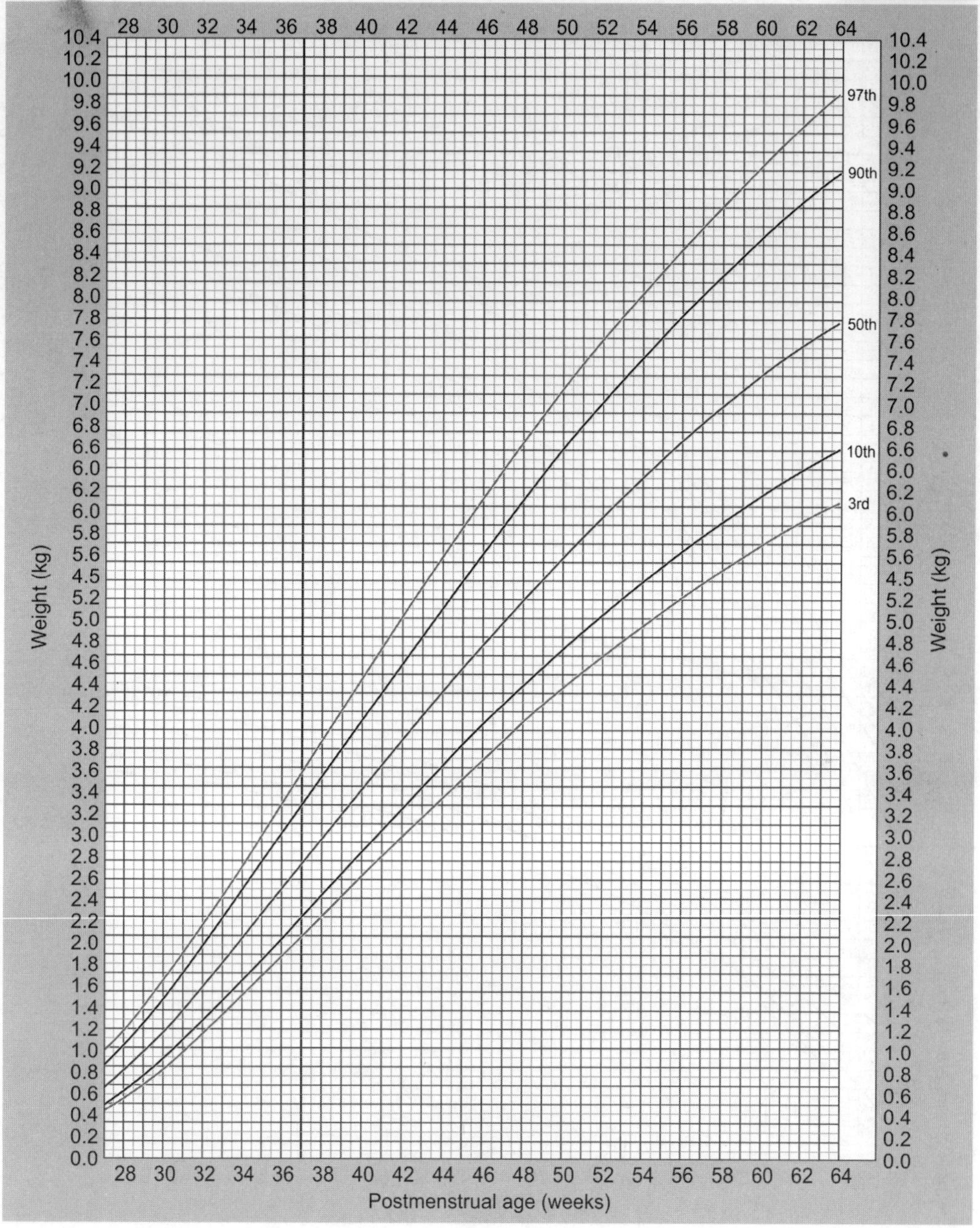

Fig. 8A

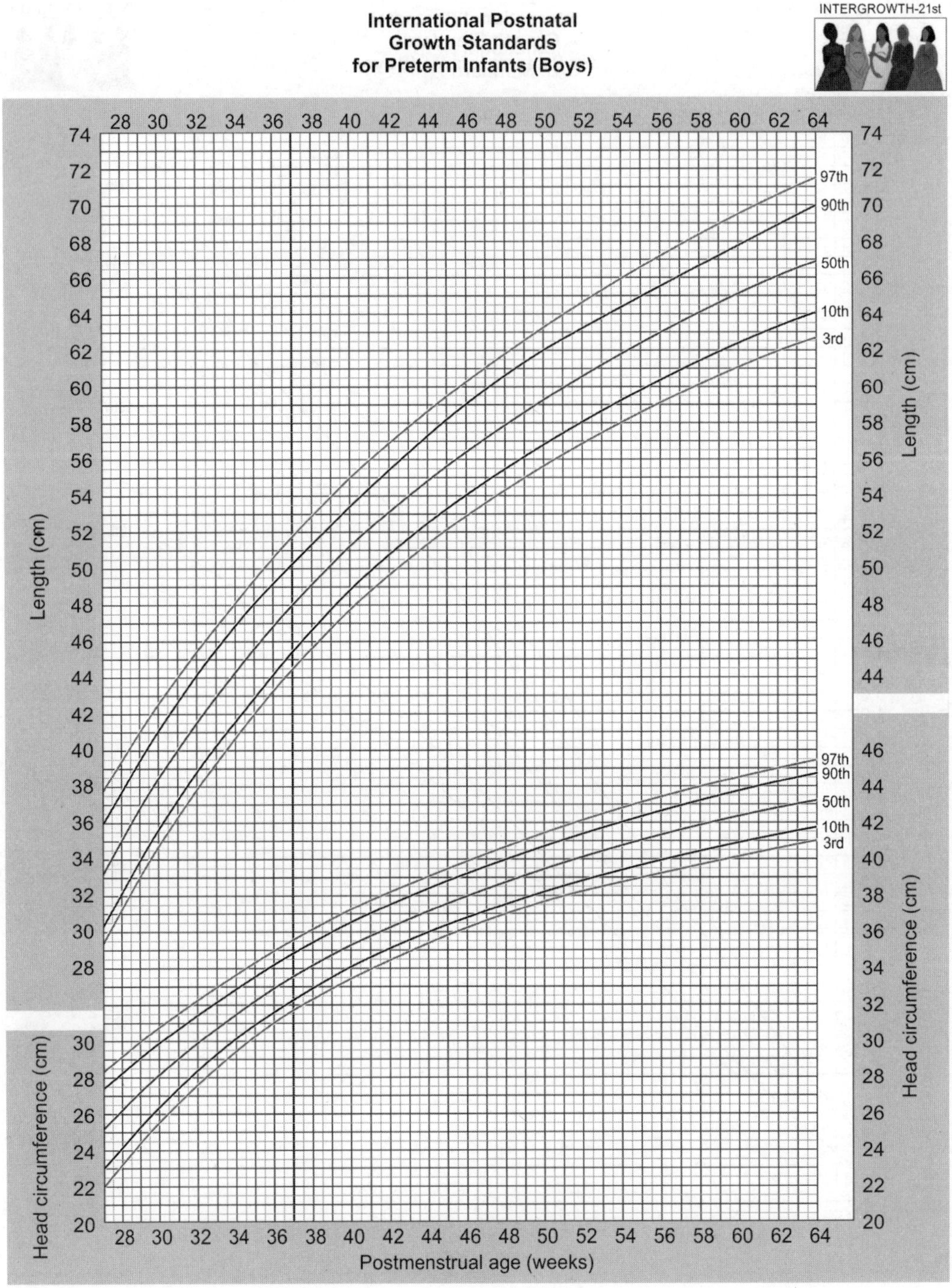

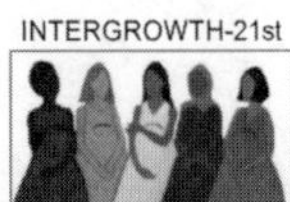

Fig. 8B

Figs. 8A and B: INTERGROWTH 21st postnatal growth standards for preterms (boys).

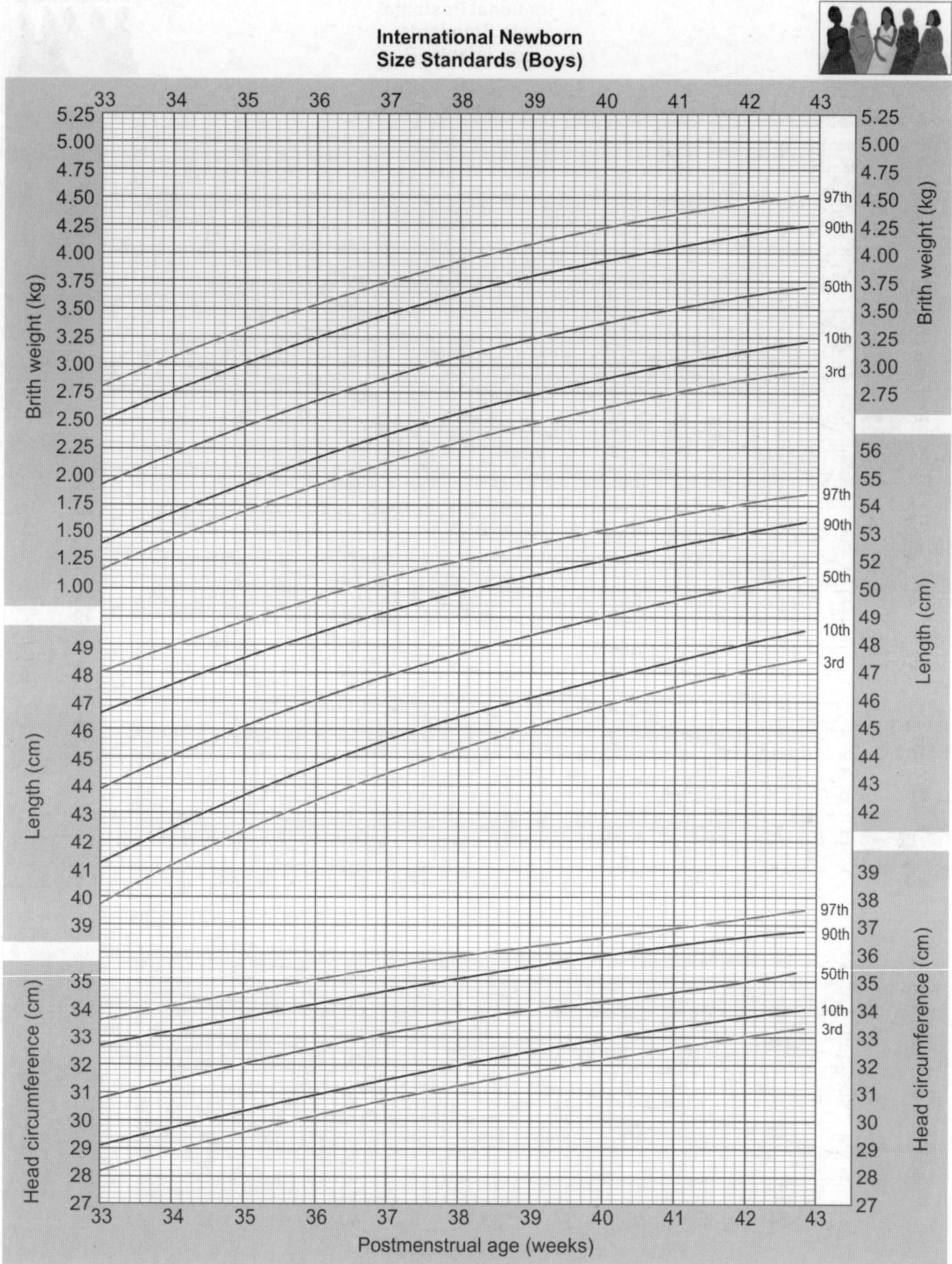

Fig. 9A

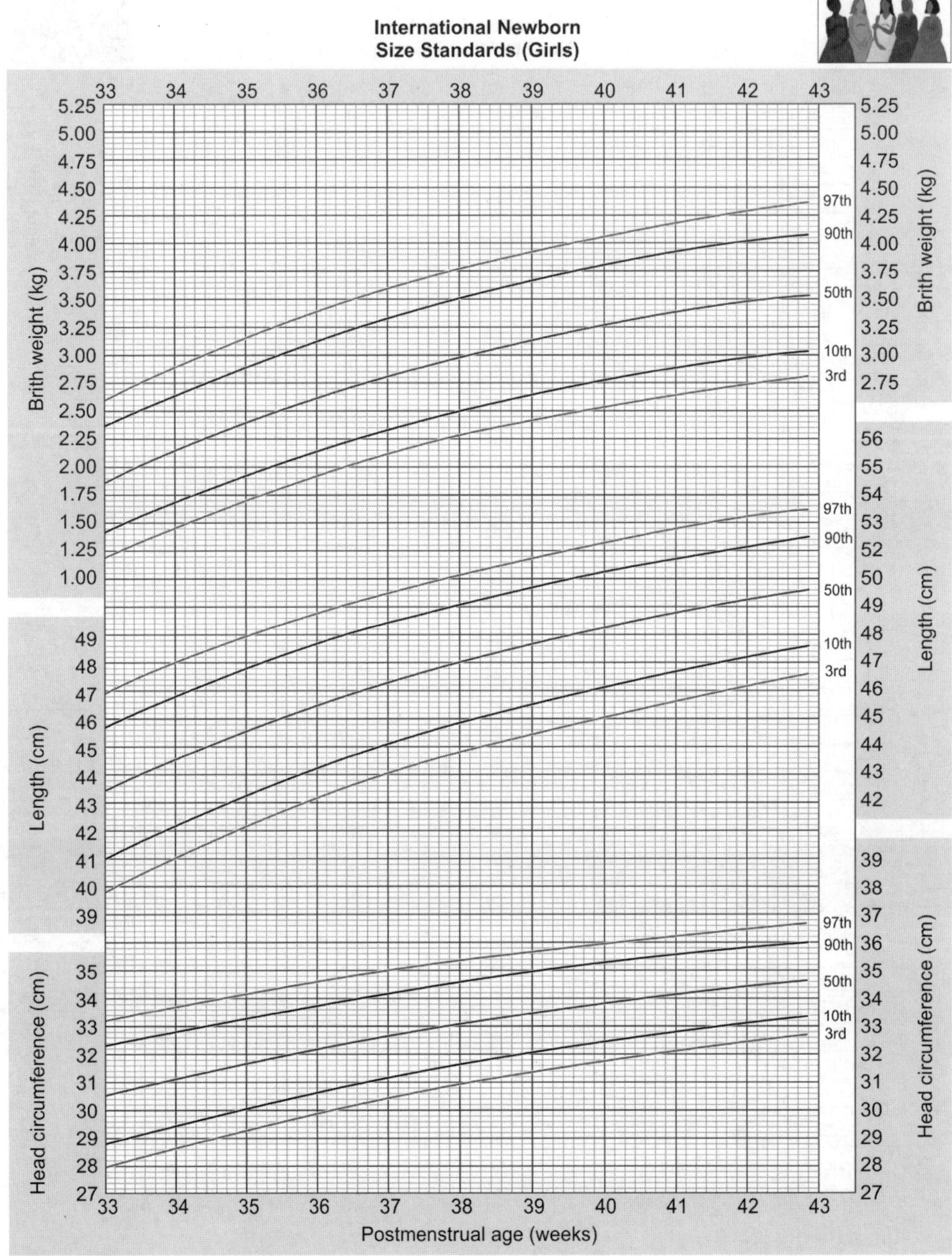

Fig. 9B

Figs. 9A and B: INTERGROWTH 21st growth standards for newborn size at birth.

Preterm Postnatal Follow-up Study

- Preterm newborns of ≥26 weeks <37 weeks followed postnatally.
- 201 preterm newborns who were eligible were included from FGLS (healthy or stable preterm).
- Followed till 64 weeks PMA.
- Growth standards for postnatal growth preterm neonates for length, HC, and weight were plotted.

Newborn Cross-sectional Study

- More than 20,000 women who were found to be eligible were enrolled.
- Study period—May 2009 and August 2013.
- Anthropometric parameters of newborn infants whose mothers were enlisted in the FGLS database were recorded.
- Centile curves were obtained according to sex and the gestational age.
- These growth standards are prescriptive international anthropometry charts to assess size of the newborn from 33 through 43 weeks gestational age.

Advantages	Disadvantages
<ul><li>Prospective study</li><li>Growth monitoring can be done continuously from early prenatal life till 5 years of age</li><li>Multiethnic, multicountry, population based, and sex-specific charts.</li></ul>	<ul><li>These charts include very few early preterms <33 weeks for the PPFS database.</li><li>The lower limit of the growth curves in the NCSS database was set at 33 weeks PMA, because it was impossible to freely enroll preterms less than this gestational age with very rigid criteria.</li><li>Hence, the growth charts available for preterms <33 weeks are still growth references</li></ul>

WHO Multicenter Growth Reference Study 2006

- Based on 1997–2003 data from the WHO MGRS.
- *India* along with six other countries from different continents was represented in this study.
- Good socioeconomic status and term gestation were the inclusion criteria.
- Growth curves for children younger than 24 months were adapted from the MGRS (longitudinal component).
- The growth curves from 24 through 59 months age were based on the cross-sectional database of MGRS.
- 125 countries use these growth standards.

Drawback

The current WHO charts do not have any representation for preterm neonates.

Fenton 2103 Versus INTERGROWTH 21st

Evidence demonstrated that incidence of EUGR is less, if we plot on Intergrowth.

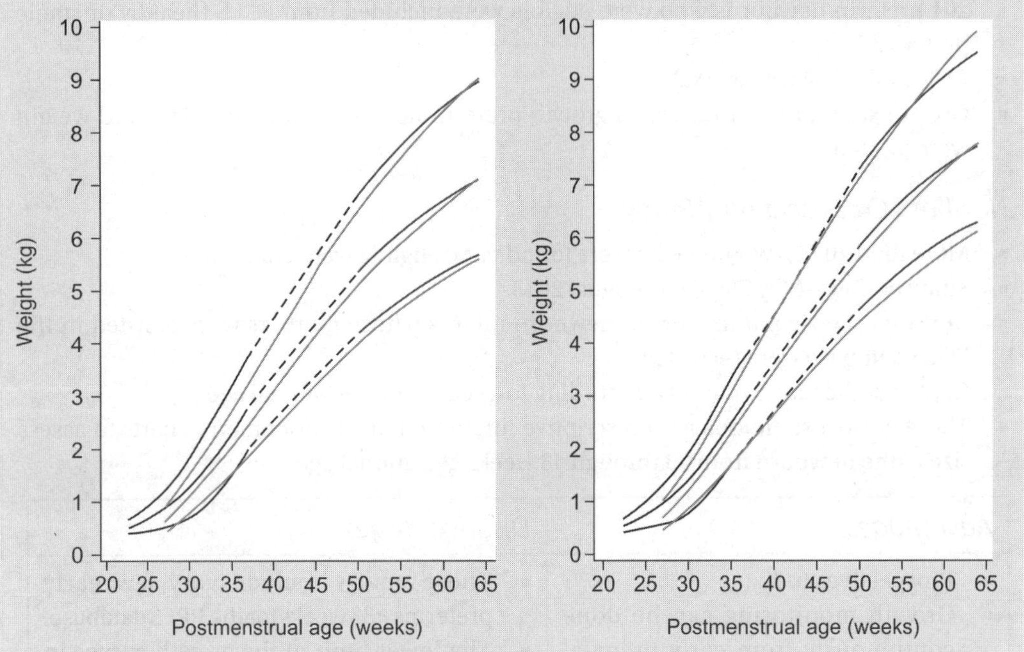

Comparison of growth centiles of the INTERGROWTH-21st with the Fenton size at birth.

Key Points to Remember

- Longitudinal growth cannot be assessed by intrauterine growth charts.
- Ehrenkranz postnatal growth charts monitor longitudinal growth but are unable to provide gestation specific patterns.
- INTERGROWTH-21st postnatal growth standards are the recommended charts for gestational ages ≥33 weeks.
- Fenton charts 2013 lack prescriptive benefits, they include data from approximately 4 million preterm infants, precise sex-specific plotting and smooth transition to WHO MGRS 2006 growth standards.
- For term infants, WHO MGRS 2006 growth charts should be used.

■ FURTHER READING

1. Babson SG, Benda GI. Growth graphs for the clinical assessment of infants of varying gestational age. J Pediatr. 1976;89(5):814-20.
2. Cole TJ. The development of growth references and growth charts. Ann Hum Biol. 2012;39(5):382-94.
3. Ehrenkranz RA, Dusick AM, Vohr BR, Wright LL, Wrage LA, Poole WK. Growth in the neonatal intensive care unit influences neurodevelopmental and growth outcomes of extremely low birth weight infants. Pediatrics. 2006;117(4):1253-61

4. Ehrenkranz RA, Younes N, Lemons JA, Fanaroff AA, Donovan EF, Wright LL, et al. Longitudinal growth of hospitalized very low birth weight infants. Pediatrics. 1999;104(2 Pt 1):280-9.

5. Fenton TR, Kim JH. A systematic review and meta-analysis to revise the Fenton growth chart for preterm infants. BMC Pediatr. 2013;13:59.

6. Fenton TR. A new growth chart for preterm babies: Babson and Benda's chart updated with recent data and a new format. BMC Pediatr. 2003;3:13.

7. Grummer-Strawn LM, Reinold C, Krebs NF, Centers for Disease Control and Prevention (CDC). Use of World Health Organization and CDC growth charts for children aged 0–59 months in the United States. MMWR Recommen Rep. 2010;59 (RR-9):1-15

8. Lubchenco LO, Hansman C, Dressler M, Boyd E. Intrauterine growth as estimated from liveborn birth-weight data at 24 to 42 weeks of gestation. Pediatrics. 1963;32:793-800.

9. Papageorghiou AT, Ohuma EO, Altman DG, Todros T, Ismail LC, Lambert A, et al. International standards for fetal growth based on serial ultrasound measurements: The Fetal Growth Longitudinal Study of the INTERGROWTH-21st Project. Lancet. 2014;384 (9946):869-79.

10. Shrestha S, Thakur A, Goyal S, Garg P, Kler N. Growth charts in neonates. Curr Med Res Pract. 2016;6:79-84.

11. The Preterm Postnatal Follow-up Study of the INTERGROWTH-21(st) Project. Lancet Glob Health. 2015;3(11):e681–91.

12. Tuzun F, Yucesoy E, Baysal B, Kumral A, Duman N, Ozkan H. Comparison of INTERGROWTH-21 and Fenton growth standards to assess size at birth and extrauterine growth in very preterm infants. J Mater Fetal Neonatal Med. 2018;31(17):2252-7.

13. Villar J, Giuliani F, Figueras-Aloy J, Barros F, Bertino E, Bhutta ZA, et al. Growth of preterm infants at the time of global obesity. Arch Dis Childhood. 2019;104(8):725-7.

14. Villar J, Ismail LC, Victora CG, Ohuma EO, Bertino E, Altman DG, et al. International standards for newborn weight, length, and head circumference by gestational age and sex: The Newborn Cross-Sectional Study of the INTERGROWTH-21st Project. Lancet. 2014;384(9946):857-68.

Embryology for Neonatologist

Prince Pareek, Sukena Susnerwala

■ CARDIOVASCULAR SYSTEM

- Heart develops from splanchnic layer of lateral plate mesoderm.
- Endoderm release vascular endothelial growth factor (VEGF) that stimulates lateral plate mesoderm to differentiate into angioblast (form blood vessels) and hemocytoblast (for blood cells).
- Lateral plate mesoderm grows to form two heart tubes and two pericardial cavities, which later fuse together to form single heart tube and single pericardial cavity (during lateral folding).
- Dorsal mesocardium connects pericardial cavity to the heart tube.
- Inner layer of heart tube is called endocardium, which is formed from angioblast. Outer layer is called myocardium formed from cardiac myocytes. Myocardium secretes cardiac jelly in between endocardium and myocardium.
- Blood enters the heart tube via two sinus venosus, then passes through primitive ventricle → primitive atrium → bulbus cordis → truncus arteriosus and exit through dorsal aortae.

Blood flow to the heart tube.	
Primitive form	*Give rise to*
Truncus arteriosus	Pulmonary artery and aortic arch
Bulbus cordis	Right ventricle and outflow tract
Primitive ventricle	Left ventricle
Primitive atria	Right and left atrium

- Veins draining into sinus venosus are common cardinal vein, umbilical vein, and vitelline veins.
- All veins draining into left sinus venosus disappears and right side umbilical vein also disappears.
- Right common cardinal vein gives rise to superior vena cava (SVC), right vitelline vein gives rise to inferior vena cava (IVC), and sinus venosus gives rise to coronary sinus.
- Sinus venosus produces cells that give rise to visceral pericardium and primitive conduction system.

- *Cardiac looping:*
    - Truncus arteriosus and bulbus cordis move toward down and right.
    - Primitive ventricle moves left of midline.
    - Primitive atria move backward and upward.
- *Septation:*
    - Neural crest cells give rise to anterior and posterior endocardial cushions, which fuse together to form septum intermedium that separates atria and ventricle into two atrioventricular (AV) canals.
    - Endocardial cells from septum intermedium give rise to AV valves.
    - *Interatrial septum:*
        - Septum primum grows from top of primitive atrium towards septum intermedium but it does not reach it. So, a small opening forms between septum primum and septum intermedium called ostium primum.
        - Later, septum primum grows further to reach septum intermedium but an opening develops in septum primum called ostium secundum.
        - Then, another tissue grows from top to block ostium secundum called septum secundum. But it does not block it completely, so a small space left in between the two called foramen ovale.
        - So, ultimately septum primum and septum secundum divide the primitive atria into right and left atrium.
    - *Interventricular septum:*
        - In between bulbus cordis and primitive ventricle, muscular septum starts to grow upward from the apex of the heart.
        - A tissue grows downward from septum intermedium to reach the muscular septum called the membranous part of interventricular septum.
        - These muscular and membranous septa separate bulbus cordis from primitive ventricle to form right and left ventricle.
    - *Separation of pulmonary artery and aorta:*
        - Neural crest cells form ridges in truncus arteriosus and bulbus cordis.
        - These ridges unite to form a septum that separates truncus arteriosus and bulbus cordis.
        - These septa twist to form an aorticopulmonary septum that separates pulmonary artery from aorta, where pulmonary artery is anterior to aorta.

Timeline of cardiac morphogenesis.	
19 days	Vasculogenesis in the cardiac region
20 days	Lateral embryonic folding brings heart tubes together
21 days	Heart tubes fuse to form primitive heart
22 days	Heart begins to beat
23 days	Cardiac looping begins
25 days	Ventricular septation begins
28 days	Cardiac looping complete
30 days	Atrial septation begins

Contd...

Contd...

6–7 weeks	• Septum intermedium is formed • Primitive atria divided into right and left atrium
8 weeks	• Coronary sinus is formed • Aorta and pulmonary artery separated
9–10 weeks	Semilunar valves formation complete
3 months	Atrioventricular valve formation complete

Aortic arch derivatives.	
1st arch	Maxillary artery
2nd arch	Stapedial and hyoid artery
3rd arch	Innominate artery and common and internal carotid arteries
4th arch	• Right 4th arch gives rise to the innominate and right subclavian arteries • Left 4th arch participates in formation of the segment of aortic arch between left carotid artery and ductus arteriosus
5th arch	Disappears
6th arch	Right 6th arch gives rise to a portion of proximal right pulmonary artery Left 6th arch gives rise to ductus arteriosus

Checklist
• Cardiac embryogenesis • Cardiac looping • Cardiac septation • Timeline of cardiac morphogenesis • Aortic arch derivatives

■ RESPIRATORY SYSTEM

- The respiratory system is anatomically divided into upper (nose, pharynx, and larynx) and lower (trachea, bronchi, bronchioles, and alveoli) and functionally conducting into the respiratory tracts.
- It has both endodermal (lining epithelium of larynx, trachea, bronchi, bronchioles, and alveoli) and mesodermal (connective tissue, cartilages, and muscles) origins.
- Retinoic acid and transcription factor TBX4 are postulated to be responsible for lung development.
- The embryologic development of the respiratory system begins in the fourth week of intrauterine life with the formation of the *lung bud or respiratory diverticulum* from the ventral wall of the primitive foregut on each side.
- *Formation of larynx and trachea:*
  - Initially, the lung buds communicate with the foregut.
  - This respiratory diverticulum expands caudally and two median ridges grow from either side medially to form the *tracheoesophageal ridges, and then the tracheoesophageal septum, which separates it from the foregut.*

- The respiratory primordium continues to communicate with the pharynx through the laryngeal orifice.
- The upper part of this diverticulum becomes the larynx while the lower part forms the trachea.
- The endothelial lining of the larynx and trachea develops from the endodermal lining of the floor of pharynx while the cartilages and muscles originate from the mesenchyme of the fourth and sixth pharyngeal arches.

- *Development of the lungs:*
  - Each lung bud consists of an endodermal tube surrounded by splanchnic mesoderm. These buds grow laterally and project into the pleural part of the embryonic coelom.
  - By 5th week, these buds enlarge to form the right and left main bronchi. The right one divides further to form three secondary bronchi and the left forms two secondary bronchi.
  - This is followed by further division till terminal bronchioles and alveoli are formed. This continues till 3–7 years of age postnatally.
  - By 27 weeks, the capillary loops are well formed and pulmonary circulation is well established.

Phases of lung maturation.	
Phases	***Characteristics of lung development during the phase***
Embryonic phase (1–6 weeks)	Formation of trachea and major airways
Pseudoglandular phase (5–16 weeks)	Branching continues to form terminal bronchioles. Primitive air sacs form
Canalicular phase (15–26 weeks)	Formation of respiratory bronchioles and alveolar ducts. Formation of primitive capillary bed and epithelial differentiation. Type 2 pneumocytes begin to develop. Some surfactant secretion begins
Saccular phase (26–36 weeks)	Terminal sacs well formed. Capillaries establish close contact with alveoli. Surfactant production well established
Alveolar phase (36 weeks–3 years)	Mature alveoli with well-established alveoli-capillary interface

Checklist
• Formation of larynx and trachea • Development of the lungs • Phases of lung maturation

GASTROINTESTINAL SYSTEM

- *Formation of the primitive gut tube:*
  - The gut tube is formed from the endoderm lining the yolk sac, enveloped by the developing coelom as a result of cranial and caudal folding.
  - During this folding, somatic mesoderm in contact with the body wall forms the parietal peritoneum while the splanchnic mesoderm wraps round the gut tube to form the suspending mesenteries.

- Initially, the gut tube is closed at both cranial and caudal end. Cranial end is closed by buccopharyngeal membrane that will later give rise to mouth and at caudal end by cloacal membrane that will give rise to anus.
- All three germ layers contribute to formation of gastrointestinal system.

Derivatives of germ layers.	
Endoderm	Mucosal epithelium, mucosal, and submucosal glands
Mesoderm	Lamina propria, muscularis mucosae, submucosal connective tissue and blood vessels, muscularis externa, and adventitia serosa
Neural crest	Neurons and nerves of submucosal and myenteric plexus

- *Subdivisions of the gut tube:*
  - The gut tube folds upon itself craniocaudally and laterally to form a definitive cranial and caudal end.
  - These form the foregut and hindgut respectively.
  - The mid gut in the center communicates with the yolk sac.
  - The three derivatives further give rise to various parts of the tract.

Various parts of gut (blood supply).	
Foregut (celiac artery)	Trachea, lungs, esophagus, stomach, liver, pancreas, gallbladder, and upper duodenum
Midgut (superior mesenteric artery)	Lower duodenum, jejunum, ileum, cecum, appendix, ascending colon, proximal two-thirds transverse colon
Hindgut (inferior mesenteric artery)	Distal one-third transverse colon, descending colon, sigmoid colon, rectum, and urogenital sinus

- *Rotation of gut:*
  - Between *6th and 10th week,* midgut loop herniates into the umbilicus, it undergoes *3 rotations* in a step-wise manner.
  - At first, it rotates by 90° in the anticlockwise direction along the axis of superior mesenteric artery. At the end of first rotation, upper limb of the midgut (future ileum) comes to lie on the fetus's right and the lower limb (future colon) lies on the left.
  - At the end of 10th week, the midgut retracts back into the abdominal cavity. The midgut undergoes an additional 180° anticlockwise rotation. The net rotation of the entire midgut is 270° anticlockwise. This brings the cecum (developed from the lower limb of the loop) to the right side.

Retroperitoneal organs.	
Primary (organs with mesentery)	*Secondary (organs which had mesentery but disappears)*
• Abdominal aorta • Inferior vena cava • Adrenal glands • Kidneys • Ureters • Bladder • Lower rectum • Esophagus	• Second, third, and fourth part of duodenum • Ascending colon • Descending colon • Head and body of pancreas

■ HEPATOBILIARY SYSTEM

- At 4 weeks of intrauterine life, the endodermal diverticulum (hepatic diverticulum) arises from the ventral wall at the junction of midgut and hindgut.
- This small diverticulum is the anlage for the development of the liver, extrahepatic biliary ducts, gallbladder, and ventral pancreas.
- Septum transversum forms the fibrous architecture of liver.
- In the 4th week, two buds arise from hepatic diverticulum. The cranial bud (pars hepatica) forms the liver and the extrahepatic biliary tree. The caudal bud develops into superior and inferior buds.
- From the superior bud, the gallbladder and cystic duct appear, and the right pancreas and left ventral pancreas develop from the inferior bud.
- Pars hepatica continues to grow to form cords of cells, these are future hepatocytes.
- These cords of cells interlace with each other to form hepatic trabeculae.
- Hepatic trabeculae invade the septum transversum containing umbilical and vitelline veins and breakdown these veins to form sinusoids.
- By 5th week, all elements of the biliary tree are recognizable.
- The development of intrahepatic duct system is completed by 10 weeks.
- Bile starts secreting around third month of intrauterine life.

Primitive structure.	
Primitive structure	*Give rise to*
Endodermal hepatic bud	• Liver parenchyma • Bile canaliculi and ductules
Vitelline and umbilical veins	Sinusoids
Septum transversum	• Fibrous stroma and capsule • Peritoneal covering • Kupffer cells • Hematopoietic cells

Checklist

• *Gastrointestinal system:*
  – Formation of primitive gut
  – Subdivisions of gut tube
  – Rotation of gut
  – Retroperitoneal organs
• *Hepatobiliary system*

■ GENITOURINARY SYSTEM

- *Urinary system:*
  - Intermediate mesoderm and splanchnic layer of lateral plate mesoderm give rise to nephrogenic cord and urogenital ridge
  - Urogenital ridge forms the urinary and reproduction system
  - *At 4 weeks:*
    - Pronephros develops from nephrogenic cord in the cervical region
    - Pronephros contains duct and nephrotome
    - Pronephros starts degenerating by the end of 4th week

- *At 5 weeks:*
  - Mesonephros develops from nephrogenic cord that extends from thoracic to lumbar region and connects with the cloaca.
  - Mesonephros contains mesonephric duct and tubules.
  - Mesonephric tubules grow to form a capsule like structure, which reaches a glomerulus like structure arise from aorta, this is the primitive urinary system till 10 weeks of gestation.
  - Mesonephros drains into cloaca, which also receives fecal matter from hind gut.
- *Collecting system development:*
  - At around 10 weeks, in pelvic region, intermediate mesoderm condenses to form metanephric blastema.
  - Metanephric blastema release growth factors that stimulate mesonephric duct to form ureteric bud.
  - Ureteric bud grows and invaginates into metanephric blastema and gives rise to renal pelvis.
  - Budding of renal pelvis gives rise to major and minor calyces and collecting tubules.
  - Ureteric bud remains attached to the mesonephric duct with a structure called ureteric stalk that will give rise to ureter.
  - Collecting tubules release growth factors that cause proliferation and condensation of metanephric mesoderm to form metanephric vesicle.
  - Metanephric vesicle grows further to form metanephric tubule, which connects with the collecting tubule.
  - Metanephric tubules give rise to distal convoluted tubule (DCT), proximal convoluted tubule (PCT), and Bowman's capsule.
  - Metanephric tubule between DCT and PCT grows to form loop of Henle.
  - Common iliac vessels give rise to vessels that form glomerulus that interact with the Bowman's capsule.
  - Later, these vessels from common iliac start degenerating and ascend of kidneys starts.
- Kidneys reach the lumbar region where renal vessels from aorta invaginates the renal parenchyma that ultimately give rise to mature kidneys.
- *Development of urinary bladder:*
  - Mesonephric duct and ureter get absorbed in the cloaca, this part will form the vesicular trigone.
  - Mesonephric duct will later form the reproductive system.
  - Urorectal septum develops in the cloaca, which divides it into urogenital sinus and anal canal.
  - Proximal portion of the urogenital sinus forms the urinary bladder, middle portion forms the urethra (prostatic and membranous), and distal portion forms the penile urethra.
- *Reproductive system:*
  - Intermediate mesoderm condenses to form urogenital ridge that give rise to the reproductive system (gonads and ductal system).

- Primitive germ cells from the yolk sac pass through the vitelline duct and reach the gonads, these give rise to sperm and ovum.
- *Male reproductive system:*
  - In male gonads, SRY gene leads to the production of testis determining factor that converts primitive testis to mature testis.
  - Testis is made up of seminiferous tubules, rete testis, leydig cells (produce testosterone), and sertoli cells (secrete Müllerian inhibitory factor).
  - Testosterone stimulates the growth of mesonephric (Wolffian duct) duct that gives rise to epididymis, vas deferens, seminal vesicle, and common ejaculatory duct.
  - Müllerian inhibitory factor inhibits the growth of paramesonephric duct (Müllerian duct).
  - 5α-reductase converts testosterone into dihydrotestosterone that stimulates the production of male external genitalia.
  - Gubernaculum guides the descent of testis into the scrotum.
- *Female reproduction system:*
  - In female gonads, in the absence of *SRY* gene, testis determining factor cannot be formed, so this will result in development of ovaries.
  - Testis is made up of follicular cells (secrete estrogen).
  - Estrogen stimulates the formation of female external genitalia.
  - In the absence of testosterone, mesonephric (Wolffian duct) duct degenerates.
  - In the absence of Müllerian inhibitory factor, paramesonephric duct (Müllerian duct) grows to form fallopian tubes, uterus, and upper two-thirds of vagina.
  - Gubernaculum guides the ovaries and ductal system into the pelvis. It also gives rise to the ovarian ligament and round ligament.

Development of external genitalia.

Male	Primitive structure	Female
• Glans penis • Corpus spongiosum • Corpus cavernosum	Genital tubercle	• Clitoris • Vestibular bulbs
Scrotum	Labioscrotal swelling	Labia majora
• Prostatic urethra • Membranous urethra • Prostate glands • Bulbourethral glands	Urogenital sinus	• Female urethra • Paraurethral glands • Bartholin glands
• Shaft of penis • Penile urethra	Urethral folds	Labia minora

Checklist

- *Urinary system:*
  - Collecting system development
  - Development of urinary bladder
- *Reproductive system:*
  - Male reproductive system
  - Female reproductive system
  - Development of external genitalia

Kamal Arora

Common Antenatal USG Findings in Fetus

77.1 ANTENATAL HYDRONEPHROSIS

- Antenatal hydronephrosis (ANH) is the enlargement or dilation of the renal pelvis.
- It can be unilateral or bilateral.
- Due to an increase in the antenatal ultrasound screening, there has been increased diagnosis of fetal hydronephrosis.
- The prevalence ranges from 0.6 to 5.4%. The condition is bilateral in 17–54% cases.

Causes of hydronephrosis:
- Transient hydronephrosis
- Pelviureteric junction obstruction
- Vesicoureteric reflux
- Multicystic dysplastic kidney
- Duplex kidneys
- Posterior urethral valves
- *Others:* Urethral atresia, urogenital sinus, and prune belly syndrome
- Tumors.

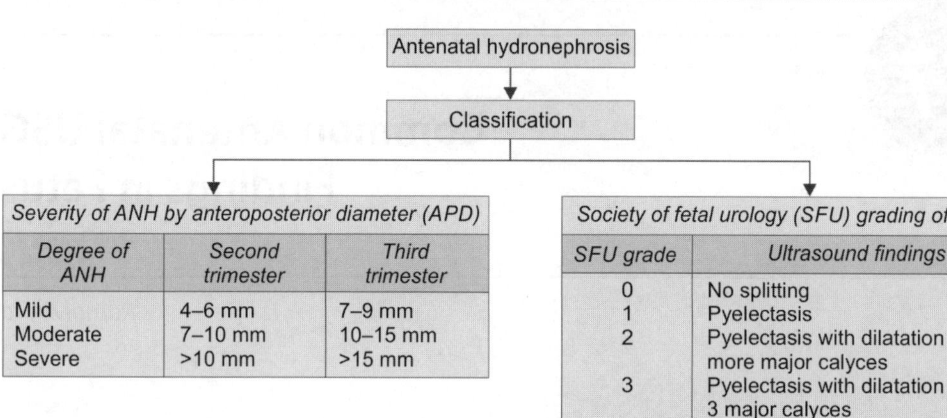

Antenatal hydronephrosis
Classification
Severity of ANH by anteroposterior diameter (APD)
Degree of ANH | Second trimester | Third trimester
Mild | 4–6 mm | 7–9 mm
Moderate | 7–10 mm | 10–15 mm
Severe | >10 mm | >15 mm
Society of fetal urology (SFU) grading of ANH
SFU grade | Ultrasound findings
0 | No splitting
1 | Pyelectasis
2 | Pyelectasis with dilatation of 1 or more major calyces
3 | Pyelectasis with dilatation of all 3 major calyces
4 | Pyelectasis with parenchymal thinning as compared to contralateral kidney

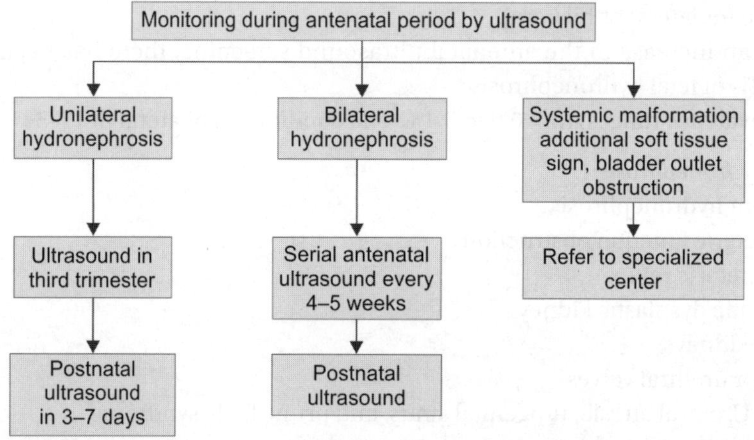

Monitoring during antenatal period by ultrasound
Unilateral hydronephrosis
Bilateral hydronephrosis
Systemic malformation additional soft tissue sign, bladder outlet obstruction
Ultrasound in third trimester
Serial antenatal ultrasound every 4–5 weeks
Refer to specialized center
Postnatal ultrasound in 3–7 days
Postnatal ultrasound

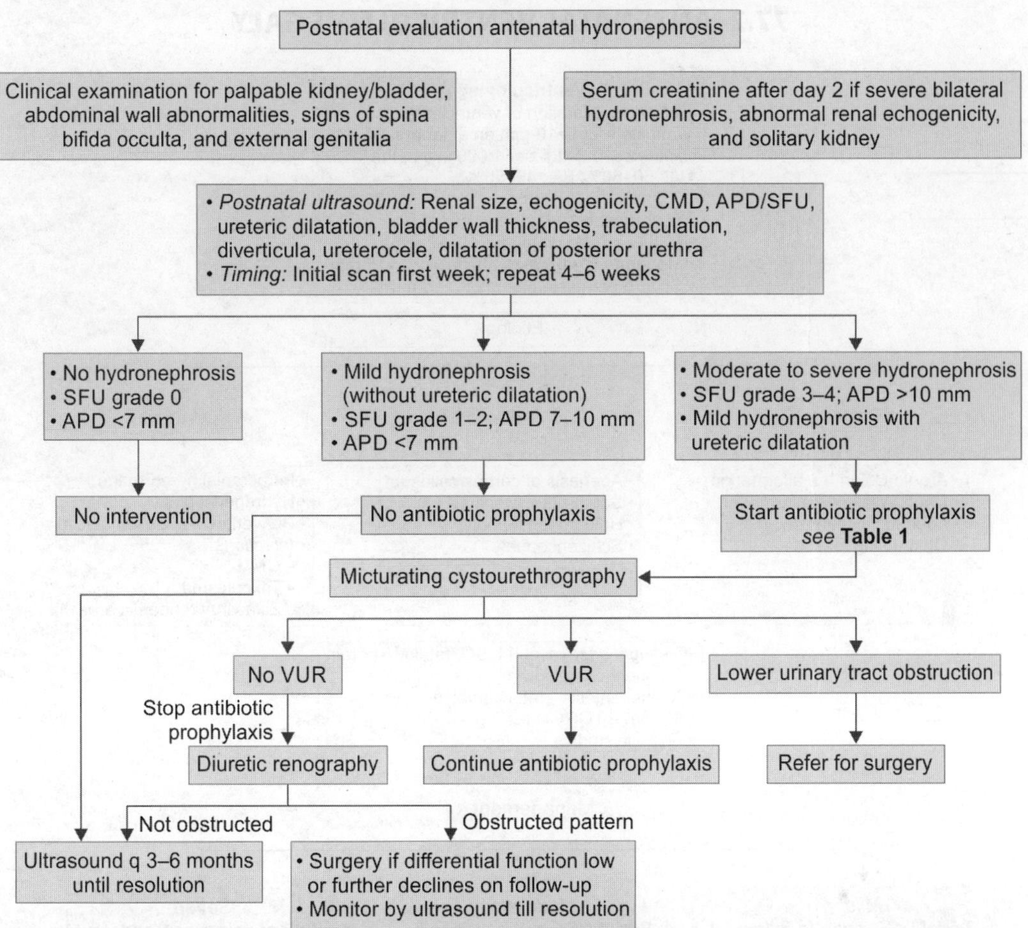

TABLE 1: Common antibiotics for prophylaxis used in ANH.	
Antibiotic	**Dose (mg/kg/day)**
Cephalexin	10
Cefadroxil	5
Cotrimoxazole[#]	1–2
Nitrofurantoin[#]	1–2
[#]Avoid in <3 months, G6PD deficiency	

77.2 ANTENATAL VENTRICULOMEGALY

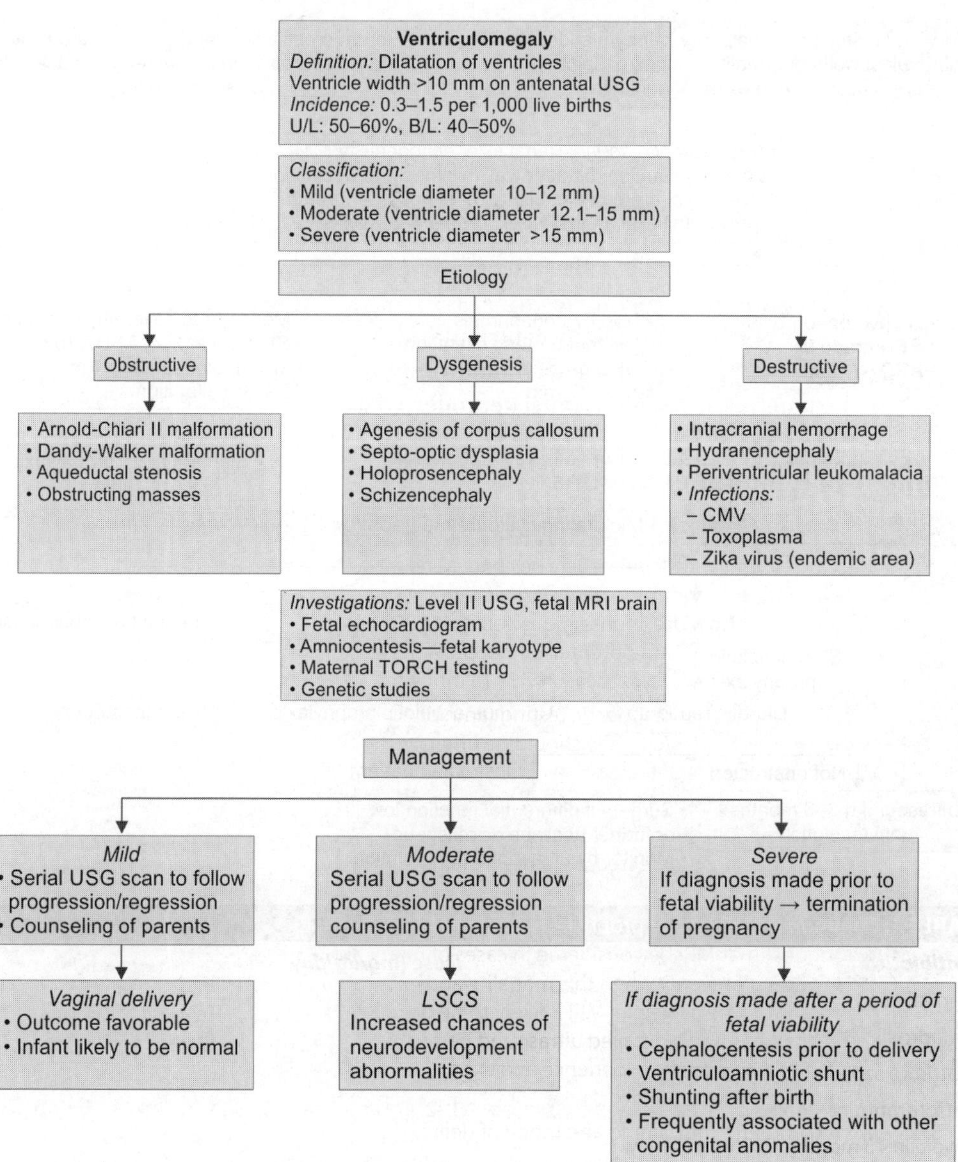

- *Fetal magnetic resonance imaging (MRI):* It may be useful for evaluating ventriculomegaly as various structural abnormalities may be missed on sonography. Diagnosis such as cortical malformations, agenesis of corpus callosum, and abnormalities of migration is often not diagnosed on ultrasound.
- Magnetic resonance imaging is most useful after 22–24 weeks of gestation as milestones of central nervous system (CNS) development become more evident as the gestation advances. MRI has a benefit as it might help to assess the extent of destructive injury in fetuses with known infection, hemorrhage, or any ischemia.

What is the Appropriate Prognosis of the Infants after the Detection of Ventriculomegaly?

Prognosis is variable in this condition and highly depends on the presence or absence of any structural or genetic abnormalities, infection, or the severity of the ventricular dilatation.

- *Isolated mild ventriculomegaly (10–12 mm):* The chances of survival of infants with mild ventriculomegaly are high and have been reported to be about 93–98% and the neurodevelopmental outcome is likely to be >90% normal. It is recommended that with isolated mild ventriculomegaly, after a complete evaluation, mother should be counseled regarding the favorable outcome of the baby.
- *Isolated moderate ventriculomegaly (13–15 mm):* The newborns with antenatal diagnosis of isolated moderate ventriculomegaly are more likely to have worse outcomes as compared to those with mild ventriculomegaly. Survival of these infants is approximately 80–97% and normal neurodevelopment is present in about 75–93%.

Summary of Recommendations

Number	Recommendations	Grade
1.	We suggest that ventriculomegaly be characterized as mild (10–12 mm), moderate (13–15 mm), or severe (>15 mm) for the purposes of patient counseling, given that the chance of an adverse outcome and potential for other abnormalities are higher when the ventricles measure 13–15 mm versus 10–12 mm	• 2B • Weak recommendation, moderate-quality evidence
2.	We recommend that diagnostic testing (amniocentesis) with chromosomal microarray should be offered when mild ventriculomegaly is detected	• 1B • Strong recommendation, moderate-quality evidence
3.	We recommend testing for CMV and toxoplasmosis when ventriculomegaly is detected, regardless of known exposure or symptoms	• 1B • Strong recommendation, moderate-quality evidence
4.	We suggest that MRI be considered in cases of mild or moderate fetal ventriculomegaly when this modality and expert radiologic interpretation are available; MRI is likely to be of less value if the patient has had a detailed ultrasound performed by an individual with specific experience and expertise in sonographic imaging of the fetal brain	• 2B • Weak recommendation, moderate-quality evidence
5.	We recommend that timing and mode of delivery be based on standard obstetric indications	• 1C • Strong recommendation, low-quality evidence
6.	We recommend that with isolated mild ventriculomegaly of 10–12 mm, after a complete evaluation, women be counseled that the outcome is favorable, and the infant is likely to be normal	• 1B • Strong recommendation, moderate-quality evidence
7.	We recommend that with isolated moderate ventriculomegaly of 13–15 mm, after a complete evaluation, women be counseled that the outcome is likely to be favorable but that there is an increased risk of neurodevelopmental disabilities	• 1B • Strong recommendation, moderate-quality evidence

Source: Society for Maternal-Fetal Medicine (SMFM), Fox NS, Monteagudo A, Kuller JA, Craigo S, Norton ME. Mild fetal ventriculomegaly: diagnosis, evaluation, and management. Am J Obstet Gynecol. 2018;219(1):B2-B9.

77.3 CHOROID PLEXUS CYSTS

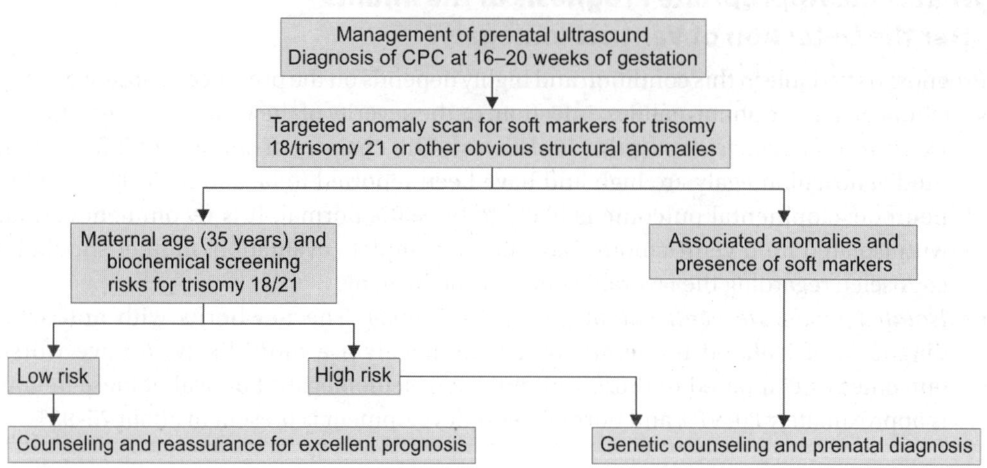

CHOROID PLEXUS CYSTS

- A CPC is a collection of fluid in the choroid plexus of the brain. They are the most common form of intraventricular cyst.
- It occurs in the second trimester, incidence is about 1%. It can be diagnosed during level II ultrasound antenatal scan showing single or multiple cystic areas in one or both choroid plexuses of the lateral cerebral ventricles.
- On ultrasound, CPC appears as echolucent cysts within the choroid plexus.
- Despite the low incidence, the cysts have clinical implications for aneuploidy mainly due to an association with trisomy 18 and trisomy 21.

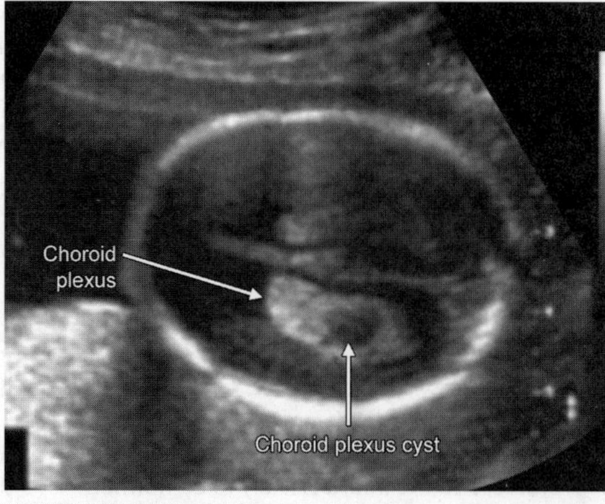

Pathophysiology

- Choroid plexus develops at about 6 weeks of gestation. A bulge from the medial wall of the lateral ventricle gets covered with pseudo-stratified epithelium and then it gets lobulated with villi.
- The cells change from cuboid to columnar epithelium. As the villi grow and become intertwined, a cystic space is formed in which the CSF gets trapped.
- By the 9th week of gestation, the choroid plexus begins producing CSF leading to expansion of the ventricular system.
- Most villi are formed at 13–18 weeks of gestation and the cysts regress by 28 weeks of gestation. Eventually, fluid accumulates and results in the cyst formation detected in sonogram.

Number	Summary of recommendations	Grade
1.	For pregnant female with no previous aneuploidy screening and isolated CPCs, counseling to estimate the probability of trisomy 18 and discussion of options for noninvasive aneuploidy screening with cfDNA or quad screen if cfDNA is unavailable or cost-prohibitive	• 1C • Strong recommendation, low-quality evidence
2.	For pregnant female with negative serum or cfDNA screening results and isolated CPCs, we recommend no further aneuploidy evaluation, as this finding is a normal variant of no clinical importance with no indication for follow-up ultrasound imaging or postnatal evaluation	• 1C • Strong recommendation, low-quality evidence

77.4 INTRACARDIAC ECHOGENIC FOCI

- Intracardiac echogenic foci (ICEF) are defined as a small (<6 mm) bright structure within the fetal heart with similar or greater echogenicity to the surrounding bone visualized in two separate planes.
- It is a soft marker detected on antenatal ultrasound during level II scan. Incidence of detection of ICEF ranges from 0.5 to 32.4% approximately.

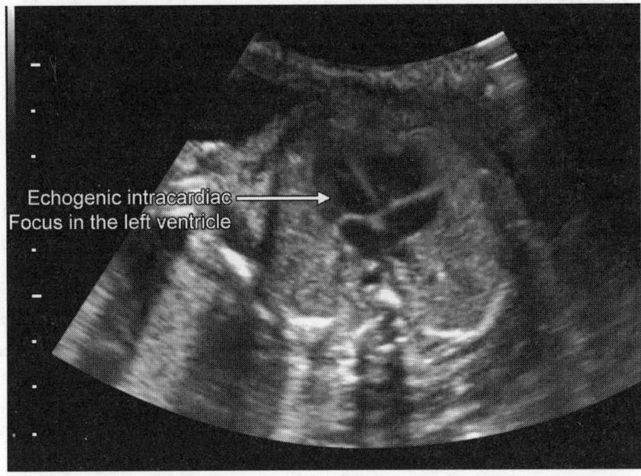

Pathogenesis

The exact cause of ICEF is unknown. It occurs due to either of the two mechanisms:

1. Small area of mineralization within the cardiac papillary muscles
2. Failure of the chordae tendinae to penetrate during cardiogenesis.

Management

- Most common time of detecting ICEF is during the ultrasound conducted around 18–22 weeks of pregnancy. ICEF may be single or occur in multiple numbers.
- The location of these foci may vary and are most commonly found in the left ventricle followed by right ventricle. ICEF is a normal variant.
- The most common chromosomal abnormalities associated with the presence of ICEF are trisomy 13 and trisomy 21. These abnormalities are usually present with other relevant signs like echogenic bowel, choroid plexus cyst (CPC), shortened long bones or renal pyelectasis, etc.
- Studies have shown that the left-sided ICEF is usually of no significance but the right sided or bilateral ICEF may have a twice-greater risk of aneuploidy.

How to Evaluate Intracardiac Echogenic Foci?

Intracardiac echogenic foci are usually a finding in antenatal routine screening sonography and hence detailed fetal echocardiography can be done to screen the fetus for any associated structural cardiac abnormality.

- For pregnant women with no previous history of aneuploidy screening and presence of an isolated ICEF, they should be counseled to estimate the probability of trisomy 21. Noninvasive techniques like aneuploidy screening of cfDNA, quadruple test should be discussed. Hence, diagnostic testing is not solely recommended for this finding.
- For pregnant women with negative serum of cfDNA screening results and an isolated ICEF, no further evaluation is recommended.

Hence, if ICEF is not associated with any structural abnormalities, invasive genetic diagnostic tests are not needed.

77.5 SINGLE UMBILICAL ARTERY

- Single umbilical artery (SUA) is a condition in which only one artery is present and the other is missing.
- The prevalence of this condition ranges from 0.2 to 11%. Various maternal as well as fetal risk factors and characteristics are associated with SUA like sex.
- Parity, multiple births, maternal age, smoking, or any other complications like preexisting diabetes, hypertension etc.

Prenatal Diagnosis

- It is difficult to visualize the vessels during the first trimester due to the small size.
- The vessels can be easily viewed during the second or the third trimester in a cross sectional image of the cord.
- As SUA might result in intrauterine growth retardation, regular ultrasounds are recommended in the third trimester to evaluate growth.
- For fetuses with isolated SUA, weekly antenatal fetal surveillance can be considered at the beginning of 36 weeks of gestation.
- Color flow Doppler imaging of the intra-abdominal portions of the umbilical arteries confirms the diagnosis.
- Prenatal diagnosis of the SUA is based on the following:
  - USG showing only two vessels in the umbilical cord, larger vessel is the vein and the smaller vessel is the artery.

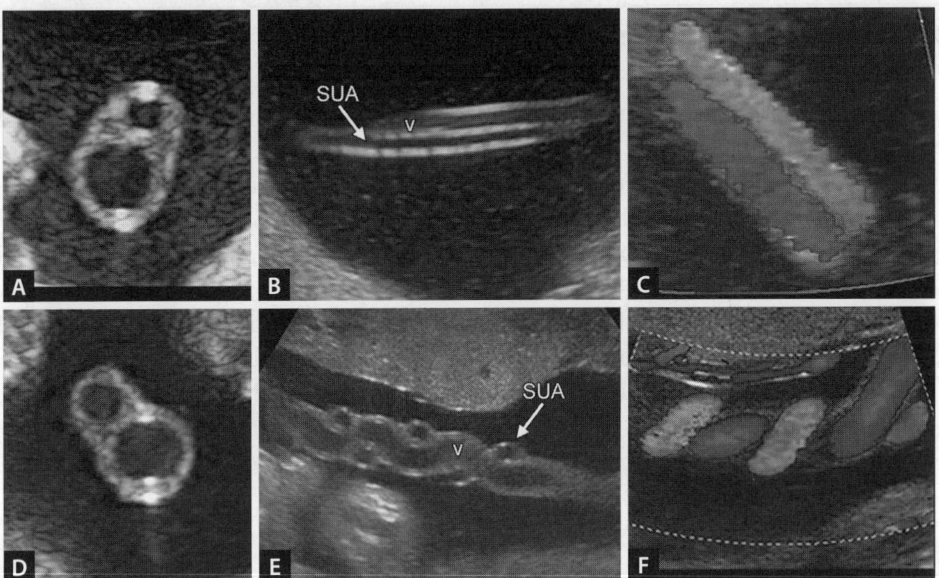

(A and D) Single umbilical artery. Transverse section of a two-vessel umbilical cord in two different fetuses shows the typical "soda can tab" sign; (B and E) Single umbilical artery. Longitudinal views of a two-vessel umbilical cord as depicted by two-dimensional ultrasound shows the single umbilical artery (SUA) and the vein (V). Image B shows fetus with a straight. Noncoiled umbilical cord. Image E shows fetus with a coiled umbilical cord; (C and F) Single umbilical artery. Color Doppler ultrasound shows a straight noncoiled, two-vessel umbilical cord; and (C) A coaled two-vessel umbilical cord (F).

  - Color flow Doppler in the region of the bifurcation of the fetal aorta showing intra-abdominal umbilical vessels only on one side of the fetal bladder (pathognomonic of SUA).

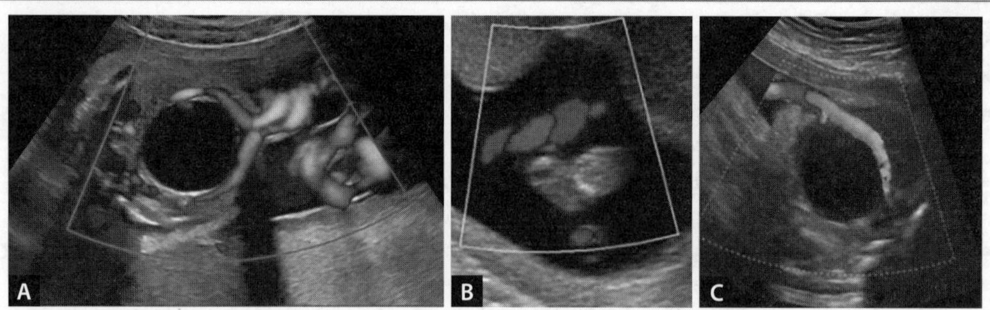

(A) Normal three-vessel umbilical cord, color Doppler shows presence of two umbilical arteries, one on each side of the bladder; (B) Two-vessel umbilical cord color Doppler images show alternating single artery and vein; (C) Two-vessel umbilical cord. Transverse view at the level of the fetal bladder shows an artery with only one side of the fetal bladder.
Courtesy: Deborah Levine, MD and Bryann Bromley, MD.

Postdiagnostic Evaluation

- Single umbilical artery has a strong association between congenital anomalies mainly in the upper and lower gastrointestinal tract (atresia or stenosis), renal agenesis, and congenital heart defects.
- Single umbilical artery might occur in trisomy 18 and 13 but rarely occurs with trisomy 21. The risk of aneuploidy ranges from 4 to 50%.
- After detecting SUA in antenatal ultrasound, a detailed fetal anatomic survey must be performed.
- A standard four-chambered view of the heart and views of the great arteries must be seen and there is no necessary indication for a fetal echocardiography.
- Detailed screening of the kidneys must be done including the number, location, and appearance of the kidneys.
- Pelvic dilation must be rule out as it a common anomaly associated with SUA.

■ FURTHER READING

1. Benn P, Borrell A, Chiu R, Cuckle H, Dugoff L, Faas B, et al. Position statement from the chromosome abnormality screening, International Society of Prenatal Diagnosis. Prenat Diagn. 2015;35(8): 725-34.
2. Van den Hof MC, Wilson RD, Diagnostic Imaging Committee, Society of Obstetricians and Gynaecologists of Canada; Genetics Committee, Society of Obstetricians and Gynaecologists of Canada. Fetal soft markers in obstetric ultrasound. J Obstet Gynaecol Can. 2005;27:592-636.

Fetal Surveillance

Chanchal

ELECTRONIC FETAL HEART RATE MONITORING

- Cardiotocograph is an indispensable tool for intrapartum fetal surveillance wherever available.
- The term nonstress test (NST) is used when CTG is done in the antenatal period. Electronic fetal heart monitoring allows for early recognition of a fetus at stress so that timely intervention can be done.
- The National Institute of Clinical Excellence (NICE) guidelines have been followed in this chapter **(Table 1)**.
- A uniform system of interpretation, classification and management of the CTG allows for effective communication **(Tables 2 and 3)**.
- Indications for continuous intrapartum electronic fetal heart rate (FHR) monitoring are given in **Box 1**.

TABLE 1: NICE classification of FHR features.

Feature	Baseline (bpm)	Variability (bpm)	Decelerations	Accelerations
Normal/ reassuring	110–160	5–25	None or Early decelerations or Variable decelerations with no concerning features lasting for <90 minutes	Present
Nonreassuring	100–109 or 161–180	<5 for >50 minutes or >25 for >25 minutes or Sinusoidal	Variable decelerations (loss of beats <60 bpm, recovery within 60 seconds) with >50% contractions for >90 minutes or Variable decelerations >60 bpm, >60 seconds up to 30 minutes or Late decelerations up to 30 minutes	Absence of accelerations with an otherwise normal trace is of unknown significance

Contd...

Contd...

Feature	Baseline (bpm)	Variability (bpm)	Decelerations	Accelerations
Abnormal	<100 or >180 or Sinusoidal pattern ≥10 minutes	<5 for ≥90 minutes	Variable decelerations >60 bpm, >60 seconds for >30 minutes or Late decelerations >30 minutes or Decelerations not responding to conservative measures or Single prolonged deceleration ≥3 minutes	

TABLE 2: Classification of CTG.

Category	Definition
Normal/reassuring	All four features are reassuring
Nonreassuring	One nonreassuring feature while rest reassuring
Abnormal	≥2 nonreassuring features or ≥1 abnormal feature

TABLE 3: Suggested management as per intrapartum CTG.

Suspicious trace	• Change maternal position
	• Correct maternal hypotension
	• Identify underlying cause:
	  – Rule out abruption, scar dehiscence, cord prolapse
	  – Siting of epidural anesthesia or top-up
	  – Tocolysis if hyperstimulation
	  – Correct maternal pyrexia
	• Maternal drugs, e.g., opioids
	• Do not give maternal oxygen

Pathological trace	• As above • Stop oxytocin • Repeat vaginal examination • "3, 6, 9, 12, and 15 minutes" action timeline • Identify antenatal and intrapartum risk factors • Consider delivery if persistently pathological trace • Mode of delivery to be guided by vaginal examination findings

BOX 1: Indications for continuous electronic fetal heart rate monitoring.

Antepartum:
- Previous caesarean section
- Pre-eclampsia
- Post-term pregnancy (>42 weeks)
- Prolonged rupture of membranes (>24 hours)
- Diabetes
- Induced labor
- Other maternal medical disease

Contd...

Contd...

Fetal:
- Growth restriction
- Prematurity
- Oligohydramnios
- Abnormal Doppler velocimetry
- Multiple pregnancy
- Meconium stained liquor
- Breech presentation

Intrapartum:
- Oxytocin augmentation
- Epidural analgesia
- Vaginal bleeding in labor
- Maternal pyrexia
- Fresh meconium stained liquor
- Chorioamnionitis
- Abnormal intermittent auscultation
- Maternal request

Features of Cardiotocograph

The intrapartum CTG has two components—(1) FHR and (2) uterine contractions. Care must be taken to accurately document patient identification and the correct date and time of recording the CTG. The calibrated paper runs at the speed of 1 cm per hour. Care must be taken to avoid "loss of contact" and get a good quality trace for correct interpretation **(Fig. 1)**.

The FHR tracing has four features:
1. Fetal heart rate
2. Variability
3. Accelerations
4. Decelerations

Each feature is classified into normal/reassuring, nonreassuring, or abnormal **(Table 1)**. The CTG is then classified into normal or reassuring, nonreassuring, or abnormal based on all four features **(Table 2)**.

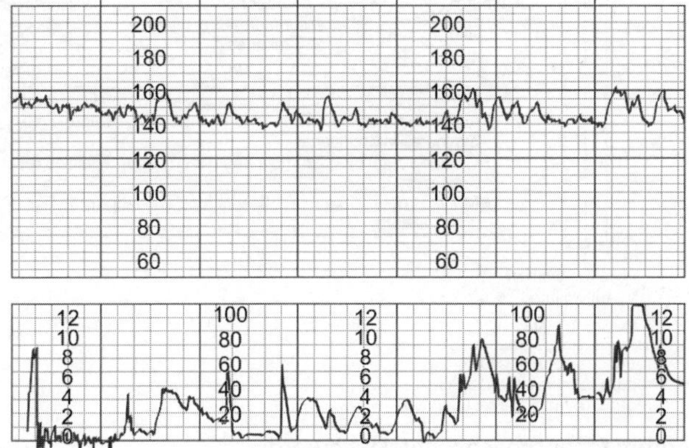

Fig. 1: Normal intrapartum CTG running at 1 cm/min. The baseline is 140 beats per minutes, variability is 10 bpm, there are accelerations and there are no decelerations. The trace also shows 3 contractions in 10 minutes. Algorithm for approach to fetal bradycardia or recurrent late deceleration on CTG.

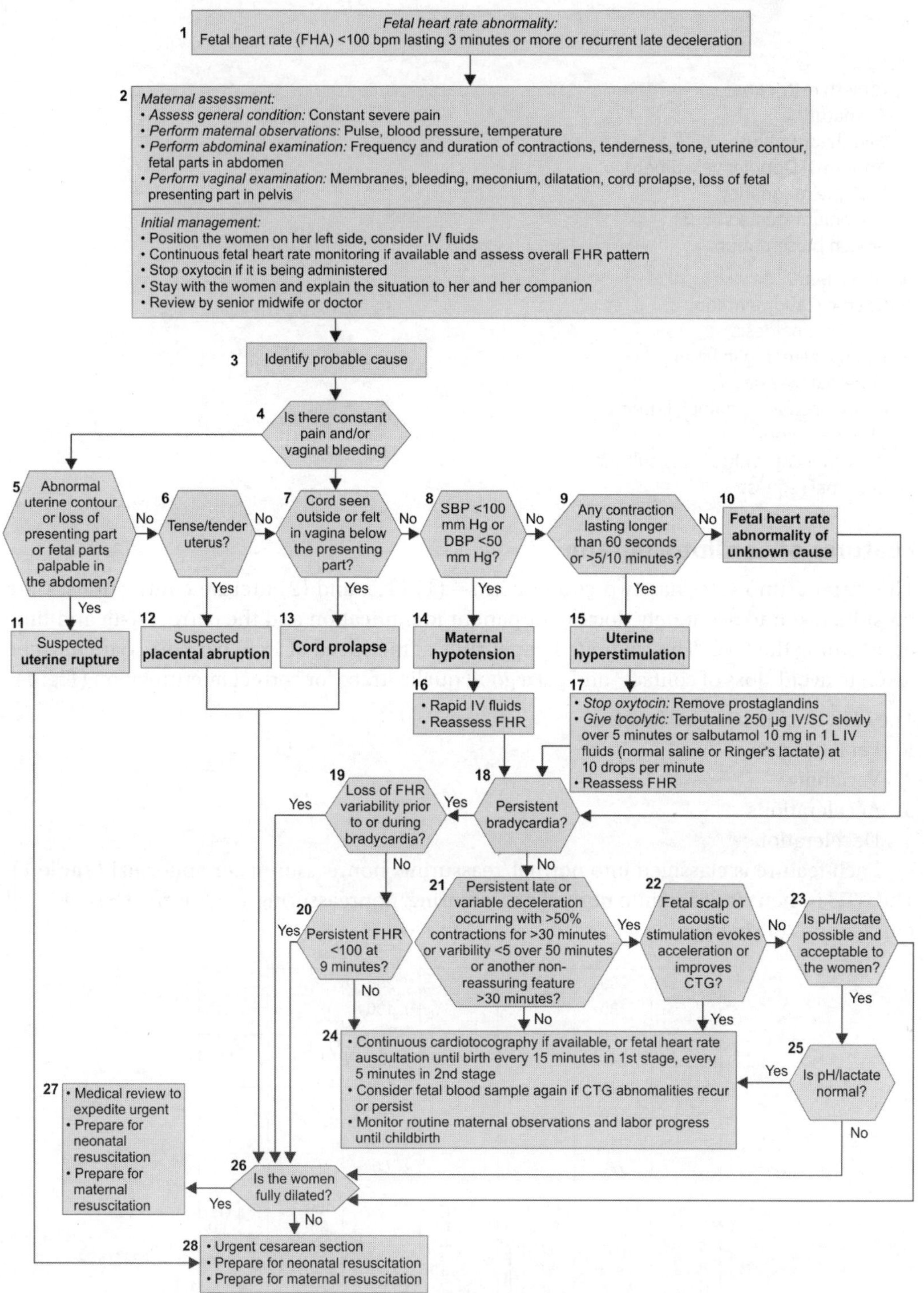

Algorithm for approach to fetal tachycardia.

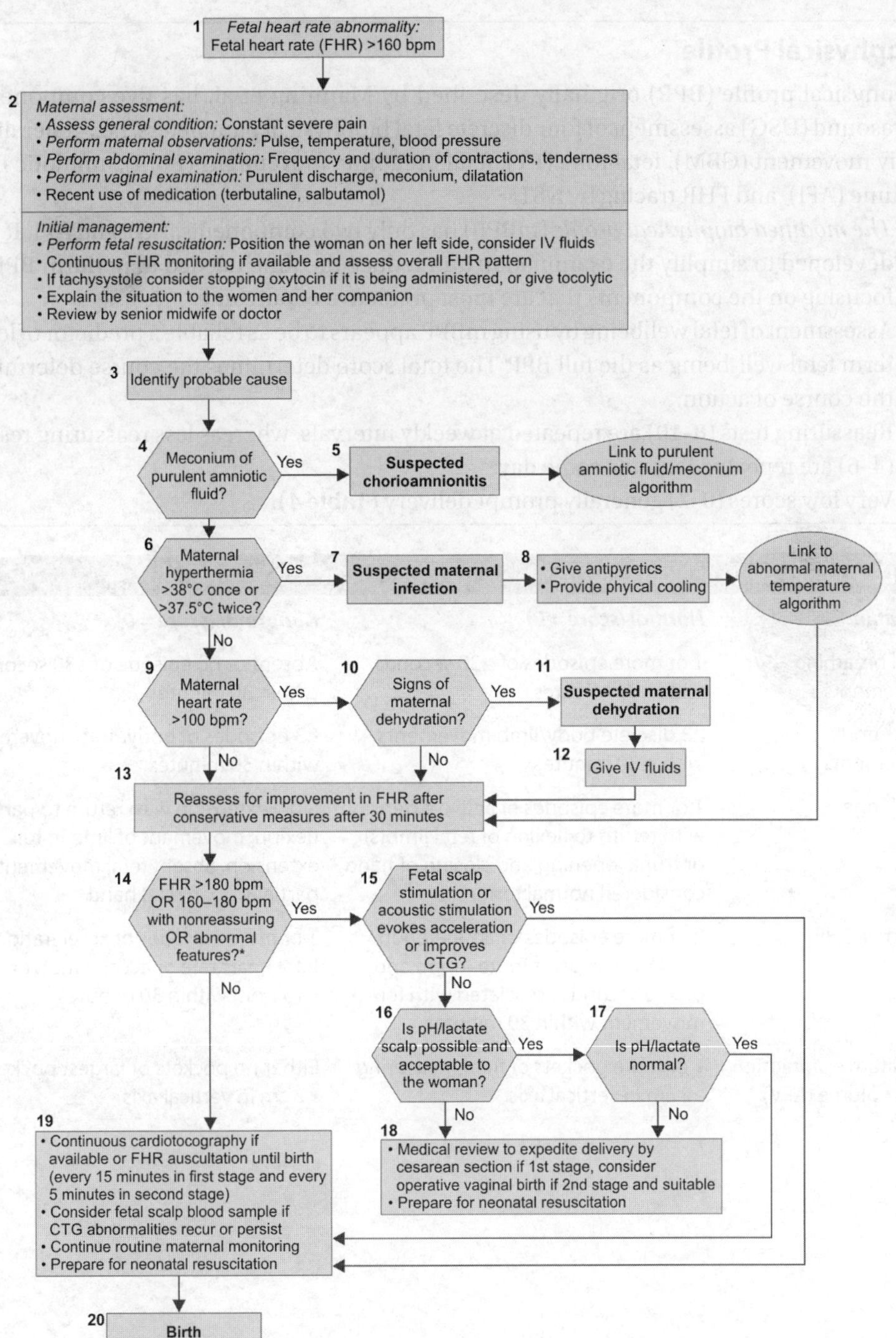

*One abnormal feature: variability <5 for 50 minutes or >25 for 25 minutes; Late decelerations or variable with abnormal features; Or two nonreassuring features: baseline >160 or <110; variability <5 for 30 minutes or >25 for 15 minutes; Variable decelerations <50% contractions or <30 minutes; late decelerations <30 minutes.

Biophysical Profile

Biophysical profile (BPP) originally described by Manning et al. has five components: ultrasound (USG) assessment of four discrete fetal biophysical parameters, i.e., generalized body movement (GBM), fetal tone (FT), fetal breathing movements (FBM), amniotic fluid volume (AFI), and FHR tracing by NST.

- *The modified biophysical profile* (mBPP) has only two components, NST and AFI. It was developed to simplify the examination and reduce the time needed to perform BPP by focusing on the components that are most predictive of outcome.
- Assessment of fetal wellbeing by using mBPP appears to be as reliable a predictor of long-term fetal well-being as the full BPP. The total score determines the course determines the course of action.
- Reassuring tests (8–10) are repeated at weekly intervals, whereas less reassuring results (4–6) are repeated later the same day.
- Very low scores (0–2) generally prompt delivery **(Table 4)**.

TABLE 4: Components of biophysical profile.

Variable	*Normal (score = 2)*	*Abnormal (score = 0)*
Fetal breathing movements	1 or more episodes of ≥30 seconds within 30 minutes	Absent or no episode of ≥30 seconds within 30 minutes
Gross body movements	≥3 discrete body/limb movements within 30 minutes	<3 episodes of body/limb movements within 30 minutes
Fetal tone	1 or more episodes of active extension with return to flexion of fetal limb(s) or trunk (opening and closing of hand considered normal tone)	Slow extension with return to partial flexion, movement of limb in full extension, absent fetal movement, or partially open fetal hand
Reactive FHR	2 or more episodes of acceleration of ≥15 beats per minute (bpm) and of >15 seconds associated with fetal movement within 30 minutes	1 or more episodes of acceleration of fetal heart rate or acceleration of <15 bpm within 30 minutes
Qualitative amniotic fluid volume (AFV)	1 or more pockets of fluid measuring ≥2 cm in vertical axis	Either no pockets or largest pocket <2 cm in vertical axis

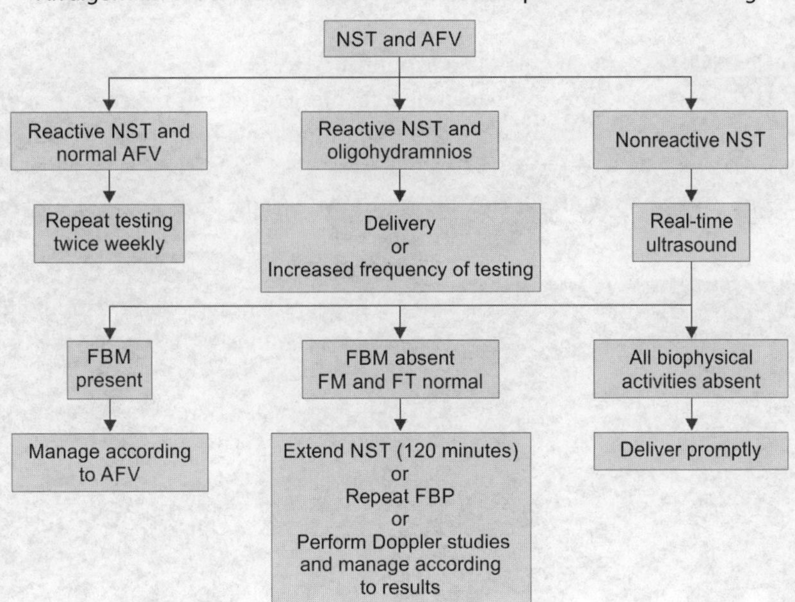

Fetal Surveillance in Growth Restriction

- Since fetal growth restriction (FGR) accounts for an overwhelming majority of perinatal morbidity and mortality, a brief outline of fetal surveillance in these high-risk pregnancies is presented here.
- It is important to correctly identify growth-restricted fetuses and differentiate these from the constitutionally small for gestational age (SGA) fetuses who will not need increased surveillance.

Diagnostic criteria for early and late fetal growth restriction (FGR) (in a structurally normal fetus).

Early FGR (diagnosed before 32 weeks)	Late FGR (diagnosed after 32 weeks)
AC[*]/EFW <3rd centile or	AC/EFW <3rd centile or
Umbilical artery – A/REDF[#] or	Any 2 of the following 3 criteria:
• AC/EFW <10th centile and • Uterine artery PI >95th centile and/or • Umbilical artery PI >95th centile	• AC/EFW <10th centile or • AC/EFW crossing centiles >2 quartiles on growth chart and • CPR <5th centile or umbilical artery PI >95th centile

[*]AC: Abdominal circumference, [#]A/REDF: Absent or reversed end diastolic flow

- Ultrasound assessment of fetal Dopplers remains the mainstay in surveillance of growth-restricted fetuses.
- The Dopplers follow a predictable pattern of deterioration in early FGR **(Fig. 2)** and the frequency of monitoring is individualized according to the gestational age and severity of maternal pre-eclampsia if present.

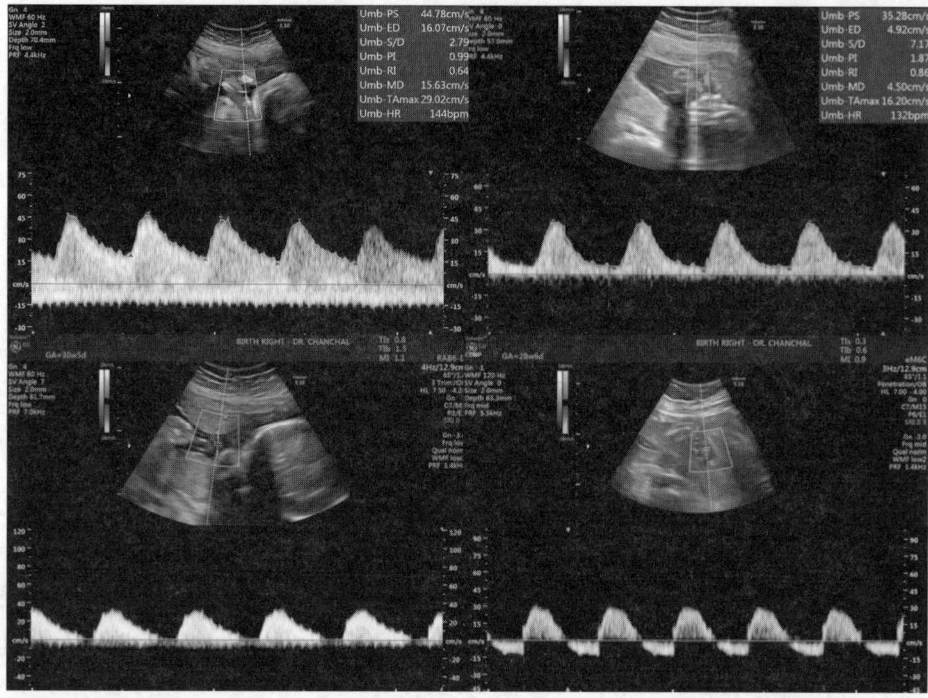

Fig. 2: Typical deterioration in umbilical artery Doppler in early FGR (clockwise): Normal waveform, increased PI, absent end-diastolic flow (AEDF) followed by reversal in end-diastolic flow (REDF).

■ SURVEILLANCE AND TIMING OF DELIVERY IN "SMALL" FETUSES

Suggested monitoring and timing of delivery in small fetuses.

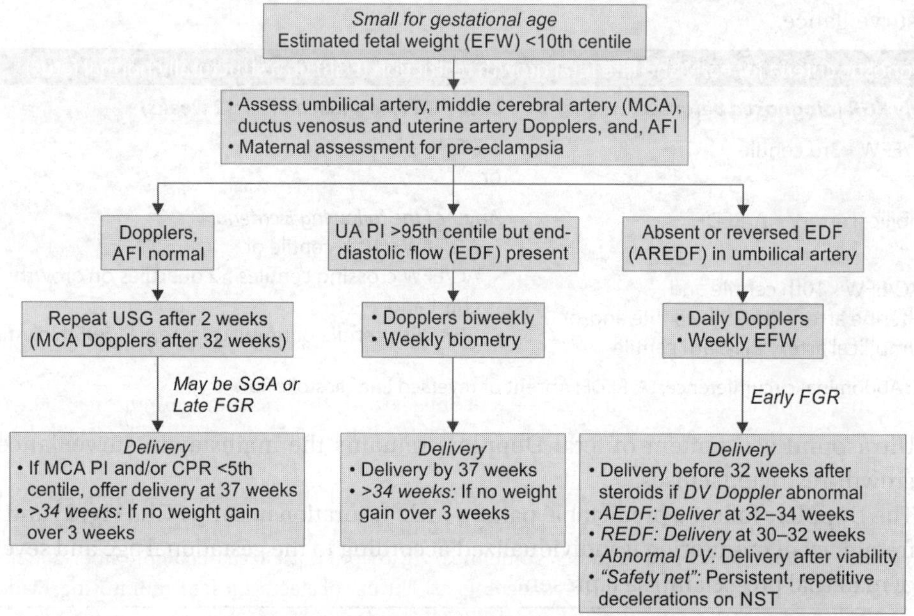

Source: Adapted from RCOG and ISUOG guidelines.

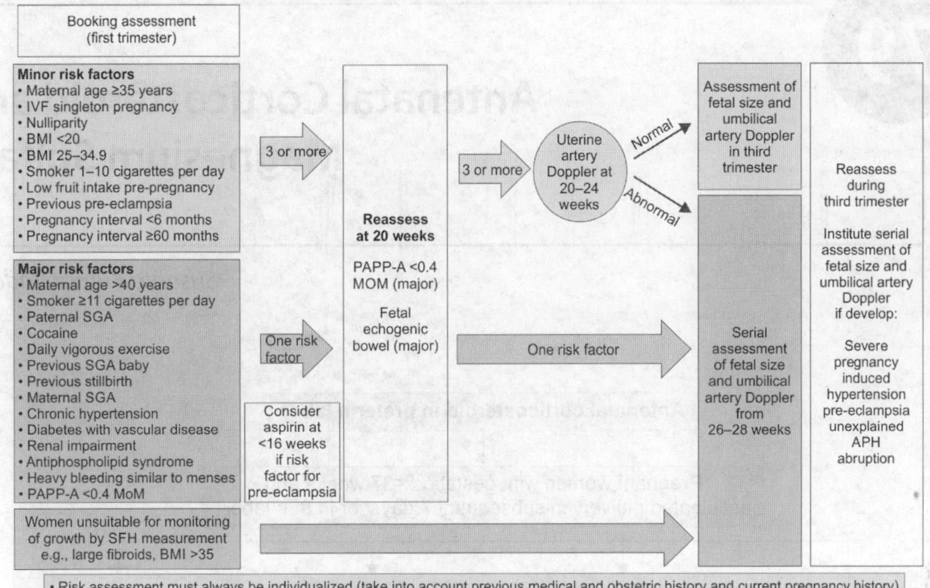

Intrauterine growth restriction.

Source: Sharma D, Shastri S, Sharma P. Intrauterine Growth Restriction: Antenatal and Postnatal Aspects. Clin Med Insights Pediatr. 2016;10:67-83.

Key Points to Remember

- The aim of fetal surveillance in the perinatal period is not only to prevent stillbirth but also to minimize neonatal morbidity secondary to fetal hypoxia.
- The most widely adopted measures are electronic fetal heart monitoring, i.e., the cardiotocograph (CTG), biophysical profile (BPP), and fetal Dopplers on ultrasound.
- Fetal Dopplers are particularly relevant in the surveillance and timing of delivery in growth-restricted fetuses.

■ FURTHER READING

1. Lees CC, Stampalija T, Baschat A, da Silva Costa F, Ferrazzi E, Figueras F, et al. ISUOG Practice Guidelines: diagnosis and management of small-for-gestational-age fetus and fetal growth restriction. Ultrasound Obstet Gynecol. 2020;56(2):298-312.

2. Nageotte MP, Towers CV, Asrat T, Freeman RK. Perinatal outcome with the modified biophysical profile. Am J Obstet Gynecol. 1994;170:1672.

3. National Institute for Health and Care Excellence. (2014). Intrapartum care for healthy women and babies [London]: NICE; Dec 2014 [updated 2017 Feb]. (Clinical guideline [CG190]). [Online] Available from https://www.nice.org.uk/guidance/cg190 [Last accessed September, 2022].

4. Royal College of Obstetricians and Gynaecologists. (2013). Small-for-Gestational-Age Fetus, Investigation and Management (Green-top Guideline No. 31). [online] Available from https:// www.rcog.org.uk/globalassets/documents/guidelines/gtg_31.pdf [Last accessed September, 2022].

5. Royal College of Obstetricians and Gynaecologists. The use of electronic fetal monitoring. Evidence-based clinical guideline, number 8. London: RCOG Press; 2001.

Antenatal Corticosteroid and Magnesium Sulfate

Susanta Kumar Badatya

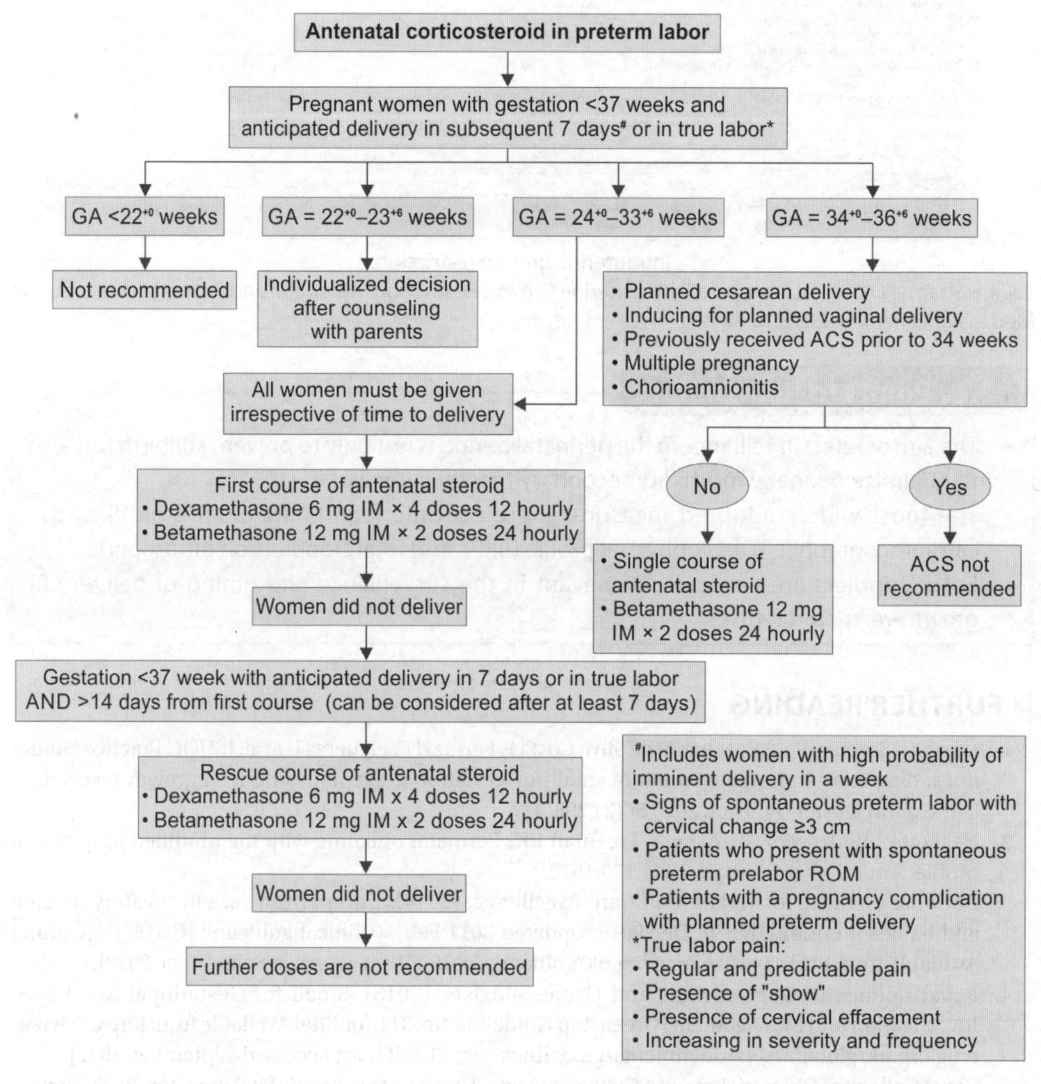

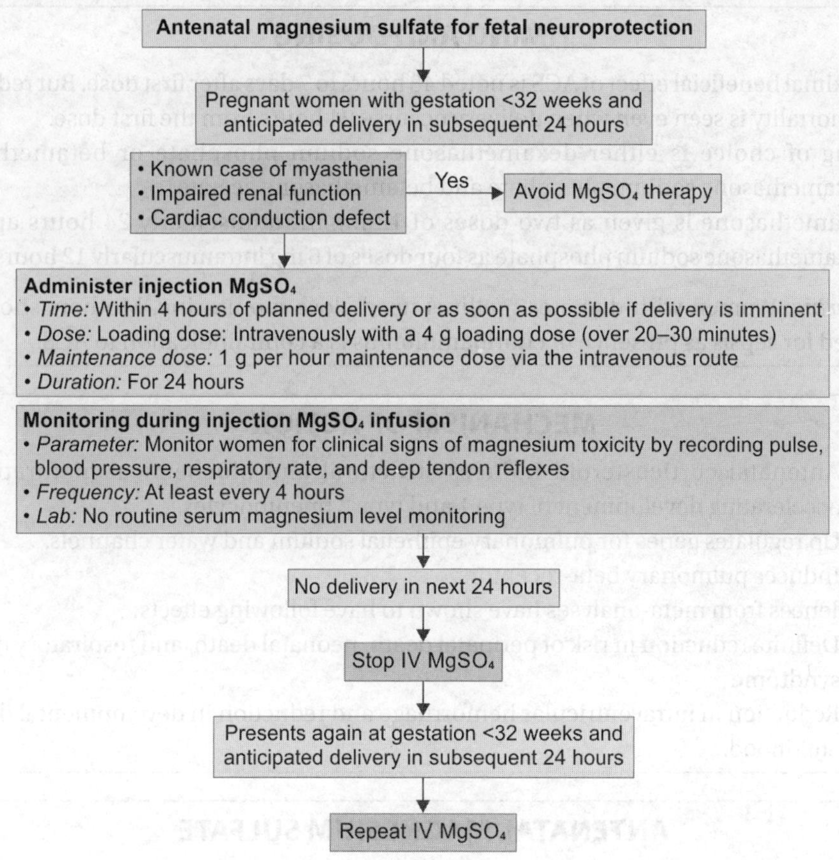

ANTENATAL CORTICOSTEROID: INDICATIONS

- Pregnant women with gestation 24–33^{+6} weeks of gestation must be given antenatal corticosteroid when delivery is anticipated either spontaneously or planned for medical reasons in subsequent 7 days. Biological effect is not seen in gestation <22 weeks, so not recommended. But for 22^{+0}–23^{+6} weeks of gestation, it should be offered when parents want aggressive neonatal intervention as it definitely offers survival benefit but long-term neurological outcome in survivors should be considered.

- For gestation between 34 and 36^{+6} weeks, the recommendation remains controversial as survival advantage and respiratory problems are easily manageable and transient. It is recommended to offer two-dose antenatal corticosteroid schedule for all women at late preterm gestation except when there is presence of chorioamnionitis, multiple pregnancy, and previously course of antenatal corticosteroids (ACS) prior to 34 weeks and the delivery is planned.

TIMING AND DOSING

- Maximal beneficial effect of ACS is noted 48 hours to 7 days after first dose. But reduction in mortality is seen even when delivery occurs <24 hours from the first dose.
- Drug of choice is either dexamethasone sodium phosphate or betamethasone (betamethasone sodium phosphate and betamethasone acetate).
- Betamethasone is given as two doses of 12 mg intramuscularly 24 hours apart or Dexamethasone sodium phosphate as four doses of 6 mg intramuscularly 12 hours apart.

Monitoring: Women with diabetes mellitus need close monitoring. Mothers should be screened for sepsis as presence of chorioamnionitis is a contraindication to ACS.

MECHANISM OF ACTION

- Antenatal corticosteroid induces structural and biochemical maturation by accelerating development of type 1 and type 2 pneumocytes.
- Up regulates genes for pulmonary epithelial sodium and water channels.
- Induces pulmonary beta-receptors.
- Evidences from meta-analyses have shown to have following effects:
  - Definite reduction in risk of perinatal death, neonatal death, and respiratory distress syndrome
  - Reduction in intraventricular hemorrhage and reduction in developmental delay in childhood.

ANTENATAL MAGNESIUM SULFATE

- *Mechanism of action:*
  - $MgSO_4$ stabilizes blood pressure and cerebral blood flow.
  - Antiexcitoxic action by blockage of glutamate like excitatory neurotransmitter
  - Antioxidant effect and anti-inflammatory effect
- Despite of heterogeneity in studies, evidence from multiple randomized control trial shows that use of magnesium sulfate for gestation <32 weeks within 24 hours of delivery reduces risk of cerebral palsy and gross motor dysfunction.
- ACOG, FIGO, and Government of India guidelines ("LaQshya" programme) endorse use of magnesium sulfate in women with preterm labor at gestation <32 weeks.
- Magnesium sulfate should be offered irrespective of number of fetuses and cause of preterm delivery.
- Only contraindication is presence of myasthenia gravis in mother. Impaired renal function and cardiac conduction defect being relative contraindications.

- *Administration protocol:* There is no single recommended protocol or dosage for magnesium sulfate infusion. It is recommended that individual institutes should adopt and follow a treatment protocol out of the available protocols from the larger randomized control trials.
  - *Protocol 1:* IV 4 g over 20 minutes, then 1 g/h until delivery or for 24 hours, whichever came first.
  - *Protocol 2:* IV 4 g over 30 minutes or IV bolus of 4 g given as single dose.
  - *Protocol 3:* IV 6 g over 20–30 minutes, followed by IV maintenance of 2 g/h.
- *Monitoring:* There is no routine need for monitoring serum magnesium level. Clinical monitoring of magnesium toxicity should be done which includes respiratory rate, blood pressure, urine out, and deep tendon reflexes.

Key Points to Remember

- Premature delivery (birth gestation <37 weeks) is one of the leading causes of neonatal and infant mortality rate worldwide.
- Only a few of antenatal interventions have been proved to be of benefit to improve immediate neonate outcome like antenatal corticosteroid and to enhance long-term neurodevelopmental outcome like antenatal magnesium sulfate.
- Antenatal corticosteroid aims to improve fetal lung maturity which in turn has been shown to decrease risk of perinatal death, neonatal death, and respiratory distress syndrome.
- Usage of antenatal magnesium sulfate decreases the chance of cerebral palsy in childhood.

■ FURTHER READING

1. Committee on Obstetric Practice. Committee Opinion No. 713: Antenatal Corticosteroid Therapy for Fetal Maturation. Obstet Gynecol. 2017;130(2):e102-9.
2. McGoldrick E, Stewart F, Parker R, Dalziel SR. Antenatal corticosteroids for accelerating fetal lung maturation for women at risk of preterm birth. Cochrane Database Syst Rev. 2020;12(12):CD004454.
3. Shennan A, Suff N, Jacobsson B; on behalf of the FIGO Working Group for Preterm Birth. FIGO good practice recommendations on magnesium sulfate administration for preterm fetal neuroprotection. Int J Gynecol Obstet. 2021;155:31-3.
4. WHO. (2015). WHO recommendations on interventions to improve preterm birth outcomes. [online] Available from https://apps.who.int/iris/bitstream/handle/10665/183037/97892415089 88_eng.pdf [Last accessed September, 2022].

Management of Neonates with Maternal Illness

Raktima Chakrabarti

MATERNAL DIABETES: INFANT OF DIABETIC MOTHER

Neonatal Complications

Short-term:

- Macrosomia or large for gestational age, i.e., birth weight ≥90th percentile or >+2SD (>97th percentile) for gestational age.
- Spontaneous preterm birth.
- Metabolic disorders such as hypoglycemia, hypocalcemia, hypomagnesemia, and hyperbilirubinemia.
- *Hematological problem:* Hyperviscosity and polycythemia.
- *Respiratory problem:* Increased incidence of respiratory distress syndrome and transient tachypnea of newborn.
- *Cardiac problem:* Hypertrophic cardiomyopathy, can affect the interventricular septum and also myocardium.
- *Neurological problem:* Perinatal asphyxia and brachial plexus injuries mostly due to shoulder dystocia due to macrosomia.
- *Gastrointestinal problem:* Poor sucking and sometimes functional lower intestinal obstruction.

Long-term:

- Myocardial dysfunction.
- Long-term risk of insulin-dependent diabetes developing by the age of 20 years.
- *Congenital abnormalities:* Like congenital heart disease, neural tube defects, caudal regression syndrome, cleft palate, and vertebral abnormalities.

Management

Follow standard treatment guidelines to manage neonatal complications.

MATERNAL HYPO AND HYPERTHYROIDISM

- Thyroid function during pregnancy plays an important role in fetal central nervous system development.
- Effects of maternal hypothyroidism on fetus: Congenital hypothyroidism:
  - Most common endocrine problem in newborns
  - Incidence—1 in 2,000–3,000 babies
  - Can be transient or permanent
  - Most common cause of permanent congenital hypothyroidism is dysgenesis
  - Most common cause for transient congenital hypothyroidism is iodine deficiency and iodine exposure.
  - Clinical signs are mostly absent at birth
  - Screening (*See* Chapter Neonatal Screening) and early treatment are the most important step (*See* Chapter Congenital Hypothyroidism).
- *Effects of maternal hyperthyroidism on fetus:*
  - This is rare
  - Mainly untreated maternal hyperthyroidism
  - Better is prevention and maternal thyroid function monitoring during pregnancy is must.
  - Risks of the fetus are hyperthyroidism and IUGR.
- Mother is having hyperthyroidism/grave's disease, neonates need monitored during first 2 weeks after birth.

MATERNAL HYPERTENSIVE DISORDER

- *Effects of maternal hypertension on newborns:*
  - Premature delivery
  - Intrauterine growth restriction
  - Increased incidence of thrombocytopenia and bleeding disorder including intracranial hemorrhage
  - Increased incidence of nucleated RBC
  - Increased incidence of patent ductus arteriosus, oxygen and assisted ventilation, and bronchopulmonary dysplasia.
- *Approach to the management:*
  - *Prevention*: Mother's blood pressure should be regularly monitored and treated at the earliest so that fetal compromise will not occur, with increase of blood pressure fetal blood supply gets compromised.
  - Timely delivery
  - Babies should be shifted to NICU whenever required and proper care to be taken.

Preeclampsia is hypertension with proteinuria and eclampsia is preeclampsia with seizure activity.

If these develop then continue till the delivery of placenta. These increase both maternal and fetal mortality.

- *Effects on newborn:*
  - Short-term sequelae of hypermagnesemia such as hypotonia or respiratory depression: proper delivery room management and resuscitation are required.
  - Small for gestational age.

Neurological disorder in pregnancy: Epilepsy, stroke, and multiple sclerosis

- Epileptic mothers need to take antiepileptic medicines, which have many teratogenic effects except most of the newer antiepileptic medicines.
- Babies are common with neurodevelopmental deficit.
- Cardiologic structural abnormality is one of the main one.
- Neonatal withdrawal symptom is also common.

Management of the Newborn

- Should be admitted in neonatal intensive care unit (NICU) and carefully monitored.
- Neonates should be monitored regularly for hypoglycemia.
- Vitamin K deficiency is common and so should be given and if required repeated.
- Benefits of breast feed out ways the risk and so mothers should feed their babies.

MATERNAL AUTOIMMUNE DISEASE ON NEWBORN

- The risk of gestational complications, including preterm delivery, intrauterine growth retardation and low birth weight is higher in autoimmune diseases than general population and probably due to maternal disorder and immunosuppressive therapy.
- The most common is maternal lupus.
- Newborns can be affected by maternal lupus and can have neonatal lupus erythematosus.
- Main symptoms are cutaneous, cardiac, and hepatic involvements. In some cases, hematologic and neurologic symptoms are also found.

Management

- Screening of infants born to mothers having SLE is very important.
- Prenatal USG to detect cardiac anomalies.
- Hematological test and skin biopsy are also required in some cases.
- Mortality and morbidity depend on degree of involvement.

MATERNAL MALNUTRITION

- The most common maternal problem in developing countries.
- Poor maternal diet can cause anemia, intrauterine growth restriction, decreased iron, iodine, folic acid, and zinc store in fetus resulting in newborn with small for gestational age.
- It can even cause stillbirth.
- Central nervous system remains immature.

Management

- Nutritional improvement before, during pregnancy and also during breastfeeding.
- Maternal multimicronutrient supplementation has a great role.

MATERNAL DRUG ABUSE ON FETUS

- Depends on the type of drugs.
- The classic signs in new born are: high-pitched cry, tremor and abnormal movement, poor sleep, increased tone, exaggerated Moro's reflex, poorly coordinated feeding, vomiting, failure to thrive, sweating, sneezing, fever, tachycardia, tachypnea, and seizures.
- *Management of the newborns:* Multidisciplinary approach, supportive care, occupational, and physical therapy.
- Withdrawal symptoms are the main effects.
- Short-term opioid therapy is given: morphine is the most common used one, methadone and buprenorphine are also used.
- Clonidine and phenobarbitone are used as second required drug.
- Finnegan and Lipsitz scoring systems are used to initiate, titrate, and weaning of opioid therapy.
- Maternal counseling is required.

■ FURTHER READING

1. Cordero L, Treuer SH, Landon MB, Gabbe SG. Management of infants of diabetec mothers. Arch Pediatr Adolesc Med. 1998;152(3):249-54.
2. Magee LA, Pels A, Helewa M, Rey E, Dadelszen PV. Diagnosis, Evaluation and Management of the Hypertensive Disorders of Pregnancy. Pregnancy Hypertens. 2014;4(2):105-45.
3. Motta M, Perez CR, Tincani A, Lojacono A, Nacinovich R, Chirico G. Neonates born from mothers with autoimmune disorders. Early Hum Dev. 2009;85(Suppl 10):S67-70.
4. Patel SI, Pennell PB. Management of epilepsy during pregnancy: An update. Ther Adv Neurol Disord. 2016;9(2):118-29.
5. Özon A, Tekin N, Siklar Z, Gülcan H, Kara C, Taştekin A, et al. Neonatal effects of thyroid diseases in pregnancy and approach to the infant with increased TSH: Turkish Neonatal and Pediatric Endocrinology and Diabetes Societies consensus report. Turk Pediatri Ars. 2018;53(Suppl1): S209-23.

Amarnath Saran, Shilpa Kalane

81

Chapter

Neonatal Clinical Case Presentation (Clinical Case Proforma for History Taking and Examination)

CHIEF COMPLAINTS

- My baby is baby of (B/O) XYZ (do not disclose the name in history), single/twin [mention birth order, type of twin conception—dichorionic diamniotic/monochorionic diamniotic (DCDA/MCDA)] female/male, born at __ weeks of gestation with a birth weight of __ g by __ (mode of delivery) due to __ [mention indication in case of assisted vaginal delivery/lower segment cesarean section (LSCS)].
- Currently baby is postnatal age (PNA) of __ hours (mention in hours till <5 days) with postmenstrual age (PMA) __ weeks (mention in preterms), is admitted with __ (mention indication for admission like respiratory distress/seizures) and is on __ (respiratory support type/room air).

ANTENATAL HISTORY (MATERNAL HISTORY, PREVIOUS OBSTETRIC HISTORY, AND CURRENT PREGNANCY)

- The baby is born to a ___ old G_P_L_A_ mother [mention previous significant history, abortion/intrauterine fetal demise (IUFD) with gestational age, if any]. This baby is a product of spontaneous/in vitro fertilization (IVF) conception.
- She was booked/unbooked at __ weeks of gestation and took periconceptional folic acid.
- During her first trimester, there is no history of any, fever, rash, or bleeding PV. In her second and third trimester, she took calcium and iron supplementation and had vaccinated with (Td/COVID-19 vaccine).
- She had no history of gestational hypertension/gestational diabetes (mention weeks of gestation at which diagnosed and number of oral medications and insulin if prescribed).
- There was no history of BPV/LPV/PROM (mention duration if present and antibiotics if administered), or history of decreased fetal movements.
- She underwent level 2 USG at 18 weeks of gestation, which was reported as normal/any significant finding (mention any history of fetal distress/oligohydramnios/polyhydramnios).

- Mother's blood group is ...().. positive/negative. The other investigations done during pregnancy like human immunodeficiency virus (HIV) enzyme-linked immune-sorbent assay (ELISA), hepatitis B, Venereal Disease Research Laboratory (VDRL), were reported as normal were reported as normal.
- Any other relevant investigation like TORCH profile, etc.

POSTNATAL COURSE

- Postnatal course should be described system wise, starting with the description of the most common system involve and initial condition and interventions done. End with concluding the present status (*See* **Table 1** for detail history).
- Always mention mother's condition and her participation in baby care at the end of history.

For example, a preterm with respiratory distress syndrome (RDS) and sepsis should be described, as follows:

- The baby developed respiratory distress soon after birth and was shifted to NICU on T-piece resuscitator. Baby was put under open care, started on continuous positive airway pressure (CPAP) with maximum setting required (mention if available) of positive end-expiratory pressure (PEEP)—7 fraction of inspired oxygen (FiO$_2$) —40%, surfactant (dose and type) was administered at 1 HOL by less invasive surfactant administration (LISA) technique.
- As the respiratory distress improved, CPAP settings were tapered and baby was weaned to room air at 48 HOL. In the last 24 hours, baby is on room air with no history of desaturations or apnea.
- In view of preterm premature rupture of the membrane (PPROM), baby was started on IV antibiotics after sending sepsis screen and blood culture. IV antibiotics were stopped after 48 hours as blood culture was suggestive of no growth.
- Baby was started on trophic feeds and total parenteral nutrition (TPN) on day 1 of life. TPN was given for 4 days. Presently baby is on full feeds by orogastric feeding, entirely on mother's own milk (MoM).
- Baby also developed jaundice on day 3 of life, requiring phototherapy for 24 hours. The maximum serum bilirubin was 14 mg/dL, mother's blood group is AB +ve and baby's blood group is B +ve.
- There were no episodes of feed intolerance or hypoglycemia. Neurosonogram done on day 1 and 3 were normal.
- Mother is doing well and visits the baby two to three times daily. Kangaroo mother care (KMC) was started on day 5 and presently baby is getting 5–6 hours of KMC daily.

LABOR AND DELIVERY DETAILS

- Presentation—vertex/breech/transverse
- Fetal distress
- She had spontaneous/induced onset of labor (mention any history of prolonged labor/ ROM duration if <24 hours and antenatal steroid and MgSO$_4$ cover if preterm).

- Amniotic fluid was clear/meconium stained/foul smelling and fetal wellbeing was monitored by cardiotocography (CTG) and intermittent fetal heart auscultation.
- The baby delivered by (mode of delivery) normal vaginal/forceps/vacuum/cesarean section under general/spinal anesthesia (...indication). The baby cried/did not cried immediately after birth and required resuscitation in the form of __ (if done) and was assigned an Apgar score of __, __ and __ at 1, 5, and 10 minutes, respectively.
- Placenta examination was __ (gross and histological). Mention placental weight for preterm/small for gestational age (SGA).

TABLE 1: Disease-specific history: Point needs to be covered during presentation.

Disease	Maternal/antenatal	Delivery details	Postnatal
Preterm/RDS	• PT labor +/- rupture of membranes • PPROM duration • IUGR/oligohydramnios/ Doppler abnormality • Steroid cover—complete/ partial, time since last dose $MgSO_4$ cover antibiotics	• Mode of delivery • Indication for LSCS/AVD • Resuscitation details • DRCPAP with FiO_2 and PEEP given • Delivery room exit temperature and NICU admission temperature (for maintaining euthermia during transport)	• Mode of ventilation— maximum settings required • Surfactant—type, time, and mode of administration, repeat dose required • Duration of respiratory support • Caffeine—when started • Colostrum • Time of starting feeds • Time to attain full feeds • Time to regain birth weight • Time of starting KMC • Features of IVH/NEC/ sepsis
Term/respiratory distress	• Previous unexplained NND/still birth • Prolonged labor • Fetal distress • MSL/foul smelling liquor/ APH • *Triple I feature:* Maternal fever, leukocytosis/fetal tachycardia/purulent fluid as cervical os • GDM • Rh isoimmunization • USG-FGR/ oligohydramnios/ polyhydramnios/CDH • *Drugs:* NSAID/SSRI (PPHN)	• AVD/LSCS (indication) • Difficult extraction • Weak cry • Resuscitation details • Worsening on bag-mask ventilation	• Time of onset and progress of respiratory distress (improving/ worsening) • Associated feed intolerance/seizures/ jitteriness/cyanosis • Maximum ventilatory requirement • Multiple intubations/ prolonged ventilation/ sedation • ECHO findings

Contd...

Contd...

Disease	Maternal/antenatal	Delivery details	Postnatal
HIE	• Postdated pregnancy • HTN/diabetes/infection/hypothyroidism/cardiac disorders • APH • MSL • FGR/multiple gestation—discordance • *Drugs:* $MgSO_4$, GA, and opioids	• *Sentinel events:* Fetal distress/placenta or cord related • Type of delivery with indication • Difficult extraction • PPV—mask/intubation • Chest compression • Drugs—$MgSO_4$, opioids • General anesthesia • Extended Apgar • Cord blood gas	• *Features of MODS:* Shock, PPHN, DIC, decreased urine output, feed intolerance • NNH • Hypoglycemia • *Progression:* Sensorium, tone, and activity • Time of onset of seizures, number of AEDs for control
Jaundice	• Family history—jaundice/anemia/repeated blood transfusion/liver disease • Previous abortion/baby with jaundice/anemia • FGR • Fever/rash during pregnancy • Diabetes • Blood group • Anti-D/Dopplers if Rh negative • Serology HBsAg/HIV	• Instrumentation/birth trauma • Precipitous delivery (polycythemia) • Resuscitation (birth asphyxia)	• Onset of jaundice • Extent of jaundice • Blood group incompatibility • Type of feeding—DBF/top fed • Excessive weight loss • Urine output (number of wet diapers/day) • Sensorium/cry/lethargy/decreased feeding/abnormal movements • Interventions—ET/TPN/NPO

GENERAL NEONATAL EXAMINATION

General condition: Sensorium—normal/drowsy/comatose, activity, and cry: Good/weak/poor and describe about the surrounding/environment:

- *Nursing:* Open care (radiant warmer)/incubator care **(Table 2)**
- Describe about the baby **(Table 3)**
- Describe about the peripheral environment **(Table 4)**

TABLE 2: Nursing: Open care (radiant warmer)/incubator care.

Radiant warmer	Incubator
Servocontrol mode	Servocontrolled (Skin temp controlled)/air mode
Set temperature	Set skin temp (servocontrolled mode)
Measured temperature	Air temperature
Heater output	Relative humidity
Thermistor probe attached	Mention excessive misting/condensation if present

TABLE 3: Describe the baby.

Position	Supine/prone, comment on nesting
Sensorium	Awake/irritable/stuporous/comatose
Pain score	Other pain scores that can be used—PIPP (premature infant pain profile), neonatal facial coding system, neonatal pain and sedation scale (NPASS), and behavioral infant pain profile *(See chapter on Management of Neonatal Pain for details)*
Respiratory support CPAP mask/nasal prongs	• Appropriate size • Snuggly fit • Indenting the nasal septum/hyperemia/blanching Grade of nasal injury (persistent erythema—grade I, superficial ulceration—grade II, and necrosis—grade III)
Tubes/lines/probes	
ETT	• Fixed at __ cm • Well secured, no soakage • Length from mouth to adapter __ cm
OG/NG tube	Fixed at __cm
UVC/UAC/PICC line/ peripheral line	Mention which limb for PICC line Fixed at __cm Mention any discharge/leakage/visible soiling/hyperemia around insertion site
Temperature/pulse oximeter probe	Position

TABLE 4: Describe the peripheral environment (respiratory support, monitor/infusions/phototherapy).

Respiratory support	*Mechanical ventilation:* • Mode • Settings • Humidification chamber—reading temperature, water level • Condensation in expiratory limb • Alarms *Bubble CPAP:* • Settings (PEEP/FiO_2/flow) • Adequate bubbling in chamber, water level • Humidification chamber—reading temperature, water level • Condensation in expiratory limb/inspiratory limb (if any)
Monitor	• Readings • Alarm limits set for SpO_2 and HR • Desaturation/bradycardia during examination
Infusions	• Total number • Mention specific infusions—dextrose, amino acid, lipid, etc. (only names) • Cumulative fluid rate
Phototherapy	• Type and number of phototherapy unit (LED/fluorescent lamp) • Switched off during examination

Vitals

- *Temperature*—set, measured, and axillary, central/peripheral temperature difference (significant/nonsignificant)
- *Heart rate*—rate, volume, femoral pulses, and alarm limit on pulse oximeter
- *Respiratory*—rate and pattern
- *Blood pressure*—systolic blood pressure (SBP), diastolic blood pressure (DBP), mean arterial pressure (MAP), pulse pressure, and mention centiles
- *Color/saturation*—fluctuations, pre-/postductal difference, alarm limit on pulse oximeter, can mention last 24 hours trend
- *Capillary refilling time (CRT)*—normal/abnormal

Anthropometry

- Weight—birth weight, present weight, % of weight loss/gain, cumulative weight loss
- Length, head circumference (HC)—compare at birth and present measurements, mention centiles
- For intrauterine growth restriction (IUGR)—ponderal index, difference between HC and chest circumference
- Plot on growth chart
- Do not perform in critically sick baby

■ GENERAL PHYSICAL EXAMINATION (HEAD-TO-TOE EXAMINATION)

Head	• Shape of skull, symmetry, and swelling • Anterior fontanel—size, level, pulsatility, fullness, and bruit, posterior fontanel, and closure • Sutures • Head circumference • Look for encephalocele, cephalohematoma, and subgaleal hemorrhage • Transillumination test of the head is performed by placing a bright light source with a dark rim on to the scalp surface in a darkened room • The normal zone of transillumination is generally 1–2 cm from the rim of light, and is somewhat larger over the frontal than the parieto-occipital regions
Eyes	• Size, position • Slant • Cataract, subconjunctival hemorrhage, periorbital edema
Ears	• Position—low set • Pre auricular tags, pits • Malformation
Face, mouth, and oral cavity	• Dysmorphism • Asymmetry • Cleft lip/palate • Tongue tie/macroglossia • Oral thrush
Skin	• Color—icterus, pallor, and cyanosis • Mottling • Neurocutaneous markers • Skin score **(Table 5)**

Contd...

Contd...

Limbs	• Position • Movements—symmetrical/asymmetrical • Polydactyly, syndactyly, clinodactyly • Palmar crease • Edema
Umbilicus	• Centrally placed, vessels (2A + 1V) • Any discharge • Umbilical hernia
Genitalia	• *Male:* Penile size, urethral opening, scrotal symmetry, rugosity, and testicular descent • *Female:* Labia majora–minora, urethral opening, hymenal tag, and blood/discharges • Hyperpigmentation
Spine	• Spine curvature • Neural tube defect
Hernial orifices	Intact/herniation

TABLE 5: Neonatal skin condition score (NSCS).

	1	*2*	*3*
Dryness	None	Visible scaling	Cracking/fissures
Erythema	None	<50% body surface	>50% body surface
Breakdown	None	Small, localized area	Extensive

■ SYSTEMIC EXAMINATION

(Describe the relevant system first, other systems if normal, should be described briefly)

RESPIRATORY SYSTEM

Focus on assessment for respiratory distress [Silverman-Anderson score and Downe's Score (SAS and DS)] and support:

- *On mechanical ventilator:*
  - Baby is intubated with endotracheal tube size __ fixed at __ cm with a mouth to adapter distance of __ cm and is kept on SIMV/AC/PSV mode with FiO_2, PEEP, Rate, PIP, Ti, and is receiving warm humidified air. Water level in the chamber is adequate with displayed temperature of __ C. There is no condensation in the inspiratory limb.
  - On these settings, baby looks comfortable/agitated, is well synchronized/asynchrony with the ventilator and has adequate/inadequate chest rise, generating a tidal volume of __mL.
  - There are minimal/significant retractions and Silverman-Andersen retraction score of __ (detail of the score if respiratory distress is significant).
  - Baby's spontaneous respiratory rate is __ min and maintaining a SpO_2 of __ % on right upper limb. On auscultation, the air entry is bilaterally equal and there are no added sounds.
- *On HFOV with nitric oxide:*
  - The baby is intubated with ET size 3.0 fixed at 8 cm with a lip to connector distance of 3 cm and is being supported on HFOV with MAP of __cm of H_2O at frequency __ Hz and amplitude of __ and FiO_2 of __ %.
  - Water level in the chamber is adequate with displayed temperature of 37°C. There is no condensation in the inspiratory limb.

- • With the above settings there is adequate chest wiggling, seen up to the level of umbilicus with saturations of __ % in right upper limb and __ % in right lower limb, receiving FiO_2 __ % and iNO of __ppm.
- *On CPAP/HFNC/NIPPV:*
  - • Baby is on bubble CPAP with PEEP, FiO_2 and flow, with mask as an interface, which is snugly fitted with no evidence of trauma.
  - • There is adequate bubbling in the chamber (or, baby is on HHHFNC with prongs fixed appropriately and leak is audible). There is no evidence of trauma due to interface.
  - • Baby is receiving flow of __L/min and FiO_2 of __%.
  - • Water level in the chamber is adequate with displayed temperature of __ C. There is no condensation in the inspiratory limb and minimal condensation in the expiratory limb.
  - • The baby looks comfortable/has respiratory distress, with respiratory rate of __ and intercostal and xiphoid retractions with SAS of __, maintaining saturation __% in the right upper limb. On auscultation air entry is equal on both sides.

CARDIOVASCULAR SYSTEM

- The baby is pink with HR is __/min with regular rhythmic and normal volume peripheral pulses.
- The femoral pulses are palpable bilaterally. The CFT is __ sec at the sternum and peripheries are warm.
- The BP is in right upper limb is at __th centile as per the Zubrow's chart. Comment on precordial pulsations. Heart sounds are normal, no murmur.
- Urine output is __/kg/h. Baby is receiving __ inotropes if present.
- *Focused examination for PDA:*
  - • *Hyperdynamic circulation*: Prominent precordial pulsations, bounding pulses (easily palpable dorsalis pedis), and wide pulse pressure (>25)
  - • Unexplained weight gain
  - • Persistent tachycardia
  - • Ejection systolic murmur (rarely pansystolic/continuous murmur)
  - • Respiratory distress/recurrent apnea
  - • Increased ventilatory requirements
  - • Hypoperfusion—cold peripheries, central peripheral temperature difference/prolonged CFT/urine output/signs of NEC/sensorium (IVH).

GASTROINTESTINAL SYSTEM

- Abdomen looks flat/moderately protuberant/distended/scaphoid. Umbilicus is centrally placed. Mention any abdominal wall defects (omphalocele/gastroschisis), erythema, meconium staining, or discharge from umbilical stump.
- Bowel sounds are normal (auscultation should be done before proceeding for palpation of abdomen in neonates).
- Abdomen is soft, nontender. Mention any hepatosplenomegaly/palpable mass (liver may be palpable up to 1–2 cm in a healthy neonate).
- Tolerating __ mL feeds every 2nd hourly. Passed stool/meconium.
- *Focused examination for NEC:*
  - • Gastric residues
  - • Abdominal distension

- Abdominal wall erythema
- Blood in stool
- Absent bowel sounds
- Tenderness
- Right lower quadrant palpable mass

■ NEUROLOGICAL EXAMINATION

S. No.	Outline of neonatal neurological examination
1.	Gestational age estimation
2.	Observation and level of alertness
3.	Cranial nerves
4.	Motor examination
5.	Sensory examination

Gestational age estimation:

Prenatal assessment:

- Naegele's rule for estimating the EDD—the EDD can be calculated by counting back 3 months from the last menstrual period (LMP) and adding 7 days
- Dating scan—crown-rump length (CRL) measured in the first trimester (up to 13^+6 weeks), if available, is the most accurate sonographic method of determining the EDD. It is accurate within ±5–7 days

Postnatal assessment:

Dubowitz method:

- Incorporates 34 physical and neurologic assessments
- Overestimates the gestation age
- Tedious and time consuming

Ballard method:

- Shortened the Dubowitz method to depend upon six physical and six neurologic criteria
- Most reliable when the examination is performed between 30 and 42 hours of age
- Easier to perform and quick
- May be inaccurate in infants who are preterm, post-term, or small for gestational age

New Ballard method:

- Modified to improve assessment of infants as preterm as 20 weeks
- Can be used in infants from 20 to 44 weeks gestation
- Correlation is best if done prior to 12 hours in infants <26 weeks
- Overestimates gestational age by 1.3–3.3 weeks

Rapid assessment of gestation age:

- Uses a few, select physical or neurologic elements of the Ballard (or Dubowitz) method

- *Eye examination:*
- The disappearance of the anterior vascular capsule of the lens occurs in an orderly sequence between 27 and 34 weeks gestation
- The disappearance of the vascular system is divided into four grades that correlate with gestational age
- The correlation between the grade and gestational age is highly significant and is independent of IUGR

Electroencephalography (EEG):
- The maturational progression of EEG background activity

MATURATIONAL ASSESSMENT OF GESTATIONAL AGE (new Ballard Score)

Name _______________________ Sex _______________________
Hospital No. _______________________ Birth weight _______________________
Race _______________________ Length _______________________
Date/time of birth _______________________ Head CIRC. _______________________
Date/time of exam _______________________ Examiner _______________________
Age when examined _______________________
APGAR score: Minute __________ 5 minutes __________ 10 minutes __________

NEUROMUSCULAR MATURITY

Neuromuscular maturity sign	Score							Record score here
	-1	0	1	2	3	4	5	
Posture								
Square window (wrist)	>90°	90°	60°	45°	30°	0°		
Arm recoil		180°	140–180°	110–140°	90–110°	<90°		
Popliteal angle	180°	160°	140°	120°	100°	90°	<90°	
Scarf sign								
Heel to ear								

Total neuromuscular maturity score

PHYSICAL MATURITY

Physical maturity sign	Score							Record score here
	-1	0	1	2	3	4	5	
Skin	Sticky friable transparent	Gelatinous red translucent	Smooth pink visible veins	Superficial peeling and/or rash, few veins	Cracking pale areas rare veins	Parchment deep cracking no vessels	Leathery cracked wrinkled	
Lanugo	None	Sparse	Abundant	Thinning	Bald areas	Mostly bald		
Plantar surface	Heel-toe 40–50 mm: -1 <40 mm: -2	>50 mm no crease	Faint red marks	Anterior transverse crease only	Creases ant. 2/3	Creases over entire sole		
Breast	Imperceptible	Barely perceptible	Flat areola no bud	Stippled areola 1–2 mm bud	Raised areola 3–4 mm bud	Full areola 5–10 mm bud		
Eye/ear	Lids fused Loosely: -1 Tightly: -2	Lids open pinna flat stays folded	Sl. curved pinna; soft; slow recoil	Well-curved pinna; soft but ready recoil	Formed and firm instant recoil	Thick cartilage ear stiff		
Genitals (male)	Scrotum flat, smooth	Scrotum empty faint rugae	Testes in upper canal rare rugae	Testes descending few rugae	Testes down good rugae	Testes pendulous deep rugae		
Genitals (female)	Clitoris prominent and labia flat	Prominent clitoris and small labia minora	Prominent clitoris and enlarging minora	Majora and minora equally prominent	Majora large minora small	Majora cover clitoris and minora		

Total physical maturity score

Score
Neuromuscular ___
Physical __________
Total __________

Maturity rating

Score	Weeks
-10	20
-5	22
0	24
5	26
10	28
15	30
20	32
25	34
30	36
35	38
40	40
45	42
50	44

Gestational age (weeks)

By dates__________
By ultrasound__________
By exam__________

Source: Ballard JL, Khoury JC, Wedig K, Wang L, Eilers-Walsman BL, Lipp R. New Ballard score, expanded to include extremely premature infants. J Pediatr. 1991;119(3):417-23.

OBSERVATION AND LEVEL OF ALERTNESS

- It is important to first determine the neonate's baseline state of consciousness or behavioral state.
- Reactions to stimulation can vary depending on the neonate's state of consciousness.
- Observation is considered by some experts to be the most important neonatal neurological examination technique.
- Observation is best performed when the neonate is in a *quiet alert state*, which most frequently occurs between feedings.
- Ideally, the neonate should be *lying supine, unclothed in a warm room with the head in midline with no confining rolls or boundaries.*
- This position allows for the accurate assessment of a neonate's resting posture, spontaneous movements, and limb position.
- Lighting should be adequate to facilitate observation; excessive light should be avoided as this may cause agitation.

Questions to be Consider during Observation

- What is the neonate's state of consciousness (awake/sleep state)?
- What is the neonate's level of alertness (e.g., normal, stupor, and coma)?
- Are there dysmorphic features?
- What is the neonate's eye position?
- Are eye movements symmetrical?
- Is there facial symmetry?
- What position are the limbs in at rest?
- Are there spontaneous limb movements?
- Do the limb movements appear similar on each side?
- Are skin lesions present?

Features of Neonatal Behavioral State—Prechtl and O'Brien

State	Eyes open	Respiration regular	Gross movements	Vocalization
1. (Deep or quiet sleep)	−1	+1	−1	−1
2. (Light or REM sleep)	−1	−1	0	−1
3. (Awake, drowsy, and dozing)	+1	+1	−1	−1
4. (Quiet, eyes open)	+1	−1	+1	−1
5. (Alert, vigorous movement)	0	−1	+1	+1
6. (Cry)	+1	−1	+1	+1

+1, present; −1, absent; 0, present or absent.

Level of Alertness Description

- *Normal neonate* responds normally to arousal and this arousal response is associated with normal motor movements of the limbs and face.

> - *Slight to moderate stupor neonate* is sleepy (slight) or asleep (moderate) with diminished or absent arousal and motor responses (slight or moderate).
> - *Deep stupor or coma neonate* cannot be aroused; motor responses are diminished or absent (coma).
> - *Irritable neonate* cannot be soothed, is agitated, and cries with minimal stimulation.
> - *Lethargic neonate* is unable to maintain an alert state.

Items Assessing Behavior

Eye appearances	Does not open eyes		Full conjugated eye movements	*Transient:* • Nystagmus • Strabismus • Roving eye movements • Sunset sign	*Persistent:* • Nystagmus • Strabismus • Roving eye movements • Abnormal pupils
Auditory orientation: Infant awake; Wrap infant; Hold rattle 10–15 cm from ear	No reaction	Auditory startle; brightens and stills; no true orientation	Shifting of eyes; head might turn towards source	Prolonged head turn to stimulus; search with eyes; smooth	Turns head and eyes towards noise every time; jerky abrupt
Visual orientation: Wrap infant, wake-up with rattle if needed or rock gently. Note if baby can see and follow red ball (B) or target (T)	Does not follow or focus on stimuli B T	Stills, focuses, follows briefly to the side but loses stimuli B T	Follows horizontally and vertically; no head turns B T	Follows in a circle B T	
Alertness: Tested as response to visual stimuli (B or T)	Will not respond to stimuli	When awake, looks only briefly	When awake, looks at stimuli but loses them	Keeps interest in stimuli	Does not tire (hyperreactive)
Irritability: In response to stimuli	Quiet all the time, not irritable to any stimuli	Awakes, cries sometimes when handled	Cries often when handled	Cries always when handled	Cries even when not handled
Consolability Ease to quiet infant	Not crying; consoling not needed	Cries briefly; consoling not needed	Cries; becomes quiet when talked to	Cries; needs picking up to console	Cries cannot be consoled
Cry	No cry at all	Whimpering cry only	Cries to stimuli but normal pitch		High pitched cry; often continuous

Source: Dubowitz L, Ricciw D, Mercuri E. The Dubowitz neurological examination of the full-term newborn. Ment Retard Dev Disabil Res Rev. 2005;11(1):52-60.

■ CRANIAL NERVE EXAMINATION

Cranial nerve	Function	Testing in the newborn	Normal neonatal response
Olfactory (I)	Smell	• Rarely tested • If tested, nutrient (breast milk or formula) odor exposure via a pacifier	• Change in behavior such as grimacing, startle, and sucking • Response present >32 weeks' gestation
Optic (II)	Vision	• Shine light in peripheral visual field • Fundoscopic examination • Move a bright object side to side (e.g., red ball) • 10–12 inches from neonate's eyes	• ≥28 weeks' gestation: blinks in response to light • Optic disk is pale whitish grey • ≥34 weeks' gestation: Able to fix and follow
Oculomotor (III)	Pupillary response and extraocular movements (EOMs)	• Check pupillary light reflex • Assess spontaneous eye movements and symmetry	• Pupil size 3–4 mm • Pupillary reaction • 30 weeks—light reaction begins • 30 weeks to term gestation—the amplitude of the pupillary response increases • EOMs as described with IVth and VIth cranial nerves
Trochlear (IV) and abducent (VI)	EOMs	Assess spontaneous eye movements and symmetry	• *Eye position*—observe the light reflected off each pupil with the light source in the midline at approximately 2 feet from the face • *Doll's eye maneuver test* (demonstrable by 25 weeks)—moving the head and neck from side to side, which leads to eye deviation to the opposite side • *Vertical spin*—spin the baby held upright; the eyes will deviate in a direction opposite to the spin • *Caloric stimulation test* (demonstrable by 30 weeks)—caloric stimulation with cold water leads to deviation of the eyes toward the side of the stimulated ear

Contd...

Contd...

Cranial nerve	Function	Testing in the newborn	Normal neonatal response
Trigeminal (V)	Facial sensation, sucking	• Rooting reflex • Sucking reflex	Rooting reflex and suck present
Facial (VII)	Facial motility, sucking	• Observe facial symmetry at rest and with crying • (Forehead wrinkling, nasolabial folds, deviation of angle of mouth, lagophthalmos)	Symmetry present
Vestibulocochlear (VIII)	Hearing	• Assess response to loud noises (e.g., clapping, bell, and crumpled paper)	≥28 weeks' gestation: Blink or startle
• *Glosso-pharyngeal (IX)* • *Vagus (X)*	Swallowing, gag	• Observe for swallowing • Test gag with a small tongue blade or during suctioning	• Gag reflex, swallowing present • ≥34 weeks' gestation: breathing, sucking, and swallowing synchrony begins
Spinal accessory (XI)	Sternocleido-mastoid muscle function	• Gently turn head side to side • Compare shoulder height	• Head turns side to side without difficulty • Symmetrical shoulder height
Hypoglossal (XII)	Tongue function	Assess for tongue symmetry and fasciculations	Tongue symmetry present without fasciculation

Summary:
• Olfaction (I)
• Vision (II)
• Optic fundi (II)
• Pupils (III)
• Extraocular movements (III, IV, and VI)
• Facial sensation and masticatory power (V)
• Facial motility (VII)
• Audition (VIII)
• Sucking and swallowing (V, VII, IX, X, and XII)
• Sternocleidomastoid function (XI)
• Tongue function (XII)
• Taste (VII and IX)

■ MOTOR EXAMINATION

- Predominantly includes muscle tone and the posture of limbs, motility and muscle power, and the tendon reflexes and plantar response.
- Pioneers in the field of neonatal neurological examination were Saint-Anne Dargassies and Amiel-Tison in the 1960's.

Methods of assessment of tone	Approach
Amiel-Tison (tone and reflexes)	• It consists of assessing the infant in terms of spontaneous posture (assessed when the baby lies undisturbed), passive tone (by applying certain maneuvers to an extremity and the resistance is measured as adductor angle, popliteal angle, scarf sign), and active tone (examined with the infant moving spontaneously in response to a given stimulus, e.g., pull to sit) • It consists of assessing the infant in terms of (1) head growth and cranial sutures, (2) alertness evaluated on visual fixation and track, (3) passive tone in limbs and axis, and (4) axial motor activity (active tone)
Prechtl method (generalized movements)	
Brazelton scale (behavioral assessment)	
Dubowitz	• Does not need training. The bedside examination consists of 34 items organized into six groups: Tone, tone patterns, reflexes, movements, abnormal signs, and behaviors • An abbreviated screening tool based on the full Dubowitz examination has been proposed for use in screening all term infants, with a modified screening tool developed for screening all preterm infants at term age
The Hammersmith neonatal neurological examination (HNNE) **(Table 6)**	• It is a quick, practical, and easy to perform examination encompassed in 34 items assessing tone, motor patterns, observation of spontaneous movements, reflexes, visual, auditory attention, and behavior • It is best used for evaluation of term born "normal" neonates in maternity ward/first follow-up in a busy follow-up clinic • If two items are in "blocked/shaded area", the neonate should have a detailed assessment

TABLE 6: Hammersmith neonatal neurological examination.

- Hammersmith neonatal neurological examination (HNNE) is a quick, practical, and easy to perform examination encompassed in 34 items assessing tone, motor patterns, observation of spontaneous movements, reflexes, visual and auditory attention, and behavior.
- Short HNNE Proforma for newborn term infants and preterm infants at term equivalent age.

	Warning signs				*Warning signs*
Posture	Arms and legs extended or very slightly flexed	Less slightly flexed (for 25–27 weeks only)	Leg well flexed but not adducted	Leg well flexed and adducted near abdomen	*Abnormal posture:* Opisthotonos Arm flexed legs extended
Arm traction	Arms remain straight, no resistance	Arms flex slightly or no resistance felt	Arms flex well till shoulder lifts, then straighten	Arms flex at approximately 100 degree and maintained as shoulder lifts	Flexion of arms 100 degree, maintained when body lifts up
Leg traction	Legs straight— no resistance	Knees flex slightly or some resistance felt	Knees flex well till bottom lifts up	Knees flex and remain flexed when bottom up	Knee flexion stays when back and bottom up
Head control (1)	No attempt to raise head	*Infant tries:* effort better felt than seen	Raises head but drops forward or back	*Raises head:* Remains vertical; it may wobble	
Head control (2)	No attempt to raise head	*Infant tries:* Effort better felt than seen	Raises head but drops forward or back	*Raises head:* Remains vertical; it may wobble	Head remains upright or neck extended; cannot be passively flexed
Head lag	Head drops and stays back	Tries to lift head but it drops back	Able to lift head slightly	Lifts head in line with body	Head in front of line of body

Contd...

Contd...

Ventral suspension	Back curved, head and limbs hang straight	Back curved, head hang straight, limbs slightly flexed	Back slightly curved, limbs flexed	Back straight, head in line with back, limbs flexed	Back straight, head above line of body
Spontaneous movement (quality)	Only stretches	Stretches and random abrupt movements, some smooth movements	Fluent movements but monotonous	Fluent alternating movements of arms + legs; good variability	• Cramped synchronized • Mothing • Jerky or other abnormal movements
Tremor		No or only when crying	Only after Moro or occasionally when awake	Frequent tremors when awake	Continuous tremors
Moro's reflex	No or opening of hands only	Full abduction at shoulder and extension of arms; no adduction	Full abduction but only delayed or partial adduction	Partial abduction at shoulder and extension of arms followed by smooth adduction	• No abduction or adduction • Only forward extension of arms from the shoulder • Marked adduction only
Visual orientation	Does not follow or follows briefly to the side but loses stimuli **B T**	Follows horizontally and vertically, no head turn **B T**	Follows horizontally and vertically; turns head **B T**	Follows in a circle **B T**	
Abnormal signs	Facial palsy **Y N**	Abn eye movements **Y N**	Sunset sign **Y N**	Fisted hand (s) **Y N**	Clonus **Y N**

A modified screening tool based on the Dubowitz neonatal neurological examination. This tool may be used for neonates at term equivalent age, regardless of gestational age at birth. Normal findings are indicated by the middle gray columns. "Warning" signs are in the unshaded columns at each far side.
Source: Wusthoff CJ. How to use: The neonatal neurological examination. Arch Dis Child Educ Pract Ed. 2013;98(4):148-53. http://www.hammersmith-neuro-exam.com/

■ MODIFIED DUBOWITZ NEUROLOGICAL EXAMINATION

Item to be assessed

Posture assessment:

- Posture is tone at rest. Passive tone, which influences the posture a neonate assumes, increases with gestational age and follows a caudocephalic direction (e.g., flexion in the lower extremities is followed by flexion in the upper extremities).
- Placing the neonate in a supine position on a flat surface with no confining rolls or boundaries.
- Placing the head in midline position to avoid stimulating asymmetries associated with the tonic neck reflex.
- Uncovering the neonate to allow for full visualization.
- Carefully observing limb position, the number and quality of spontaneous movements, and symmetry of movements.
- Assessing the neonate's thumb positioning. A thumb-in-fist posture is the predominant hand position in term neonates.
- The hands should intermittently loosely open spontaneously. Over the first few months of life, the fists gradually become loosely closed to allow for voluntary grasping.

Posture Infant supine, look mainly at position of legs but also note arms. *Score predominant posture*	Arms and legs extended or very slightly flexed	Legs slightly flexed	Leg well-flexed but not adducted	Leg well flexed and adducted near abdomen	*Abnormal posture:* Opistotonus

Assessing limb tone

Arm recoil Take both hands, quickly extend arms parallel to the body, count to three. Release. Repeat × 3	Arms do not flex	Arms flex slowly, not always; not completely	Arms flex slowly, more complete	Arms flex quickly and complete	Arms difficult to extend; snap back forcefully
Arm traction Hold wrist and pull arm upwards. Note flexion at elbow and resistance while shoulder lifts off table *Test each side separately*	Arms remain straight; no resistance felt R L	Arms flex slightly or some resistance felt R L	Arms flex well till shoulder lifts, then straighten R L	Arms flex at approx 100° and maintained as shoulder lifts R L	Flexion of arms <100° and maintained when body lifts up R L

Contd...

Contd...

	No flexion 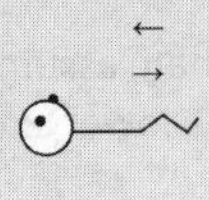	Incomplete or variable flexion 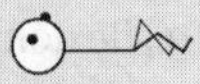	Complete but slow flexion 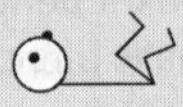	Complete fast flexion 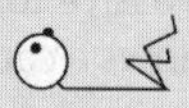	Legs difficult to extend; snap back forcefully
Leg recoil Take *both* ankles in one hand, flex hips+ knees. Quickly extend. Release. Repeat × 3					
Leg traction Grasp ankle and slowly pull leg upwards. Note flexion at knees and resistance as buttocks lift *Test each side separately*	Legs straight; no resistance felt	Legs flex slightly or some resistance felt	Legs flex well till bottom lifts up	Knee flexes remains flexed when bottom up	Flexion stays when back+bottom up
	R L	R L	R L	R L	R L
Popliteal angle Fix knee on abdomen, extend leg by gentle pressure with index finger behind the ankle. Note angle at knee. *Test each side separately*	180°	= 150°	= 110°	= 90°	< 90°
	R L	R L	R L	R L	R L

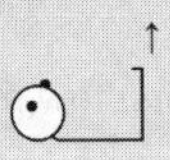

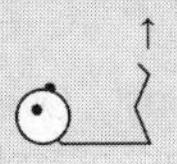

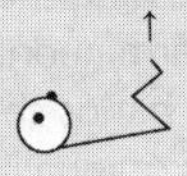

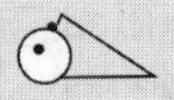

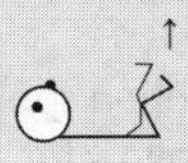

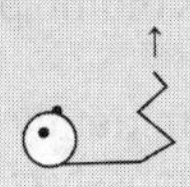

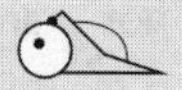

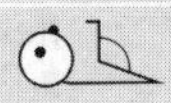

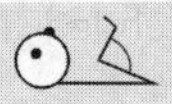

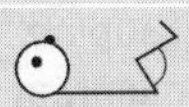

Assessing axial tone

	No attempt to raise head 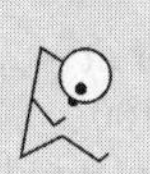	Infant tries: Effort better felt than seen 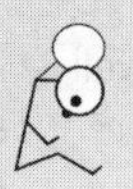	Raises heads but drops forward or back 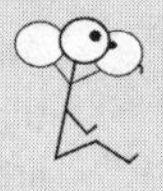	Raise head: Remains vertical; it may wobble 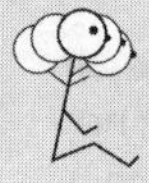	
Head control (1) *(extensor tone)* Infant sitting upright; Encircle chest with both hands holding shoulders Let head drop forward					
Head control (2) *(flexor tone)* Infant sitting upright Encircle chest with both hands holding shoulders Let head drop backward	No attempt to raise head 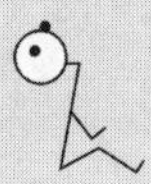	Infant tries: Effort better felt than seen 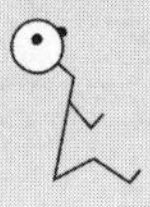	Raises heads but drops forward or back 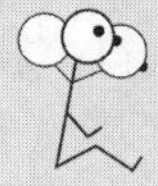	Raises head: Remains vertical; it may wobble 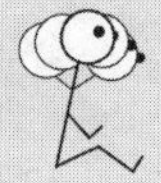	Head upright or extended; cannot be passively flexed

Contd...

Contd...

Head lag Pull infant to towards sitting posture by traction on both wrists and support head slightly. Also note arm flexion	Head drops and stays back	Tries to lift head but it drops back	Able to lift head slightly	Lift head in line with body	Head in front of body
Ventral suspension Hold infant in ventral suspension; observe back, flexed of limbs and relation of head to trunk. If it looks different DRAW	Back curved, head and limbs hang straight	Back curved, head ↓, limbs slightly flexed	Back slightly curved, limbs flexed	Back straight, head in line, limbs flexed	Back straight, head above body

Source: Dubowitz L, Ricciw D, Mercuri E. The Dubowitz neurological examination of the full-term newborn. Ment Retard Dev Disabil Res Rev. 2005;11(1):52-60.

Interpretation of:
The Dubowitz screening tool consists of 12–14 items on a one-page proforma. It is best performed when the newborn is calm and awake, ideally between feeds.
- *Two or more abnormal findings*—consider "warning signs", warranting full neurological examination
- *Multiple abnormal findings on examination*—need for further evaluation for neurological abnormality
- *A normal full Dubowitz examination or one with 1–2 abnormal single exam items*—rules out 1-year neurological outcome for an individual child with very good accuracy.

Prechtl system:
First 8 weeks—writhing movements are prominent
- 8–20 weeks CA—fidgety movements prominent
- >20 weeks CA—fidgety movements evolve concurrent with neuromaturation and resolve by 20 weeks of age (swipes and swats)
- Absence of fidgety movements at a time when they should be normally present is predictive of major long-term neurologic sequelae

■ NEONATAL REFLEXES

Deep tendon reflexes (an examiner's finger that is placed over the tendon to be tested can be lightly struck with a percussion hammer to elicit the reflex)	• Can be elicited in the newborn infant generally after 33 weeks gestation • *Jaw*—tapping the chin with the mouth slightly open leads to slight jaw closure • *Biceps*—with the elbow flexed, tapping the biceps tendon in the antecubital fossa leads to flexion at the elbow • *Brachioradialis (supinator)*—tapping above the wrist on the radial aspect of the forearm leads to flexion at the elbow • *Knee (patellar)*—tapping the quadriceps tendon below the patella leads to extension of the knee • *Ankle clonus* of 5–10 beats also should be accepted
Superficial reflexes	• *Abdominal reflexes*—in each of the four quadrants of the abdomen are elicited by gentle stroking in an axial to peripheral direction, resulting in contraction of the abdominal wall • *Cremasteric reflex*—stroking the inner thigh area in an anterior to posterior direction, which results in ipsilateral scrotal retraction and testicular rise due to contraction of the scrotal dartos muscle • *Anal wink reflex*—gentle stroking of the perianal region, which results in contraction of the perianal muscle • *Corneal reflex*—gentle, tactile stimulation of the cornea with a tissue paper results in an ipsilateral and consensual blink response • *Extensor plantar response (Babinski)*—physiologic. Elicited by stroking the lateral plantar surface of the foot with a pointed but not sharp object

Primitive reflexes (developmental reflexes):
- They are mediated at the brainstem or spinal cord level and are generally present at birth
- Persist beyond the age by which they should have normally disappeared
- Abnormal if:
  - Absent during the neonatal period
  - Asymmetric (suggesting hemiplegia or monoplegia).

Reflex	Onset (in utero in weeks)	How to elicit reflex	Integrates (i.e., suppressed/ inhibited
Palmer grasp	28	Place finger in palm	5–6 months Allows for voluntary grasping
Asymmetric Tonic Neck Reflex (ATNR)	35	Neonate in the supine position, the head is turned to one side	6 months Allows for rolling over and reaching or grasping
Moro	28	Sudden drop of the neonate's head and shoulders a few inches in relation to their trunk into the examiner's hands	6–8 months Allows for sitting
Plantar grasp	28	Touch ball of foot with thumb causing toes to curl down	• 7–9 months • Allows for standing and walking
Rooting	28	Stroke cheek near mouth causing head to turn toward stimulus	3 months
Sucking	26–28	Touch lips with gloved finger or soother	10–12 months
Swallowing	12	Observe for swallowing	• 32–34 weeks • Stronger synchronization with sucking

■ ITEMS ASSESSING REFLEXES

	Absent	Felt, not seen	Seen	'Exaggerated'	Clonus
Tendon reflex Test biceps, knee and ankle jerks					
Suck/gag Little finger into mouth with pulp of finger upwards	No gag/no suck	• Weak irregular suck only • No stripping	Weak regular suck Some stripping	*Strong suck:* (a) Irregular (b) Regular Good stripping	No suck but strong clenching
Palmar grasp Put index finger into the hand and gently press palmar surface. Do not touch dorsal surface	No response R　　　L	Short, weak flexion of fingers R　　　L	Strong flexion of fingers R　　　L	Strong finger flexion, shoulder ↑ R　　　L	Very strong grasp; infant can be lifted off couch R　　　L
Plantar grasp Press thumb on the sole below the toes	No response R　　L	Partial plantar flexion of toes R　　L	Toes curve around the examiner's finger R　　L		
Placing Lift infant in an upright position and stroke the dorsum of the foot against a protruding edge of a flat surface. *Test each side separately*	No response R　　　L	Dorsiflexion of ankle only R　　L	Full placing response with flexion of hip, knee and placing sole on surface R　　　L		
Moro One hand supports infant's head in midline, the other the back. Raise infant to 45° and when relaxed, let his head fall through 10°. Note if jerky. Repeat 3 time	No response or opening of hands only	Full abduction at shoulder and extension of the arms; no adduction	Full abduction but only delayed or partial adduction	Partial abduction at shoulder and extension of arms followed by smooth adduction	• No abduction of adduction • Only forward extension of arms from the shoulders • Marked adduction only or

Source: Dubowitz L, Ricciw D, Mercuri E. The Dubowitz neurological examination of the full-term newborn. Ment Retard Dev Disabil Res Rev. 2005;11(1):52-60.

SENSORY SYSTEM

- The neonatal assessment of sensation is challenging because it is difficult to accurately determine an infant's response to sensory stimuli.
- As a result, sensory assessment is limited or not generally performed as part of the neonatal neurologic examination.
- Perioral tactile sensation can be evaluated by the rooting response.

DIAGNOSIS ON ADMISSION

Single/multiple/gestation in weeks/weight in grams/SGA or AGA or LGA/sex/add neonatal disease as per system involvement.

MANAGEMENT PLAN (INVESTIGATION AND TABCFMC)

- Temperature
- Airway
- Breathing
- Circulation
- Fluid and feeding
- Medication and monitoring
- Communication and follow-up

FREQUENTLY ASKED QUESTIONS (FAQS) DURING CLINICAL CASE PRESENTATION IN EXAMINATION

WHAT IS CONSOLABILITY?

- Consolability is easiest to assess in a crying infant.
- Number of techniques are used to try to calm the infant within 15 seconds are infant sucking on a pacifier or the examiner's finger, holding, rocking, placing a hand on the infant's belly, restraining one or both arms of the infant, soothing by voice, or a combination of a soothing voice and the examiner's face approaching the infant.

WHAT IS HABITUATION?

- Habituation is a marker of cortical inhibitory function and measures the infant's ability to learn to diminish his/her response to repetitive stimuli. The use of repeating light or auditory stimuli are used to test for habituation.
- The shining of a soft light initially elicits a blinking response that diminishes in intensity over the first four to five trials, and afterward ceases with subsequent trials.
- Similarly, auditory stimuli, such as handclaps, elicit a startle response to the first four or five stimuli, after which there is little to no response.

WHAT ARE NEONATAL NEUROLOGICAL ALARM SIGNS?

- Persistent irritability
- Difficulty in feeding
- Persistent deviation of head and/or eye
- Persistent asymmetry in posture and movement
- Persistently abducted thumbs in a fisted hand
- Persistent posture of flexed arm and extended legs
- Opisthotonos posture
- Floppiness, severe generalized hypotonia
- Convulsion
- Abnormal cry
- Sun setting signs (hydrocephalous)

Key Points to Remember

Before history taking and clinical examination:
- Obtain basic information about the mother and baby.
- Introduce yourself to the mother and explain what you are doing.
- Purpose of the examination is to answer any question that the mother may raise.
- Examination, if possible should be always be done in her presence
- Observe the mother's attitude toward baby and whether she is confident, happy, tense, or withdrawn.

Clinical case presentation before the examiner, revise your history and examination and it is useful to have a mental checklist of the following information:
- Baby's sex, birth weight, and GA
- Mother's age and social background
- Is there any chronic maternal disease? If so, what treatment is the mother receiving?
- Is there any possibly relevant family history?
- The outcome of any previous pregnancies.
- Was the pregnancy normal? Were there any complications?
- Any pregnancy screening tests, e.g., 20-week ultrasound scan?
- Were any special diagnostic procedures, e.g., amniocentesis performed?
- Were there any signs of fetal distress during labor?
- What drugs and/or anesthesia were given during labor and delivery?
- How was the baby delivered?
- Was there a breech presentation after 36 weeks (an indication for a hip scan)?
- What was baby's condition at birth (Apgar scores at 1 and 5 minutes, cord pH)?
- Was any resuscitation needed? After how long-sustained respiration was established?
- Was the baby in the neonatal unit? If so, why?
- How is the mother planning to feed the baby, and how is the feeding going?

Demonstration of clinical examination before the examiner:
- The order of the examination performed is largely a matter of personal preferences. However, a proposed order of examination is given below.

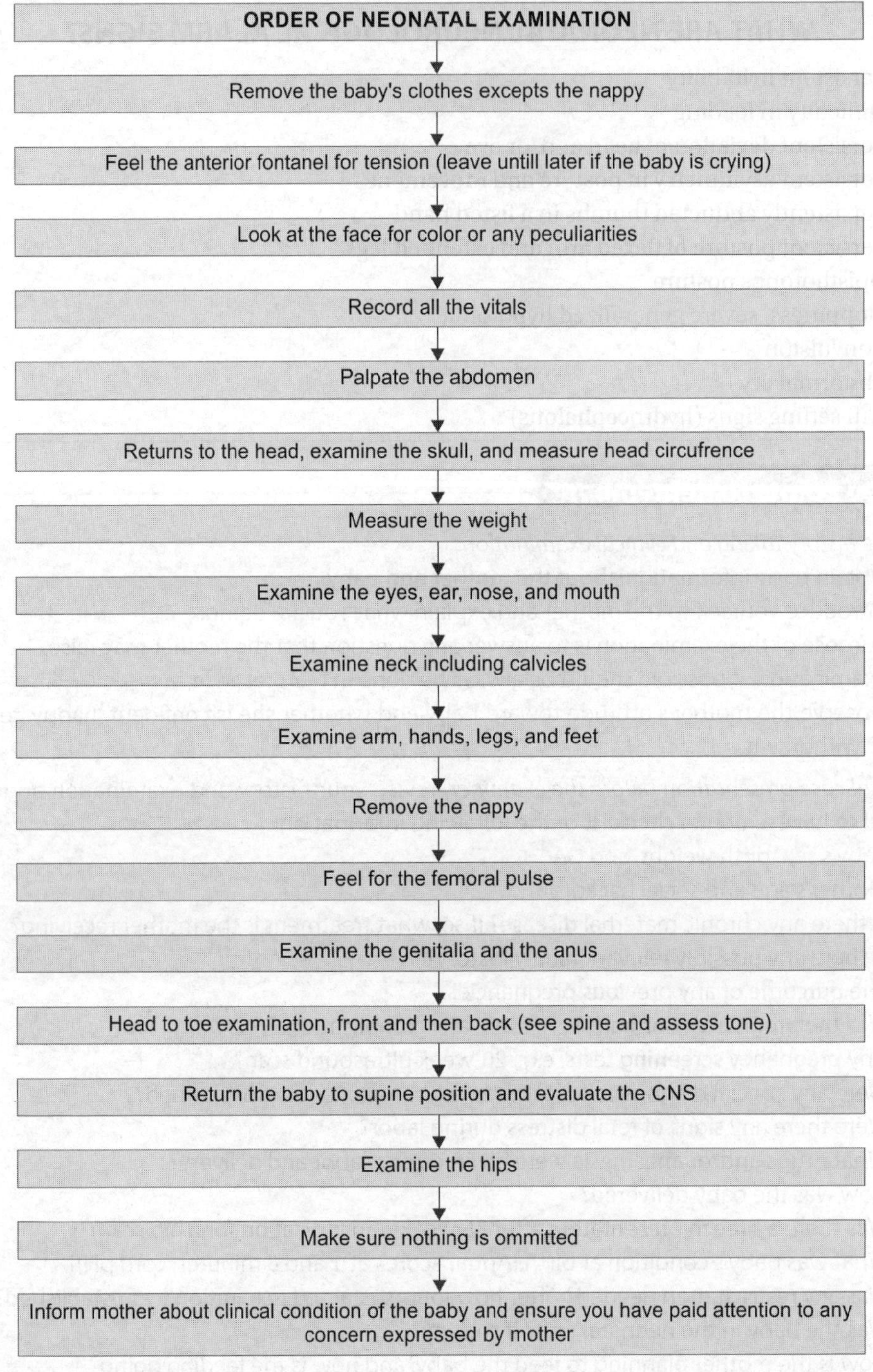

ORDER OF NEONATAL EXAMINATION
Remove the baby's clothes excepts the nappy
Feel the anterior fontanel for tension (leave untill later if the baby is crying)
Look at the face for color or any peculiarities
Record all the vitals
Palpate the abdomen
Returns to the head, examine the skull, and measure head circufrence
Measure the weight
Examine the eyes, ear, nose, and mouth
Examine neck including calvicles
Examine arm, hands, legs, and feet
Remove the nappy
Feel for the femoral pulse
Examine the genitalia and the anus
Head to toe examination, front and then back (see spine and assess tone)
Return the baby to supine position and evaluate the CNS
Examine the hips
Make sure nothing is ommitted
Inform mother about clinical condition of the baby and ensure you have paid attention to any concern expressed by mother

S. No.	Checklist of neonatal examination		Yes	No
1.	Chief complaints			
2.	Antenatal history			
3.	Labor and delivery history			
4.	Post-natal history/course during hospital stay			
5.	General examination	General condition of the baby		
		Vitals		
		Anthropometry		
		General physical examination (head to toe)		
6.	Systemic examination	Respiratory system		
		Cardiovascular system		
		Gastrointestinal system		
		Neurological system		
		Any other system: Only relevant based on case		
7.	Diagnosis on admission/differential diagnosis (DD)			
8.	Management plan including investigation			
9.	Final outcome			

■ FURTHER READING

1. Gleason CA, Devaskar SU. Examination of the normal newborn. Avery's Diseases of the Newborn, 9th edition. Philadelphia: Elsevier; 2012.
2. Martin RJ, Fanaroff AA, Walsh MC. Physical examination of the newborn, Neonatal and perinatal medicine. Fanaroff & Martin's Neonatal-Perinatal Medicine, 11th edition. Philadelphia: Elsevier; 2019.
3. Rennie JM. Rennie and Roberton's Textbook of Neonatology, 5th edition. Edinburgh: Churchill Livingstone Elsevier. London, UK; 2012.
4. Volpe J, Inder T, Darras B, de Vries L, du Plessis A, Neil J. Neurological examination. Volpe's Neurology of the Newborn, 6th edition. Philadelphia: Elsevier; 2017.

Neonatal Screening

Varun Vij

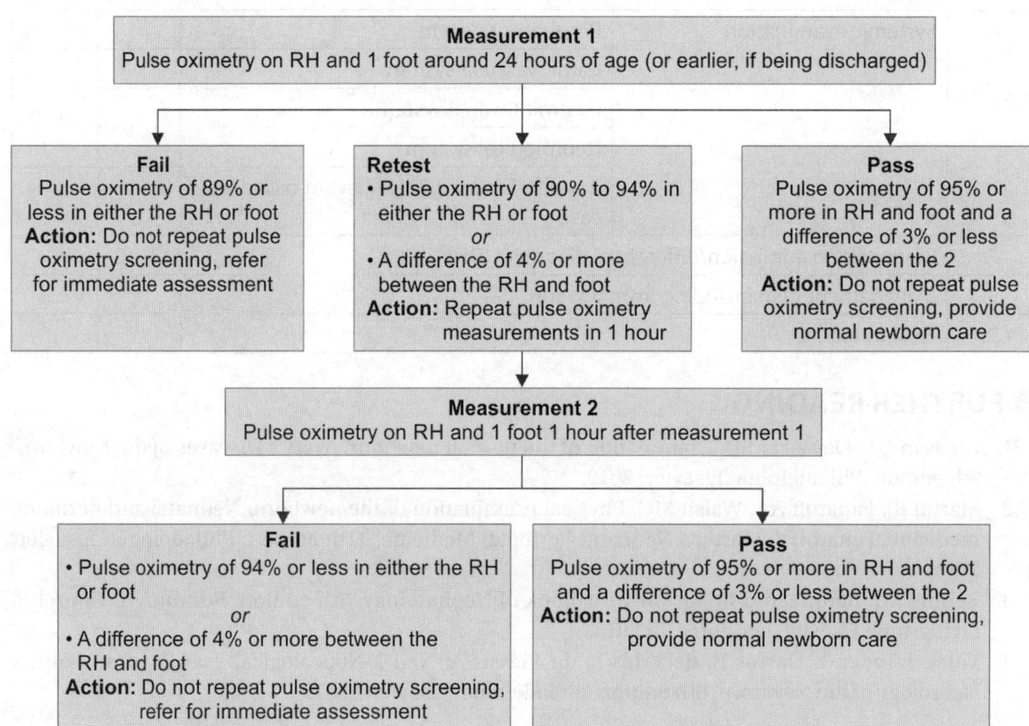

SCREENING FOR CRITICAL CONGENITAL HEART DISEASE

- Congenital heart disease (CHD) is common birth defects, occurring in approximately 1% of newborns, i.e., 8/1,000 births.
- Critical congenital heart disease (CCHD) is heart lesions for which early surgical interventions are required for the baby to survive.
- It is of paramount importance to screen all the newborns for these critical heart conditions around birth preferably between 12 and 24 hours of life.
- Since 2010, pulse oximetry screening (POS) of the newborns has been included in the list of uniform screening programs before discharge in many countries.

- In neonatal intensive care unit (NICU) pulse, oximetry has become standard of care and is often regarded as the "fifth vital sign".
- The seven defects classified as CCHD are:
  1. Hypoplastic left heart syndrome (HLHS)
  2. Pulmonary atresia with intact septum (PA/IVS)
  3. Tetralogy of Fallot (TOF)
  4. Total anomalous pulmonary venous return (TAPVR)
  5. Transposition of the great arteries (TGA)
  6. Tricuspid atresia (TA)
  7. Truncus arteriosus communis (TAC)
- *Whom to screen:* All newborn babies before they are discharged home.
- *When to screen:* Preferably around 24 hours of life or before discharge, whichever is earlier.
- *How to screen:* See algorithm below
- Babies with positive screen should be further evaluated by doing thorough clinical evaluation as well as 2D ECHO by pediatric cardiologist in the hospital or transfer to a medical facility with pediatric cardiology services.
- Infants who pass POS test are clinically well without signs concerning possible critical CHD (e.g., cardiac murmur, weak femoral pulses) and do not require additional evaluation.
- However, screening with pulse oximetry cannot "rule out" the presence of a CCHD or noncritical acyanotic heart defects.
- If there is antenatal suspicion or postnatally clinical suspicion for CCHD, additional evaluation should be pursued even in the setting of a normal POS.

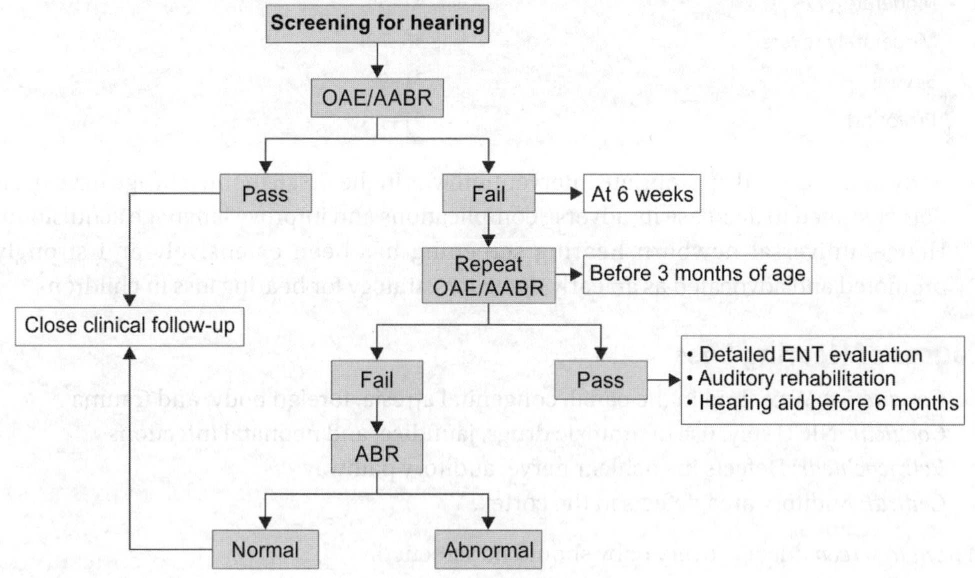

SCREENING FOR HEARING

- Hearing impairment can cause a massive impact on child development, in form of delayed language or speech development, poor academic performance, personal-social maladjustments, and emotional disturbances.
- In India, hearing impairment in neonates ranged between 1.59 and 8.8/1,000 births. Among "at risk" neonates, it ranged from 7 to 49.18/1,000 births (ten times more in at-risk babies).
- Worldwide reporting of hearing loss finds that the prevalence of moderate and severe bilateral hearing deficit (>40 dB) is 1–3/1,000 live births in well baby nursery population and 2–4 in 100 infants in an intensive care population.
- Vocabulary of a 3-year-old child with hearing impairment if remediated at birth is 300–700 words; if remediated at 6 months is 150–300 words and if remediated at 2 years is 0–50 words, respectively; as compared to vocabulary of a 3-year-old child with typical hearing which is 500–900 words.
- The extent of hearing loss is defined by measuring the hearing threshold in decibels (dB) at various frequencies. Normal hearing has a threshold of –10–15 dB. Hearing loss ranges from slight to profound.

Degree of hearing loss	Hearing loss range (db)
Normal	−10–15
Slight	16–25
Mild	26–40
Moderate	41–55
Moderately severe	56–70
Severe	71–90
Profound	91+

- Early detection and appropriate intervention within the first 6 months of age have been demonstrated to decrease its adverse complications and improve language acquisition. Hence, universal newborn hearing screening has been extensively and strongly promoted and advocated as an early detection strategy for hearing loss in children.

Causes of Hearing Loss

- *Conductive:* Wax, fluid in the canal, congenital atresia, foreign body, and trauma
- *Cochlear:* NICU stay, use of ototoxic drugs, jaundice, and neonatal infections
- *Retrocochlear:* Defects in cochlear nerve, auditory pathway
- *Central:* Auditory area defects in the cortex.

Whom to screen: Ideally, every baby should be screened.

Screening methods: Otoacoustic emissions (OAE) and automated auditory brainstem response (AABR) can be used for newborn hearing screening.

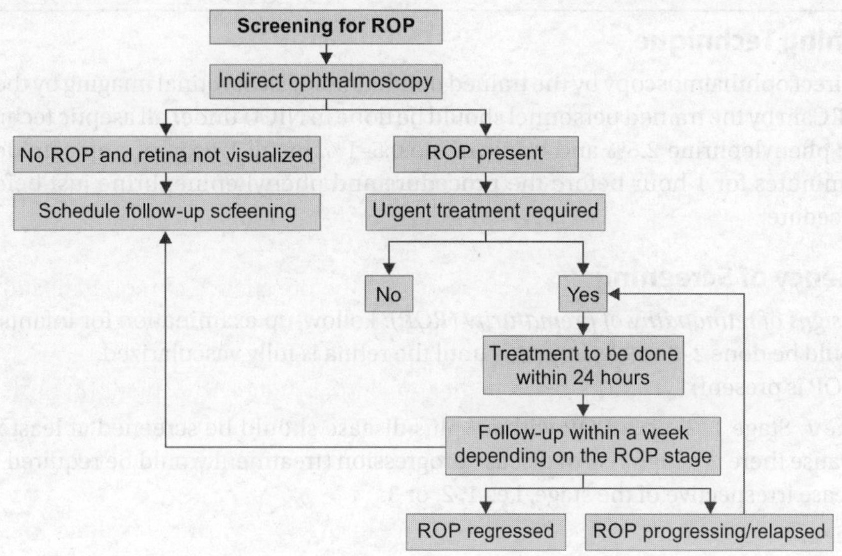

SCREENING RETINOPATHY OF PREMATURITY

- The prevalence of childhood blindness in India is 6.5/10,000 children based on a population-based study from Southern India.
- It is one of the leading preventable causes of blindness in India. Approximately, half of all the childhood blindness can be avoided or treated.
- Eye examination proforma that needs to be carried out in all the babies constitutes the following:
  - Ocular history
  - External examination of eyes
  - White reflex with a torch
  - Red reflex examination with an ophthalmoscope
  - Retinal examination where indicated.

Whom to Screen (As per RBSK Operational Guideline)

- Birth weight <2,000 g
- Gestational age <34 weeks
- Gestational age between 34 and 36 weeks but with risk factors such as (1) cardiorespiratory support, (2) prolonged oxygen therapy, (3) respiratory distress syndrome, (4) chronic lung disease, (5) fetal hemorrhage, (6) blood transfusion, (7) neonatal sepsis, (8) exchange transfusion, (9) intraventricular hemorrhage, (10) apneas, (10) poor postnatal weight gain.
- Infants with an unstable clinical course who are at high risk (as determined by the neonatologist or pediatrician).

When to Screen

- Preterm neonates >28 weeks of gestation to be screened at 4 weeks of life.
- Extreme preterms <28 weeks should be evaluated early at 3 weeks of age.

Screening Technique

- Indirect ophthalmoscopy by the trained ophthalmologist or retinal imaging by the use of RET Cam by the trained personnel should be done in NICU under all aseptic techniques.
- Use phenylephrine 2.5% and tropicamide 0.5–1%. Instill 1 drop of tropicamide every 15 minutes for 1 hour before the procedure and phenyl epinephrine just before the procedure.

Frequency of Screening

- *No signs of retinopathy of prematurity (ROP):* Follow-up examination for infants at risk should be done 2–3 weeks intervals until the retina is fully vascularized.
- If ROP is present:

  Zone 1: Stage 1, 2, or 3; ROP without plus disease should be screened at least weekly because there is a high risk of disease progression (treatment would be required in plus disease irrespective of the stage, i.e., 1, 2, or 3.

  Zone 2:
  - Immature vasculature should be screened once in 2–3 weeks.
  - Zone 2 stage 1 ROP should be screened once in 2 weeks.
  - Zone 2 stage 2 ROP without plus should be screened once in 1–2 weeks.
  - Zone 2 stage 3 ROP without plus should be screened at least weekly.

If there is pre-plus disease, baby should be screened at 3–4 day interval.

Treatment Modalities

- Type 1 ROP—peripheral retinal ablation by laser
- Stage 4 or 5 ROP—vitreoretinal surgical intervention
- Retinal detachment—a high risk of irreversible blindness.

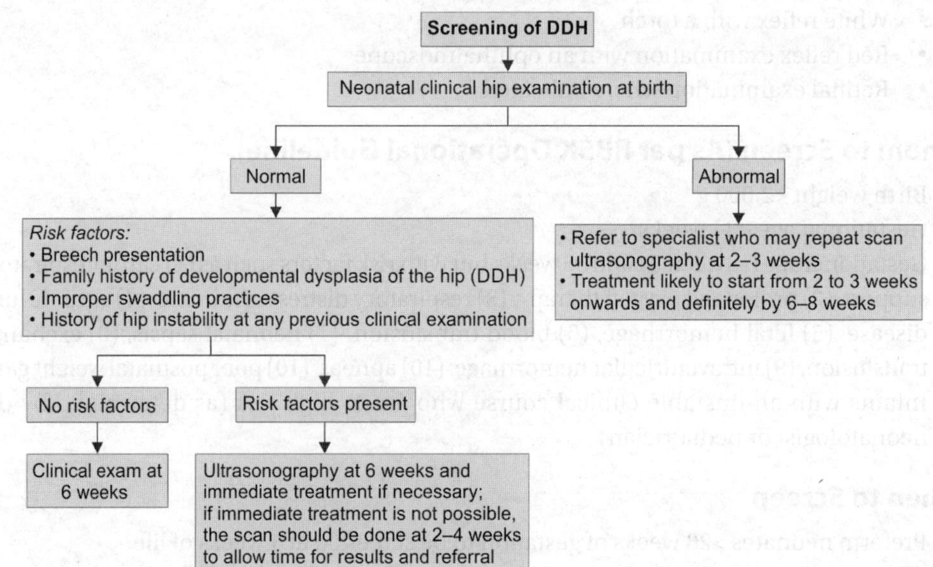

NEONATAL SCREENING

- It is recommended to include CAH screening in all newborn screening programs, if feasible. It helps in early diagnosis, timely treatment, and correct gender assignment of babies with classical CAH. Steroid therapy can be life-saving in babies with salt-losing CAH where adrenal crisis may be misdiagnosed as sepsis especially in male babies who go undetected in the absence of genital ambiguity.
- *Two-tier screening* is recommended, the first-tier screen should use 17-OHP fluoroimmunoassay on dried blood spots (DBS) obtained by heel prick. The cut-off based on gestational age rather than weight should be used. Second tier confirmatory testing should be done by LC-MS on venous sample.
- As the level of 17-OHP is high in the immediate postnatal period due to birth stress and immature metabolism in newborns, the blood sample should be obtained *after 24–72 hours* of life when it decreases rapidly. The use of cord blood is not recommended as the level of 17-OHP is significantly high immediately after birth.

Antenatal Screening

- Prenatal dexamethasone administration to pregnant woman a prior CAH affected child for prevention of virilization of a female fetus is considered experimental.
- It is started from 9 weeks of gestation and is required to be continued throughout pregnancy with good compliance.
- There are maternal adverse effects, variable genital outcome and unknown long-term side effects of dexamethasone therapy.

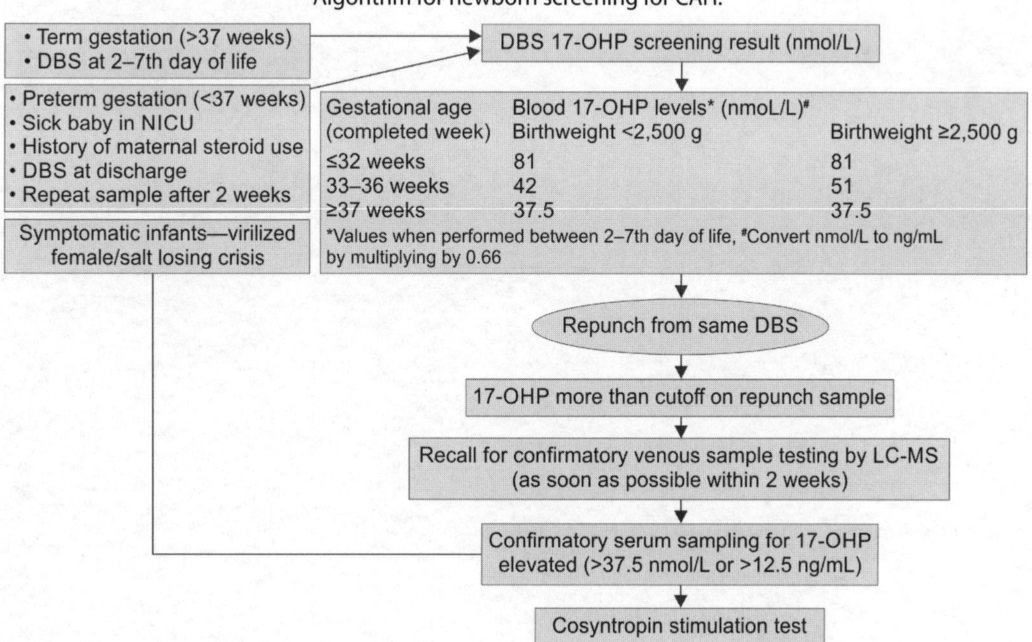

Algorithm for newborn screening for CAH.

■ FURTHER READING

1. Aroojis A, Anne RP, Li J, Schaeffer E, Ananda Kesavan TM, Shah S, et al. Surveillance for Developmental Dysplasia of the Hip in India: Consensus Guidelines From the Pediatric Orthopaedic Society of India, Indian Academy of Pediatrics, National Neonatology Forum of India, Indian Radiological and Imaging Association, Indian Federation of Ultrasound in Medicine and Biology, Federation of Obstetric and Gynaecological Societies of India, and Indian Orthopaedic Association. Indian Pediatr. 2022;59(8):626-35.
2. Martin GR, Ewer AK, Gaviglio A, et al. Updated Strategies for Pulse Oximetry Screening for Critical Congenital Heart Disease. Pediatrics. 2020;146(1):e20191650. doi:10.1542/peds.2019-1650.
3. From National Consultation Meeting for Developing IAP Guidelines on Neurodevelopmental Disorders under the aegis of IAP Childhood Disability Group and the Committee on Child Development and Neurodevelopmental Disorders; Paul A, Prasad C, Kamath SS, Dalwai S, Nair MKC, et al. Consensus Statement of the Indian Academy of Pediatrics on Newborn Hearing Screening. Indian Pediatr. 2017;54(8):647-51.
4. National Neonatology Forum of India. (2020). Screening and Management of Retinopathy of Prematurity. Clinical Practice Guideline. [online] Available from http://www.nnfi.org/assests/pdf/cpg-guidelines/ropp.pdf [Last accessed September, 2022].
5. RBSK, MOHFW, GOI. (2017). Universal eye screening in newborn. [online] Available from https://www.nhm.gov.in/images/pdf/programmes/RBSK/Resource_Documents/Revised_ROP_Guidelines-Web_Optimized.pdf [Last accessed September, 2022].
6. Saxena A, Mehta A, Ramakrishnan S, Sharma M, Salhan S, Kalaivani M, et al. Pulse oximetry as a screening tool for detecting major congenital heart defects in Indian newborns. Arch Dis Child Fetal Neonatal Ed. 2015;100:F416–21.

Communication in Newborn Care

Ramesh Choudhary

PRINCIPLES OF EFFECTIVE COMMUNICATION

- Help families to arrive at crucial informed decisions.
- Alleviates parental anxiety and conflicts.
- Help to maintain healthy association between healthcare providers (HCPs) and families.
- Builds trust and credibility.
- Helps healthcare providers to understand about problems of family and barriers to practice optimally, prevailing healthcare myths, care-givers misconceptions, knowledge gaps identification, and remediation thereof.
- Reduces chances of medico-legal issues.

ESSENTIAL ASPECTS OF COMMUNICATION (VERBAL) (GALPAC)

- *Greeting family:* Senior most family member to senior most HCP. Talk in respectful, gentle friendly manner. Start with general discussion on well-being then come to situation/problem. HCP may be doctor or nurse (talking points may be decided by units). Use appropriate verbal and *nonverbal language* (correct body posture, gesture, eye contact, touch, and facial expression).
- *Ask and listen:* Listen carefully to find out what the baby's problems are and what the parent/mother is already doing for her baby. Remember to ask open-ended questions.

  Open-ended questions are more likely to identify harmful beliefs than closed-ended questions. For example:

  Do not say: "Does the baby sleep well?"

  Instead say: "How is the baby sleeping?" (Open question)

  Use "body language" to show that you are listening to the family.

  Reflect back what the mother or caregiver says.

  Empathize—show that you understand what she/he feels.

  Avoid judgmental sounding words.
- *Praise:* Praise the mother and family if they are doing something well or if they have understood correctly.
  - Praising the family for this will strengthen their confidence to maintain the beneficial behavior and to adopt other beneficial behaviors.

- Make sure that praise is genuine, and only praise actions that are indeed helpful to the baby.
  - You can always find something to praise.
  - Praise can be given throughout the counseling process when appropriate.
- *Advice:* Limit your advice to what is relevant to the parents/mother at this time (depending upon when you are talking like immediate postadmission/daily progress/outcome)
  - Use simple, easily understandable and nontechnical language.
  - Use technical words only, if commonly used.
  - Use pictures (*mother cards* or similar) or real objects to explain.
  - Advise against any harmful practices that the parent/mother may have used.

Explain why the practice is harmful.

Some advice requires that you teach the mother how to do a task; like feeding with cup and spoon or any baby care skill (may be done in group) using three basic steps:

1. Tell them how to do task.
2. Demo/show them how to do it correctly.
3. Let them practice while you watch and recorrect them (if needed).

- *Check understanding:* Find out what a mother has learned. Ask questions that require the mother to explain what, how, how much, how many, when, or why.
  - Do not ask questions that can be answered with just a "yes" or "no".
  - Give the time to think and then answer.
  - Praise the mother/family for correct answers.
  - If she needs it, give more information, examples or practice.

NONVERBAL COMMUNICATION (BODY LANGUAGE)

- Sit opposite the person you are listening to at same head level and appropriate distance.
- Lean a bit toward the person to show interest in what they are saying.
- Maintain eye contact as appropriate.
- Look relaxed and open, show you are at ease with them—arms should not be crossed.
- Do not be in rush or show as if you are in a hurry.
- Gestures, such as nodding and smiling, or saying "mmm" or "ah".
- Touch, as appropriate.

Reflect Back

- When a person states how they are feeling (afraid, worried, happy, etc.), let them know that you hear them by repeating it.
- This is called reflecting feelings and is a tool to show you are listening. An example would be "so you say you are worried."

Empathy

- Showing empathy is putting yourself in someone else's place and understand how they feel in a situation.
- It builds trust.

LEVEL OF COMMUNICATION

- At the time of admission
- During hospital stay (as per unit protocol)
- At the time of discharge
- At the time of death
- At the time of referral
- Any time when clinical condition not improving.

Key Points to Remember

- Good communication is an integral part of comprehensive patient care.
- Information should be practical and in simple language easily understood by parents. Avoid technical jargon.
- Do not flood with too much of information.
- Healthcare workers should be formally trained in counseling of parents and families of sick, hospitalized neonates.
- Counseling by HCP for parents of sick neonates should be individualized and structured.
- One-to-one counseling should be preferred over group counseling for updating infant condition, prognosis, or decision-making. Individual counseling protects parents' privacy and is especially important while breaking bad news or sharing complex information.
- A designated area should be used for counseling. It offers privacy during complex or difficult situations, allows parents to share their emotions, and improves their confidence to ask questions.
- Additional family support or peer-to-peer support groups should be encouraged. It offers unique support through experience sharing.
- Written documentation must for all procedural.

■ FURTHER READING

1. Clinical Practice guidelines, National Neonatology Forum of India, 2021.
2. Facility based new born care. MoHFW, GoI; 2022.

Purvi Patel

BRIEFING

A briefing is a detailed discussion among the team members to review the clinical situation using available perinatal information to anticipate potential complications and plan further management to reduce the risk of failure or harm.

Preresuscitation Team Briefing

- Assess antepartum or intrapartum risk factor
- Team leader identification
- Possible scenario team may encounter are discussed.
- Anticipate potential complications and plan a team response.
- Delegate task optimally.
- Assigning the roles and settings clear, detailed expectations for each role via closed loop communication.
- Identify who will document events as they occur and communicate with parents.
- Determine what supplies and equipment will be needed.
- Identify how to call for additional help.
- Positioning each team member within the resuscitation environment.

Closed-loop Communication

Closed-loop communication is a technique to avoid misunderstanding as it ensures that instructions are received and understood.

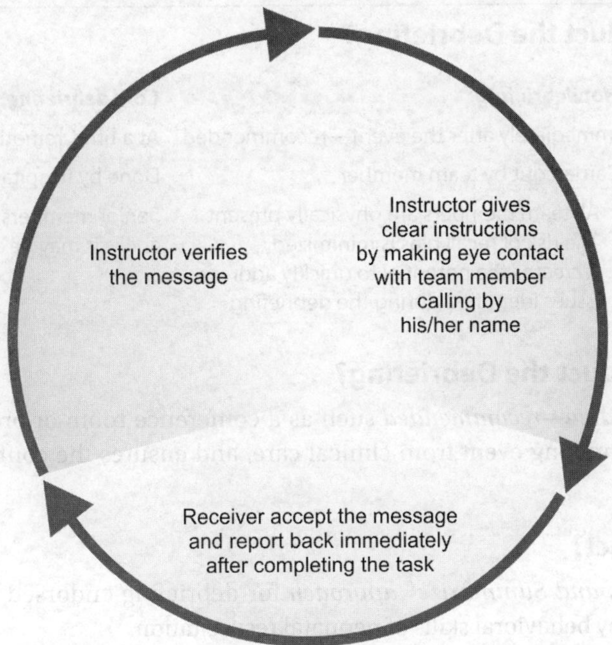

DEBRIEFING

- Debriefing is a *facilitated discussion* among team members about events that just occurred.
- Multidirectional both between and among the leader(s)/facilitator of the debriefing and those being debriefed. Preassigned facilitator ensures consistent debriefing and able to self-discover about the events which happened.

Effective Debriefing Questions

- Tell me in a few sentences what happened to this baby?
- What did the group do well and why?
- What key behavioral skills did you use? When did you use (a key behavioral skill?)
- What was the most distressing and satisfying aspect?
- What could have been handled differently?
- What could have gone better and how?
- What did you learn?
- Is there anything else you would like to discuss?

When to Conduct the Debriefing?

Type	Hot debriefing	Cold debriefing
Time of delivery	Immediately after the event—recommended	At a time, remote from the event
Conducted by	Carried out by team member	Done by hospital committee
Benefits	• All team members are physically present • The risk of recall bias is minimized • It creates the potential to quickly address issues identified during the debriefing	Senior members capable of proper analysis may be available

Where to Conduct the Debriefing?

Nonpatient care area—recommended such as a conference room or break room, which separates the debriefing event from clinical care, and ensures the confidentiality of the discussion.

How to Conduct?

"Gather, Analyze, and Summarize" approach for debriefing endorsed by the AHA and includes the 10 key behavioral skills of neonatal resuscitation.

Key Behavioral Skills

1. Knowledge of environment
2. Anticipation and planning
3. Use available information
4. Identify a team leader
5. Effective communication
6. Delegation of task
7. Attention allocation
8. Use of available resources
9. Calling for help when needed
10. Professional behavior

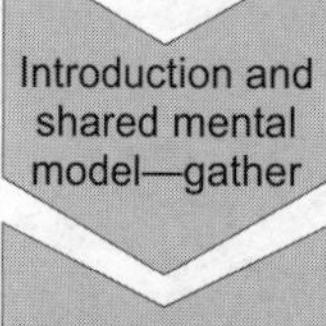

Introduction and shared mental model—gather
- Quick debriefing of that event within few minutes having a goal of improving our performance as a team and the care that we provide
- Review the clinical event and share the information

Analyze and summarize
- *What went well and what did not?*
- Did the team follow the established guidelines and protocols if not why?
- Any technical, equipment, procedural issues?
- Discuss 2–3 key behavioral skills?
- *What will the team do differently next time?*

Conclude
- *Follow-up issues:* Record issues to be discussed
- *Conclusion:* 'Thank you for taking time in debriefing'

COMMUNICATION WITH PARENTS WHILE RESUSCITATION

- Attentive communication gives the parents relief in their difficult time. In contrast, lack of communication leads to feelings of neglect and loneliness which adds burden to the family.
- It is a two-way street as treating physician needs to transmit the information which should be understood by parents and at the same time parents want to share their anxieties and feelings so both should support each other.
- Communicating with parents in these circumstances is difficult but clinicians are needed to communicate with families in an empathetic and effective way.

How to Communicate with Parents

Before the resuscitation:
- Self-introduction
- Mention resuscitation can be difficult and so may not be able to communicate during resuscitation

During the resuscitation:
- Allow father to approach the bedside and acknowledge his presence
- Encourage father to go back to mother
- Acknowledge mother's presence
- Prepare parents for the death in two to three steps
- Take the decision to stop the resuscitation (do not ask parents)
- State clearly about infant's death
- Note time of death

After the death:
- State that everybody has put sufficient efforts including parents
- Placed the infant in the mother or the father's arms
- Sit down
- Allowed opportunity for parents to ask questions (30 s silence)
- Know what happens to the body after death
- Allow them to create memories
- Offer to call family or spiritual supports
- Provide future support

BREAKING BAD NEWS

Giving bad news is a complex and challenging task for health professionals and receiving it is very difficult for the family.

Some basic principles (SPIKES) should be kept in mind when SPIKES for breaking bad news consists of six steps which creates suitable environment to deliver news in a gentle, informative, and consoling way with proper eye contact.

1. *Setting:* An appropriate room or place for the conversation in the presence of professionals and family members.
2. *Perception:* Understand what parents know about the clinical condition as they should be regularly updated regarding the progress of the patient.
3. *Invitation:* Respond gently to questions asked by parents regarding their child's health.

4. *Knowledge:* Passing on information using clear terms gradually, using pauses and repeat when necessary.
5. *Emotions, empathy:* Showing support and understanding by welcoming their feelings; allow them to perform last religious rituals after cleaning the baby.
6. *Strategy, summary:* Closing the conversation and including a care plan.
- Breaking bad news is an important but difficult clinical skill but via integration of empathetic communication makes it more comfortable for the health professional and helps in gaining confidence and satisfaction of the family.
- These skills can be learned in continuing education programs.

Key Points to Remember

- Communication is defined as the sharing information and providing emotional support verbally or nonverbally between people.
- Communication during resuscitation includes both with the team members including briefing, debriefing, and with the parents also.
- The neonatal resuscitation requires rapid decision-making skills within dynamic situations in unpredictable circumstances.
- It is a constructive review of actions and thought processes that promotes reflective learning.
- To improve performance and confidence of a team to facilitate the acquisition and maintenance of the skills necessary for effective neonatal resuscitation.
- *Outcome:* Briefing or debriefing may improve short-term clinical and performance outcomes for infants and staff.

FURTHER READING

1. Fawke J, Stave C, Yamada N. Use of briefing and debriefing in neonatal resuscitation, a scoping review. Resusc Plus. 2020;5:100059.
2. Halamek LP, Cady RAH, Sterling MR. Using briefing, simulation and debriefing to improve human and system performance. Semin Perinatol. 2019;43(8):151178.
3. Lizotte MH, Barrington KJ, Sultan S, Pennaforte T, Moussa A, Lachance C, et al. Techniques to communicate better with parents during end-of-life scenarios in neonatology. Pediatrics. 2020;145(2):e20191925.
4. Marçola L, Zoboli I, Polastrini RTV, Barbosa SMM. Breaking bad news in a neonatal intensive care: the parent's evaluation. Rev Paul Pediatr. 2020;38:e2019092.
5. Saugstad OD, Robertson NJ, Vento M. A critical review of the 2020 International Liaison Committee on Resuscitation treatment recommendations for resuscitating the newly born infant. Acta Paediatr. 2021;110(4):1107-12.
6. Weiner GM, Zaichkin J, American Academy of Pediatrics, American Heart Association. Textbook of Neonatal Resuscitation, 8th edition. United States: American Academy of Pediatrics; 2021.

Point of Care Quality Improvement

Suprabha Patnaik

■ STEPS IN QUALITY IMPROVEMENT

- Quality improvement is a systematic approach to address the gaps in the delivery of healthcare services and coming up with changes in the functionality of the system and various processes at the point of care.
- This involves series of steps in sequential order to achieve the outcome.

Step 1: Identify the problem	Analyze the existing data in the unit and identify the gaps in care delivery. Discuss with the stakeholders and identify the existing problems. Identify the issues with processes and outcomes	• *Stakeholders*: All the multidisciplinary persons including the patient and care-provider, involved in the care delivery • *Process*: The activities carried out by the healthcare provider • *Outcome*: The result of the various processes carried out by the healthcare provider
Step 2: Prioritize the problems	The problems have to be prioritized based on factors like relevance to patient outcome, ease of measurement, within existing resources	
Step 3: Formation of the team to address the problem	A team has to be formed comprising of representatives of various stakeholders Team members should have roles assigned. The various roles identified are team leader, data collector, communicator	

Contd...

Contd...

Step 4: Formation of aim statement	The team has to formulate aim regarding the problem to be addressed. This has to be SMART (specific, measurable, achievable, relevant to patient outcome, timely)	For example, We aim to increase the *exclusive breastfeeding rates* of *term healthy babies* in the *postnatal ward* from the current *80–90%* in next *6 weeks*
Step 5: Analysis of the problem	Using various tools, team has to analyze the various contributing factors toward the problem	*Tools include*: • Root cause analysis • Five WHYS • Pareto chart • Process flow *Root cause analysis*: Enumerate all the factors related to *people, policy, place, and procedure*, contributing to existing problem
Step 6: Formulating indicators of processes and outcomes	*Indicator* is the calculated data depicting the percentage of occurrence of an event (process or outcome), in a defined cohort This indicator has to be plotted on a time series chart or run chart	For example, process or outcome indicator (numerator/denominator × 100) *Numerator*: Number of times a process/outcome is happening *Denominator*: Number of times a process/outcome should be happening *Run chart*: Plot time in days/weeks or months on X-axis and the indicator on Y-axis
Step 7: Developing change ideas	After identifying the contributing factors toward a problem, the team should think of alternative ways of functioning, which address the contributing factors, and discuss the prediction for success or failure of these alternative working	
Step 8: Test the change ideas	Using *Plan-Do-Study-Act* (PDSA) cycle, test the change idea on a small scale	*Plan*: Plan what has to be done, who has to do, where it has to be done, for how long it has to be tested *Do*: Do the planned testing of the alternative way of functioning *Study*: Analyze the results of the testing carried out *Act*: As per the analysis, decide whether the test idea can be adapted, adopted, or abandoned

Contd...

Contd...

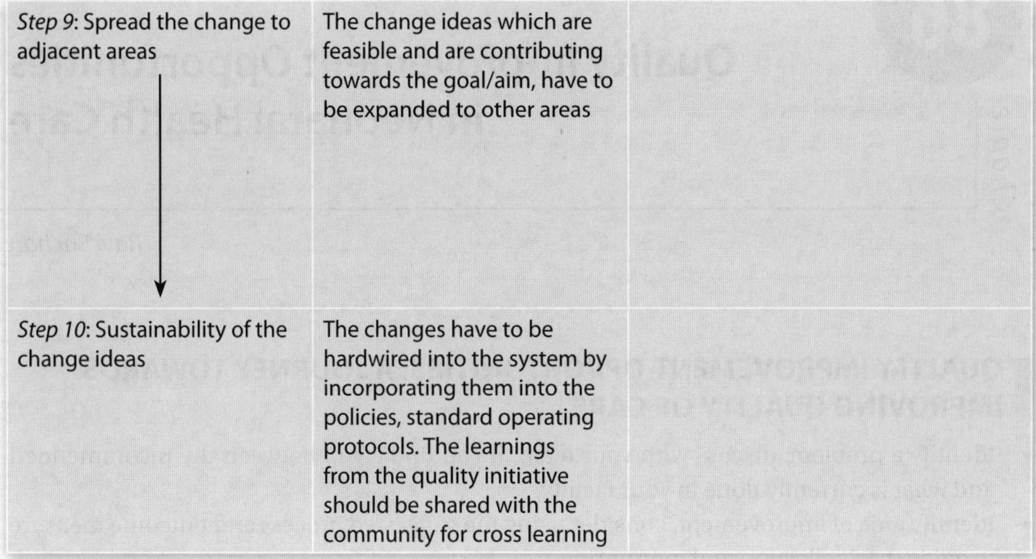

Step 9: Spread the change to adjacent areas	The change ideas which are feasible and are contributing towards the goal/aim, have to be expanded to other areas	
Step 10: Sustainability of the change ideas	The changes have to be hardwired into the system by incorporating them into the policies, standard operating protocols. The learnings from the quality initiative should be shared with the community for cross learning	

■ FURTHER READING

1. Point of Care Quality Improvement. (2017). Improving the quality of care for mothers and newborns in health facilities. Learner's Manual: version 2. [online] Available from https://www.healthynewbornnetwork.org/hnn-content/uploads/POCQI-Learner-Manual-1-1.pdf [Last accessed September, 2022].

Quality Improvement Opportunities in Neonatal Health Care

Ravi Sachan

QUALITY IMPROVEMENT OPPORTUNITIES: A JOURNEY TOWARDS IMPROVING QUALITY OF CARE

- Identify a problem, discuss with your team, if you find a gap between the recommended and what is currently done in your facility.
- Identify area of improvement, consider using the suggested process and outcome measure to guide data collection and monitoring.
- Quality indicators (rate/ratio or event) measure different domains of quality, used for comparison and improvement.
- *Process indicator (measure of process):* Action that are taken in delivery of care.
- *Outcome indicator (measure of outcome):* The result of action taken.

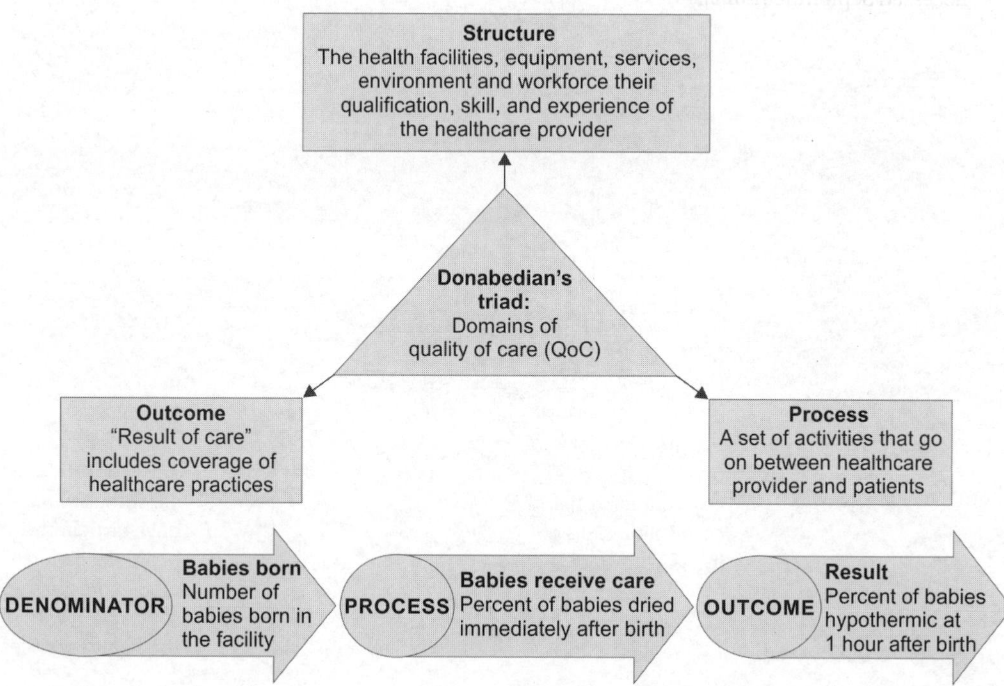

■ MEASURING THE QUALITY OF CARE: NEONATAL QUALITY INDICATORS

S. No.	Standards of care	Structure (input measure)	Process (output measure)	Outcome (outcome measure)
1.	For every newborn, competent and motivated healthcare for providing routine care and management of complication	• A written policy for QI and patient safety • A designated QI team and responsible personnel • All standard policies and protocols are in place and accessible • Skilled birth attendants available at all times, in sufficient numbers to meet the anticipated work load • A program for continuing professional and skills development for all skilled birth attendants and conducts regular training in Neonatal Resuscitation Program (NRP) • The health facility provides an enabling, supportive environment for professional staff development, with regular supportive supervision and mentoring	• Proportion of staff oriented to their roles and responsibilities • Number of visits to support clinical competence and performance at regular interval • The proportion of monthly meetings on the quality of care that were actually held in the preceding 12 months • Proportion of all newborns in the health facility with congenital abnormalities who are correctly referred to an appropriate referral center according to standard operating procedures	• Proportion of newborns who were delivered by a skilled birth attendant who have completed NRP course • The proportion of all women who gave birth at the health facility who were satisfied with the care and support from facility staff
2.	All women and their families receive information about the care and have effective interactions with staff	• Easily understood health education materials, in an accessible written or pictorial format, are available in the local languages • The health facility has a written, up-to-date policy that outlines clear goals, operational plans, and monitoring mechanisms to promote the interpersonal communication and counseling skills of healthcare staff	The proportion of all women discharged who received written and verbal information and counseling before discharge on the exclusive breastfeeding and danger signs	• The proportion of all women who gave birth in the health facility who reported that their needs and preferences were taken into account during labor, childbirth and postnatal care • The proportion of all women who gave birth in the health facility who expressed satisfaction with the health services

Contd...

Contd...

S. No.	Standards of care	Structure (input measure)	Process (output measure)	Outcome (outcome measure)
3.	Every Newborns receive routine care immediately after birth	• Health facility has written equipment checklist and clinical protocols for essential newborn care • All essential supplies of clean towels, sterile cord clamps, and scissors available in sufficient quantities at all times for the expected number of births • All healthcare provider in the labor and childbirth areas trained in NRP or regular refresher sessions in essential newborn care and breastfeeding support at least once every 12 months • The health facility has local arrangements and a mechanism to maintain a documented room temperature in the labor and childbirth areas at or above 25°C and free of draughts • Healthcare staff in the labor and childbirth areas receive at least monthly drills or simulation exercises and supportive supervision in essential newborn care and supporting breastfeeding	• The proportion of all newborns who were breastfed within 1 hour of birth • The proportion of all newborns who were kept in skin-to-skin contact with their mothers for at least 1 hour after birth • The proportion of all newborns whose umbilical cord was clamped 1–3 minutes after birth • The proportion of all newborns who were dried immediately and thoroughly at birth • The proportion of all newborns who received all four elements of essential newborn care—immediate drying, immediate skin-to-skin contact, delaying cord clamping (DCC), and early initiation of breastfeeding in the first hour • Proportion of newborns who was shifted with the mother	• The proportion of all neonates with hypothermia at 1 hour • The proportion of all very low birth weight neonates with hypothermia at admission to neonatal intensive care unit (NICU) • Percentage of skin-to-skin care given = Total nos. of normal delivery given skin to skin care within 1 hour of birth / Total numbers of normal deliveries in labor room × 100 • Percentage of delayed cord clamp = Total numbers of normal deliveries with cord clamp after one minute/ Total numbers of normal deliveries in labor room × 100 • Percentage of normal newborn receiving breast feed within one hour of birth = Total numbers of newborns breast fed within one hour of birth/ Total nos. of normal newborn delivery × 100

Contd...

Contd...

S. No.	Standards of care	Structure (input measure)	Process (output measure)	Outcome (outcome measure)
4.	Newborns who are not breathing spontaneously receive appropriate stimulation and resuscitation with a bag-and-mask within 1 minute of birth, chest compression and medication as per standard guidelines	• The health facility has a suction device, at least two sizes of neonatal mask and a self-inflating bag in the childbirth and neonatal areas of the labor room • The health facility has written, up-to-date clinical protocols for managing newborns who are not breathing spontaneously in the childbirth areas • All healthcare workers providing care for newborns in the health facility are skilled in basic newborn resuscitation, as demonstrated by simulating positive-pressure ventilation with a bag-and-mask on a manikin • Healthcare staff in the childbirth and neonatal areas of the maternity unit receive in-service training and regular refresher sessions in basic newborn resuscitation at least once every 12 months • Healthcare staff in the childbirth and neonatal areas of the LR receive monthly drills or simulation exercises and supportive supervision in basic newborn resuscitation	• The proportion of all newborns who were not breathing spontaneously after additional stimulation at the health facility who were resuscitated with a bag-and-mask • The proportion of newborn who required ventilatory corrective steps • The proportion of newborn with meconium-stained amniotic fluid still undergoes direct laryngoscopy and tracheal suction • The proportion of the newborn intubated in the delivery room • The proportion of the newborn intubated in the delivery room by a skilled provider trained in advance NRP • The proportion of newborn who required chest compression and medication	• The proportion of all newborns who were not breathing spontaneously after additional stimulation who were resuscitated with a bag-and-mask within 1 minute of birth • The proportion of all newborns who developed HIE • Proportion of neonates who failed resuscitation • The proportion of all live babies born at term ($\geq$37 weeks) with no major congenital malformations in the health facility who died within 7 days of birth (early neonatal mortality
5.	Every newborns receive routine postnatal care	• The health facility has written, up-to-date clinical protocols for postnatal care in the postnatal care areas of the maternity unit that are consistent with standard guideline	• The proportion of all newborns who received vitamin K and full vaccination as per national guidelines	• *Neonatal mortality rate in the health facility:* Number of neonatal deaths in the total number of neonates

Contd...

Contd...

S. No.	Standards of care	Structure (input measure)	Process (output measure)	Outcome (outcome measure)
		• The health facility practices and enables rooming-in to allow mothers and babies to remain together 24 hours a day • The health facility has local arrangements for alternative feeding methods, including cup or cup-and-spoon feeding • The health facility has local arrangement to inform pregnant women and their families about the benefits and management of breastfeeding	• The proportion of all stable newborns in the health facility who are fed exclusively on breast-feeding from birth to discharge • The proportion of all newborns in the health facility who received a full clinical examination before discharge • Proportion of all |newborns on post-natal care wards for whom there is documented information on the newborn body temperature, respiratory rate, feeding behavior, and the absence or presence of danger signs • The proportion of all healthy mothers on postnatal wards or areas in the health facility who received breastfeeding counseling and support from a skilled healthcare provider • The proportion of all women who gave birth in the health facility who were allowed to room-in with their newborn 24 hours a day	• The proportion of all newborns in the health facility who were exclusively breastfed at the time of discharge from hospital

Contd...

Contd...

S. No.	Standards of care	Structure (input measure)	Process (output measure)	Outcome (outcome measure)
6.	Preterm and small babies receive appropriate care as per standard guidelines	• The health facility has written, up-to-date clinical protocols for the care of small and preterm babies • The health facility has a 24-hour triage system and a designated emergency care area, room or trolley equipped with appropriate neonatal equipment, supplies and essential medicines for emergency resuscitation and initial treatment • The health facility has supplies and materials to provide optimal thermal care to stable and unstable preterm babies, including kangaroo mother care (support binders, baby hats, and socks), clean incubators and radiant warmers • The health facility has the supplies and materials to provide optimal feeding to preterm babies and support for breastfeeding or alternative feeding • Healthcare staff in the health facility who work in LR receive training and regular refresher sessions in appropriate care of preterm and low-birth-weight babies at least once every 12 months	• Proportion of newborns admitted to NICU with no indication for NICU admission • Proportion of newborns under a radiant warmer without a temperature probe for monitoring • Proportion of newborns admitted to the health facility who receive intravenous fluids with no clear indication • Proportion of eligible small and sick newborns who are screened for retinopathy of prematurity and the findings are documented • Proportion of newborns admitted to the health facility for whom there were proven medication errors • Proportion of eligible newborns (<2,000 g or preterm) who receive nearly continuous kangaroo mother care • The proportion of all low-birth-weight newborns born in the health facility whose mothers received additional support to establish breastfeeding	• The proportion of all preterm babies (<28 weeks, 28–32 weeks and 32–37 weeks of gestational age) born in the health facility who died within the first 7 days of life • The proportion of all low birth weight newborns born in the health facility who were exclusively fed on their mother's milk during their stay in the health facility • The proportion of all live preterm babies born in the health facility who had severe neonatal morbidity (respiratory distress syndrome, intraventricular hemorrhage, and necrotizing enterocolitis) • Proportion of all newborns treated for respiratory conditions in the health facility who are oxygen-dependent at 28 days of age (as a proxy of bronchopulmonary dysplasia)

Contd...

Contd...

S. No.	Standards of care	Structure (input measure)	Process (output measure)	Outcome (outcome measure)
				• The proportion of low birth weight baby deaths in the facility attributed to sepsis • Proportion of discharged small and sick newborns who are referred for follow-up who attend scheduled follow-up appointments
7.	Newborns with suspected infection or risk factors for infection are promptly given antibiotic treatment	• The health facility has essential supplies of all injectable antibiotics • The health facility has a written, up-to-date clinical protocol for early diagnosis and management of neonatal infection • Healthcare staff in the health facility know the signs of newborn sepsis and how to treat it as per standard guidelines	• Proportion of newborns in the health facility for whom a blood culture was requested before antibiotic treatment was started • The proportion of all newborns in the health facility with signs of infection who received injectable antibiotics • Proportion of staff in the neonatal unit who practice hand hygiene according to WHO standards • Proportion of reusable neonatal equipment disinfected by standard procedures • Number of times the neonatal clinical area and neonatal equipment are cleaned according to standard operating procedures	• The proportion of newborns treated for sepsis in the health facility who died (case fatality rate) • Proportion of newborns admitted to the health facility who received antibiotics when not indicated • The proportion of all severe neonatal morbidity in the health facility that was due to neonatal sepsis • Proportion of newborns admitted to the health facility with infections proven to be healthcare-associated infection

■ FURTHER READING

1. Ministry of Health & Family Welfare, Government of India. (2017). LaQshya, labour room, and quality improvement initiative. [online] Available from https://nhm.gov.in/index1.php?lang=1&level=3&sublinkid=1307&lid=690 [Last accessed September, 2022].
2. World Health Organization. Improving the quality of care for mothers and newborns in health facilities: point of care quality improvement. Facilitator Manual. New Delhi, India: World Health Organization; 2020.
3. World Health Organization (WHO). Standards for improving quality of maternal and newborn care in health facilities. Geneva: WHO; 2016.
4. World Health Organization (WHO). Standards for improving the quality of care for small and sick newborns in health facilities. Geneva: WHO; 2020.

Quality Improvement in NICU: An Experience

Deepika Kainth, Meena Joshi, Anu Sachdeva

APPLICATION IN NEONATOLOGY: OUR EXPERIENCE

The neonatal intensive care unit is a complex and highly error prone environment. In presence of such complexity, the development of safety culture needs to be fostered as the first step toward the journey of QI. The presence of safety culture and cohesive team work improves the overall performance of the unit. Further, increasing generation of medical evidence, rapid advances and striking differences in mortality and morbidity across units (especially low-and-middle-income countries) portray a great case for the need of context specific interventions through the methodology of QI. It helps to pinpoint why best evidence-based interventions fail to perform in a certain scenario, usually due to prevailing practices, behaviors, and beliefs in the unit.

Understanding of the same encouraged us to identify problems in our unit at AIIMS, New Delhi and solve those using simple interventions as a QI initiative. This initiative was started in 2015 and has expanded over the years. Currently, we are continuing multiple QI projects with involvement of faculty, nursing officers, staff, and neonatal fellows **(Table 1)**. By virtue of these activities, we strive to improve the care that we provide to neonates (and their families) not only in terms of mortality and morbidity, but also patient satisfaction.

During this QI journey at AIIMS, many leaders and unit champions surfaced who continue to lead many more QI projects outside of the unit, pushing new fronts for this movement for change. Our nurse educator is the QI champion of our unit has been pivotal in leading and supervising small teams of each QI project and in the process, identifying many more QI champions like her.

AIIMS, a WHO Collaborating Center for Newborn health disseminates QI to other organizations through its face-to-face workshops, online resource material and the Point of Care Continuous Quality Improvement (POCQI) module. A dedicated website (*www. pocqi.org*) on QI provides free resources for teaching and learning QI, and as a platform for capacity building of teams and sharing QI work.

TABLE 1: Quality initiatives in NICU at AIIMS, New Delhi.

S. No.	Problem statement	Indicators	Processes and change ideas	Result	Challenges
1.	Compliance to hand hygiene	Percentage compliance to hand hygiene moments	• Training using educational videos • CCTV monitor	Improvement in rates from 61.8 to 77% over 16 weeks	• Possible Hawthorne effect • Retraining • Behavioral factors for low compliance
2.	Hypothermia at admission to NICU	• Incidence of moderate hypothermia • Incidence of hyperthermia (as a balancing outcome)	• Strengthening warm chain • Use of plastic bags • Delivery room thermometer	Moderate hypothermia reduced from 50 to 12.5% over a period of 11 months	• Complex with use of bundles • Involvement of labor room staff • Need for multiple PDSA cycles
3.	Rates of exclusive human milk feeding	• Proportion of neonates receiving MOM on day 7 • Milk expression within the first 6 hours	• Postnatal counseling • Motivation of staff by incentives and awards	• Time to first expression of breast milk reduced from 48 hours to 3 hours • Proportion of neonates on MOM increased from 12.5 to 81% • Sustenance at 1 year	Constant motivation and training
4.	Frequent breakage of warmer probes	• Average life span of a probe in days • Time interval between two probe breakdown	• Refresher course for equipment care • Tracking probe breakage • Mother's involvement	• Life span increased from 9 to 40 days • Minimum time interval between two probe breakdown increased to 60 days	• Understanding the resistance to change • Training and retraining of stakeholders
5.	Duration of KMC	Median daily duration of KMC	• Training using educational videos • Daily written instruction	Increase of daily duration from 5 to 11 hours	• Disruption due to restricted entry in COVID pandemic • Dependence on maternal health and availability of attendant

Contd...

Contd...

S. No.	Problem statement	Indicators	Processes and change ideas	Result	Challenges
6.	Excessive noise in NICU	Incidence of false alarms in multipara monitor	• Educational videos • Tracking of alarm limits for admitted neonates	• Incidence decreased for 35 to <2% over 6 weeks • Attained sustenance	Need for retraining
7.	Medication (prescription and transcription) error	• Percentage of prescription error • Percentage of transcription error	• Sensitization of nurses and doctors • Creation of WhatsApp group for reporting and feedback	Reduction in medication error from 30 to 4%	• Continued motivation and sensitization • Lapses during busy months
8.	Universal thyroid screening	Percentage of babies being screened for hypothyroidism using cord TSH	• Development and revision of unit protocol • Tracking using a register • Monthly reporting	• Establishment of universal thyroid screening for all deliveries • 95% of the babies being screened	• Changing residents almost every month • Monthly orientation sessions for new residents
9.	*Other ongoing projects*: • Reduction in periprocedural pain • Streamlining and proofreading of neonatal-perinatal database • HAI surveillance • Increasing the amount of pooled and pasteurized donor human milk • Improving breastfeeding rates at discharge				

IMPLEMENTATION OF QUALITY IMPROVEMENT: CHALLENGES AND SOLUTIONS

Despite the great results achieved by the QI initiatives, there are various barriers to its implementation. A major challenge is the difficulty to sustain a change that led to improvement. Frequent change in managing personnel (both doctors and nurses), need for constant motivation, regular training and retraining, requirement for change in behavior, presence of a strong team, and champions with leadership skills are some of the factors that pose as hurdles to sustained improvement. These can be addressed by the following solutions:

- Start with a small and simple problem. Gradually shift toward bigger and complex problems with one step at a time.
- Understand your system and the processes involved for the particular problem in context.

- Choosing a change idea that is inherent to the system and not personnel or patient specific, to ensure sustenance.
- Identify solutions to eliminate redundancy and replication of one or multiple steps in a process.
- A *"bottom up"* approach is preferred where the frontline workers identify opportunities and implement change ideas for improvement in their workplace with guidance from the senior members of the unit, rather than senior leaders (faculty or head of organization) directing the change through frontline staff (*"top down"* approach).
- A written policy for the unit to ensure awareness and orientation to the new members of the unit.
- Regular meetings for constant motivation of the members, celebration of successes, and learning from failures.

  Inculcating patience in team members is the key to sustenance!

  To summarize, quality is everyone's responsibility. Practically, all healthcare units are error prone and suffer from inherent challenges and problems. Identification and initiating a QI initiative for small problems with simple solutions at the start can go a long way to create future leaders with a great team, along with producing clinical dividends for betterment of the neonatal care.

Key Points to Remember

- Providing good quality of care is the prime responsibility of the healthcare providers.
- Good quality care abides to principles of safety, efficacy, efficiency, timeliness, and has patient centered approach. With explosion of scientific knowledge and research, practicing evidence-based medicine (EBM) is the need of the hour.
- Despite presence of evidence-based guidelines and recommendations for ideal healthcare standards, their application at bedside and translation into clinical dividends remains challenging.
- To bridge this know-do gap, the concept of quality improvement (QI) was first proposed by William E Deming. QI focuses on changing behaviors, approaches, and systems to improve the quality of care that patients receive.
- Unlike conventional research, it implements (rather than discover) the knowledge relevant to problem in context, using multiple short improvement cycles with no control group, blinding, or randomization and uses simple tools, with immediate results.
- The QI methodology entails a systematic and scientific approach to identify, prioritize, and solve problems by working as teams.

■ FURTHER READING

1. Chandra P, Tewari R, Dolma Y, Das D, Kumawat D. Reducing preoperative waiting-time in a pediatric eye operation theater by optimizing process flow: a pilot quality improvement project. Indian Pediatr. 2018;55(9):773-5.

2. Gopalakrishnan S, Chaurasia S, Sankar MJ, Paul VK, Deorari AK, Joshi M, et al. Correction: stepwise interventions for improving hand hygiene compliance in a level 3 academic neonatal intensive care unit in north India. J Perinatol Off J Calif Perinat Assoc. 2021;41(12):2847.
3. Institute of Medicine (US) Committee on Quality of Health Care in America. Crossing the Quality Chasm: A New Health System for the 21st Century. Washington (DC): National Academies Press (US); 2001.
4. Sahoo T, Joshi M, Madathil S, Verma A, Sankar MJ, Thukral A. Quality improvement initiative for reduction of false alarms from multiparameter monitors in neonatal intensive care unit. J Educ Health Promot. 2019;8:203.
5. Sivanandan S, Sethi A, Joshi M, Thukral A, Sankar MJ, Deorari AK, et al. Gains from quality improvement initiatives—experience from a tertiary-care institute in India. Indian Pediatr. 2018;55(9):809-17.

88

Quality Improvement in Delivery Room: Improving Newborn Care Immediately after Birth (Routine Care): An Experience

Ravi Sachan

EXTENT OF THE PROBLEM AND ANALYSIS AT GTB HOSPITAL, DELHI

- Labor room of public sector tertiary care teaching hospital at Delhi, with annual delivery load of 20,000 approximately.
- The quality improvement (QI) team analyzed the causes of lack of compliance of care around birth (CAB) practices [predelivery counseling (PDC), SSC, DCC, and EIBF]
- Healthcare workers both doctors and nurses form the NICU and LR, who were enthusiastic and willing to improve were included in the QI team.
- We formed our team, defined aim objectives. Analysis of the problem was done using various tools for QI as per the point of care quality improvement (POCQI) methodology.
- Multiple change ideas were tested using the PDSA (plan-do-study-act) cycle approach and successful change ideas were adopted based on the feasibility and scalability, in the given context.
- Process measure, outcome indicator-balancing indicators were developed to monitor progress and compliance.

The changes ideas that resulted in improvements in quality of care are:
- Change in the existing process flow of receiving normal newborn delivery.
- Structured PDC
- Defining and integrating the protocol for steps of keeping newborn over mother's abdomen.

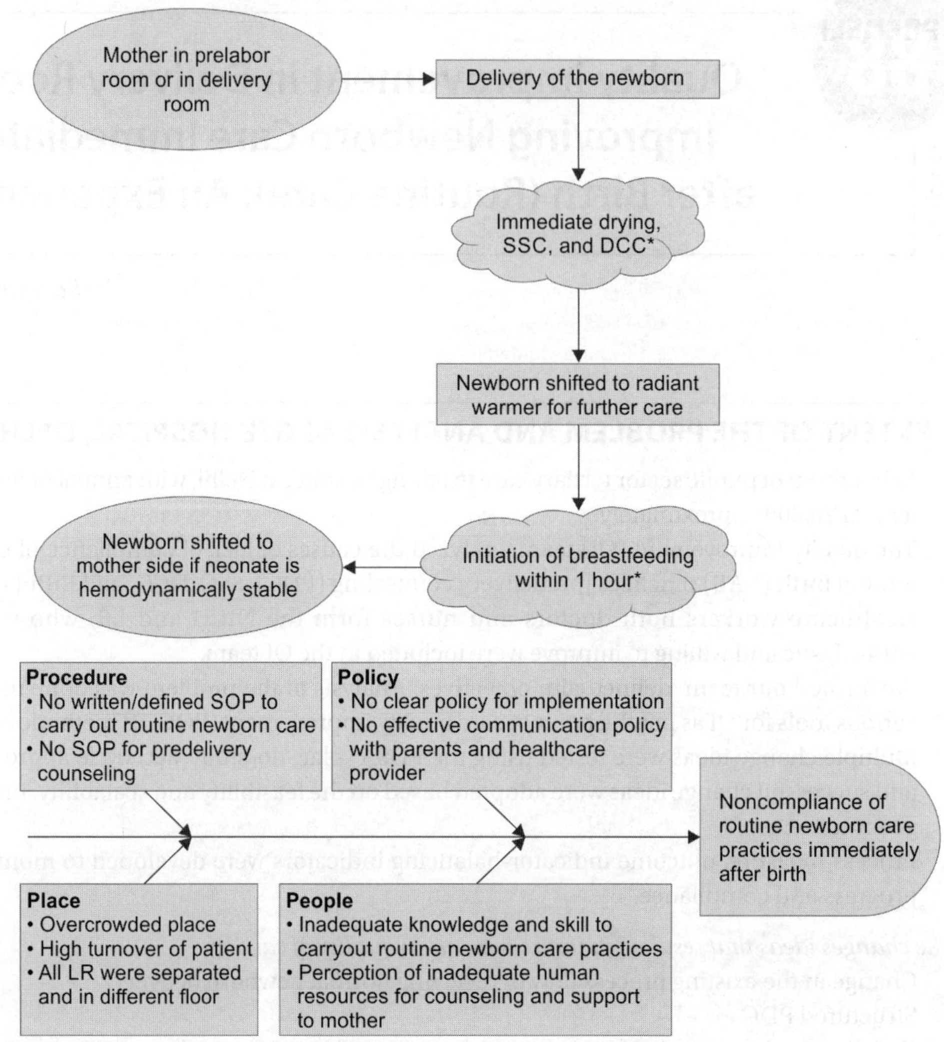

*Clouds represent: No clear-cut policy/guideline.

Source: Sachan R, Srivastava H, Srivastava S, Behera S, Agrawal P, Gomber S, et al. Use of point of care quality improvement methodology to improve newborn care, immediately after birth, at a tertiary care teaching hospital, in a resource constraint setting. BMJ Open Qual. 2021;10(Suppl 1):e001445.

■ PREDELIVERY COUNSELING

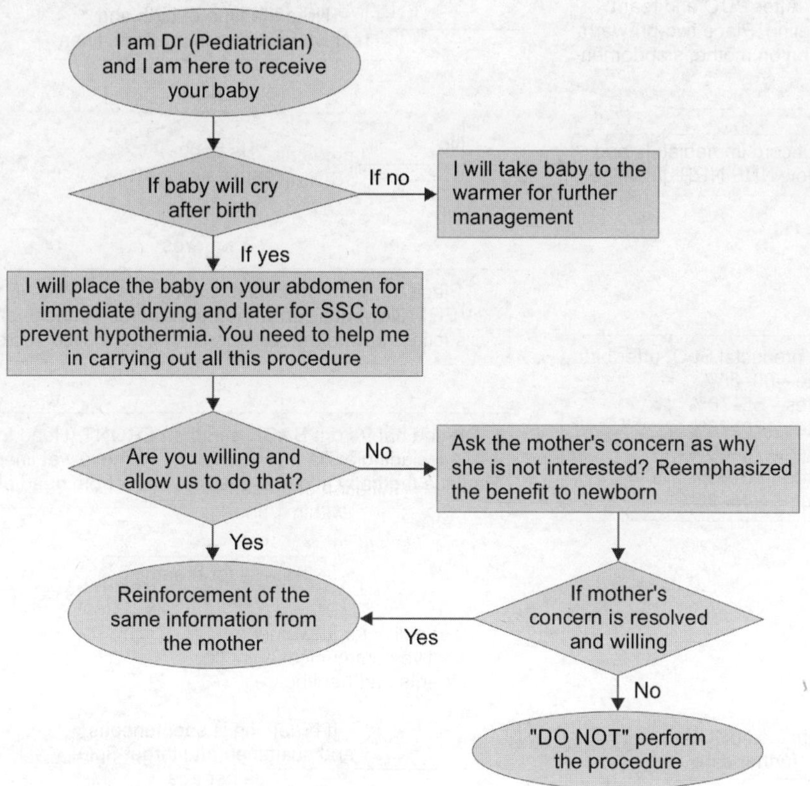

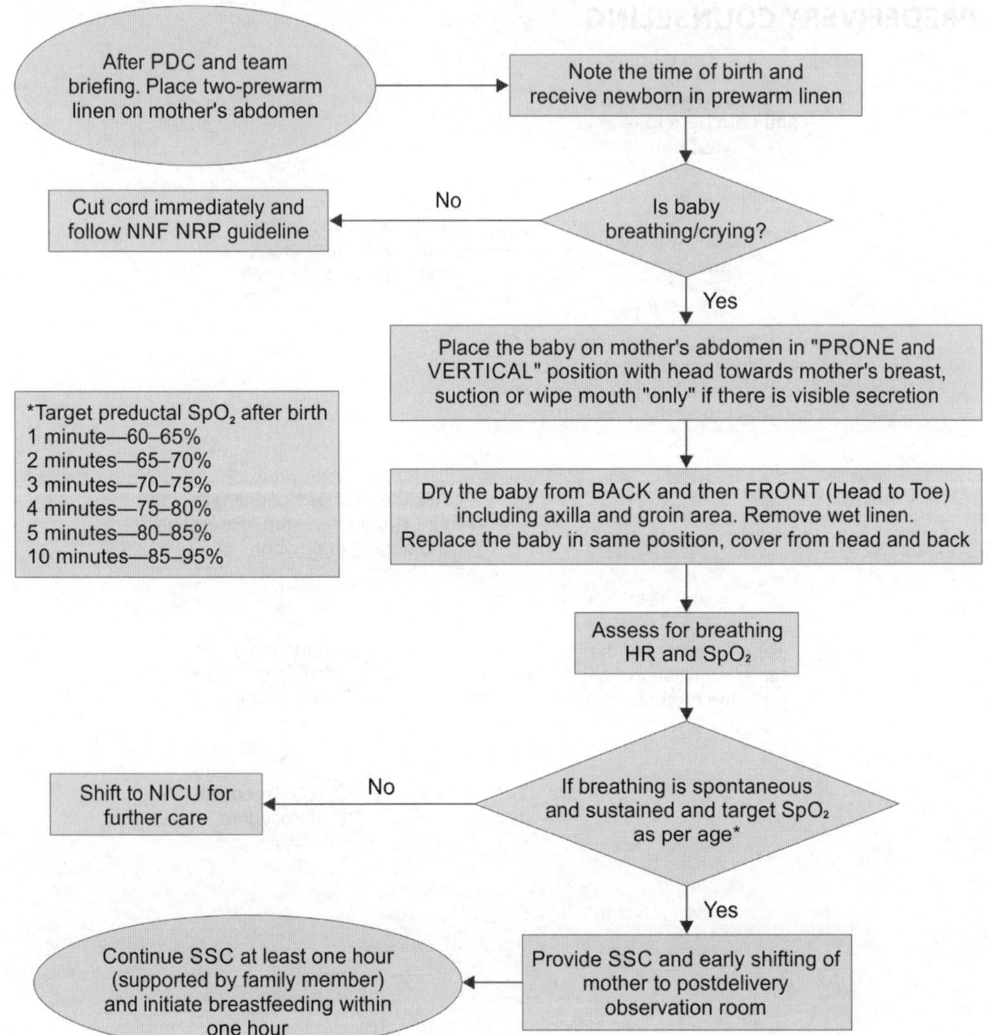

Integration of successful charge idea and hard wiring of the system leads to sustenance.

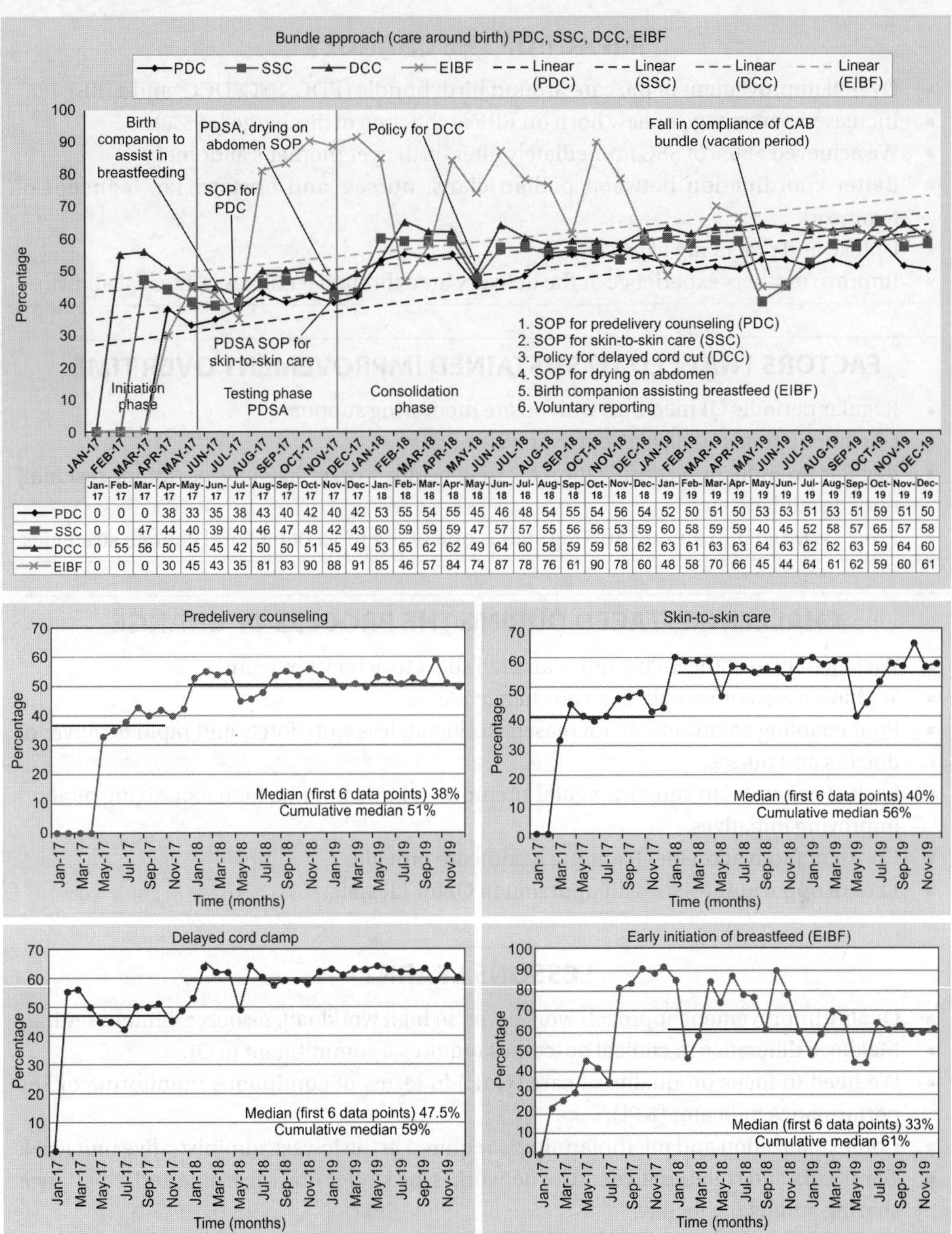

	Jan-17	Feb-17	Mar-17	Apr-17	May-17	Jun-17	Jul-17	Aug-17	Sep-17	Oct-17	Nov-17	Dec-17	Jan-18	Feb-18	Mar-18	Apr-18	May-18	Jun-18	Jul-18	Aug-18	Sep-18	Oct-18	Nov-18	Dec-18	Jan-19	Feb-19	Mar-19	Apr-19	May-19	Jun-19	Jul-19	Aug-19	Sep-19	Oct-19	Nov-19	Dec-19
PDC	0	0	0	38	33	35	38	43	40	42	40	42	53	55	54	55	45	46	48	54	55	54	56	54	52	50	51	50	53	53	51	53	51	59	51	50
SSC	0	0	47	44	40	39	40	46	47	48	42	43	60	59	59	59	47	57	57	55	56	56	53	59	60	58	59	59	40	45	52	58	57	65	57	58
DCC	0	55	56	50	45	45	42	50	50	51	45	49	53	65	62	62	49	64	60	58	59	59	58	62	63	61	63	63	64	63	62	62	63	59	64	60
EIBF	0	0	0	30	45	43	35	81	83	90	88	91	85	46	57	84	74	87	78	76	61	90	78	60	48	58	70	66	45	44	64	61	62	59	60	61

Time series care around birth bundles.

IMPACT OF THE CHANGES

- Overall improvement of the care around birth bundle (PDC, SSC, DCC, and EIBF)
- Increased percentage of new born on EBF at the time of discharge (>95%)
- We achieved >60% of SSC immediately after birth over mother's abdomen
- Better coordination between pediatricians, nurses, and obstetrician, concept of teamwork
- Uptake and practicing of QI skills
- Improve mothers experience at the delivery area through feedbacks (internal audit).

FACTORS THAT LED TO SUSTAINED IMPROVEMENT OVER TIME

- Regular periodic QI meetings with onsite mentoring support
- Documentation and display of new revised SOPs
- Regular preinduction sensitization for new health worker like interns, junior resident, nursing student, etc.
- Process ownership among nursing staff is one of the most behavioral change strategies.

CHALLENGES FACED DURING THE PROCESS OF CHANGE

- We failed measurably many times and fall short to achieve our aim.
- We have tested more than 25 to 30 change ideas.
- Poor enabling environment, increased workload, less work force, and rapid turnover of doctors and nurses.
- Lack of resources to support regular mentoring, hand holding for encouraging quality-improving initiatives.
- Constant motivation for QI among healthcare provides.
- Lack of opportunities for skill updation in QI for LR staff.

LESSONS LEARNT

- Quality improvement approach works even in high workload, resource-limited setting.
- Making a difference in clinical outcomes requires a commitment to QI.
- We need to focus on quality of care (QoC) in terms of continuous monitoring of key performance indicator (KPI).
- Contextualization and microplanning is required at the lowest administrative unit level.
- Team work and collaborative care of network is the key for quick learning and experience sharing among the facility.

ABOUT THE STUDY

- Single largest QI study published which incorporated all routine newborn care practices immediately after birth.
- Simultaneous balancing indicators were also monitored.
- Sustenance of changed process flow with improvement was observed for >2 years.

Key Points to Remember

- As per World Health Organization (WHO) standards for improving quality of maternal and newborn care in health facilities, every newborn receives routine care immediately after birth.
- Because it facilitates adaptation of the newborn to the new environment, meets immediate needs in the best possible way, and avoids preventable complications.
- After birth, immediate drying followed by skin-to-skin contact (SSC) prevents hypothermia, promotes physiologic stability, increases colonization with protective family bacteria, and facilitates early initiation of breastfeeding (EIBF) within 1 hour.
- Clamping of the umbilical cord is delayed until 1–3 minutes after birth. Delayed cord clamping (DCC) decreases anemia in neonate and prevents brain hemorrhage.
- Translation of these evidence-based practices into clinical practice is a challenge in the public healthcare systems especially in low-resource settings.

◼ FURTHER READING

1. Sachan R, Srivastava H, Srivastava S, Behera S, Agrawal P, Gomber S, et al. Use of point of care quality improvement methodology to improve newborn care, immediately after birth, at a tertiary care teaching hospital, in a resource constraint setting. BMJ Open Qual. 2021;10:e001445.

National Health Program

National Neonatal Health Program

Smriti Saryan, Arti Uniyal

1. LAQSHYA: THE NATIONAL LABOUR ROOM QUALITY IMPROVEMENT INITIATIVE

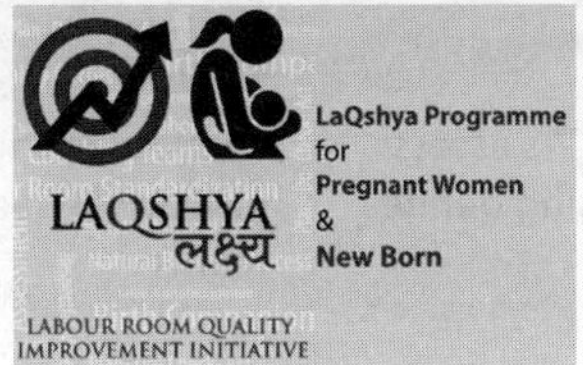

It was launched by the Ministry of Health and Family Welfare in the year 2017.

Goal

Reduce preventable morbidity and mortality, and stillbirth associated with care around the delivery room and operation theater.

Objectives

- To reduce maternal and newborn mortality and morbidity

- To improve quality of care during the delivery and immediate postpartum care, stabilization of complications and ensure timely referrals and enable an effective two-way follow-up system

- To enhance the satisfaction of beneficiaries visiting the health facilities and provide Respectful Maternity Care (RMC) to all pregnant women attending the public health facility

Beneficiaries

Pregnant women and newborns delivering in a public health institution.

Strategies

01	Labor room and Maternity Operation Theater layout and workflow	As per 'Labor Room Standardization Guidelines' and 'Maternal and Newborn Health Toolkit' issued by the MoHFW Government of India
02	Dedicated obstetric HDUs in at least all medical colleges and high caseload district hospital	For managing complicated pregnancies (as per GOI guidelines) that require life-saving critical care
03	Ensure strict adherence to clinical protocols	For management and stabilization of the complications before referral to higher centers

Targets

Immediate (0–4 months)

80%	80%
Selected labor rooms and maternity OTs assess their quality and staff competence using defined NQAS checklists and OSCE	Of labor rooms and maternity OTs have set up functional quality circles and facility-level quality teams

Short-term (up to 8 months)

80%	60%	50%	30%
Labor room and OT • Follow latest protocol, respectful maternal care (RMC) and quality improvement processes • Monthly micro-biological sampling	Deliveries conducted using: • Real time partographs • Safe birth checklist and safe surgery checklist in labor room and maternity OT respectively	Deliveries take place in presence of the birth companions	• Increase in breast-feeding within 1 hour of delivery • Reduction in surgical site infection rate in the maternity OT

Immediate-term (up to 8 months)

100%	80%	60%	30%	30%
• Maternal death, neonatal death audit, and discussion on near-miss/maternal and neonatal complications • Administration of Oxytocin, immediately after birth	• All beneficiaries are either satisfied or highly satisfied • Labor rooms have staffing as per defined norms • Labor rooms and OTs are reporting zero stock-outs drugs and consumables	Labor rooms are reorganized as per 'Guidelines for Standardization of Labor Rooms at Delivery Points'	• Reduction in pre-eclampsia, eclampsia, and PIH, APH/PPH-related mortality • Increase in antenatal corticosteroid administration in case of preterm labor	Reduction in stillbirth rate, newborn sepsis, asphyxia-related admissions in SNCUs for inborn deliveries

Long-term (up to 18 months)

60%	50%	15%
Labor room achieve quality certification against the NQAS	Labor room are linked to obstetrics HDU/ICU	Improvement in short-term and Intermediate targets

After 18 months, this initiative would be continued through sustained mentoring.

Intervention

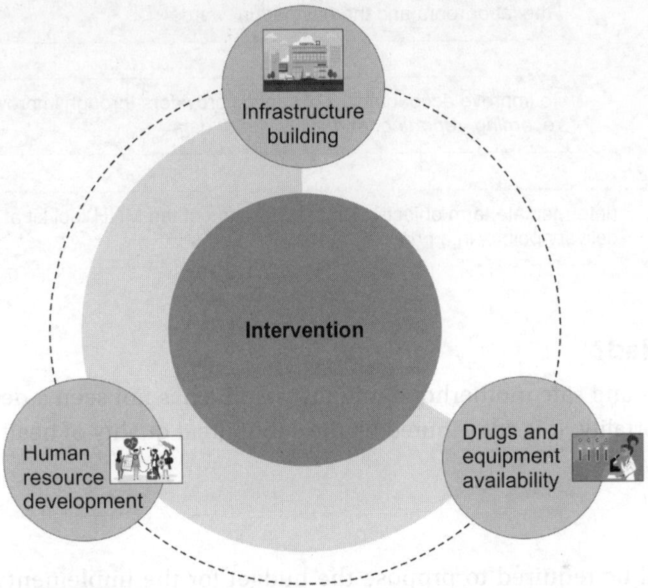

2. Dakshata

An initiative by the Ministry of Health and Family Welfare was launched in April 2015.
It is an important pillar of India Newborn Action Plan (INAP).

Goal

The goal of Dakshata is to improve the quality of maternal and newborn care during the intra- and immediate postpartum period through providers who are competent and confident (Dakshata) to decrease infant and maternal mortality.

Objectives

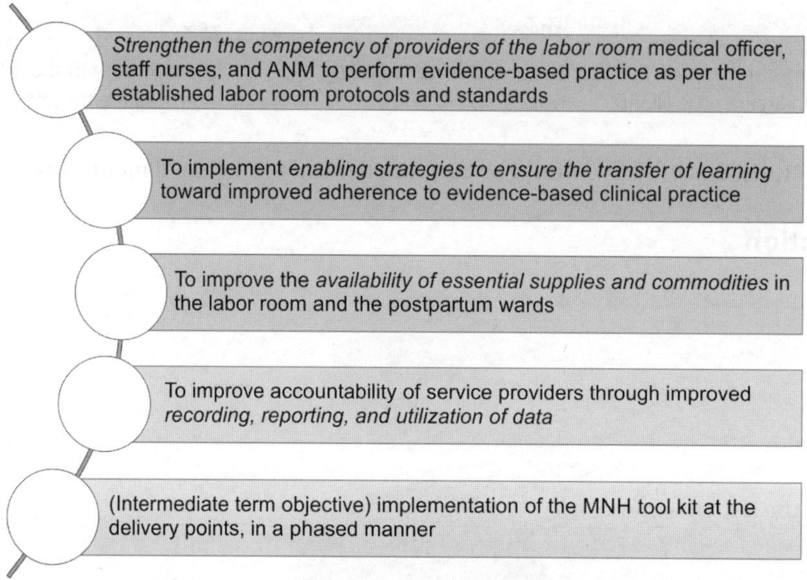

Why It is Needed?

Despite all efforts and safe motherhood initiatives, India has not seen a decline in maternal and newborn mortality. It is contributed by the suboptimal quality of health services during institutional deliveries.

Budget

The states would be required to propose the budget for the implementation of program activities.

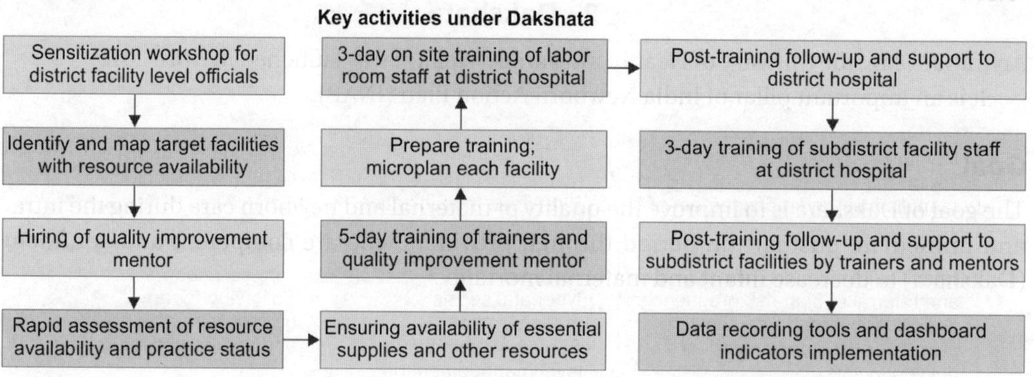

3. SURAKSHIT MATRITVA AASHWASAN

It is an initiative for zero preventable maternal and newborn deaths. It was launched on 10th October, 2019 by Ministry of Health and Family Welfare (MoHFW).

Vision

To create a responsive healthcare system which strives to achieve zero maternal and infant deaths through quality care provided with dignity and respect.

Goal

To end all preventable maternal and newborn deaths.

Beneficiaries

- All pregnant women
- All mothers up to 6 months postdelivery
- All sick infants.

Objectives

- To provide high quality medical, surgical, and emergency care services in a dignified and respectful manner as per Surakshit Matritva Aashwasan (SUMAN) service package at no cost to the beneficiaries.
- To leverage institutional and community-based platforms to help create awareness in the community on the entitlements under SUMAN.
- To strengthen Grievance Redressal Mechanism by incorporating client feedback.
- To orient service providers and build their capacity for delivering SUMAN package.
- To ensure reporting and review of all maternal and infant deaths.

Institutional Framework

National	National level Committee
State	State Level Committee
District	District Level Committee
Block	Block Level Committee

Basic Package HWC-SC/HWC-PHC/PHC/UPHC		
Maternal: • Routine ANC (4+ one PMSMA) • PNC • Identification and management of basic complications • Management of breast conditions • Identification basic management and referral of high-risk pregnancies • Skilled birth attendance (only in subcenter (SC) designated as delivery points) • Prereferral management for obstetric emergencies (eclampsia, PPH, and shock)	*Newborn:* • ENBC including resuscitation (NCC) • Birth dose immunization • Identification and prompt referral of "at risk" or "sick" newborn • Neonatal sepsis management • For infant, community level management of diarrhea and pneumonia	*Family planning:* • Provision of condoms, OCPs and pregnancy testing kits • Confidential counseling • Referral for safe abortion care services • Follow-up for any complication after abortion and appropriate referral

All in BEmONC Package, plus the following:

SUMAN SERVICE GUARANTEE—BEmONC
Non-FRU CHC/UCHC/HWC-PHC/Other Hospitals

Maternal:	*Newborn:*	*Family planning:*
• Management of basic complications • Assisted vaginal deliveries • Referral after initial management if required • Episiotomy and suturing • Stabilization of obstetric emergencies and assured referral to CEmONC facilities • Postnatal maternal care • Package including 48 hours stay	• Antibiotics for preterm or PROM for prevention of sepsis of newborns • Newborn Stabilization Units (non-FRU CHC) • Identification and Management of LBW infants ≥ 1,800 g with no other complications • Phototherapy for newborns • Stabilization and referral of sick and VLBW newborns • Facility level management of sick infant • Breastfeeding (expressed) and KMC	• Sterilization services (if available) • CAC services for medical methods (MMA) in PHCs • Both manual vacuum aspiration (MVA) and MMA in CHCs as per provisions of MTP Act (depending on the availability of trained provider/s in facility)

All in basic package, plus the following:

SUMAN SERVICE GUARANTEE—CEmONC
Medical College/DH/SDH/CHC-FRU/UCHC

Maternal:	*Newborn:*	*Family planning:*
• Elimination of mother to child transmission (EMTCT) services for HIV and syphilis including early infant diagnosis • Link ART at DH • Delivery of HIV positive women • CEmONC services including signal functions • Comprehensive management of all obstetric emergencies, e.g., PIH/eclampsia, sepsis, PPH, retained placenta, and shock • Cesarean section and other surgical interventions • Blood grouping and cross-matching	• Management of LBW infants • Managing all sick newborns (except those requiring mechanical ventilation major surgical interventions) • Management of newborn sepsis • Stabilization and referral of sick newborns for level III care • Follow-up of all babies	• Medical and surgical methods of abortion up to 20 weeks as per provisions of MTP act • Treatment of incomplete/spontaneous abortions • Management of all postabortion complications (depending on the availability of trained provider/s in facilities)

Grievance Redressal Mechanism

- The existing 104 GR mechanisms and health helpline will be integrated under SUMAN.
- All "urgent" grievances need to be resolved preferably within 24 hours.
- If a facility cannot resolve a grievance (within 7 days), it would be escalated to district/state level.
- Synopsis of grievances to be presented before the "SUMAN" committees.

4. JANANI SHISHU SURAKSHA KARYAKRAM (JSSK)

It was launched by the MoHFW under National Health Mission (NHM) on 1st June, 2011 in Mewat Haryana.

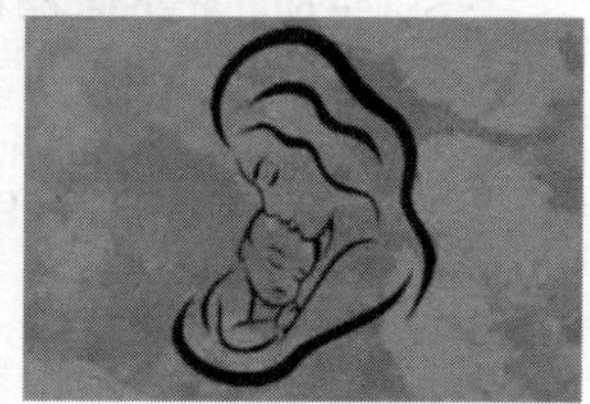

Goal

It was an intervention launched in order to decrease maternal and infant mortality rates.

Objectives

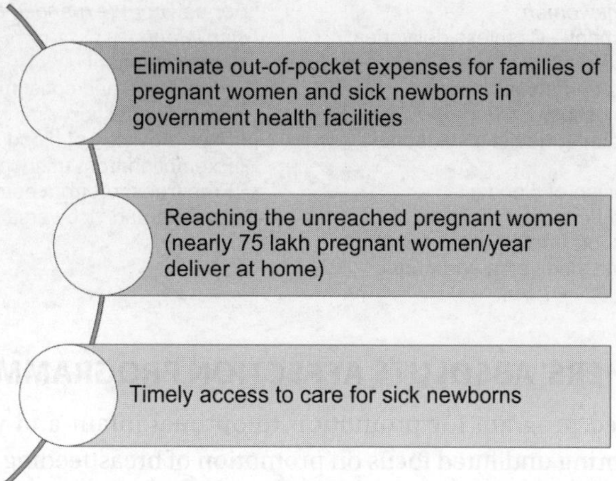

Intervention

Providing completely free and cashless services.

Beneficiaries

- Pregnant women for normal deliveries and cesarean operations.
- Sick newborns up to 30 days of life. In 2014, it was expanded to cover all the sick infants.

Components of Janani Shishu Suraksha Karyakram

- Early registration
- Identification of complicated cases
- Three antenatal care and postnatal care (ANC and PNC) visits
- Organizing referral services and transport
- Convergence with ICDS (integrated child development services)
- Transparent and timely disbursement of cash
- 24 × 7 delivery services at primary health center (PHC)
- Making FRU (first referral units) functional.

There are *free entitlements* given to pregnant women and infants.

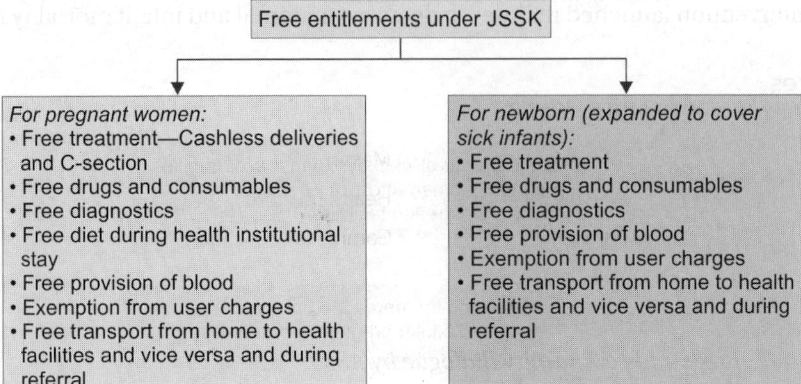

5. MOTHERS' ABSOLUTE AFFECTION PROGRAMME (MAA)

- It is an intensified program for promotion to optimal infant and young child feeding practices and to bring undiluted focus on promotion of breastfeeding practices.
- It was launched on 5th August, 2016.
- It covers all States and Union Territories.
- Targets around 3.9 crore pregnant and lactating mothers.
- 8.8 lakh ASHAs conduct mobilization.
- 18,000 birthing facilities skilled in lactation management.

Goal

To revitalize efforts toward promotion, protection, and support of breastfeeding practices through health systems to achieve higher breastfeeding rates.

Current rates (RSOC 2013–2014):
- *Early initiation of breastfeeding (within 1 hour of birth):* 46.5%
- *Exclusive breastfeeding (first 6 months):* 64.9%
- *Timely initiation of complementary feeding (6–8 months):* 50.5%

Objectives

- Building an enabling environment for breastfeeding and demanding generation of awareness through mass media and mid media targeting pregnant and lactating mothers, family members, and society.
- Capacity building of community health workers on breastfeeding. Breastfeeding to be positioned as an important intervention for child survival and development.
- Capacity building of auxiliary nurse midwife (ANM)/nurses/doctors in lactation support and management at facilities and reinforcement on breastfeeding at delivery points facilities through trained healthcare providers and through skilled community health workers.

■ Monitoring and recognition to incentivize and recognize those health facilities that show high rates of breastfeeding along with processes in place for lactation.

Implementation

It will be implemented at three levels:

Macrolevel	Mass media
Mesolevel	Health facilities
Microlevel	Communities

Community Level Activities

■ *Capacity building and community dialogue by ASHA:*
  • Orientation and equipping ASHA for optimal messaging (first information link on BF in the community).
  • ASHA's will promote BF at community level and counsel regarding management of breast engorgement and inverted nipples.
  • ASHA conducts quarterly meetings with mothers for which ASHA are given an incentive of ₹ 100, i.e., ₹ 300 for three quarters.
■ *Skilling of ANM and lactation support:*
  • Dedicated training for ANMs in IYCF in a phased manner over the year
  • Lactation support and management at subcenter.
■ *Capacity building of healthcare providers:*
  • Reinforcing roles and responsibilities regarding breastfeeding/infant and young child feeding
  • Emphasis on counseling on 9th of every month, under PMSMA—Pradhan Mantri Surakshit Matritva Abhiyan
  • One-day sensitization of all ANM/nurse/doctors at delivery points
  • Four-day training of ANMs/nurse/doctor in phased manner
  • Room for breastfeeding with proper space and information on breastfeeding.

Award and Recognition

■ Award for delivery point demonstrating breastfeeding processes—*Mothers' Absolute Affection (MAA) award*
■ Cash prize of ₹ *10,000* per district for one facility/district
■ Criterion for awards to be laid out—following 10 steps of BFHI (baby friendly hospital initiative) for at least 6 months.
■ Facility monitoring by certified assessor.

6. FACILITY-BASED NEWBORN CARE (FBNC)

Facility-based newborn care is one of the key components to improve the status of newborn health.

The various components of FBNC are given here.

Newborn Care Corners (NBCCs)

Newborn care corner is established at delivery points to provide essential newborn care at birth soon after delivery.

These are dedicated spaces within the delivery room where essential care as well as lifesaving care including resuscitation is provided to the newborn.

This area is mandatory for all health facilities where deliveries take place.

Services provided in the newborn care corner include:

- Essential Care at birth
- Resuscitation
- Provision of warmth
- Early initiation of breastfeeding
- Weighing the neonate.

Newborn Stabilization Units

Facility located within or in close proximity to the maternity ward where sick and low birth weight newborns are cared for short periods.

All FRUs/CHCs need to have a NBSU in addition to NCC.

Special Newborn Care Units

A neonatal unit in the vicinity of the labor room to provide special care (all care except assisted ventilation and major surgery) to the sick newborns.

Special newborn care unit (SNCU) at the district hospital is expected to provide the following services:

- Care at birth
- Resuscitation of asphyxiated newborns
- Managing sick newborns (except those requiring mechanical ventilation and major surgical interventions)
- Kangaroo mother care
- Post-natal care
- Follow-up of high risk newborns
- Referral services
- Immunization services.

Human Resources for Newborn Care Service

- *Newborn Care Corners:*
  - One doctor and one staff nurse. Trained in Navjaat Shishu Suraksha Karyakram (NSSK)
  - Newborn care corners at subcenter: ANM must also receive NSSK training.
- *Newborn stabilization units (NBSUs):* One trained doctor, four-time nurse, trained in facility-based integrated management of neonatal and childhood illness (f-IMNCI).

- *Special newborn care units:*
  - One pediatrician trained in neonatology, three to four trained doctors, medical officers trained in FBNC.
  - Trained support staff for cleaning nursery, part time lab technician and data operator.

7. INDIA NEWBORN ACTION PLAN (INAP)

- Response to global Every Newborn Action Plan (ENAP)- June 2014
- Implemented under existing RMNCH+A
- India Newborn Action Plan is guided by the principles of integration, equity, gender, quality of care, convergence, accountability, and partnerships.

Goals

- Ending preventable newborn deaths to achieve "Single Digit NMR" by 2030 with all the states to individually achieve this target by 2035.
- Ending preventable stillbirths to achieve "Single Digit SBR" by 2030, with all the states to individually achieve this target by 2035.

Targets

Targets	Current	2017	2020	2025	2030
Impact targets					
NMR (per 1000 live births)	29	24	21	15	<10
SBR (per 1000 live births)	22	19	17	13	<10
Coverage targets					
Safe delivery (institutional + home delivery by SBA (%)	76	90	95	95	95
Initiation of breastfeeding within one hour of birth (%)	–	75	90	90	90
Women with preterm labor receiving at least one dose of antenatal corticosteroids (%)	–	75	90	95	95
Babies born in health facilities with birth asphyxia received resuscitation (%)	–	75	90	95	95
Babies received complete schedule of home visits under HBNC by ASHA (%)	–	50	75	95	95
Newborn with sepsis in the community received Gentamicin by ANM (%)	–	50	75	75	75
Newborn discharged from SNCU followed until age one (%)	–	35	50	75	75
Newborn with low birth weight/l Prematurity managed with KMC at facility (%)	–	35	50	75	90

Strategic Intervention Packages

- *Impact on neonatal mortality:*
  - Antenatal screening for high-risk pregnancies
  - Complications and their management

- Immediate newborn care
- Care during labor and childbirth
- Care of healthy newborn especially in the first week
- Care of small and sick newborn
- Care beyond newborn survival
- *Impact on stillbirths:*
  - Care during labor and childbirth
  - Preconceptional and ANC

Preconceptional and Antenatal Care

Community	Subcenter	Health facility
• Reproductive health and family planning • Nutrition-related interventions • Counseling and birth preparedness • Prevention against malaria	• Antenatal screening for anemia and hypertensive disorders • Prevention and management of mild-moderate • Anemia • Tetanus immunization • Adolescent friendly health services • Intrauterine contraceptive device (IUCD) insertion	• Screening and management of severe anemia, hypertensive disorders • Gestational diabetes, HIV • Adolescent friendly health clinic • Postpartum family planning services • Prevention of Rh disease

Care During Labor and Childbirth

Community	Subcenter	Health facility
• Skilled birth attendant • Clean birth practices	• Timely referral • Prereferral dose by ANM • Antenatal corticosteroids, antibiotics in case of PROM	• Emergency obstetric care • Management of preterm labor

Immediate Newborn Care

Community	Subcenter	Health facility
• Early cord clamping • Skin-to-skin contact • Early initiation of breastfeeding • Hygiene	• Vitamin K at birth • Neonatal resuscitation	Advanced neonatal resuscitation

Care of Healthy Newborn

Community	Subcenter	Health facility
• Home visits by ASHA • Exclusive breastfeeding • Hygiene	Immunizations	All interventions

Care of Small and Sick Newborn

Community	Subcenter	Health facility
Thermal care and feeding support	• IMNCI • Injectable gentamicin by ANMs—prereferral completion if referral is refused (after intimation to medical officer)	• Skin-to-skin contact • NBSU/SNCU • NICU for assisted ventilation, surfactant, and surgery

Care beyond Newborn Survival

Community	Subcenter	Health facility
• Screening for birth defects, failure to thrive, and developmental delays • Follow-up visits	As before	• Newborn screening • Management of birth defects • Follow-up

8. RASHTRIYA BAL SWASTHYA KARYAKRAM (RBSK)

The "Child health screening and EARLY intervention services" program under NHM initiated by MoHFW.

The service covers all children of 0–6 years of age in rural and urban slums in addition to older children up to 18 years of age enrolled in classes 1st to 12th in government and government-aided schools.

Beneficiaries

Children from birth to 18 years of age.

Aim

To reduce child mortality and enable a systematic approach to child health screening and early intervention.

Objective

Early identification and early intervention for children to cover 4D's, viz.:
1. *D*efects at birth
2. *D*iseases in children
3. *D*eficiency conditions
4. *D*evelopment delays including disabilities.

Defects	Deficiencies	Childhood diseases	Developmental delays
• Neural tube defect • Down's syndrome • Cleft lip and palate/cleft palate alone • Talipes (club foot) • DDH • Congenital cataract • Congenital deafness • CHD • ROP	• Anemia • Vitamin A deficiency (Bitot spot) • Vitamin D deficiency (Rickets) • SAM • Goiter	• Skin conditions (scabies, fungal infection, and eczema) • Otitis media • RHD • Reactive airway disease • Dental caries • Convulsive disorders	• Vision impairment • Hearing impairment • Neuromotor impairment • Motor delay • Cognitive delay • Language delay • Behavior disorder (autism) • Learning disorder • ADHD • Congenital hypothyroidism, sickle cell anemia, beta-thalassemia (optional)

Program Implementation

> - *For newborn:*
>   - Facility-based newborn screening at public health facilities, by existing health manpower
>   - Community-based newborn screening at home through ASHAs for newborn till 6 weeks of age during home visits
> - *For children 6 weeks to 6 years:* Anganwadi center-based screening by dedicated mobile health teams at least twice a year
> - *For children 6 years to 18 years:*
>   - Government and government-aided school-based screening by mobile health teams at least once a year
>   - At least 3 mobile health teams per block to conduct screening, each consist of four members—2 doctors (AYUSH) 1 male and 1 female, 1 ANM/ Staff nurse, and 1 pharmacist
>   - Then arrangements for the provision of free management for these children will be made at District Early Intervention Center (DEIC) or existing tertiary level institutions.
>   - Birth defect surveillance system (BDSS) is being established, with at least 1 center in each state preferably in medical colleges, as a tool for identifying congenital anomalies.

9. BABY-FRIENDLY HOSPITAL INITIATIVE (BFHI)

This initiative by WHO and UNICEF was established in the year 1991. It was updated in 2006 and relaunched in 2009.

Aim

To give every baby the best start in life.

Objectives

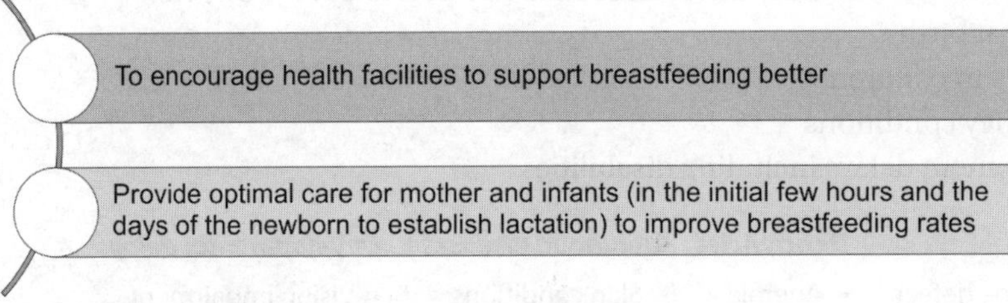

Ten Steps to Successful Breastfeeding (Revised in 2018 by WHO)

Clinical Management Procedure

- *Hospital policies* support mother for breastfeeding by:
  - Not promoting human milk substitutes such as formula feeds, bottles, or teats (following the international code of marketing of breast milk substitutes).

- Making breastfeeding standard practice (by making written policies)
- Keeping track of breastfeeding support (by ongoing monitoring and data management)
- *Ensure staff competency*—training staff and assessing their knowledge and skills.

Key Clinical Practice

- *Antenatal care*—discuss the importance of breastfeeding with the mother and the family; prepare women on how to feed the baby.
- *Care right after birth*—after birth immediate and uninterrupted skin-to-skin contact; support mother in order to initiate breastfeeding as soon as possible after birth.
- *Support mother with breastfeeding*—for initiation and maintenance of breastfeeding and managing common difficulties.
- *Supplementing*—promote breast milk unless there are medical reasons; prioritize donor human milk for supplementation.
- *Rooming-in*—letting mother and babies stay together 24 hours a day.
- *Responsive feeding*—recognize and respond to infant feeding cues.
- *Feeding bottles, teats, and pacifiers*—use and risk should be counseled.
- *Coordinate discharge*—parents and their infants have timely access to ongoing support and care.

Ten steps to successful breastfeeding

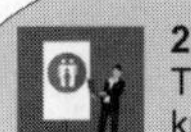

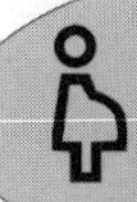

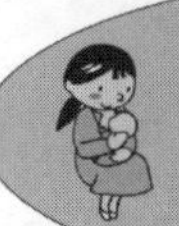

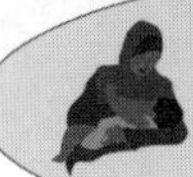

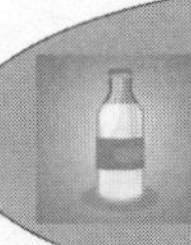

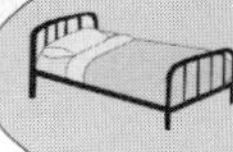

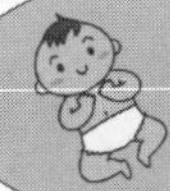

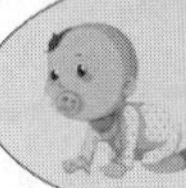

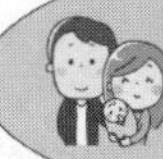

10. INTEGRATED MANAGEMENT OF NEONATAL AND CHILDHOOD ILLNESS (IMNCI)

An IMNCI clinical guideline is an Indian adaptation of the integrated management of childhood illness (IMCI) protocol to target children <5 years of age by the MoHFW.

- The guideline is an evidence-based, syndromic approach to case management.
- It determines the severity of the disease, classification (green, yellow, and pink), and the actions required.
- It supports the rational, effective, and affordable use of drugs and diagnostic tools hence promoting maximum use of the health system; and actively involving family members and the community in the healthcare process.
- It was updated in the year 2018 to include low birth weight and breastfeeding problems.

Objectives

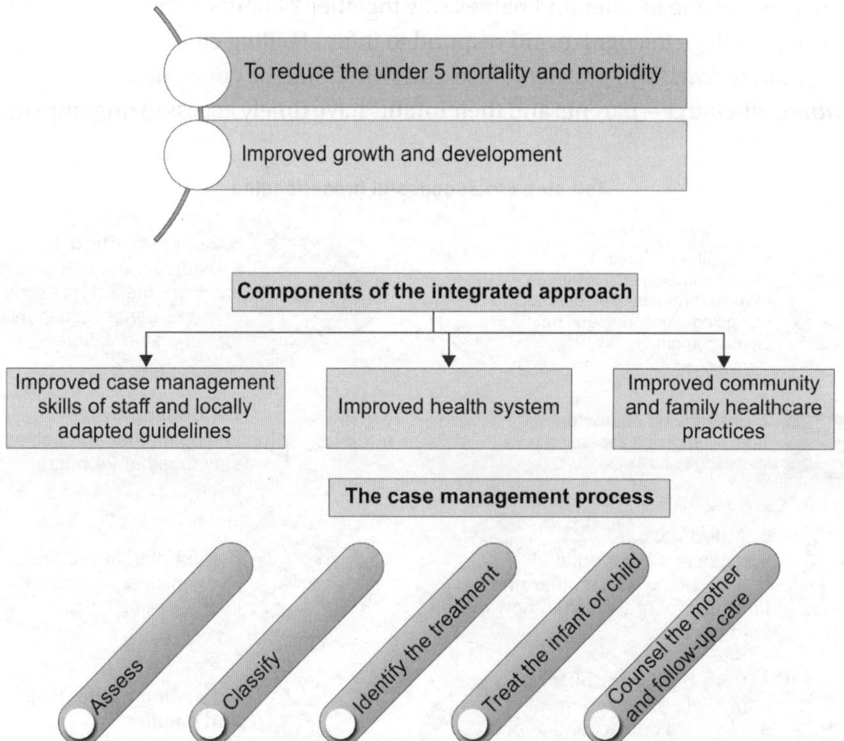

The charts of IMNCI are enclosed in the annexure.

Annexures

1. Procedure
   Sana Ibad Khan, Garima Saxena, Sanjeev Chetry, Amit Yadav, Souradip Banik, Bhavya Kukreja, Anunaya Katiyar, Anuradha Bansal, Nidhi Jain, Gunjan Srivastava, Neha Jain

2. Equipment
   Manish Diwedi, Swati Upadhyay, Mrinal Sinha, Swati Jangra, Anantika Garg, Boby Varghese, Arun Gautam, Neha Jain, Jubilant James, Garima Saxena

3. Medication
   Richa Malik

4. Common Laboratory Reference Value
   Sachin Garg

5. Biostatistics
   Ramji Bhardwaj, Amit Yadav, Aparna Prasad

6. OSCE
   Swati Upadhyay, Sidharth Nayyar, Naveen Prakash Gupta

Procedure

Sana Ibad Khan, Garima Saxena, Sanjeev Chetry, Amit Yadav, Souradip Banik, Bhavya Kukreja, Anunaya Katiyar, Anuradha Bansal, Nidhi Jain, Gunjan Srivastava, Neha Jain

1.1 UMBILICAL VENOUS CATHETERIZATION

Sana Ibad Khan

Objective

One should be able to catheterize umbilical vein in newborn.

Indications

- During resuscitation as an emergency vascular access
- For exchange transfusion
- For monitoring of central venous pressure
- For administration of intravenous fluids, drugs, TPN, and blood products.

Equipment and Supplies

- Umbilical catheter—<1,500 g –3.5 Fr, >1,500 g –5 Fr, 6 Fr, 7 Fr
- Dressing set—sterile drapes/gauze/scissors
- Measuring tape
- Sterile cap/mask/gowns/gloves
- Chlorhexidine solution
- *Instruments:* Nontooth forceps, iris forceps, artery forceps, towel clamps, sterile blade
- Syringe 5 mL, 10 mL
- Three way/octopus
- Tegaderm/DuoDERM
- Sucrose/dextrose gel/25% dextrose/EBM for analgesia
- Normal saline or sterile water
- Length from shoulder to umbilical length chart
- Tri way or octopus connector
- Neo bridge or transparent dressing or goalpost adhesive
- Sutures.

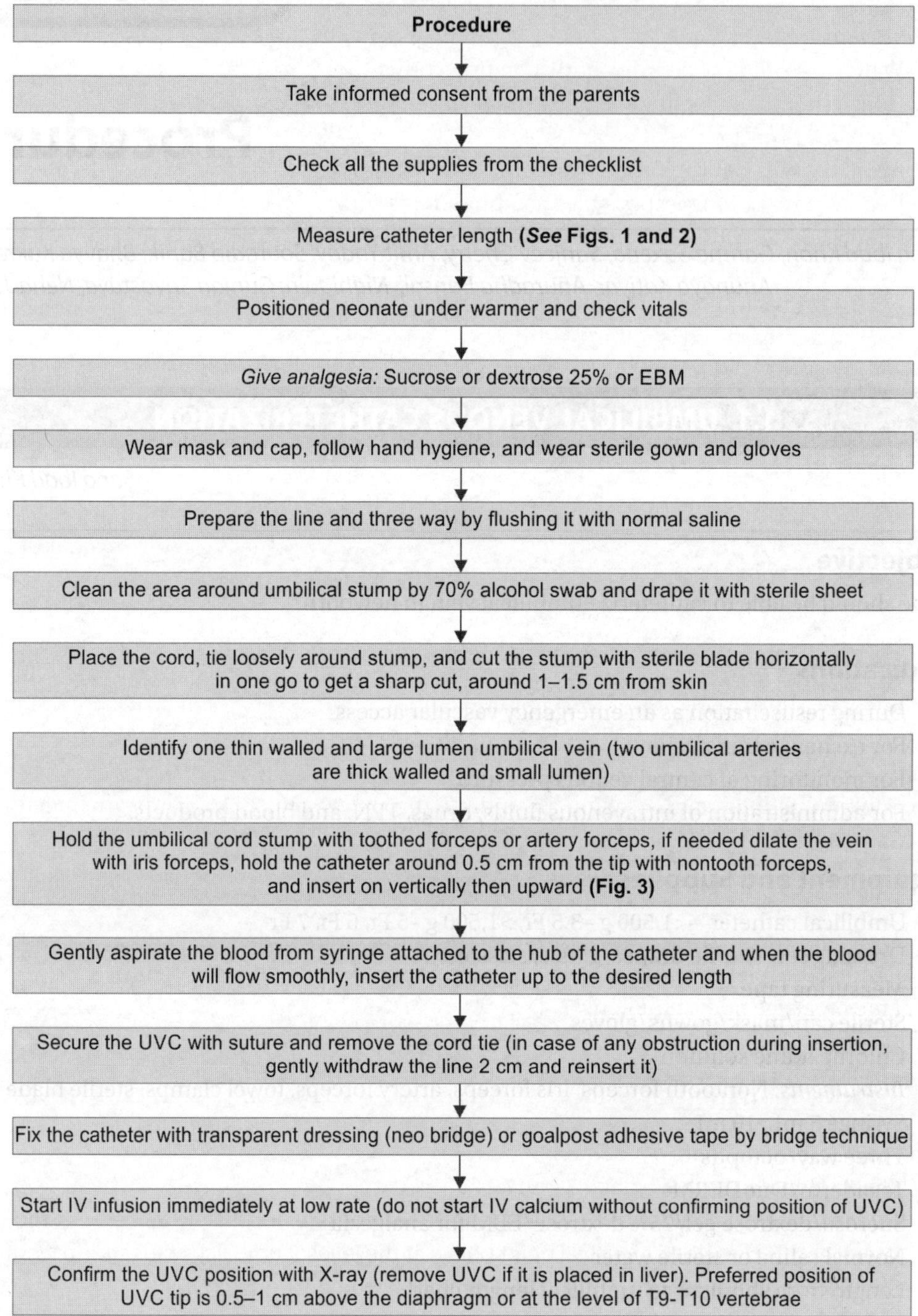

Procedure

Take informed consent from the parents

Check all the supplies from the checklist

Measure catheter length (*See* Figs. 1 and 2)

Positioned neonate under warmer and check vitals

Give analgesia: Sucrose or dextrose 25% or EBM

Wear mask and cap, follow hand hygiene, and wear sterile gown and gloves

Prepare the line and three way by flushing it with normal saline

Clean the area around umbilical stump by 70% alcohol swab and drape it with sterile sheet

Place the cord, tie loosely around stump, and cut the stump with sterile blade horizontally in one go to get a sharp cut, around 1–1.5 cm from skin

Identify one thin walled and large lumen umbilical vein (two umbilical arteries are thick walled and small lumen)

Hold the umbilical cord stump with toothed forceps or artery forceps, if needed dilate the vein with iris forceps, hold the catheter around 0.5 cm from the tip with nontooth forceps, and insert on vertically then upward (Fig. 3)

Gently aspirate the blood from syringe attached to the hub of the catheter and when the blood will flow smoothly, insert the catheter up to the desired length

Secure the UVC with suture and remove the cord tie (in case of any obstruction during insertion, gently withdraw the line 2 cm and reinsert it)

Fix the catheter with transparent dressing (neo bridge) or goalpost adhesive tape by bridge technique

Start IV infusion immediately at low rate (do not start IV calcium without confirming position of UVC)

Confirm the UVC position with X-ray (remove UVC if it is placed in liver). Preferred position of UVC tip is 0.5–1 cm above the diaphragm or at the level of T9-T10 vertebrae

Maintenance of UVC:
- Watch for soiling of dressing and change accordingly.
- Gauze should not be put over the umbilical vein.
- Keep line away from diaper.
- Avoid keeping baby in prone position.
- Remove line as soon as possible (recommended duration 14 days).
- Follow CLASBI bundle approach.
  - Perform hand hygiene before and after assessing catheter or using catheter.
  - Access insertion site daily for any soiling of site.
  - Use standardized IV tubing set ups.
  - Always scrub the hub for 15 seconds before using line.
  - Keeps catheter connection sterile.
  - Establish sterile field under access port.

Removal of line:
- Remove line as soon as possible.
- Grasp the catheter and gently remove the line.
- Measure length of catheter after removing it.
- Cover the site with sterile dressing, press it for few seconds if there is bleeding from the site.
- If resistance is felt while removing dressing then do not remove the dressing forcefully, apply warm compress over the vein tract and reattempt after 30 minutes (one to two attempts can be done 12–24 hours apart), do X-ray to locate catheter.

Complication:
- Look the redness and swelling around the umbilicus, which may indicate infection. Stop the infusion and remove the UVC.
- *Catheter-related sepsis and infections:* Omphalitis, endocarditis, cellulitis, liver abscess.
- *Vascular complication:* Air embolism, thrombosis.
- *Line migration:* Leads to cardiac arrhythmia, pericardial effusion, pericardial tamponade, pleural effusion, NEC, hepatic necrosis
- Line breakage or dysfunction.

Key Points to Remember

How to measure the length of insertion:
- *Shukla formula:* (Birth weight × 3 + 9) / 2+1
- *Dunn's formula:* Shoulder to umbilical length normogram, for this distance from top of lateral end of clavicle to a vertical point below at the level of umbilicus plus stump length.
- Shoulder-umbilical length (cm) × 0.66 + umbilical stump length (cm).

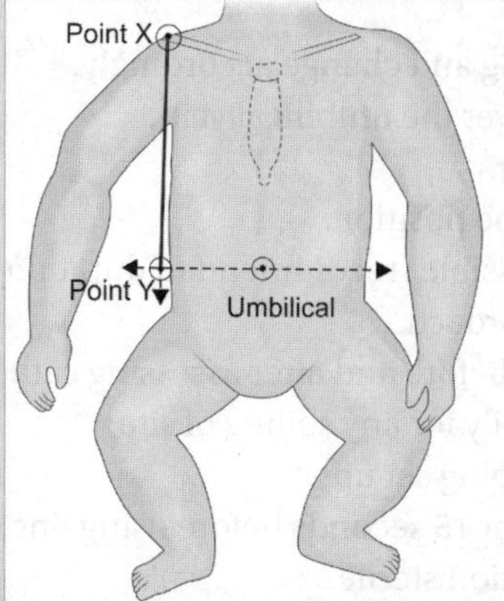

Fig. 1: Shoulder–umbilicus length—the distance measured in an inferior vertical direction from the shoulder tip (*X*) to the level of the umbilicus (*Y*)—as measured by Dunn.

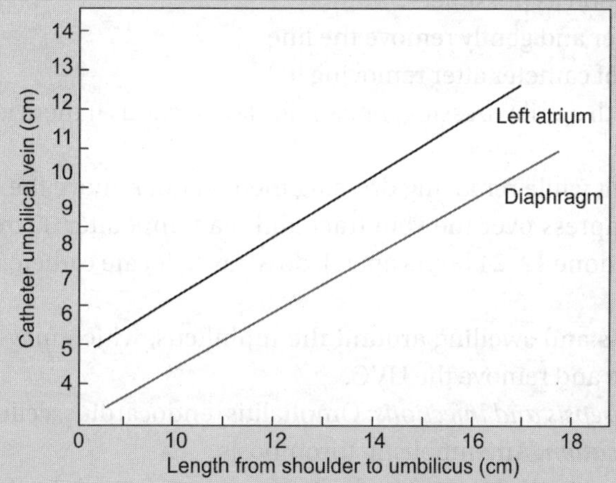

Fig. 2: Graph showed the measurement of the shoulder–umbilicus length to the estimated insertion depth for umbilical venous catheters, the solid lower line indicates the depth that estimates insertion to the diaphragm.

Note: There is no consensus evidence regarding the authenticity of any formula for optimal UVC length, UVC tip position is confirmed by X-ray or ultrasound after procedure is required.

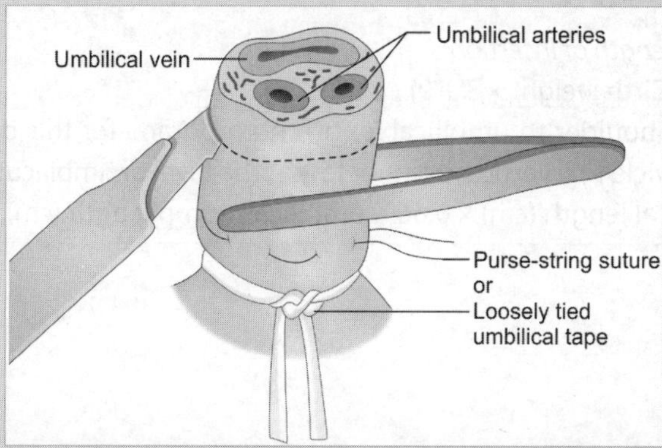

Fig. 3: Hold the umbilical cord stump with toothed forceps or artery forceps.

OSCE/Checklist: Procedure—Insertion of UVC			
*Name of the participants:*____			
S. No.	*Performance steps*	*Yes*	*No*
1.	Check records and identify neonates		
2.	Gather all the supplies and prepare solution to be infused		
3.	Perform hand washing		
4.	Wear sterile gloves		
5.	Assistant opens all supplies aseptically and put them in a sterile tray		
6.	Prepare the umbilical and the surrounding skin with spirit swab in outward circular motion and allow to dry		
7.	Repeat the procedure with betadine swab, using same technique		
8.	Place cut sterile drapes over the baby's body so that only umbilical area is exposed		
9.	Fill the umbilical catheter with NS using closed syringe attached to the end of the catheter		
10.	Place the cord tie or suture around the base of the umbilicus to control bleeding and cut the cord to a length of 1–2 cm using a sterile blade		
11.	Identify single umbilical vein (and two umbilical arteries)		
12.	Hold the catheter in one hand and insert the catheter into the UV and advance further toward head of the baby and to the baby's right side		
13.	Advance the catheter gently until blood flows back freely into the catheter. Do not advance further		
14.	Suture around the stump using purse string suture to hold the catheter in place		
15.	Remove the syringe and connect the infusion set to the catheter. Ensure there is no air bubble		
16.	Secure the catheter with adhesive tape/transparent dressing to prevent it from dislodged		
	Total score		

▮ FURTHER READING

1. Hermansen MC, Hermansen MG. Intravascular catheter complications in the neonatal intensive care unit. Clin Perinatol. 2005;32(1):141-56, vii.
2. Lewis K, Spirnak PW. (2022). Umbilical vein catheterization. [online] In: StatPearls [Internet]. Treasure Island (FL): StatPearls Publishing. Available from https://pubmed.ncbi.nlm.nih. gov/31751059/ [Last accessed October, 2022].
3. Shukla H, Ferrara A. Rapid estimation of insertional length of umbilical catheters in newborns. Am J Dis Child. 1986;140(8):786-8.

1.2 UMBILICAL ARTERIAL CATHETERIZATION

Sana Ibad Khan

Objective

One should be able to catheterize umbilical artery in newborn.

Indications

- Arterial blood pressure monitoring in sick and ventilated neonates.
- To perform frequent arterial blood gas monitoring.
- To perform isovolumetric exchange transfusion.

Equipment and Supplies

- Umbilical catheter—<1500 g –3.5 Fr, >1500 g –5 Fr, 6 Fr, 7 Fr
- Dressing set—sterile drapes/gauze/scissors
- Measuring tape
- Sterile cap/mask/gowns/gloves
- Chlorhexidine solution
- *Instruments:* Nontooth forceps, iris forceps, artery forceps, towel clamps, sterile blade
- Syringe 5 mL, 10 mL
- Three way/octopus
- Tegaderm/DuoDERM
- Sucrose/dextrose gel/25% dextrose/EBM for analgesia
- Normal saline or sterile water
- Length from shoulder to umbilical length chart
- Tri way or octopus connector
- Neo bridge or transparent dressing or goalpost adhesive
- Sutures

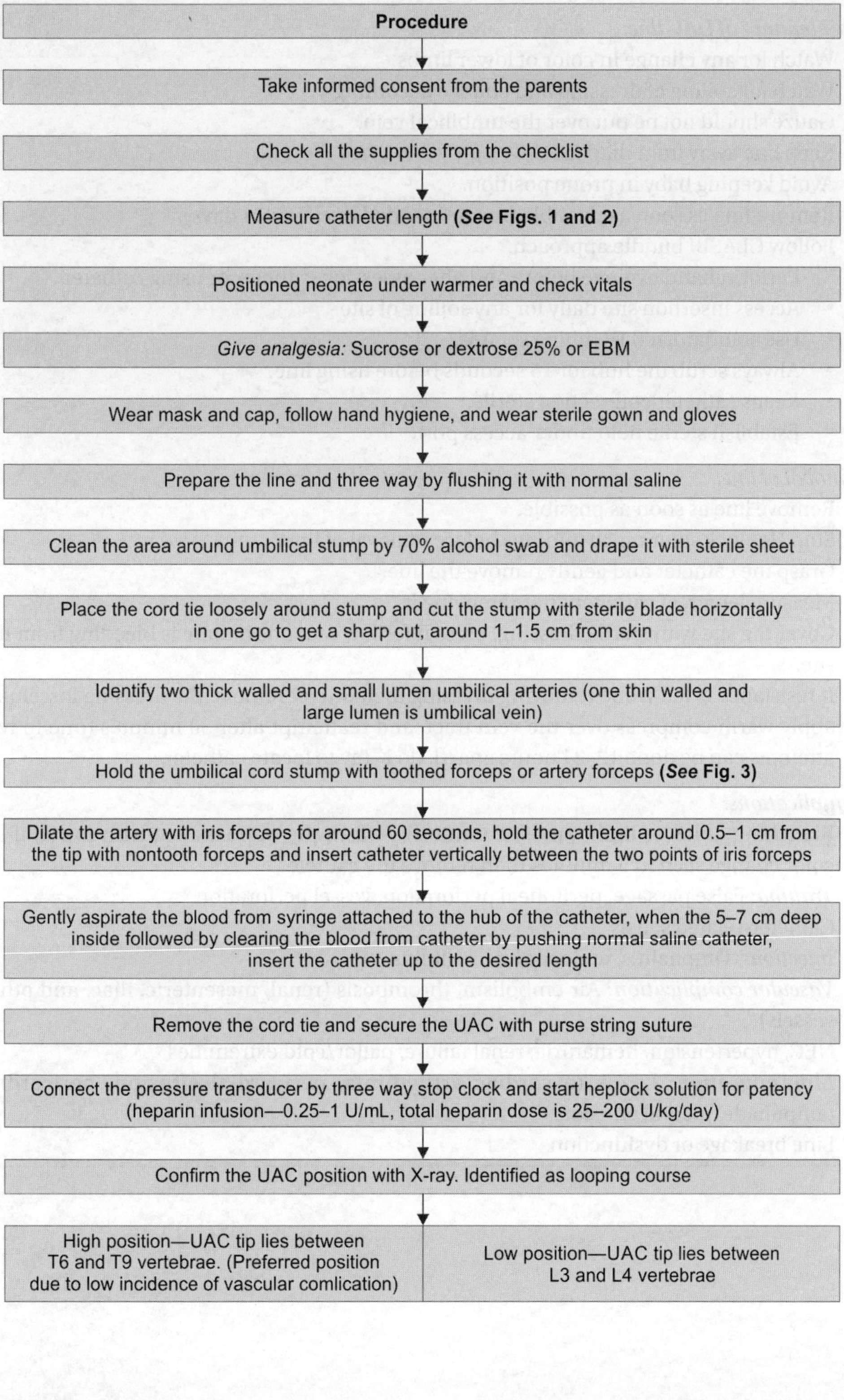

Procedure

↓

Take informed consent from the parents

↓

Check all the supplies from the checklist

↓

Measure catheter length (*See* **Figs. 1 and 2**)

↓

Positioned neonate under warmer and check vitals

↓

Give analgesia: Sucrose or dextrose 25% or EBM

↓

Wear mask and cap, follow hand hygiene, and wear sterile gown and gloves

↓

Prepare the line and three way by flushing it with normal saline

↓

Clean the area around umbilical stump by 70% alcohol swab and drape it with sterile sheet

↓

Place the cord tie loosely around stump and cut the stump with sterile blade horizontally in one go to get a sharp cut, around 1–1.5 cm from skin

↓

Identify two thick walled and small lumen umbilical arteries (one thin walled and large lumen is umbilical vein)

↓

Hold the umbilical cord stump with toothed forceps or artery forceps (*See* **Fig. 3**)

↓

Dilate the artery with iris forceps for around 60 seconds, hold the catheter around 0.5–1 cm from the tip with nontooth forceps and insert catheter vertically between the two points of iris forceps

↓

Gently aspirate the blood from syringe attached to the hub of the catheter, when the 5–7 cm deep inside followed by clearing the blood from catheter by pushing normal saline catheter, insert the catheter up to the desired length

↓

Remove the cord tie and secure the UAC with purse string suture

↓

Connect the pressure transducer by three way stop clock and start heplock solution for patency (heparin infusion—0.25–1 U/mL, total heparin dose is 25–200 U/kg/day)

↓

Confirm the UAC position with X-ray. Identified as looping course

↓

High position—UAC tip lies between T6 and T9 vertebrae. (Preferred position due to low incidence of vascular comlication)	Low position—UAC tip lies between L3 and L4 vertebrae

Maintenance of UAC line:
- Watch for any change in color of lower limbs.
- Watch for soiling of dressing and change accordingly.
- Gauze should not be put over the umbilical vein.
- Keep line away from diaper.
- Avoid keeping baby in prone position.
- Remove line as soon as possible (recommended duration 14 days).
- Follow CLASBI bundle approach.
    - Perform hand hygiene before and after assessing catheter or using catheter.
    - Access insertion site daily for any soiling of site.
    - Use standardized IV tubing set ups.
    - Always scrub the hub for 15 seconds before using line.
    - Keeps catheter connection sterile.
    - Establish sterile field under access port.

Removal of line:
- Remove line as soon as possible.
- Stop Heplock solution 30 minutes before removal of line.
- Grasp the catheter and gently remove the line.
- Measure length of catheter after removing it.
- Cover the site with sterile dressing, press it for few seconds if there is bleeding from the site.
- If resistance is felt while removing dressing then do not remove the dressing forcefully, apply warm compress over the vein tract, and reattempt after 30 minutes (one to two attempts can be done 12–24 hours apart), do X-ray to locate catheter.

Complications:
- Blanching of lower limbs (most common)—warm the opposite leg with towel, if no color change seen in 5 minutes then remove the catheter.
- *Trauma:* False passage, peritoneal perforation, vessel perforation
- Catheter-related sepsis
- *Infections:* Omphalitis, endocarditis, cellulitis
- *Vascular complication:* Air embolism, thrombosis (renal, mesenteric, iliac, and other vessels)
- NEC, hypertension, hematuria, renal failure, pallor/cold extremities
- *Line migration:* Leads to cardiac arrhythmia, pericardial effusion, pericardial tamponade, pleural effusion
- Line breakage or dysfunction

Key Points to Remember

How to measure the length of insertion:

- Shoulder–umbilical length—shoulder to umbilical length normogram, for this distance from tip of lateral end of clavicle to a vertical point below at the level of umbilicus plus stump length plus stump length.
- Infants 31,500 g = (birth weight in kg × 3) + 9 cm + umbilical stump length
- Infants <1,500 g = (birth weight in kg × 4) + 7 cm + umbilical stump length

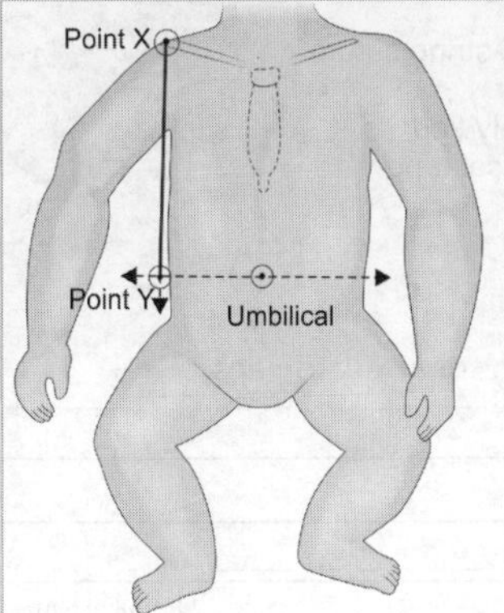

Fig. 1: Shoulder–umbilicus length—the distance measured in an inferior vertical direction from the shoulder tip (*X*) to the level of the umbilicus (*Y*)—as measured by Dunn.

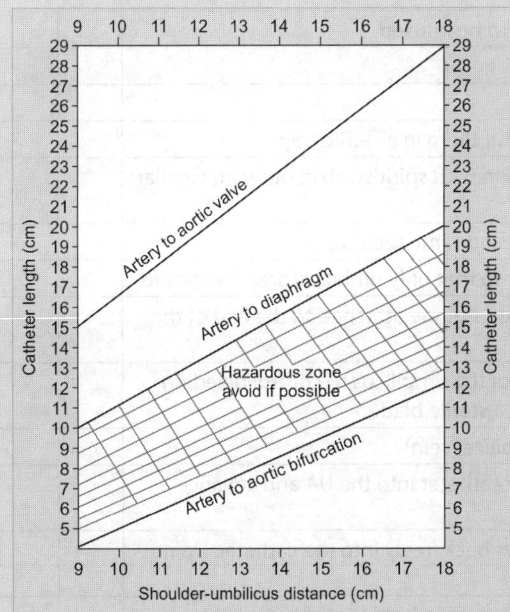

Fig. 2: Graph showed the measurement of the shoulder–umbilicus length to the estimated insertion depth for umbilical venous catheters, the solid middle line indicates the depth that estimates insertion to the diaphragm.

Note: There is no consensus evidence regarding the authenticity of any formula for optimal UAC length, UAC tip position is confirmed by X-ray or ultrasound after procedure is required.

- Attempt UAC insertion first followed by UVC insertion (in case of emergency need for venous access UVC is attempted first).

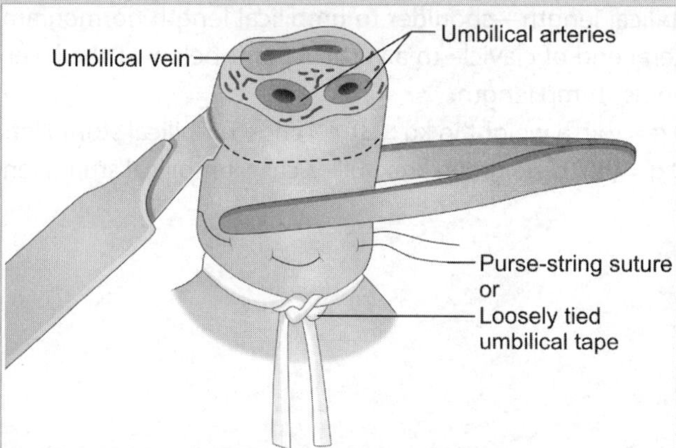

Fig. 3: Hold the umbilical cord stump with toothed forceps or artery forceps.

OSCE/Checklist: Procedure—Insertion of UAC			
Name of the participants:			
S. No.	*Performance steps*	*Yes*	*No*
1.	Check records and identify neonates		
2.	Gather all the supplies and prepare solution to be infused		
3.	Perform hand washing		
4.	Wear sterile gloves		
5.	Assistant opens all supplies aseptically and put them in a sterile tray		
6.	Prepare the umbilical and the surrounding skin with spirit swab in outward circular motion and allow to dry		
7.	Repeat the procedure with betadine swab, using same technique		
8.	Place cut sterile drapes over the baby's body so that only umbilical area is exposed		
9.	Fill the umbilical catheter with NS using closed syringe attached to the end of the catheter		
10.	Place the cord tie or suture around the base of the umbilicus to control bleeding and cut the cord to a length of 1–2 cm using a sterile blade		
11.	Identify two umbilical artery (and single umbilical vein)		
12.	Hold the catheter in one hand and insert the catheter into the UA and advance further		
13.	Advance the catheter gently until blood flows back freely into the catheter. Do not advance further		
14.	Suture around the stump using purse string suture to hold the catheter in place		
15.	Remove the syringe and connect the infusion set to the catheter. Ensure there is no air bubble		
16.	Secure the catheter with adhesive tape/transparent dressing to prevent it from dislodged		
	Total score		

■ FURTHER READING

1. Hermansen MC, Hermansen MG. Intravascular catheter complications in the neonatal intensive care unit. Clin Perinatol. 2005;32(1):141-56, vii.
2. Lewis K, Spirnak PW. (2022). Umbilical vein catheterization. [online] In: StatPearls [Internet]. Treasure Island (FL): StatPearls Publishing. Available from https://pubmed.ncbi.nlm.nih.gov/31751059/ [Last accessed October, 2022].
3. Shukla H, Ferrara A. Rapid estimation of insertional length of umbilical catheters in newborns. Am J Dis Child. 1986;140(8):786-8.

1.3 SURFACTANT REPLACEMENT THERAPY

Sana Ibad Khan

Objective

One should be able to perform exogenous surfactant replacement therapy under all aseptic conditions.

Indications

- Respiratory distress syndrome
- Meconium aspiration syndrome
- Persistent pulmonary hypertension of the newborn
- Neonatal pneumonia
- Pulmonary hemorrhage

Methods of Delivery

- *EINSURE (Enhanced INSURE):* This is an updated technique for surfactant administration, as INSURE does not have clear guideline on duration, monitoring, sedation, and ventilation technique used after surfactant. EINSURE consist of all these points. It can be used as a reference technique.
- *INSURE:* INtubate-SURfactant administration-Extubate
- *INRECSURE:* It has been seen that lung recruitment method before surfactant administration showed better outcomes in extremely premature neonates.
- *LISA (less invasive surfactant administration):* LISA is performed through a catheter [feeding tube (4–5 Fr) or suction catheter or umbilical catheter] introduced into trachea using Magill Forceps under direct laryngoscopy. LISA helps in avoiding mechanical ventilation and also improved outcomes of preterm in preventing BPD and intracranial hemorrhage. The disadvantages with LISA are surfactant reflux and catheter-induced bradycardia.
- *MIST (minimally invasive surfactant technique):* There are four different MIST methods, viz., pharyngeal surfactant administration, aerosolized surfactant administration, laryngeal mask-guided surfactant administration, and surfactant administration via Angiocath.

Equipment and Supplies

- Surfactant
- Syringes—2 mL, 5 mL, 10 mL
- Infant feeding tube—5 Fr, 6 Fr
- Surgical blade
- Laryngoscope with miller blades of size 00, 0, and 1 (prechecked)
- Endotracheal tubes—2, 2.5, 3, and 3.5
- T-piece resuscitator/self-inflating bag (prechecked)
- Mask of different size
- Suction catheter
- Oxygen connection tubes
- Sterile mask, gloves, gown, cap
- Midazolam

- Tegaderm or Durapore
- Stethoscope
- Pulse oximeter
- Scissors

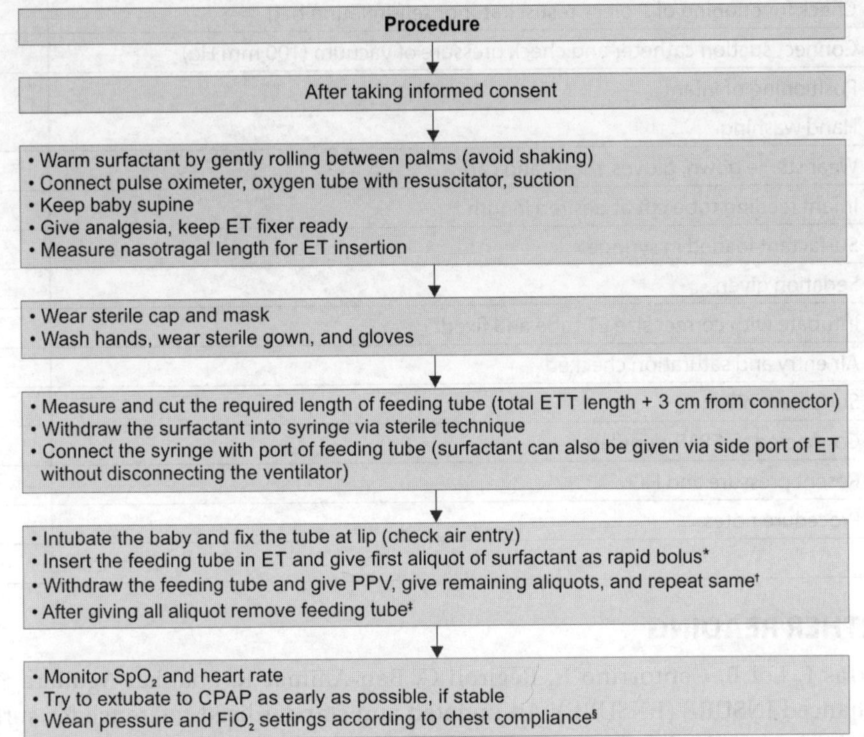

*If neonate is already ventilated, assistant should disconnect the ET tube from ventilator port.

†Increase PIP by 10% and rate at 50–60/min after surfactant administration for 5 minutes for uniform administration of surfactant.

‡If the neonate is already ventilated then reconnect the ventilator and wean pressure and FiO₂ after 5–10 minutes accordingly.

§Second dose of surfactant to be planned according to work of breathing, pressure, and FiO₂ requirement.

Key Points to Remember

- Types of surfactant

Surfactant	Surfactant dose (mL/kg)	Phospholipids dose (mg/kg)
Survanta	4	100
Curosurf	2.5	200
Neosurf	5	135

- Identification of neoate with ID and MR/IPN No.
- Presurfactant ventilation/CPAP setting.
- Postsurfactant change in ventilation/CPAP setting.
- Documentation of procedure in the record file.

OSCE/Checklis: Procedure—Surfactant Replacement Therapy		
Name of the participants:_______________________________________		
S. No.	Performance steps	Yes	No
1.	Functioned laryngoscope with blade		
2.	Check functioning of T-piece resuscitator or self-inflating bag		
3.	Connect suction catheter and check pressure of vacuum (100 mm Hg)		
4.	Positioning of infant		
5.	Hand washing		
6.	Wear sterile gown, gloves, mask, and cap		
7.	Infant feeding tube cut at desired length		
8.	Surfactant loaded in syringe		
9.	Sedation given		
10.	Intubate with correct size ET tube and fixed		
11.	Air entry and saturation checked		
12.	Surfactant given		
13.	Connected to CPAP/ventilator		
14.	Resent pressure and FiO_2		
15.	Procedure notes		
	Total score		

■ FURTHER READING

1. Fortas F, Loi B, Centorrino R, Regiroli G, Ben-Ammar R, Shankar-Aguilera S, et al. Enhanced INSURE (ENSURE): An updated and standardised reference for surfactant administration. Eur J Pediatr. 2022;181(3):1269-75.

2. Gupta BK, Saha AK, Mukherjee S, Saha B. Minimally invasive surfactant therapy versus InSurE in preterm neonates of 28 to 34 weeks with respiratory distress syndrome on non-invasive positive pressure ventilation—a randomized controlled trial. Eur J Pediatr. 2020;179(8):1287-93.

3. Herting E, Härtel C, Göpel W. Less invasive surfactant administration: best practices and unanswered questions. Curr Opin Pediatr. 2020;32(2):228-34.

4. Jena SR, Bains HS, Pandita A, Verma A, Gupta V, Kallem VR, et al.; On Behalf of Sure Group. Surfactant therapy in premature babies: SurE or InSurE. Pediatr Pulmonol. 2019;54(11):1747-52.

5. Shim GH. Update of minimally invasive surfactant therapy. Korean J Pediatr. 2017;60(9): 273-81.

1.4 PERIPHERALLY INSERTED CENTRAL CATHETER

Sana Ibad Khan

Objective

One should be able to perform in section of peripherally inserted central catheter (PICC) under all aseptic conditions.

Indications

- Requirement for long-term IV access (usually >5–7 days).
- Need to infuse hyperosmolar medications that tends to place veins at risk. (For example, >12.5% dextrose, injection calcium gluconate)
- Need to infuse parenteral nutrition
- Difficult intravenous access

Equipment and Supplies

- PICC line—28G (<1,000 g), 24G (>1,000 g)
- Dressing set—sterile drapes/gauze/scissors
- Measuring tape
- Sterile cap/mask/gowns/gloves
- Chlorhexidine solution
- Nontooth forceps
- Syringe 5 mL
- Tri way/octopus
- Heparinized solution (0.5–1 U/mL NS)
- Tegaderm/DuoDERM
- Sucrose/dextrose gel/25% dextrose/EBM for analgesia
- Normal saline

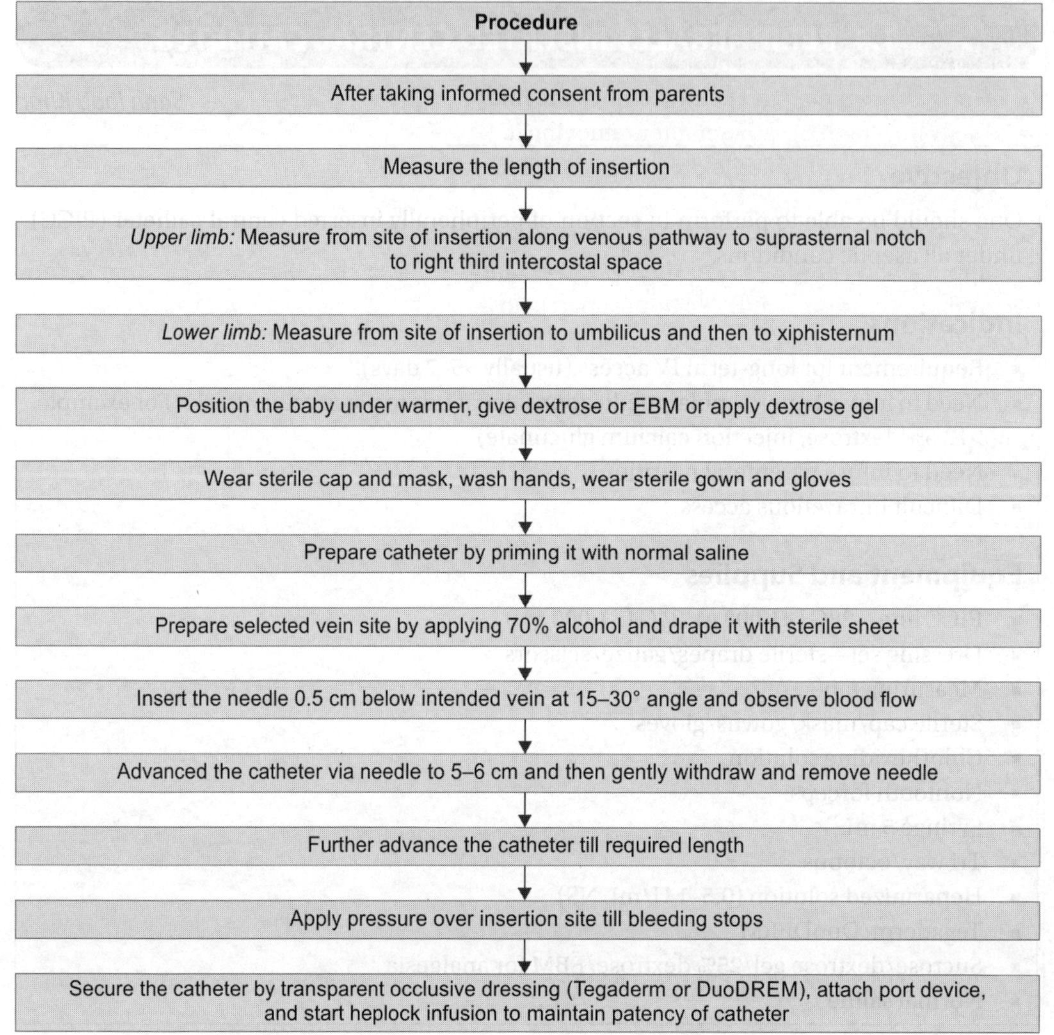

Maintenance of PICC line:

- Watch for soiling of dressing and change accordingly.
- Dressing should not be put tightly.
- Do not measured BP at PICC line site.
- Avoid flushing line forcefully and with syringe <5 mL.
- Follow CLASBI bundle approach.
  - Perform hand hygiene before and after assessing catheter or using catheter.
  - Access insertion site daily for any soiling of site.
  - Use standardized IV tubing set ups.
  - Always scrub the hub for 15 seconds before using line.
  - Keeps catheter connection sterile.
  - Establish sterile field under access port.

Removal of line:

- Remove line as soon as possible.
- Grasp the catheter and gently remove the line.
- Measure length of catheter after removing it.
- Cover the site with sterile dressing, press it for few seconds if there is bleeding from the site.
- If resistance is felt while removing dressing then do not remove the dressing forcefully, apply warm compress over the vein tract, and reattempt after 30 minutes (one to two attempts can be done 12–24 hours apart), do X-ray to locate catheter.

Complications:

- Catheter-related sepsis
- Hemorrhage
- Phlebitis
- Air embolism
- *Line migration:* Leads to cardiac arrhythmia, pericardial effusion, pericardial tamponade, pleural effusion
- Extravascular fluid collection
- Line breakage or dysfunction

Key Points to Remember

- Vein selection antecubital fossa—basilic vein (preferred), leg—femoral vein, great saphenous, scalp veins—superficial temporal, posterior auricular
- Secure the catheter by transparent occlusive dressing (Tegaderm or DuoDERM), attached port device, and start heplock infusion to maintain patency of catheter.
- Confirm position of PICC line tip radiologically (X-ray AP-view and both AP- and lateral view for lower limb).
- *Upper limb:* Line should have crossed first rib with tip lying between T3 and T6 vertebrae. Tip should be outside the cardiac chamber (1 cm in preterm and 2 cm in term neonates).
- *Lower limb:* Line should be in inferior vena cava just below the diaphragm (T9-T10) and above the L4-L5.

OSCE/Checklist: Procedure—Insertion of PICC Cannula			
Name of the participants:_______________________________________			
S. No.	Performance steps	Yes	No
1.	Gather all supplies		
2.	Perform hand washing		
3.	Wear sterile gloves		
4.	Assistant opens all supplies aseptically and put them in a sterile tray		
5.	Prepare the skin with spirit swab for 30 seconds		
6.	Pricks skin surface at 30–45° to skin		
7.	Backflow of blood ensured		
8.	Flushes cannula with normal saline		
9.	Fixes cannula with transparent dressing like Tegaderm		
	Total score		

■ FURTHER READING

1. Gleason CA, Devaskar SU. Avery's Diseases of the Newborn, 9th edition. Philadelphia: Elsevier; 2012.

2. Rennie JM. Rennie & Roberton's Textbook of neonatology, 5th edition. United Kingdom: Churchill Livingstone; 2012.

1.5 INTRA-ARTERIAL BLOOD PRESSURE MONITORING

Sana Ibad Khan

Objective

One should be able to monitor the intra-arterial blood pressure.

Indication

Blood pressure monitoring in hemodynamically unstable neonates.

Equipment and Supplies

- UAC (if umbilical artery is preferred)
- Cannula (if peripheral artery is preferred)—22–24 gauge
- Alcohol swab/70% alcohol
- Sterile gloves, gown, head cap, mask
- Pressure transducer
- Three way
- Heplock solution
- Multichannel monitor
- Stopcock
- IV stand
- Transilluminator torch
- Transparent dressing

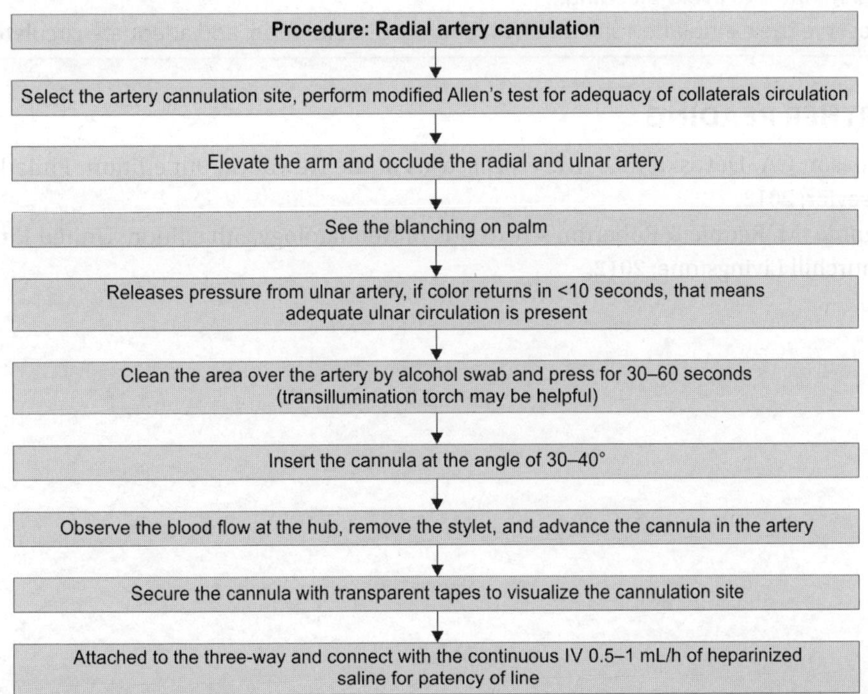

For Assembly of Monitor

- Fix monitor assembly on IV stand, place transducer at the level of neonate's heart.
- Flush whole system with saline to remove air bubble and connect stopcock of monitor assembly with syringe pump.
- Another flushed line is connected with upper port of stopcock, connect this line UAC.
- Connect transducer to multichannel monitor.

Zeroing of Assembly

- Turn off the stopcock connecting UAC and transducer.
- Calibrate arterial pressure in monitor to zero.
- Open the stopcock from the neonate's side.

Key Points to Remember

- Umbilical artery (most commonly used).
- *Peripheral arteries:* Radial, ulnar, dorsalis pedis.
- Proper positioning of catheter tips is checked by X-ray or USG.
- *For errors in BP reading:* Check for air bubbles, blood clots, and kinking in the circuit.
- Zeroing should be ensured.
- Avoid long tubing.
- Monitor for arterial vasospasm.
- *Removal of arterial line:* Stop the infusion before removal of catheter and turn of the stopcock. Remove the dressings and gently remove the cannula, apply pressure for 3–5 minutes to avoid bleeding.
- Observe the cannulation site for any bleeding, discoloration, and adequate circulation.

■ FURTHER READING

1. Gleason CA, Devaskar SU. Avery's Diseases of the Newborn, 9th edition. Philadelphia: Elsevier; 2012.
2. Rennie JM. Rennie & Roberton's Textbook of Neonatology, 5th edition. United Kingdom: Churchill Livingstone; 2012.

1.6 PREVENTION OF VENTILATION-ASSOCIATED PNEUMONIA IN NEONATES

Garima Saxena, Sanjeev Chetry

Definition

The Centers for Disease Control and Prevention defines ventilation-associated pneumonia (VAP) as a nosocomial infection diagnosed in a patient undergoing mechanical ventilation for at least 48 hours.

Diagnosis

Diagnosis of VAP requires a combination of radiological, clinical, and laboratory criteria.

Radiological Signs

CXR with one or more (patients with underlying disease two or more):

- New or progressive and persistent infiltrates
- Consolidation
- Cavitation
- Pneumatocele.

Clinical Signs and Symptoms

Worsening of gas exchange, increased oxygen requirements or increased ventilation, and three of the following:

1. Temperature instability with no other recognized cause.
2. Leukopenia (<4,000 WBC/mm or leukocytosis >15,000 WBC/mm and left shift (>10% band forms)
3. New onset of purulent sputum or change in character of sputum or increase in respiratory secretions or increased suctioning requirements
4. Apnea tachypnea, nasal flaring with chest wall retraction, or grunting
5. Wheezing, rales, or rhonchi
6. Cough
7. Bradycardia (<100/min) or tachycardia (>170 beats/min).

Microbiological Findings

At least one of the following:

1. Positive growth in blood cultures not related to any source of infection.
2. Positive growth pleural fluid cultures
3. Positive quantitative cultures from minimally contaminated LRT specimen (BAL (>10 CFU/mL or protected specimen brushing (>10 CFU/mL).
4. >5% BAL obtained cell contain intracellular bacteria on direct microscopic examination (Gram stain).

5. Histopathological shows at least one of the following:
    Abscess formation or foci of consolidation with intense PMN accumulation in bronchioles and alveoli, positive quantitative cultures of lung parenchyma or evidence of lung parenchyma (>/10 CFU/g tissue) or evidence of lung parenchyma invasion by fungal hyphae or pseudohyphae.

Risk Factors

- Prematurity
- VLBW
- Duration of ventilation
- Primary bloodstream infection
- Prior antibiotic use
- Sedation
- Enteral feeds
- Parenteral nutrition
- Endotracheal suctioning

Diagnostic Biomarkers

- Procalcitonin
- Calcitonin
- Interleukins

Management

- Initiation of empirical antibiotic according to nosocomial flora and resistance pattern.
- Aerosolized antibiotic, alternative route and reduce systemic antibiotic.
- Duration of antibiotic is still not sure.

Bundle Care for Prevention of VAP

- *Hand hygiene:*
    - Wash hands with soap and water.
    - Wear mask, cap, and gloves.
    - Do not touch baby or baby's environment with gloves.
    - Handwash or use alcohol-based hand sanitizer.
- *Endotracheal tube care:* Aseptic condition to be maintained during intubation.
- *Humidification:*
    - Heated humidifier at 37°C with 100 relative humidity.
    - Auto refill technique to fill water for humidifier.
    - No condensation in inspiratory limb.
    - Drain condensate in water trap.
    - Condensate to be considered as infectious waste.

- *Respiratory equipment care:*
  - Ventilator circuits should be changed when visibly soiled.
  - Ventilator circuits should be used only once if disposable and if reusable they should be sterilized after each use.
  - The respiratory case instrument should be handled under strict sepsis.
  - Endotracheal suction should be done preferably by health personnel with one person assisting handling suction catheter.
  - CPAP should not be allowed to be standby for 12 hours.
  - Resuscitation bags not to be kept on bed and bags should be replaced once in a week.
  - The circuit to be positioned parallel to the baby and its development position.
- *Position of infant:*
  - 30–45° elevation head end.
  - Lateral decubitus is preferred.
  - Frequent change in positions.
- *Stress ulcer prophylaxis:*
  - Acidic gastric content prevents bacterial contamination.
  - Avoid using antacids like ranitidine.
- *Oral hygiene:*
  - Oral suctioning to prevent pooling of secretions.
  - Moisten lips with saline.
  - Avoid reusable tunes for oral suction.
  - Promote oral colostrum care.
- *Enteral feeds:*
  - Encourage oral feeds through orogastric feeds.
  - Prefer EBM (expressed breast milk) over formula.
  - Trophic feeds if not enteral feeds.
- *Shorter duration of intubation and ventilation:*
  - Daily consideration of extubation in morning and shift to noninvasive mode.
  - Use of noninvasive ventilation should be preferred.
  - Wean off ventilator as soon as possible.
  - Prevent unplanned extubation.
  - Avoid unnecessary reintubation.
- *Postextubation:*
  - Frequent change in position.
  - Oral and nasal suctioning as indicated.
  - Nebulization if required.
  - Watch for respiratory distress.

OSCE/Checklist: Prevention of VAP			
Name of the participants:______________________________			
S. No.	Performance steps	Yes	No
	Hand hygiene		
1.	Wash hands with soap and water		
2.	Wear mask, cap, and gloves		
3.	Do not touch baby or baby's environment with gloves		
4.	Hand wash or use alcohol-based hand sanitizer		
	Endotracheal tube care		
1.	Aseptic condition to be maintained during intubation		
2.	Oral intubation must be preferred over nasal		
	Humidification		
1.	Heated humidifier at 37°C with 100 relative humidity		
2.	Auto refill technique to fill water for humidifier		
3.	No condensation in inspiratory limb		
4	Drain condensate in water trap		
5.	Condensate to be considered as infectious waste		
	Respiratory equipment care		
1.	Ventilator circuits should be changed when visibly soiled		
2.	Ventilator circuits should be used only once if disposable and if reusable they should be sterilized after each use		
3.	The respiratory case instrument should be handled under strict sepsis		
4.	Endotracheal suction should be done preferably by health personnel with one person assisting handling suction catheter		
5.	CPAP should not be allowed to be standby for 12 hours		
6.	Resuscitation bags not to be kept on bed and bags should be replaced once in a week		
7.	The circuit to be positioned parallel to the baby and its development position		
	Position of infant		
1.	30–45° elevation head end		
2.	Lateral decubitus is preferred		
3.	Frequent change in positions		
	Stress ulcer prophylaxis		
1.	Acidic gastric content prevents bacterial contamination		
2.	Avoid using antacids like ranitidine		
	Oral hygiene		
1.	Oral suctioning to prevent pooling of secretions		
2.	Moisten lips with saline		

Contd...

Contd...

3.	Avoid reusable tunes for oral suction		
4.	Chlorhexidine oral application is optional		
	Enteral feeds		
1.	Encourage oral feeds through orogastric feeds		
2.	Prefer EBM (expressed breast milk) over formula		
3.	Trophic feeds if not enteral feeds		
	Shorter duration of intubation and ventilation		
1.	Daily consideration of extubation in morning and shift to noninvasive mode		
2.	Use of noninvasive ventilation should be preferred		
3.	Wean off ventilator as soon as possible		
4.	Prevent unplanned extubation		
5.	Avoid unnecessary reintubation		
	Postextubation		
1.	Frequent change in position		
2.	Oral and nasal suctioning as indicated		
3.	Nebulization if required		
4.	Watch for respiratory distress		

1.7 CENTRAL LINE-ASSOCIATED BLOODSTREAM INFECTION (CLABSI) AND IV CARE BUNDLE

Amit Yadav, Souradip Banik

Definition

- Primary blood stream infection in a baby who had a central line within the 48 hours period before development of infections.
- Infections must not be related to an alternative cause.

Criteria

Primary BSI with symptoms of:

- Fever (>38°C), hypothermia (<36°C), apnea, or bradycardia
- BSIs caused by a recognized pathogen (e.g., *Escherichia coli*) isolated from ≥1 blood culture

or

- Common skin commensal [e.g., coagulase-negative staphylococci (CoNS)] cultured from ≥2 blood cultures drawn on separate occasions.

Pathogenesis of Central Line-associated Bloodstream Infection

Source

- Catheter insertion site
- During catheter hub preparation
- Contamination of fluids or drugs
- Can be due to secondary infection.

Pathology of Infection

Biofilm formation extraluminally and intraluminally (composed of bacteria embedded within an extracellular polysaccharide matrix on the catheter surface)

↓

- It develop within 24 hours of catheter insertion and are mainly formed on the external surface of the catheter
- Over time a biofilm is formed in the inner surface of the catheter

↓

Occurs when a catheter is placed for a long time >10 days

↓

These biofilms are highly impenetrable to antibiotics

Blood Specimen

- Two or more blood specimen collected on separate days means:
  - Blood culture from two separate site is collected on the same or consecutive calendar days.

- Two separate site preparations (decontamination steps) are performed during specimen collection.
- The blood cultures are assigned separate accession numbers, processed individually, and are reported separately in the final laboratory report.
- Blood collected from central line can have higher rate of contamination than peripheral line sample but any positive result must be included for CLABSI surveillance.
- Catheter tip cultures cannot be used in place of blood specimens for meeting criteria.

Prevention of Central Line-associated Bloodstream Infection

- Education and training of the stuff.
- Choose the central line type like UVC, PICC based on the clinical needs of the NICU patients not only the basis of CLABSI.
- Intervention bundle for CVC insertion and maintenance.
- Skin antiseptic in infant and neonates—70% alcohol, tincture of iodine or alcoholic chlorhexidine gluconate (CHG) solution recommended.
- Choose the insertion site of central line based on the clinical needs of the NICU patients not only the basis of CLABSI.
- Choose fewest number of lumen based on the clinical needs of NICU patients.
- Minimize number of central line hubs and minimize blood sampling through central line to prevent infection.
- Remove the central line (PICC) as soon as possible when no longer needed.
- Consider removal of UVC/UAC at or before 7 days of dwell time.
- Consider dedicated catheter care team to present CLABSI in NICU.
- Do not use prophylactic antimicrobial infusion routinely to present CLABSI.
- Do not use prophylactic anticoagulant infusion.
- Replacement of administration sets—minimum after 96 hours, but surely after 7 days.

IV Care Maintenance

Insertion bundle:
- Establish a central line kit or cart to consolidate all necessary items for the procedure.
- Hand hygiene with hospital approved alcohol-based product or antiseptic containing soap before and after palpating insertion site and before and after inserting central line.
- Barrier precaution during insertion including sterile gown, gloves, mask, cap, and larger sterile drape.
- Skin preparation with antiseptic before catheter insertion.
- Minimize the number of access.
- Keep connecting ports with UVC/UAC away from diaper area.
- Use either sterile transparent semipermeable dressing or sterile gauze to cover the insertion site.
- Prefer upper limb vein over lower limb.

- Ensure catheter tip is at proper position.
- No blood stains around the insertion site.
- The insertion should preferably be done by a skilled trained healthcare person and should always be assisted by another person while inserting.

Maintenance bundles:

- Hand hygiene with hospital approved disinfectant before and after changing the dressing.
- Evaluate the catheter insertion site daily for signs of infection and dressing integrity.
- If dressing is damp, soiled, or loose, change the dressing and disinfect the skin around the insertion site with appropriate antiseptic.
- Develop and use standardized tubing setup and changes.
- Maintain aseptic technique when changing intravenous tubing and when entering the catheter including "scrub the hub".
- Maintenance bundle card to be displayed on the infant warmer for daily audit.
- Any creak in the circuit of central line should be done in the presence of two healthcare personnel to maintain asepsis.
- Daily review of catheter necessity with prompt removal when no longer needed.

Hub care bundle:

- Cleanse hands with soap and water.
- Put on gloves.
- Establish sterile field under access port.
- Place syringes on edge of sterile field.
- Scrub access port with alcohol-based solution/antiseptic being used in the NICU as per protocol, for 15 seconds and allow it to dry.
- Pick up syringe keeping in the tip sterile.
- Attach the syringe to hub, keeping connections sterile.

Removal bundle:

- Review the need of the central line daily and remove as early as possible.

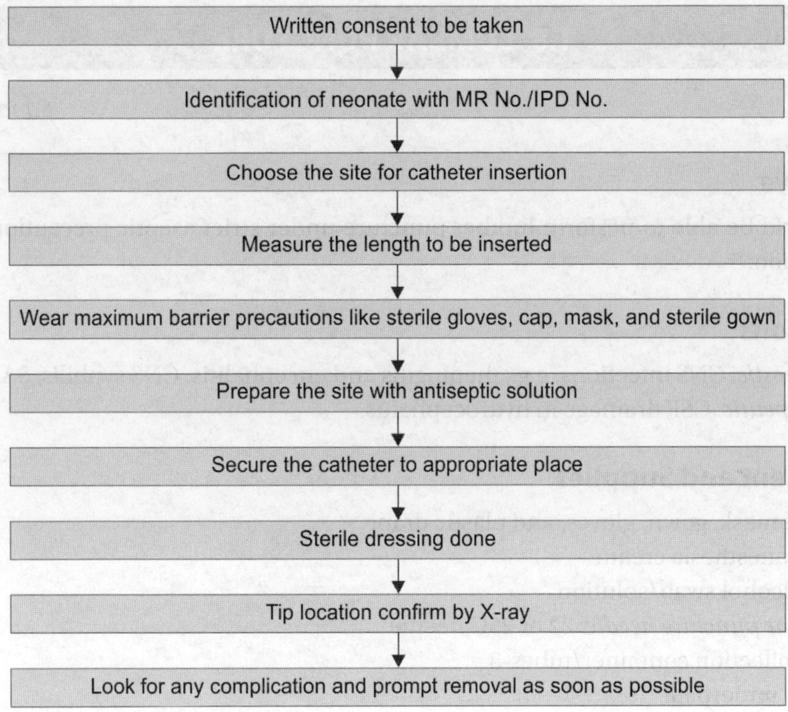

■ FURTHER READING

1. Centers for Disease Control and Prevention. (2022). National healthcare safety network (NHSN) patient safety component manual: bloodstream infection event. US Government. Atlanta.
2. Cho HJ, Cho HK. Central line-associated bloodstream infections in neonates. Korean J Pediatr. 2019;62(3):79-84.

1.8 LUMBAR PUNCTURE

Sana Ibad Khan

Objective

One should be able to perform lumber puncture under strict aseptic precaution for CSF examination.

Indications

- *Diagnostic:* CNS infections, e.g., meningitis and encephalitis, CNS syphilis, SAH.
- *Therapeutic:* CSF drainage in hydrocephalus.

Equipment and Supplies

- Sterile mask, gown, gloves, and plastic drape
- Local anesthesia cream
- 70% alcohol swab/solution
- *Lumbar puncture needle:* 22 or 25G needle
- CSF collection container/tubes-3
- Sterile underpad
- Resuscitation tray.

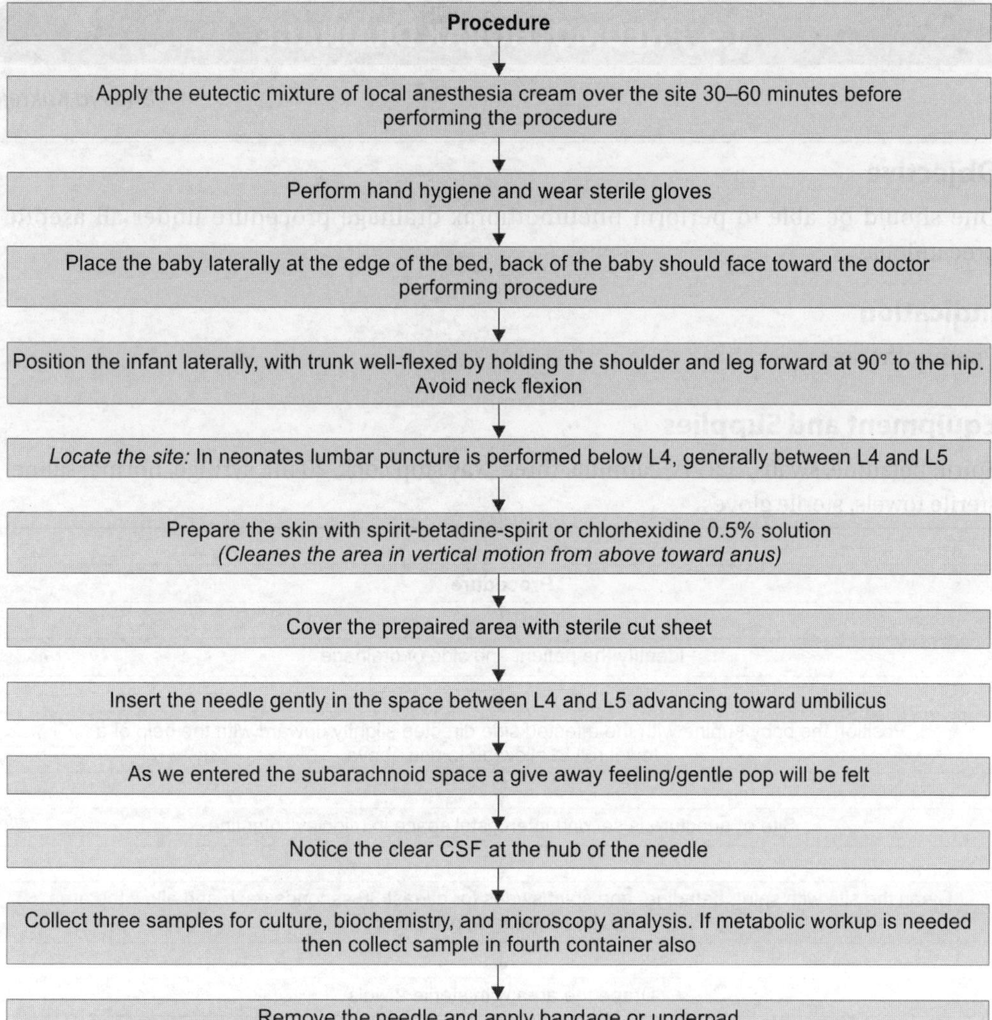

Key Points to Remember

- In case of traumatic LP blood generally clears as CSF flow.
- Blood stained CSF can be sent for culture in case of traumatic tap and procedure need to be repeated after 48 hours.
- Send first sample for culture and gram stain, second for glucose and protein, and third for cell count.
- Remove the bandage after 30 minutes of procedure and check for any staining and CSF leak.
- Document the dry or traumatic tap.

1.9 PNEUMOTHORAX DRAINAGE

Bhavya Kukreja

Objective

One should be able to perform pneumothorax drainage procedure under all aseptic precautions.

Indication

Pneumothorax.

Equipment and Supplies

Spirit, betadine, swabs, 22G IV cannula, three-way stop cock, 20 mL syringe, normal saline, sterile towels, sterile gloves

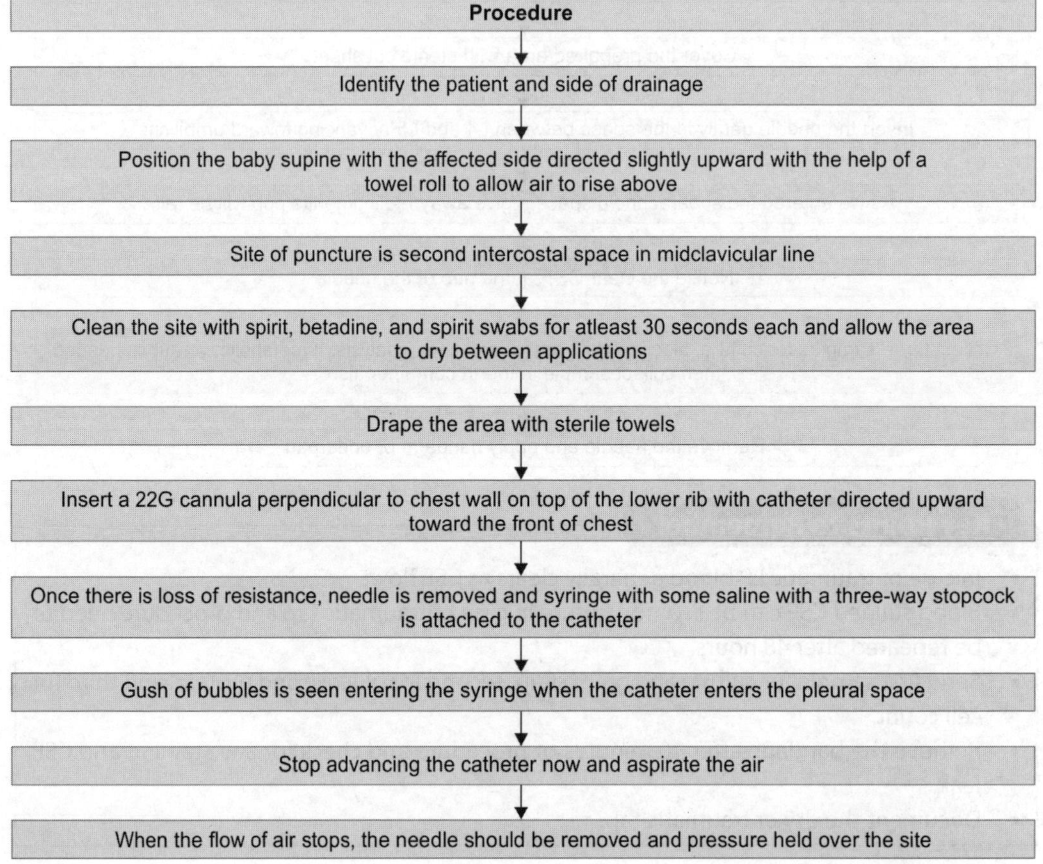

OSCE/Checklist: Procedure—Estimation of Blood Glucose		
*Name of the participants:*____		
S. No.	*Performance steps*	*Yes*	*No*
1.	Identifies patient and laterality		
2.	Arranges all supplies		
3.	Proper hand washing		
4.	Wears sterile gloves		
5.	Assistant opens all supplies in a sterile tray		
6.	Positions patient in supine and slightly upward on side of pneumothorax		
7.	Prepares area with spirit, betadine, spirit for 30 seconds each and let dry between applications		
8.	Drape with sterile towels		
9.	Insert 22G cannula in second intercostal space in midclavicular line perpendicular to skin		
10.	Stop inserting once loss of resistance is felt		
11.	Remove the needle and attach to syringe with stopcock		
12.	Aspirates air into the syringe till bubbles come		
13.	Removes cannula and patches it up with gauze		
	Total score		

1.10 VENTRICULAR TAP

Bhavya Kukreja

Objective

One should be able to perform ventricular tap under all aseptic precautions.

Indications

- To drain CSF in noncommunicating hydrocephalus.
- To diagnose ventriculitis.

Equipment and Supplies

- Sterile gloves, sterile sheets, razor, lumbar puncture needle, spirit, betadine, sterile swabs, specimen bottles.
- To administer intraventricular drugs.

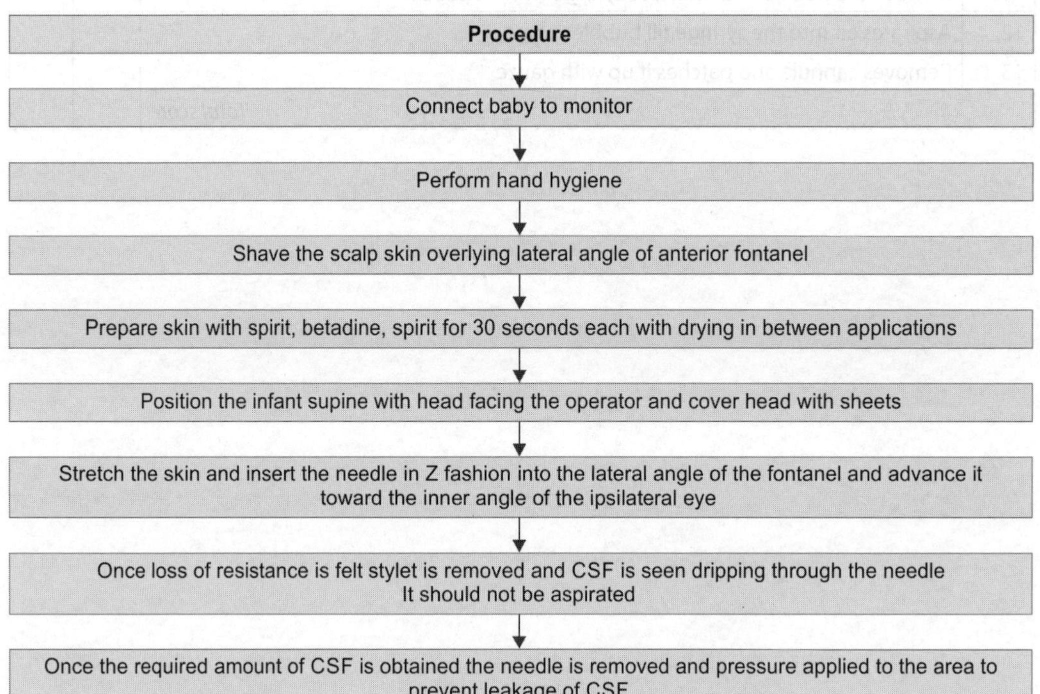

Prior to tapping, an ultrasound should be obtained to confirm ventriculomegaly and measurement taken to ascertain depth and direction of needle insertion.

OSCE/Checklist: Procedure—Ventricular Tap			
*Name of the participants:*____			
S. No.	*Performance steps*	*Yes*	*No*
1.	Obtains informed consent from parents		
2.	Ascertains the depth and direction of needle insertion by ultrasound		
3.	Performs hand hygiene		
4.	Shaves scalp without any injury to skin		
5.	Prepares skin overlying anterior fontanel		
6.	Maneuvers the needle in Z fashion into the lateral angle of anterior fontanel with needle directed toward inner canthus of ipsilateral eye		
7.	Removes stylet and let CSF drain		
8.	Removes needle once the required amount of CSF is removed		
	Total score		

1.11 NEONATAL PERITONEAL DIALYSIS

Anunaya Katiyar

Objective

To optimally perform dialysis in neonates allowing for the slow removal of fluid and solutes while avoiding hemodynamic instability.

Indications

Indications for renal replacement in neonates include:

- Fluid overload
- Hyperkalemia
- Refractory metabolic acidosis
- Congestive heart failure
- Hypertension
- Metabolic abnormalities
- Uremic symptoms
- Creating space for nutrition.

Contraindications

- Recent abdominal surgery or trauma
- Extensive intra-abdominal adhesions
- Necrotizing enterocolitis
- Large intra-abdominal mass
- Diaphragmatic hernia
- Ventriculoperitoneal shunt
- Prune belly syndrome

Types of Peritoneal Dialysis Based on Catheter Type

- A *"permanent soft catheter"* is preferred when it is anticipated that the need for PD will be longer than a few days, this catheter can be inserted bedside by physician or by a surgeon (peritoneoscopic/laparoscopic/open method) in an OT.
- *"Temporary rigid catheter"* come with a metal stylet and is a lifesaving procedure in patients with AKI in regions with limited resources. It is inserted bedside by physician.

Equipment and Supplies

- *Peritoneal dialysis catheter:*
  - Neonatal rigid PD catheter kit
  - Neonatal Tenckhoff PD catheter with single cuff
  - A 10F neonatal chest drain tube can be used in newborn.
- *PD fluid:*
  - Lactate buffered electrolyte balanced dextrose solution (PD 1.7): Routinely used
  - Special bicarbonate-based PD fluids
  - Special chloride-based PD fluid

- ■ *Sterile dressing tray containing:*
  - Suture materials
  - Sterile surgical blade number 11
  - Hypodermic sterile needle 18G
  - Urobag
  - IV sets
  - Two- and three-way connectors
  - Y connector set
  - 2% lidocaine injection
  - Dressing adhesive

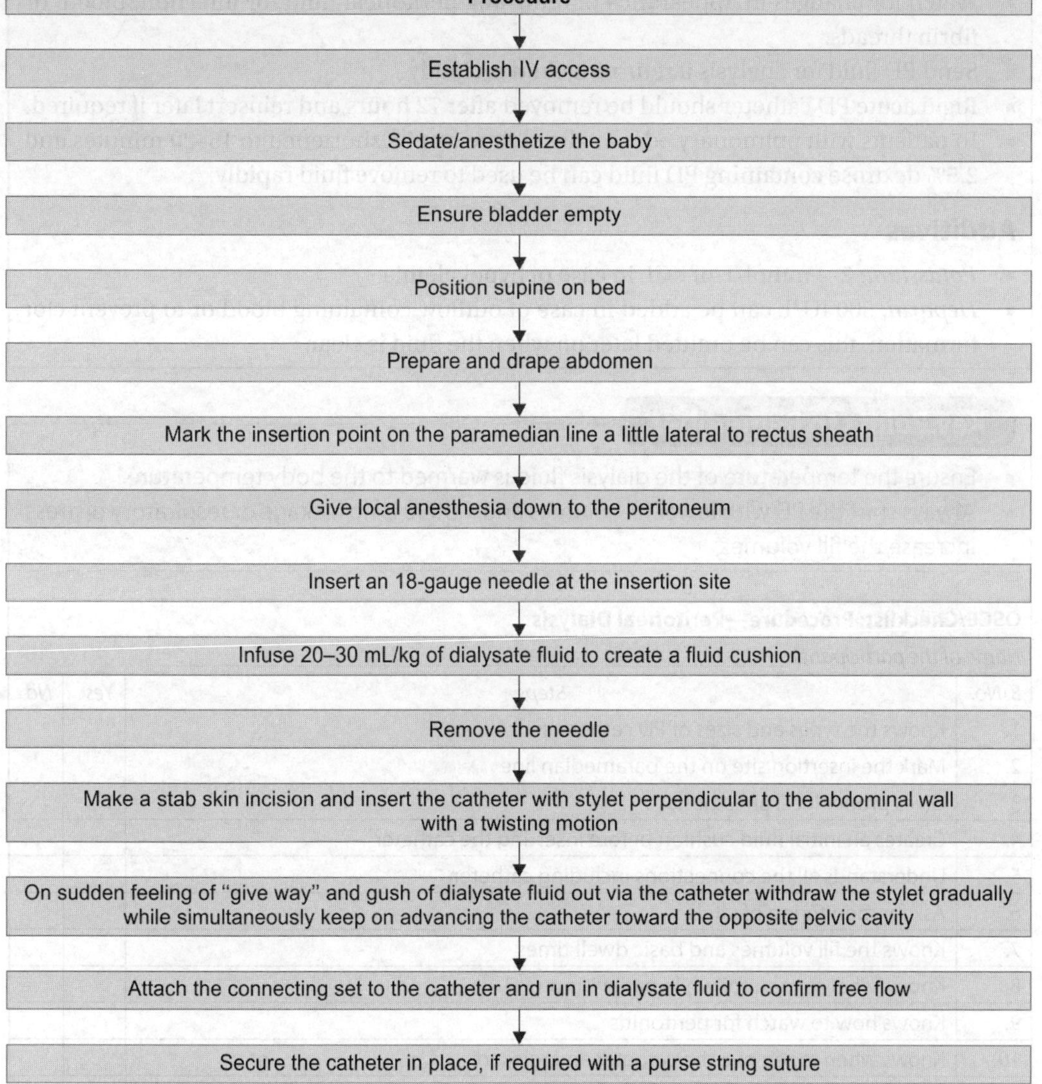

Peritoneal Dialysis Prescription and Monitoring

Fill volume	30–50 mL/kg
Run in time	5–10 minutes
Dwell time	20–30 minutes
Outflow time	10–20 minutes

- Ensure continuous monitoring of pulse, blood pressure, respiratory rate, and saturation.
- Strict intake/output hourly chart
- Serum electrolytes and blood sugar every 8 hourly
- Blood urea and creatinine every 24 hourly
- Watch for changes in appearance of returning peritoneal fluid for infection, blood, or fibrin threads.
- Send PD fluid for analysis if returning fluid is cloudy.
- Rigid acute PD catheter should be removed after 72 hours and reinsert later if required.
- In patients with pulmonary edema, dwell time can be shortened to 15–20 minutes and 2.5% dextrose containing PD fluid can be used to remove fluid rapidly.

Additives

- *Potassium:* 2-4 mmol/L of KCL in case of hypokalemia
- *Heparin:* 500 IU/L can be added in case of outflow containing blood or to prevent clot formation, this can be omitted later on when the fluid is clear.

Key Points to Remember

- Ensure the temperature of the dialysis fluid is warmed to the body temperature.
- Always start the PD with lower fill volumes and if there is no leakage or respiratory distress increase the fill volumes.

OSCE/Checklist: Procedure—Peritoneal Dialysis

*Name of the participants:*____

S. No.	Steps	Yes	No
1.	Knows the types and sizes of PD catheters		
2.	Mark the insertion site on the paramedian line		
3.	Gives proper local anesthesia		
4.	Creates an initial fluid cushion before inserting the catheter		
5.	Understands all the connections including catheter		
6.	Ask for monitoring of vitals		
7.	Knows the fill volumes and basic dwell times		
8.	Knows what to monitor while patient is on PD		
9.	Knows how to watch for peritonitis		
10.	Knows when to remove the catheter and reinsert		
	Total score		

1.12 PHOTOTHERAPY

Anuradha Bansal

Mechanism of phototherapy: First-line treatment for neonatal jaundice—
- Reduces bilirubin by photo-isomerization, structural isomerization, and photo-oxidation
- Noninvasive, easily available, cost-effective, and safe
- Most effective lights for phototherapy—lights with high-energy output near maximum adsorption peak of bilirubin, i.e., 450–460 nm.
- A phototherapy unit with alternating two blue and two white tubes (20 W each) is sufficient to provide adequate irradiance of 4–8 µw/cm^2/nm.
- A combination of four blue and two white lights is used to increase the irradiance to 12 µw/cm^2/nm.
- Intensive phototherapy: Irradiance in blue–green spectrum (wavelength of ~430–490 nm) of at least 30 µw/cm^2/nm and delivered to as much of infant's surface area as possible.

Risk assessment for phototherapy:
- *Bedside clinical method:* Modified Kramer's staging

Area of body	Serum bilirubin (mg/dL)
• Face	• 4–6
• Upper trunk	• 8–10
• Lower abdomen and thighs	• 12–14
• Arms and lower legs	• 15–18
• Palms and soles	• 15–20

- *Laboratory method:* Bhutani's nomogram for hour-specific-serum-bilirubin values.

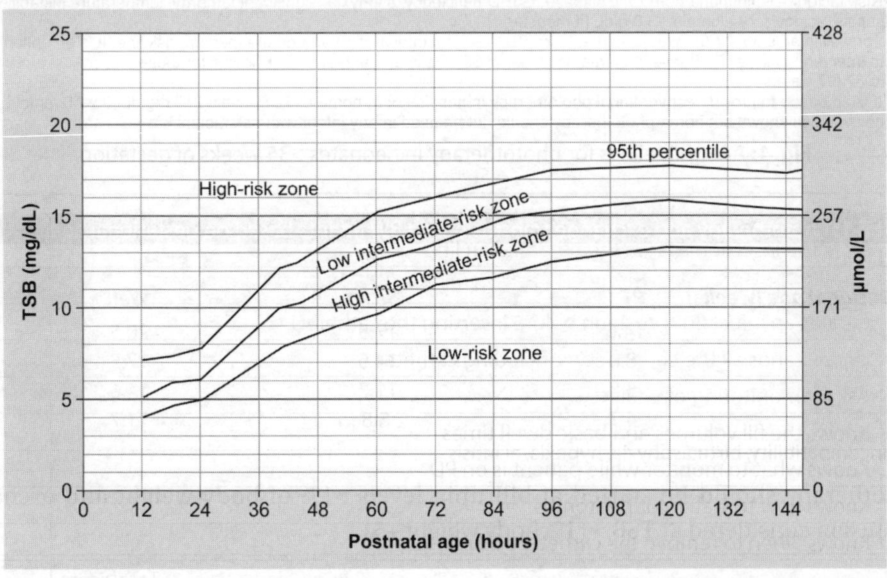

- *When to start phototherapy:*
  - Jaundice appearing within first 24 hours
  - Staining of palms and soles
  - Serum bilirubin in phototherapy range as per AAP guidelines (**Fig. 1 and Table 1**).
- *When to stop phototherapy:* Bilirubin levels 2–3 mg/dL below the phototherapy range.
- *Rebound bilirubin:* Preterm babies, those with hemolytic disease and with onset of jaundice in <60 hours are at highest risk of bilirubin rebound and hence should have rebound bilirubin levels after 24 hours of stopping phototherapy.

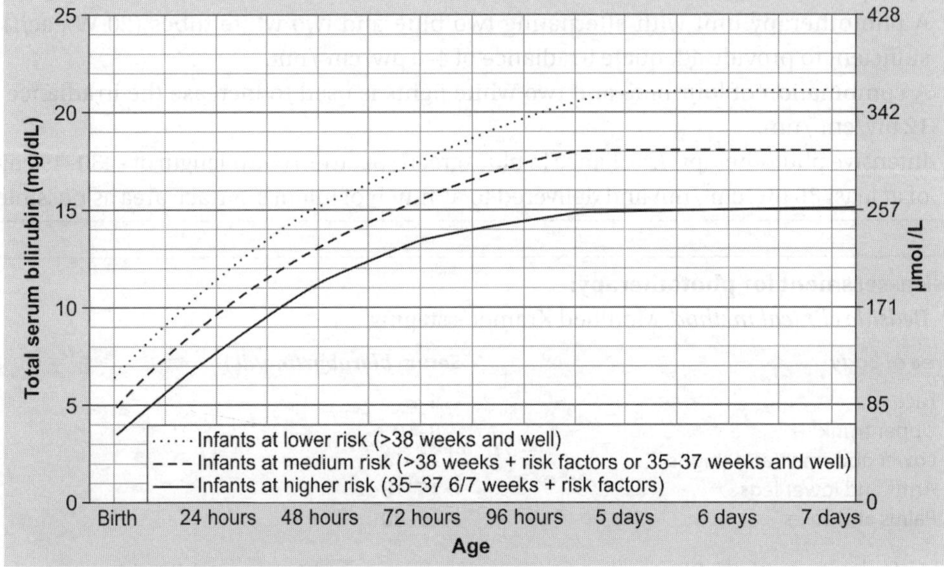

- Use total bilirubin. Do not subtract direct reacting or conjugated bilirubin
- Risk factors = isoimmune hemolytic disease, G6PD deficiency, asphyxia, significant lethargy, temperature instability, sepsis, acidosis, or albumin <3.0 g/dL (if measured)
- For well infants 35–37 6/7 weeks can adjust TSB levels for intervention around the medium risk line. It is an option to intervene at lower TSB levels for infants closer to 35 weeks and at higher TSB levels for those closer to 37 6/7 weeks
- It is an option to provide conventional phototherapy in hospital or at home at TSB levels 2–3 mg/dL (35–50 mmol/L) below those shown but home phototherapy should not be used in any infant with risk factors

Fig. 1: AAP guidelines for phototherapy in neonates >35 weeks of gestation.

TABLE 1: Phototherapy and exchange transfusion in LBW infants based on gestational age.

Gestational age (weeks)	PT	ET	
		Sick*	Well
36	14.6	17.5	20.5
32	8.8	14.6	17.5
28	5.8	11.7	14.6
24	4.7	8.8	11.7

*Rh incompatibility, birth asphyxia, hypoxia, acidosis

Phototherapy should be started at bilirubin levels >1% of body weight and exchange transfusion considered at TSB > (1% body weight +5).

Key Points to Remember

- Do not expose the baby to sunlight, it does not help in the treatment of jaundice.
- Discontinuation of breastfeeding is not recommended either for diagnosis or for treatment of breast milk jaundice in neonates.
- The baby under phototherapy may pass loose green stool, develop skin rashes, increased insensible water loss, etc. Continue phototherapy and breastfeeding as these side effects are harmless and are reversible.
- *Bronze baby syndrome:* Discontinue phototherapy if baby has conjugated hyperbilirubinemia.
- Do not use drugs like phenobarbitone or steroids to prevent or treat jaundice.
- Prophylactic phototherapy is not recommended for management of neonates with Rh immunization or ABO incompatibility.
- Stable neonates with hyperbilirubinemia requiring phototherapy should be initiated in them by their mothers' side.
- Provide intensive phototherapy by using single or multiple phototherapy devices in neonates requiring phototherapy.
- There is no role of routine fluid supplementation in neonates under phototherapy.
- Routine periodic changes in body position—from supine to prone and vice versa—are not recommended.
- In neonates with bilirubin value near exchange transfusion threshold, TSB should be measured every 4–6 hours after initiation of intensive phototherapy; once TSB starts declining, subsequent TSB may be measured every 8–12 hours.
- A follow-up TSB measurement may be done 12–24 hours after discontinuation of phototherapy in neonates with features of hemolysis.
- TSB is preferred over transcutaneous bilirubin (TcB) for monitoring of hyperbilirubinemia during phototherapy or in the first 24 hours after discontinuing phototherapy in term and preterm neonates.
- Phototherapy can be discontinued when TSB value is at least 2.9 mg/dL (nearly 50 µmol/L) below the treatment threshold.
- A single value below this threshold is sufficient to discontinue phototherapy in neonates with nonhemolytic jaundice; two consecutive values below the threshold are usually required in neonates with hemolytic jaundice.
- Albumin priming prior to or during exchange transfusion is not recommended in neonates with hyperbilirubinemia.

1.13 EXCHANGE TRANSFUSION

Bhavya Kukreja

Objective

One should be able to perform exchange transfusion under all aseptic precautions.

Indications

- Failure of response to phototherapy.
- Initial bilirubin levels in exchange range as per the AAP chart **(Fig. 1)**

Equipment and Supplies

- Sterile gloves, cap, mask, gown, cross-matched blood, umbilical lines, spirit, betadine, swabs, sterile sheets, IV infusion sets, stop cocks, syringes, saline, transparent dressing, surgical blade

Volume of blood to be exchanged = 2 × Blood volume (80–90 mL/kg) × Weight

Types of blood for exchange transfusion:
- Fresh whole blood (<7 days old)
- If whole blood is not available, packed cells reconstituted in plasma in ratio of 7:3.
- *Rh hemolytic disease: Rh-ve* blood cross matched against baby. Best choice: *O-ve* packed cells suspended in *AB-ve* plasma.
- *ABO incompatibility:* O blood group Rh compatible with the baby. Best choice: O group (Rh compatible) packed cells suspended in AB plasma.
- *Other indications:* Baby's blood group cross matched with maternal plasma.

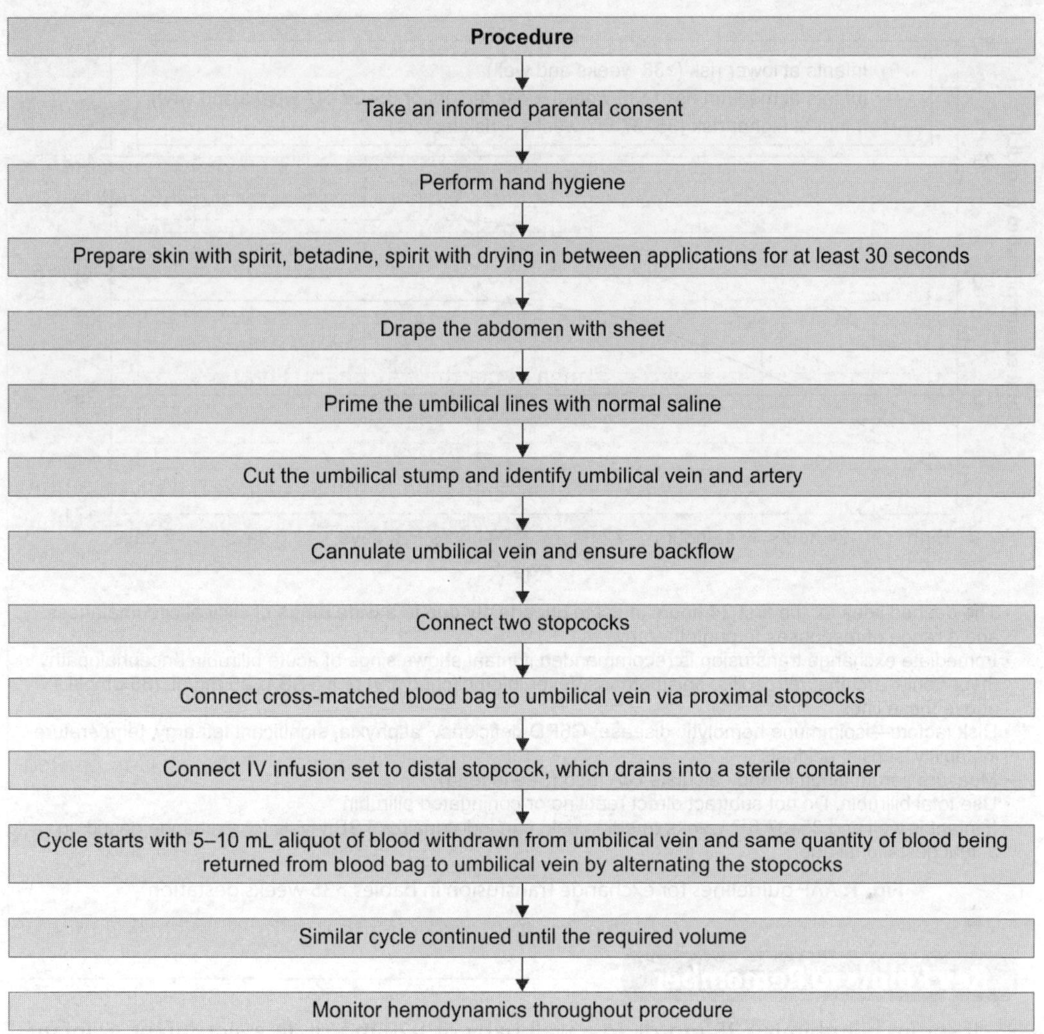

Procedure
Take an informed parental consent
Perform hand hygiene
Prepare skin with spirit, betadine, spirit with drying in between applications for at least 30 seconds
Drape the abdomen with sheet
Prime the umbilical lines with normal saline
Cut the umbilical stump and identify umbilical vein and artery
Cannulate umbilical vein and ensure backflow
Connect two stopcocks
Connect cross-matched blood bag to umbilical vein via proximal stopcocks
Connect IV infusion set to distal stopcock, which drains into a sterile container
Cycle starts with 5–10 mL aliquot of blood withdrawn from umbilical vein and same quantity of blood being returned from blood bag to umbilical vein by alternating the stopcocks
Similar cycle continued until the required volume
Monitor hemodynamics throughout procedure

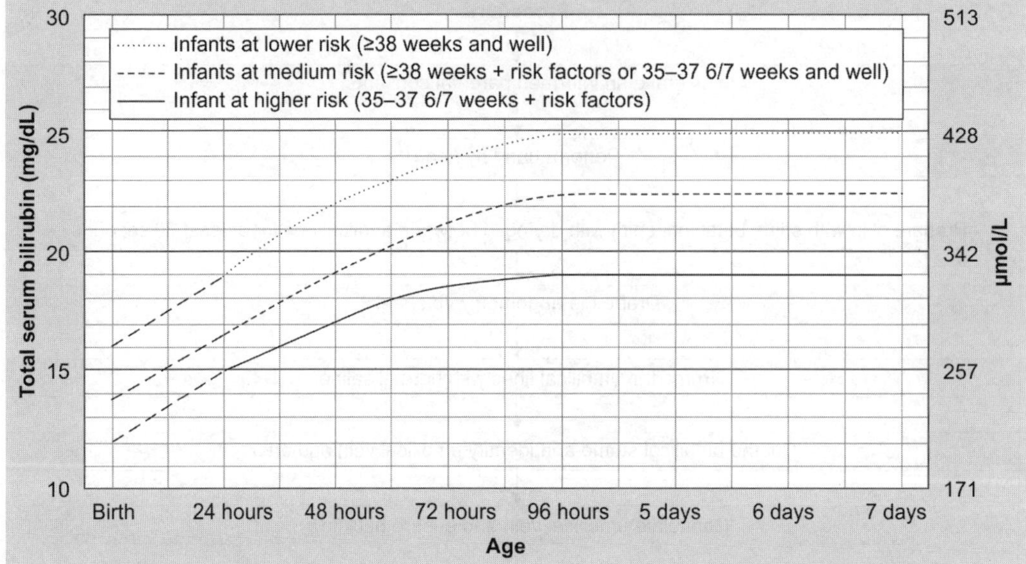

- The dashed lines for the first 24 hours indicate uncertainty due to a wide range of clinical circumatances and a range of responses to phototherapy
- Immediate exchange transfusion is recommended if infant shows sings of acute bilirubin encephalopathy (hypertonia, arching, retrocollis, opisthotonos, fever, high pitched cry) or if TSB is ≥5 mg/dL (85 µmol/L) above these lines
- Risk factors—isoimmune hemolytic disease, G6PD deficiency, asphyxia, significant lethargy, temperature instability, sepsis, acidosis
- Measure serum albumin and calculate B/A ratio (See legend)
- Use total bilirubin. Do not subtract direct reacting or conjugated bilirubin
- If infant is well and 35–37 6/7 weeks (median risk) can individualize TSB levels for exchange based on actual gestational age

Fig. 1: AAP guidelines for exchange transfusion in babies >35 weeks gestation.

Key Points to Remember

- If serum bilirubin is ≥25 mg/dL in a well baby or >20 mg/dL in a sick infant or infant <38 weeks gestation, take sample for cross match and request blood for exchange transfusion.
- In babies with isoimmune hemolytic disease, if bilirubin levels are rising despite intensive phototherapy or fall within 2–3 mg/dL of exchange levels, administer IVIG 0.5–1 g/kg over 2 hours.
- If the baby is clinically dehydrated or has >12% weight loss, dehydration correction with quantified expressed breast milk or formula is recommended. Give IV fluids only if oral intake is poor.

OSCE/Checklist: Procedure—Exchange Transfusion		
*Name of the participants:*____		
S. No.	*Performance steps*	*Yes*	*No*
1.	Takes informed consent		
2.	Calculates total blood volume required and volume of each aliquot		
3.	Records start time		
4.	Cross-matched blood bag		
5.	Perform hand washing and wears gloves		
6.	Prepares skin with spirit, betadine, spirit		
7.	Drapes the prepared area		
8.	Prepare a sterile tray with all supplies		
9.	Primes umbilical catheter with normal saline		
10.	Identify umbilical vein and cannulates it, ensures backflow		
11.	Connects two stopcock to catheter		
12.	Connects proximal stopcock to blood bag and distal one to infusion set connected to waste container		
13.	Pulls out an aliquot of blood from baby and same volume is pushed into baby		
14.	Monitors hemodynamics during procedure		
15.	Records end time		
	Total score		

1.14 BLOOD PRODUCT TRANSFUSION IN NEONATES

Nidhi Jain

Objective

To know when and how to use blood product judiciously and safely.

Equipment and Supplies

- Peripheral IV line insertion tray
- Blood group bag to be transfused and cross checked.
- Infusion pump
- Blood transfusion set
- Keep few paedipacks to reduce multiple donor exposure for multiple transfusion.

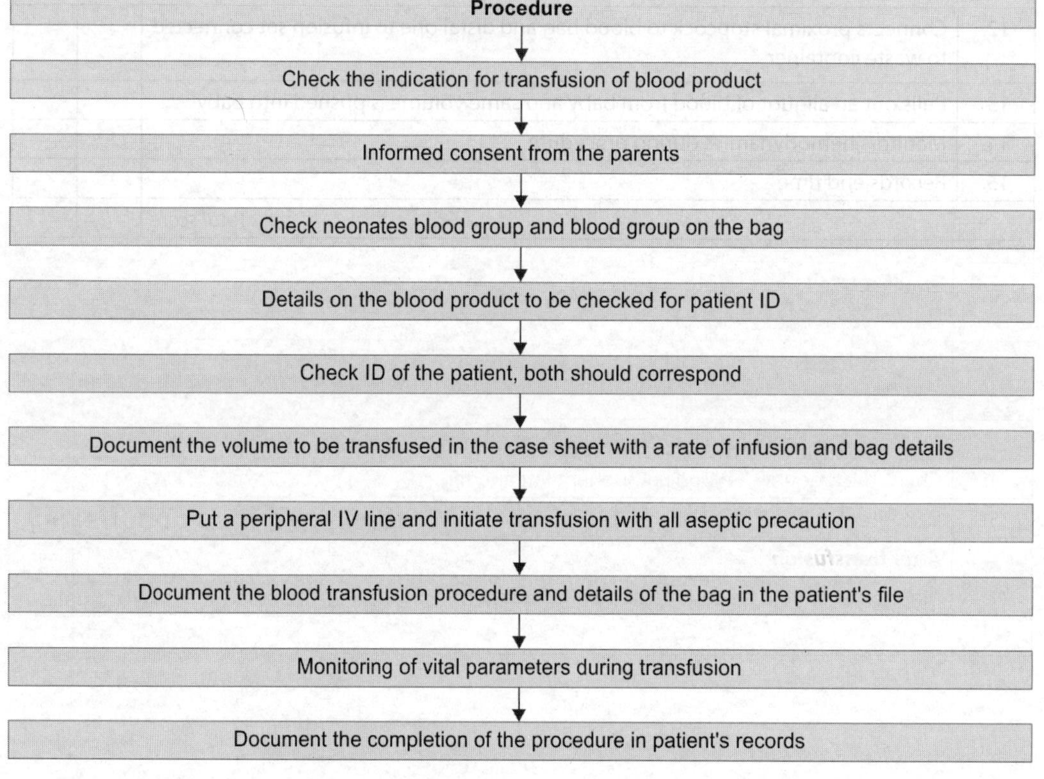

Key Points to Remember

- Strictly follow the guidelines for blood transfusions.
- Platelet transfusion should be always cross-matched and should be given immediately (<30 minutes).
- Stop maintenance fluid, unless treated for hypoglycemia.
- Use of *paedipacks* reduces donor exposure for multiply transfused preterm.
- A blood count should be performed 1 hour and 24 hours after completion of the transfusion in order to evaluate the efficacy of the transfusion.
- Do not routinely withhold feeding during transfusion unless hemodynamically unstable.
- Do not give diuretics routinely after blood transfusion.

OSCE/Checklist: Procedure—Blood Product Transfusion in Neonates			
Name of the participants:________________________________			
S. No.	Performance steps	Yes	No
	Before transfusion		
1.	Look for indication of transfusions		
2.	Check all the supplies		
3.	Informed consent taken from parents		
4.	Check patients details identification and blood product		
5.	Check for neonates' blood group and blood product		
6.	Document the volume to be transfused with rate		
7.	Take extra sample for further workup		
	During transfusion		
1.	Put peripheral IV line with all aseptic precautions		
2.	Look for any local site reactions		
3.	Monitor vitals (HR, RR, SpO_2, perfusion) during transfusion		
4.	Check the amount of blood component left and time elapsed		
5.	Document completion of the procedure in the patients records		
	After transfusion		
1.	Monitoring should be continued post-transfusion for 2–4 hours		
	Total score		

1.15 HANDWASHING

Gunjan Srivastava

Objective: To provide an overview of steps of handwashing.

Indications

- When hands are visibly dirty or soiled with blood or other body fluids and after using the toilet
- If suspected or proven exposure to a potential spore forming pathogen.

Supplies: Liquid handwash, running water source.

HOW TO HANDWASH?

Wash Hands when Visibly Soiled: Otherwise, Use Handrub

Duration of the entire procedure: 40–60 seconds

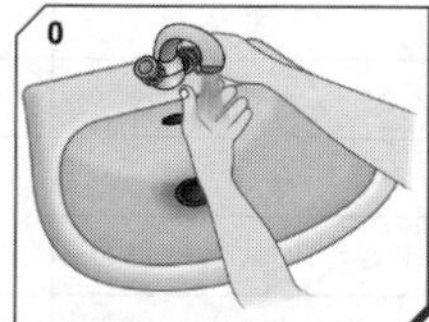
Wet hands with water

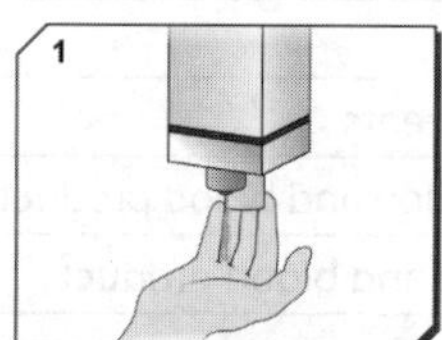
Apply enough soap to cover all hand surfaces

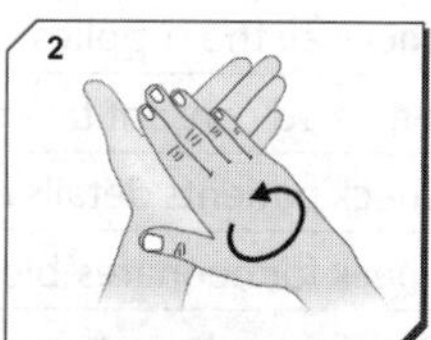
Rub hands palm to palm

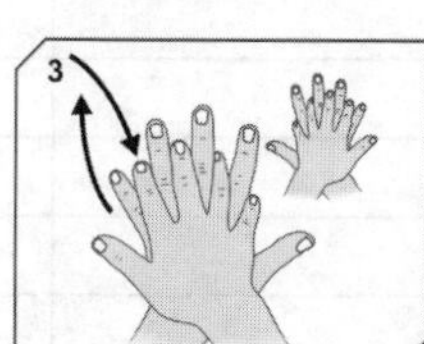
Right palm over left dorsum with interlaced fingers and vice versa

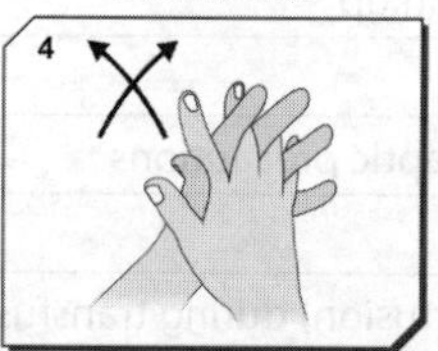
Palm to palm with fingers interlaced

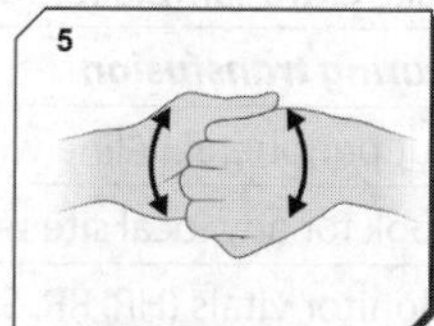
Backs of fingers to opposing palms with fingers interlocked

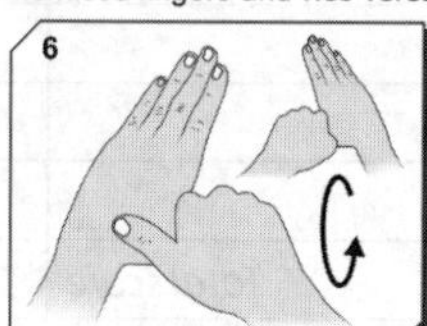
Rotational rubbing of left thumb clasped in right palm and vice versa

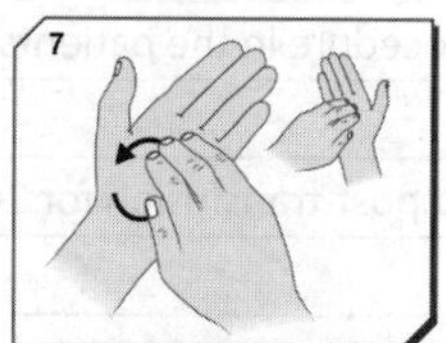
Rotational rubbing, backwards and forwards with clasped fingers of right hand in left palm and vice versa

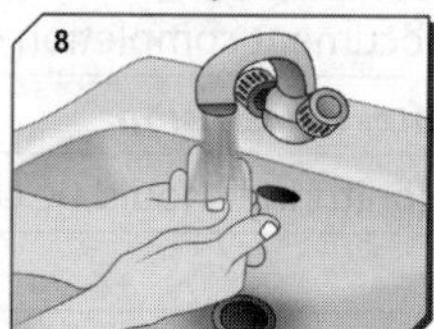
Rinse hands with water

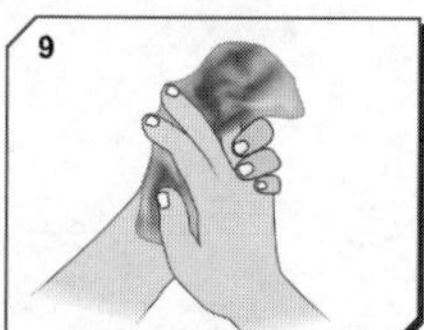
Dry hands thoroughly with a single use towel

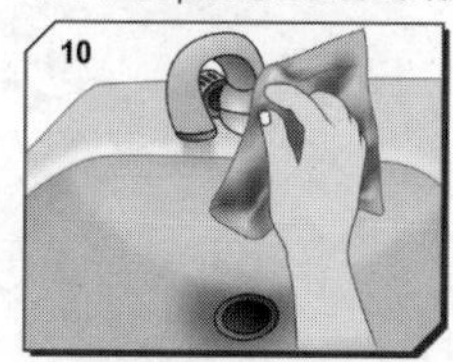
Use towel to turn off faucet

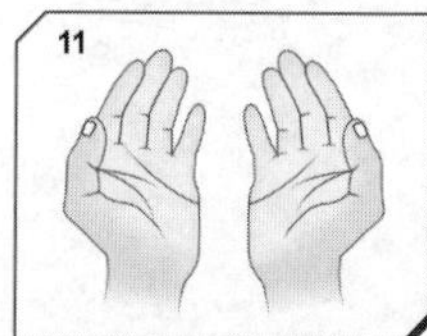
Your hands are now safe

Source: WHO

HOW TO HANDRUB?

Rub Hands for Hand Hygiene: Wash Hands When Visibly Soiled

Duration of the entire procedure: 20–30 seconds

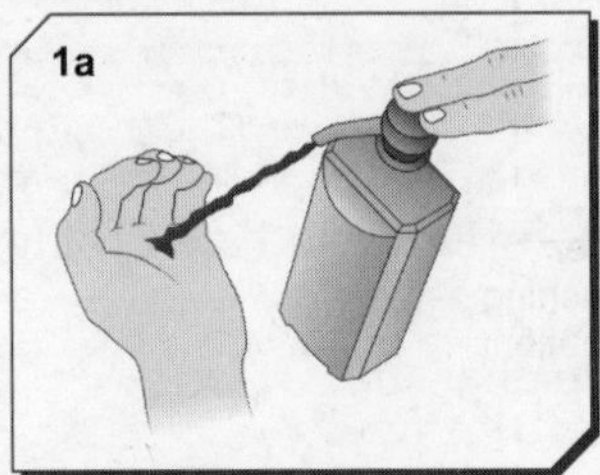

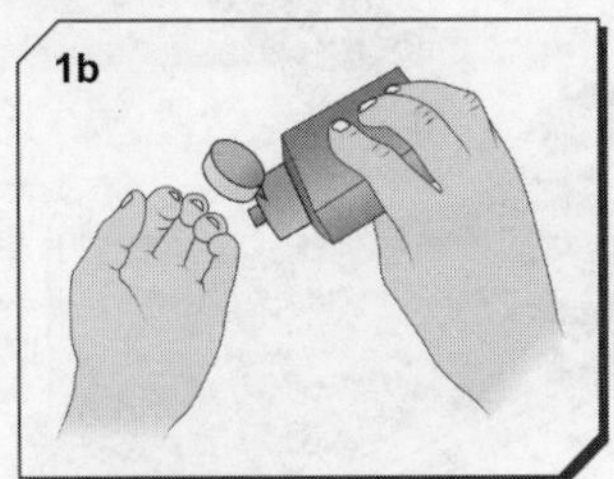

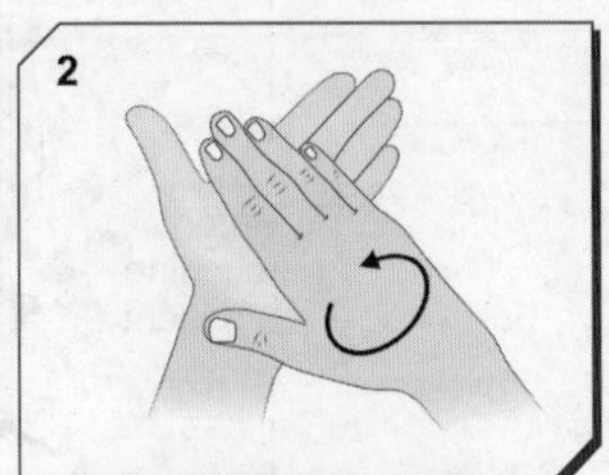

Apply a palmful of the product in a cupped hand, covering all surfaces

Rub hands palm to palm

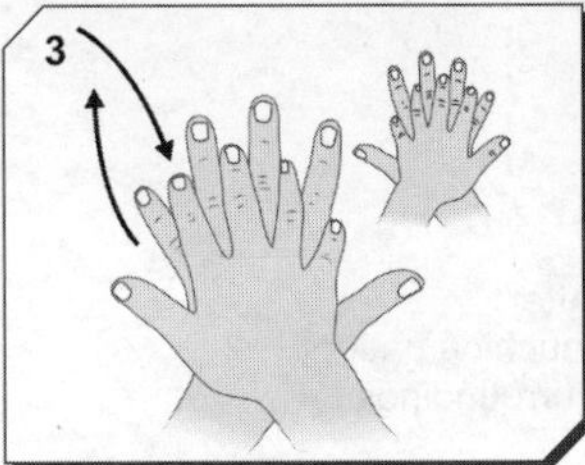

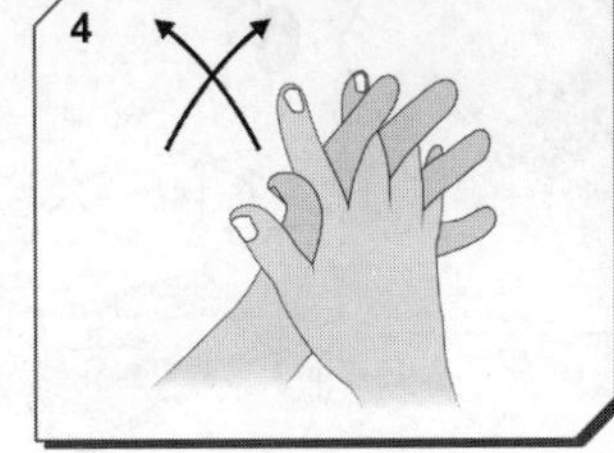

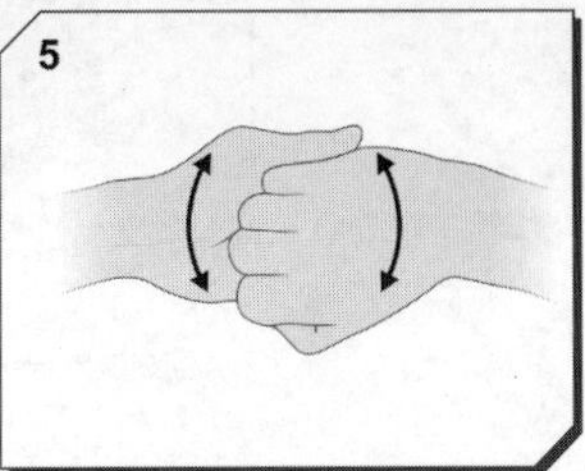

Right palm over left dorsum with interlaced fingers and vice versa

Palm to palm with fingers interlaced

Backs of fingers to opposing palms with fingers interlocked

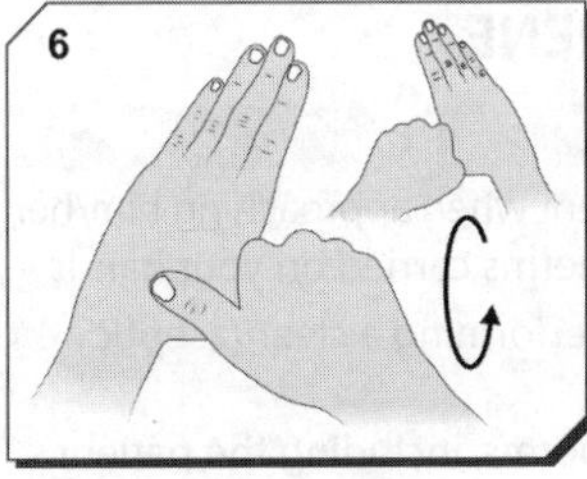

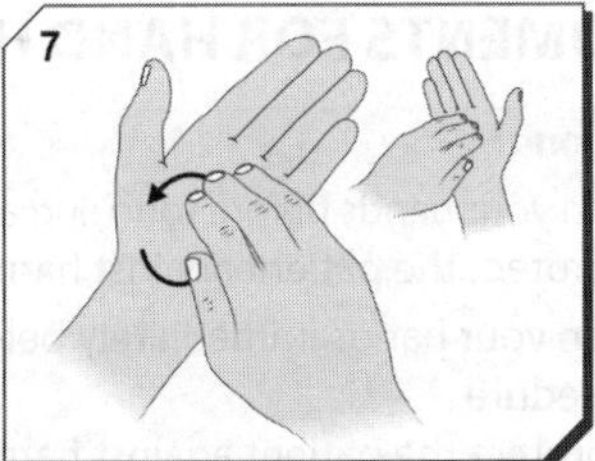

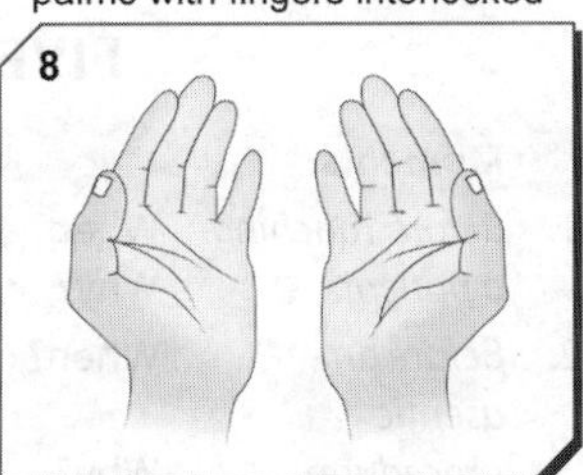

Rotational rubbing of left thumb clasped in right palm and vice versa

Rotational rubbing, backwards and forwards with clasped fingers of right hand in left palm and vice versa

Once dry, your hands are safe

Source: WHO

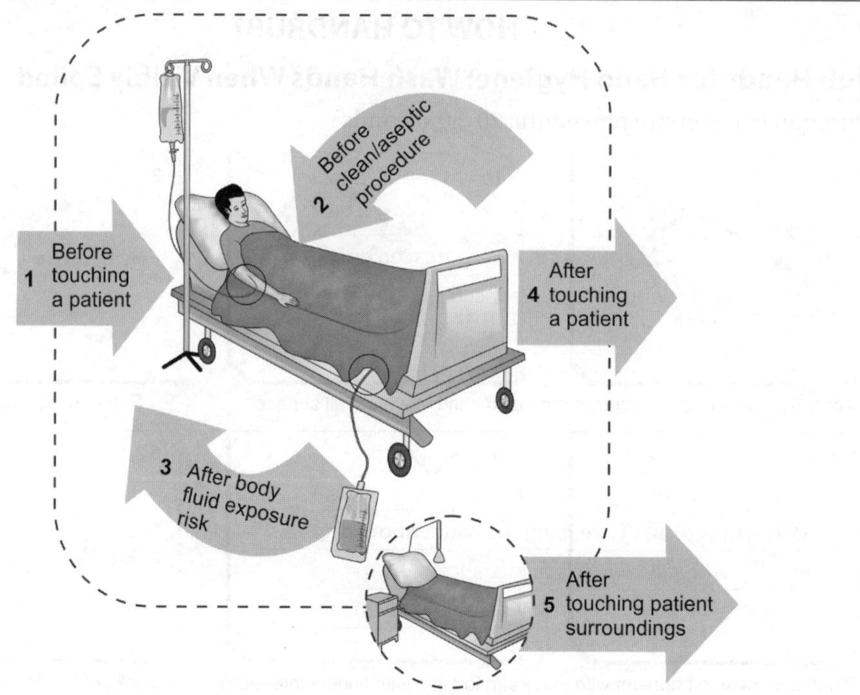

FIVE MOMENTS FOR HAND HYGIENE

	Moments		Rational
1.	Before Touching a patient	When?	Clean your hands before touching a patient when approaching him/her
		Why?	To protect the patient against harmful germs carried on your hands
2.	Before an aseptic procedure	When?	Clean your hands immediately before performing a clean/aseptic procedure
		Why?	To protect the patient against harmful germs, including the patient's own, from entering his/her body
3.	After exposure to patient's body fluid	When?	Clean your hands immediately after an exposure risk to body fluids (and after glove removal)
		Why?	To protect yourself and the health care environment from harmful patient germs
4.	After touching a patient	When?	Clean your hands after touching a patient and her/his immediate surroundings, when leaving the patient's side
		Why?	To protect yourself and the health care environment from harmful patient germs
5.	After touching patient surroundings	When?	Clean your hands after touching any object or furniture in the patient's immediate surroundings, when leaving—even if the patient has not been touched
		Why?	To protect yourself and the health care environment from harmful patient germs

- Alcohol rub can be used if hands are not visibly soiled with blood or any other secretions.
- Alcohol hand rub is to be used on both sides of hands for a duration of 20–30 seconds.
- The steps are same as handwashing.

OSCE/Checklist: Procedure—Handwashing Technique			
Name of the participants:_______________________________________			
S. No.	Performance steps	Yes	No
1.	Remove rings, bracelet, watch, etc.		
2.	Wet hands in clean running water and apply enough soap to cover hand surface		
3.	Rub hands palm to palm		
4.	Right palm over left dorsum with interlaced fingers and vice versa		
5.	Palm to palm with fingers interlaced		
6.	Back of fingers to opposing palms with fingers interlocked		
7.	Rotational rubbing of both thumb alternately		
8.	Rub the fingertips and creases		
9	Rub wrist and forearm		
10.	Rinse hands in running water		
11.	Dry hands to air dry keeping the hands above the waist level		
12.	Use towel or elbow to close the faucet		
13.	Steps of handwashing—total duration (40–60 seconds)		
	Total score		

▪ FURTHER READING

1. Hand hygiene—World Health Organization (WHO). Available from https://www.who.int/teams/integrated-health-services/infection-prevention-control/hand-hygiene. [Last accessed November, 2022].

1.16 INSERTION OF OROGASTRIC TUBE AND GAVAGE FEEDING

Gunjan Srivastava

Objective

One should be able to insert orogastric (OG) tube insertion and provide gavage feeding. Under all aseptic precautions.

Indications

- *Feeding:* For sick, preterm, or low birth weight babies who cannot accept orally.
- *Gastric decompression:* For babies with abdominal distension, CPAP belly, during prolong PPV, ventilations, suspected intestinal obstruction and to ruleout TEF.

Equipment and Supplies

Sterile OG tube (6F or 8F), 2–5 mL syringe (for aspiration), sterile 10 mL/20 mL syringe (for feeding), stethoscope, scissors, adhesive tape, normal saline, measuring tap and expressed MOM (mother's own milk).

Procedure: Insertion of orogastric tube

↓

Arrange necessary supplies and wash hands, air dry, wear clean/sterile gloves

↓

Measurement sterile with tap: From angle of mouth to tragus and then mid point between the xiphisternum and umbilicus

↓

Ask your assistant to remove OG tube from sterile back. Note the marking of this length as this length of tube should be inserted through the mouth

↓

Moisten the tip of tube with normal saline and gently insert it through mouth pointing toward back of throat to desired length has been introduced

↓

Check position: Place a stethoscope below xiphisternum slightly left over upper abdomen, push 2–3 mL of air into the OG tube and auscultate to hear sound of gush of air in the stomach

↓

Secure the tube in place gently with tape at the angle of mouth and the single loop on the cheek and note the point of insertion. Document the procedure in baby's record file

Key Points to Remember

- *Feeding tube size:* 8F for babies >1,500 g and 6 F for babies <1,500 g.
- While inserting the tube closely observe the baby for any color change or difficulty in breathing, if this happens remove the OG tube immediately as it may be in trachea.
- If resistance is felt during OG insertion remove the tube and retry.
- While feeding the baby do not push the milk in the syringe with its plunger, let it go slowly with gravity.
- There is no need to burp a gavage fed baby.
- Routine prefeed gastric aspirate is not recommended.
- Abdominal girth should be measured (just above the umbilical stump) before every feed.
- If the abdominal girth increases by >2 cm from the baseline then prefeed aspiration should be done.
- If the aspirate is >25% of the last feed or if it contains blood, feeding should be suspended.
- If OG tube inserted for abdominal decompression then the tube should be left uncapped.
- Remove the tube by kinking if it is not required.
- Dispose the tube as per BMW management protocol.

OSCE/Checklist: Procedure—Steps of Gavage Feeding			
*Name of the participants:*____			
S. No.	*Performance steps*	*Yes*	*No*
1.	Gather all supplies and wash hands		
2.	Choose appropriate size feeding tube as per gestational weight of the baby		
3.	Insert the feeding tube with proper measurement		
4.	*Secure the feeding tube:* By taping at angle of mouth		
5.	Check the position of feeding tube before feeding (to be checked every time before feeding)		
6.	Attach a 10 mL syringe to the end of feeding tube without the plunger		
7.	Pinch the end of feeding tube and put required amount of milk in the syringe		
8.	Let the feed run in by gravity keeping above the baby's head (do not push the plunger to push feed)		
9.	Observe the infant for any breathing difficulty, change in color/looks blue, apnea and vomiting		
10.	Cap the end of feeding tube after feeds or hang up with thread (except when baby is on CPAP therapy, where it should be left open half an hour after feeds)		
11.	Check abdominal girth at next feeding session and proceed to feed if no increase in girth. If the girth increased by 2 cm, do a prefeed gastric aspirate and analyse the amount and content to decide about next feed		
	Total score (maximum score:12)		

1.17 EXPRESSION OF BREAST MILK AND KATORI-SPOON/PALADAI FEEDING

Boby Varghese

Objective

One should be able to give katori-spoon/paladai feeding.

Indication

Feeding: For sick, preterm (>34 weeks) or LBW and who cannot suck.

Equipment and Supplies

Katori and spoon, paladai (a small bowl with long pointed tip used for feeding low birth weight babies) expressed MOM.

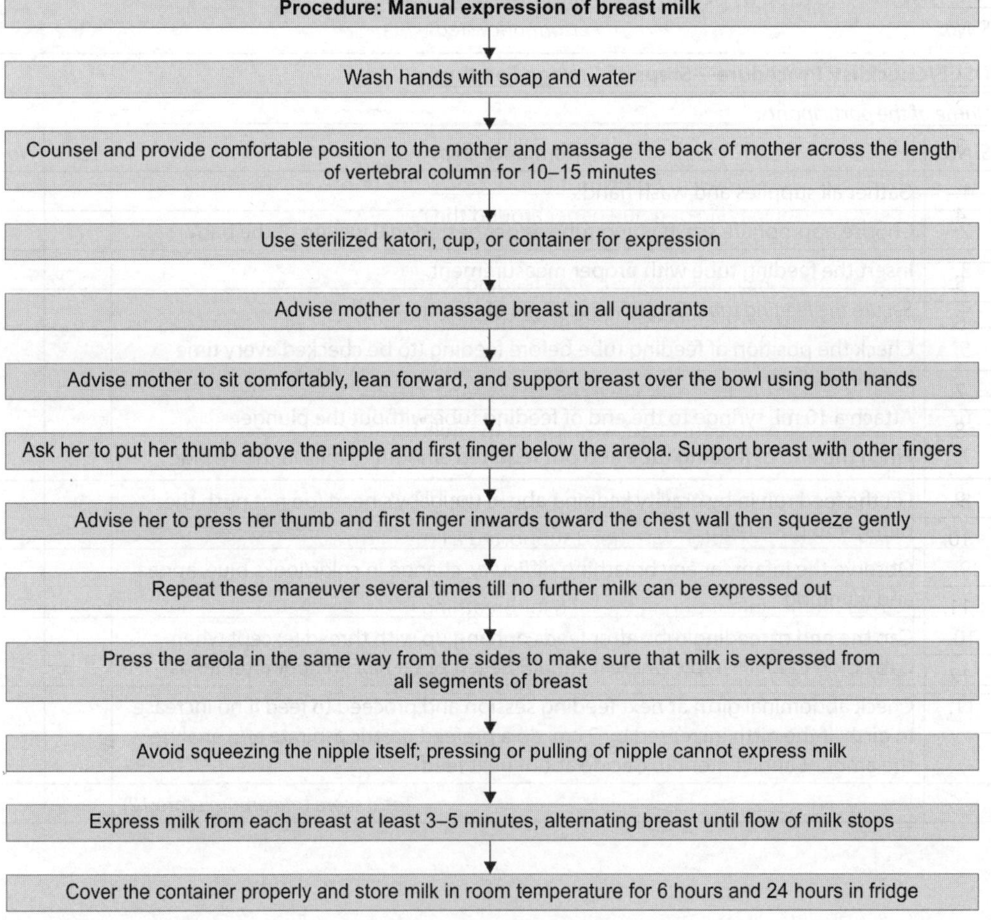

Key Points to Remember

- If the baby dose not accept and swallow the feed, try gentile stimulation. If he is still sluggish, do not feed further. It is better to switch back to gavage feed till the baby is ready again.
- *Advantages:*
    - Simple and effective method to feed babies not able to suck directly from breast
    - Easy to follow
    - Socially acceptable
    - Reduces infection
- *Disadvantages:*
    - Caregiver should be very careful while feeding.
    - To avoid pouring large amount of feed to the baby's mouth

OSCE/Checklist: Procedure—Steps of Katori-Spoon/Paladai Feeding

*Name of the participants:*____

S. No.	Performance steps	Yes	No
1.	Washed hands properly		
2.	Take sterilized utensils		
3.	Take the measured amount of breast milk/prepared formula by a sterile syringe and take it into paladai/katori		
4.	Keep a cotton napkin or tissue paper around the neck, keep the baby in semi-upright position with head well supported		
5.	Ensure the baby is fully awake before feeding so that he/she swallows properly		
6.	Hold the paladai in a manner so that pointed tip rests slightly on the baby's angle of mouth		
7.	Pour small amount of milk slowly into baby's mouth		
8.	Feed slowly; ensure that baby swallowed the milk before giving more milk to the baby		
9.	Perform burping gently by holding baby in upright position		
10.	Place in lateral position with head supported a little higher than the rest of the body		
11.	Observed the infant during the feed for breathing difficulty, change in color/looks blue, apnea, and vomiting		
12.	Wash the paladai/cup and put it for sterilization before another feed		
	Total score		

1.18 BLOOD GLUCOSE ESTIMATION

Bhavya Kukreja

Objective

One should be able to perform bedside estimation of blood glucose for prompt prevention and treatment of hypoglycemia.

Indications

Preterm, SGA, LGA sick neonates, and high-risk neonates.

Equipment and Supplies

Glucometer, glucometer test strips, lancet or 26G sterile needle, alcohol-based swab (70% isopropyl alcohol).

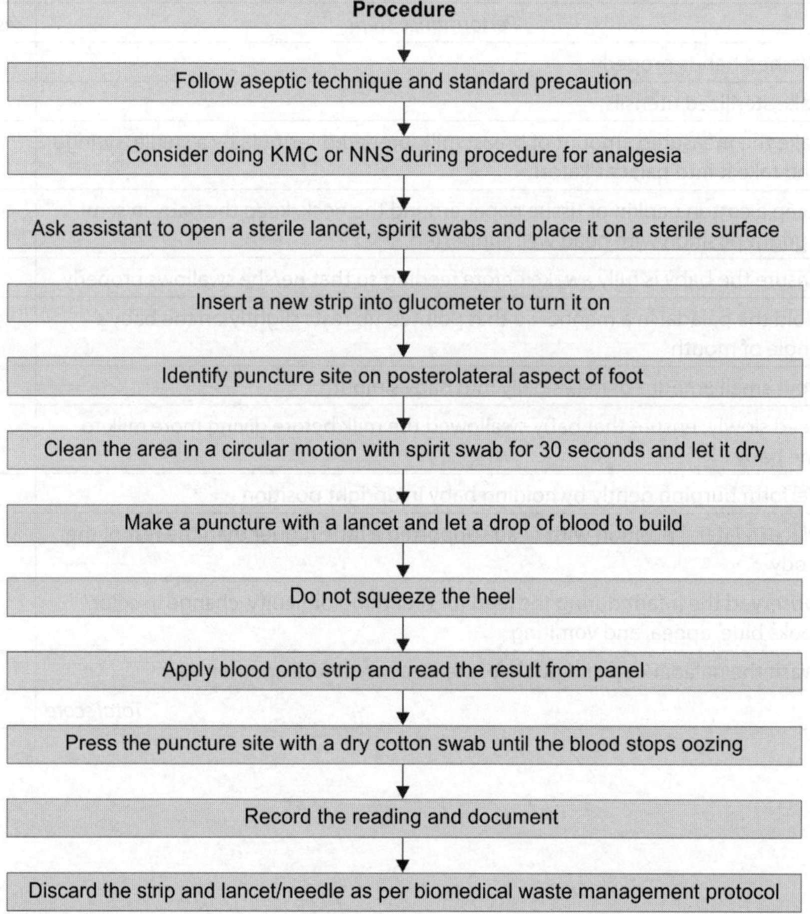

Key Points to Remember

- Keep the strip containing box tightly closed.
- Do not use povidone/betadine for cleaning the site.
- Do not prick in the middle portion of heel and avoid deep pricks. (Risk of the osteomyelitis of the heel).
- Direct prick over the vein can also be done to obtain the blood drop. It is less painful.
- For PT neonates use smaller lancet (0.85 mm).
- Rewarming the heel help in free flow of blood from the puncture site.
- Plasma glucose is 10% higher than blood glucose.
- Delay in laboratory analysis of blood sample may result in fall of plasma glucose level by 14–18 mg/dL/h.

OSCE/Checklist: Procedure—Estimation of Blood Glucose

*Name of the participants:*____

S. No.	Performance steps	Yes	No
1.	Check all supplies and equipment		
2.	Check expiry date of strips		
3.	Performs pharmacological/nonpharmacological measure to decrease pain		
4.	Performs hand hygiene		
5.	Inserts a new strip into glucometer		
6.	Identifies puncture site		
7.	Prepare area with spirit swab and let it dry		
8.	Punctures the heel with lancet and let a drop of blood to form		
9.	Apply blood to the strip and read the result from glucometer panel		
10.	Press the puncture site with a dry cotton swab		
11.	Discard the disposable as per BMW management protocol		
	Total score		

1.19 ASSESSMENT OF CAPILLARY REFILL TIME (CRT)

Neha Jain

Objective

One should be able to assess perfusion by using CRT method.

Indication

Neonates with hypothermia, sepsis and shock.

Equipment and Supplies

Stop watch/wrist watch.

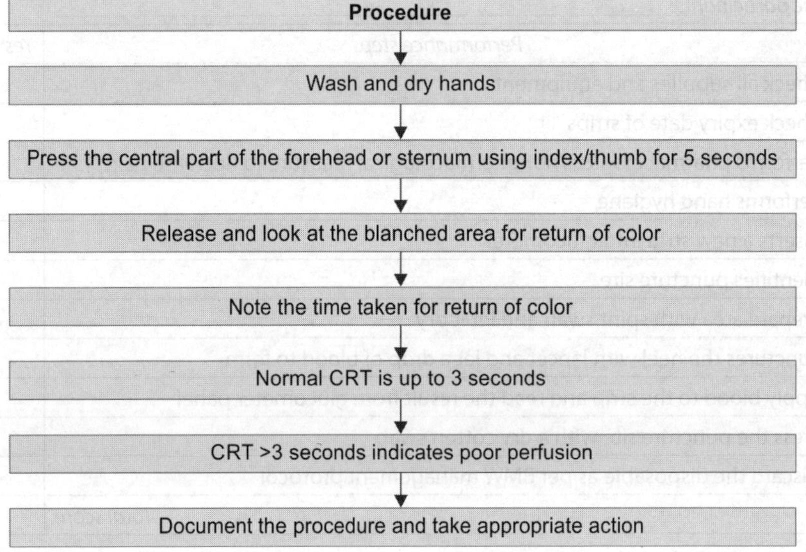

1.20 METHODS OF DELIVERING OXYGEN THERAPY IN NEONATES

Sweta Kumari

OSCE/Checklist: Procedure—Delivery of Blended, Heated, and Humidified Oxygen			
Name of the participants:__________________________			
S. No.	Performance steps	Yes	No
1.	Does hand hygiene and gather supplies		
2.	Asks for equipment and counsel (0.5 × 8) • Oxygen source • Compressed air source • Flow meter for air and oxygen (Blender) • Humidifier and device for warming gas • Appropriate size nasal prongs • Adhesive for fixation of prongs, scissors • Job aid to adjust flow		
3.	Connects flow meters to air and oxygen source (Blender)		
4.	Connects humidifier and warmifier and check its working		
5.	Connects the system to nasal prongs (Appropriate size)		
6.	Adjusts flow of oxygen and flow of air looking at the job aid		
7.	Attaches nasal prongs to neonate		
8.	Attaches baby to pulse oximeter after cleaning the probe		
9.	Applies the probe to right hand ensuring that the LED and the sensor are exactly opposite each other		
10.	Secures the probe with the attached velcro/micropore		
11.	Checks for upper and lower set alarm, if not appropriate adjusts upper alarm limit to 95% and lower limit to 90%		
12.	Positions the infant's head in the midline and keep it in neutral position by placing the shoulder roll if required		
13.	If the neonate does not improve; take corrective steps		
14.	Look at pulse oximeter probe for waveform		
15.	Increase FiO$_2$ level by adjusting flow of oxygen and air as per job aid if lower limit of alarm saturation is not achieved		
16.	If upper alarm limit of saturation is achieved, decrease FiO$_2$ by adjusting flow rate of oxygen and air (blender)		
	Total score		

OSCE/Checklist: Procedure—Oxygen Administration by Oxygen Hood		
*Name of the participants:*___________________________________		
S. No.	*Performance steps*	*Yes* | *No*
1.	Washes hands properly and gather all supplies	
2.	Attaches the flow meter to the available oxygen source	
3.	Starts the flow of oxygen by rotating the knob of flow meter	
4.	Observes for bubbles in the humidifier chamber	
5.	Sets oxygen flow rate at 2–3 L/kg/min or between 4 and 6 L/min	
6.	Positions the infant's head in sniffing position	
7.	• Keep the clean hood over the neonate's head (1 × 2) • Observes the front portion of the hood should be at the level of the neck of the neonate • Ensure that the seal is not tight	
8.	Takes new oxygen tubing and attaches one end of it to the flow meter and the other end to the oxygen hood	
9.	Records SpO_2	
10.	Interprets SpO_2 as provided by the examiner and takes action	
11.	Assesses the (1 × 4): • Temperature • Heart rate • Respiration (RR and retractions) • Capillary refill time	
12.	Counsels the parents/caretakers	
	Total score	

OSCE/Checklist: Procedure—Oxygen Administration by Nasal Prongs		
*Name of the participants:*___________________________________		
S. No.	*Performance steps*	*Marks*
1.	Washes hands properly and gather all supplies	
2.	Attaches the flow meter to the available oxygen source	
3.	Starts the flow of oxygen by rotating the knob of flow meter	
4.	Sets oxygen flow rate between 0.5 and 1 L/min	
5.	Chooses a proper size new nasal cannula	
6.	Positions the infant's head in sniffing position	
7.	Attaches appropriate end of the nasal cannula to the flow meter	
8.	Secures the nasal cannula on the cheeks near the nose with transparent adhesive	
9	Records and interprets SpO_2 as provided by the examiner and takes action	
10.	Assesses the (1 × 4): • Temperature • Heart rate • Respiration (RR and retractions) • Capillary refill time	
11.	Counsels the parents/caretakers	
	Total score	

1.21 MEASUREMENT OF AXILLARY TEMPERATURE BY DIGITAL THERMOMETER

Neha Jain

Objective

One should be able to record axillary temperature in newborn.

Indication

To ascertain the degree of hypothermia.

Equipment and Supplies

- Digital thermometer
- Alcohol-based hand rubs
- Sprit swab.

OSCE/Checklist: Procedure—Measurement of axillary temperature by digital thermometer		
*Name of the participants:*____		
S. No.	*Performance steps*	*Yes*	*No*
1.	Check all the supplies		
2.	Perform hand hygiene		
3.	Clean the bulb of thermometer with spirit swab from tip to the base and allow to dry		
4.	Ensure that the axilla is dry		
5.	Switch on the thermometer and place the bulb on the roof of baby's axilla		
6.	Check the baby's arm held close to the body to keep the thermometer in place. Wait till the beep sound		
7.	Record the temperature displayed and inform the mother (no addition or subtraction from the recorded temperature should be done)		
8.	Clean the thermometer with the spirit swab from base to the tip of the bulb, before keeping back		
	Total score		

OSCE/Checklist: Procedure—Assessment of temperature by human-touch method (Tactile assessment)			
Name of the participants:			
S. No.	Performance steps	Yes	No
1.	Perform hand hygiene and explain the mother about the procedure		
2.	Dry and rewarm the hands by rubbing together		
3.	Touch the baby's palms and sole and then the abdomen with the dorsum of the hand		
4.	If both areas warm—normothermic		
5.	If palm and soles are cold but abdomen warm-cold stress		
6.	If both palm and sole and abdomen cold-significant hypothermia		
	Total score		

1.22 ENDOTRACHEAL TUBE SUCTION OF VENTILATED NEONATES

Gunjan Srivastava

Definition

It is a process of applying negative pressure to the distal endotracheal tube and trachea by inserting a suction catheter to clear excess or abnormal secretions.

Objective

One should be able to perform ET suction in a ventilated neonate under all aseptic conditions.

Indications

Desaturation, bradycardia, tachycardia, decreased/absent chest movements, decreased breath sounds, increased work of breathing, and visible secretions in ET tube.

Equipment

Functioning suction unit, suction catheter (open suction), T-piece resuscitator/AMBU bag, suction unit for closed suction, normal saline, and sterile glove.

Appropriate Size Suction Tube (Open Suction)

ETT size (mm)	Suction catheter size
2.5	5 FG
3.0–3.5	6–7 FG
4.0–4.5	8 FG
Measuring length of suction catheter = cm markings on ETT + length of ETT adapter (1 – 1.5 cm).	

Procedure: Open suction—procedure requires two clinical personals

↓

Increase FiO₂ by 10–20% above baseline approximately 2 minutes prior to suction

↓

Determine size of suction catheter. Check suction pressure (desired pressure 80–100 cmH₂O)

↓

Perform hand hygiene and wear clean gloves, observe presuction physiological parameters

↓

- Assistant disconnects ETT from ventilator tubings
- Primary clinician passes suction catheter to desired length (as explained earlier)

↓

- Negative pressure should only be applied while withdrawing the suction catheter, suction catheter should be gently rotated while withdrawing from ETT
- Duration of negative pressure should not exceed 6 seconds to prevent hypoxemia

↓

- Use small amount of sterile water to remove secretions from suction tubings
- Turn-off vacuum pressure and perform hand hygiene
- Ensure baby is in contained and comfortable position

Procedure: Closed suction—this procedure is safe to complete with one physician

↓

- Determine suction catheter size
- Check suction pressure. Hand hygiene and gloves

↓

Remove cap from end of suction system and connect to wall suction tubing

↓

- Unlock device by rotating the suction control valve by 180°
- Introduce suction catheter to required depth (appropriate color is seen in window)

↓

Apply suction by depressing suction control valve and withdraw catheter to fully extended length

↓

- To clear secretions use sterile NaCl via lavage port
- Change the closed suction system weekly. Repeat as necessary

Key Points to Remember

- *Assessment of effectiveness:*
  - Improvement in breath sounds
  - Improvement in vital parameters (e.g., oxygen saturation and heart rate)
  - Decreased work of breathing, improved chest movements removal of secretions
- *Complications:*
  - Hypoxemia, atelectasis, and bradycardia
  - BP fluctuations, airway mucosal trauma, bacteremia
  - Fluctuations in intracranial pressure and cerebral blood flow.

1.23 ORAL SUCTION (IN NONVENTILATED NEONATES)

Gunjan Srivastava

Objective

One should be able to perform safe and effective oral and nasopharyngeal suction under all aseptic suctions.

Indications

Desaturation, bradycardia, tachycardia, increased work of breathing, and visible secretions.

Equipment and Supplies

- Pair of sterile gloves
- Appropriate size suction catheter
- Wall suction
- Sterile water

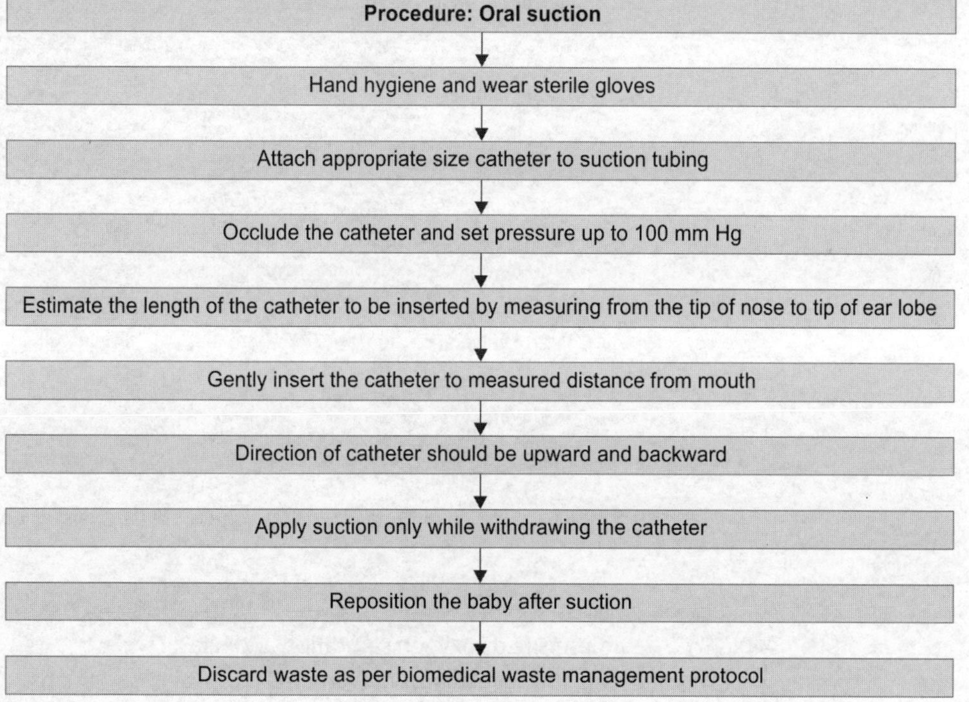

Key Points to Remember

- Limit attempts till 6 seconds.
- Monitor vitals.
- Suction mouth first then nose.
- Do not allow the tip of suction catheter to touch any unsterile area.
- Do not use excessive pressure to cause trauma.
- Do not pass the catheter completely through nares.
- Do-not disconnect noninvasive interface for oral suction.

1.24 INSERTION OF INTRAVENOUS CANNULA AND ADMINISTRATION OF IV MEDICATION

Bhavya Kukreja

Objective

One should be able to administer parenteral fluids, and medications under all aseptic conditions.

Indication

Giving emergency medication, IV fluid, and sampling.

Equipment and Supplies

Appropriate size cannula, transparent dressing, cotton swabs, spirit, gloves, syringe, and normal saline.

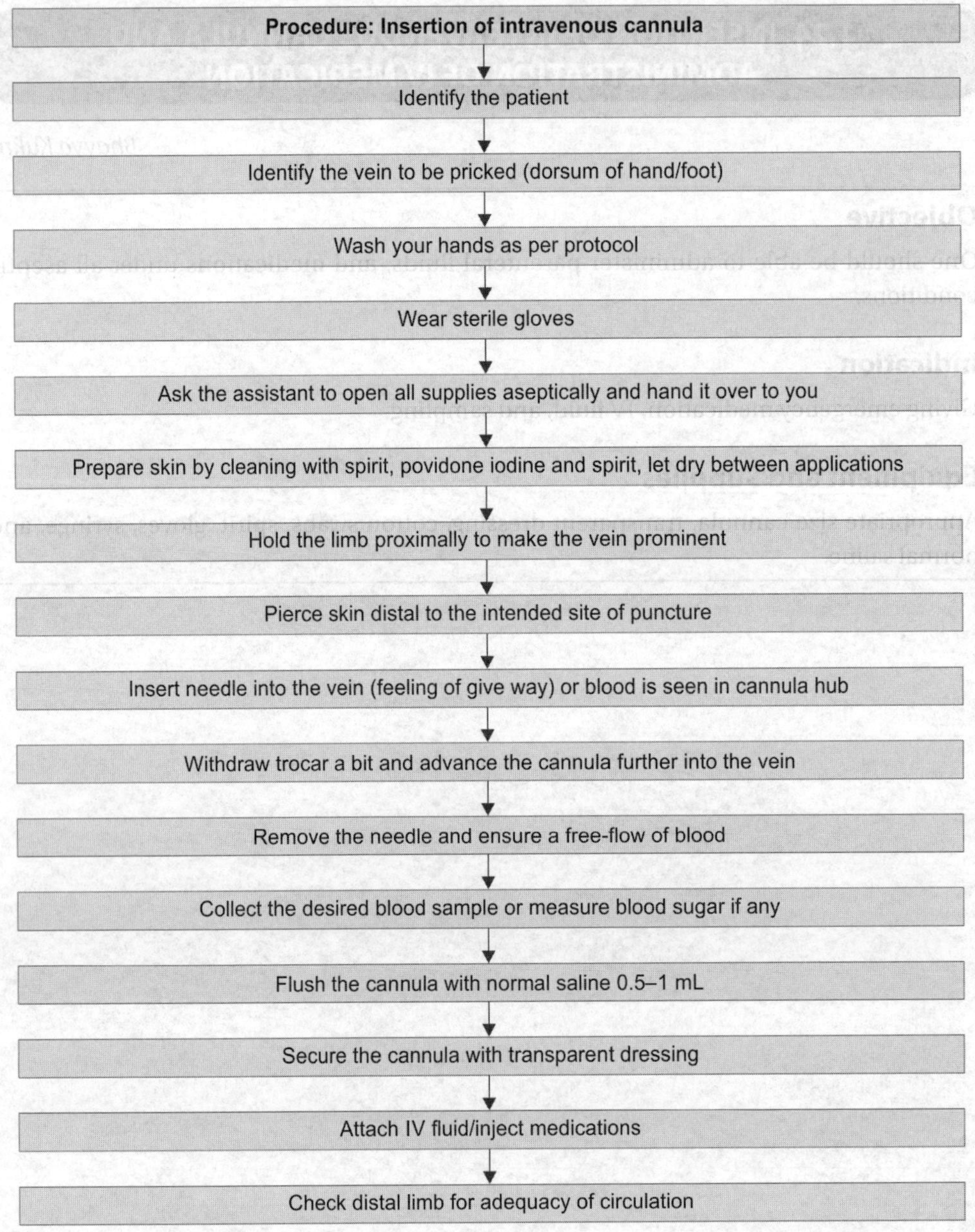

Procedure: Insertion of intravenous cannula
Identify the patient
Identify the vein to be pricked (dorsum of hand/foot)
Wash your hands as per protocol
Wear sterile gloves
Ask the assistant to open all supplies aseptically and hand it over to you
Prepare skin by cleaning with spirit, povidone iodine and spirit, let dry between applications
Hold the limb proximally to make the vein prominent
Pierce skin distal to the intended site of puncture
Insert needle into the vein (feeling of give way) or blood is seen in cannula hub
Withdraw trocar a bit and advance the cannula further into the vein
Remove the needle and ensure a free-flow of blood
Collect the desired blood sample or measure blood sugar if any
Flush the cannula with normal saline 0.5–1 mL
Secure the cannula with transparent dressing
Attach IV fluid/inject medications
Check distal limb for adequacy of circulation

OSCE/Checklist: Procedure—Insertion of IV Cannula

*Name of the participants:*____

S. No	Performance steps	Yes	No
1.	Check all supplies		
2.	Perform hand washing		
3.	Wear sterile gloves		
4.	Assistant opens all supplies aseptically and put them in a sterile tray		
5.	Prepare the skin with spirit swab for 30 seconds		
6.	Pricks skin surface at 30–45° to skin		
7.	Backflow of blood ensured		
8.	Flushes cannula with normal saline		
9.	Fixes cannula with transparent dressing like tegaderm		
	Total score		

OSCE/Checklist: Procedure—Administration of IV Drugs Through ANTT (Aseptic Non-touch Technique)

*Name of the participants:*____

S. No.	Performance steps	Yes	No
1.	Check all supplies		
2.	Perform hand washing		
3.	Wear sterile gloves		
4.	Assistant opens all supplies aseptically and put them in a sterile tray		
5.	Examine the central/peripheral line (insertion) site using visual infusion phlebitis score (known as *VIP score*)		
6.	With your sterile hands, (do not touch unsterile items or area with gloved hands. Keep gloved hands above waist level) cross-check the medicine, patient's name, name of the drug, dosage, and dilution		
7.	Take the alcohol-wipe and by spreading it fully and onto it gain access to the injection port of central line/vascular line exit port using one hand		
8.	Take another alcohol wipe, place the tip of the exit port/cannula hub into the center of the wipe with the other hand scrub, creating friction for 15–20 seconds using circular motion (progress from more clean area to less clean area)		
9.	Allow it to dry for 30 seconds before use		
10.	Discard the used wipe into the kidney tray		
11.	Take the prepared medicine and administer the flush/drug with relevant doctor's prescription and unit protocol		
12.	Take-off the syringe, close the cannula hub/exit port via sterile port cap		
13.	Gather all the used items together and discard it appropriately using biomedical-waste management		
14.	Perform hand-hygiene		
15.	Documentation to be recorded; both procedure and any untoward reaction to/surrounding the vascular-line site		
	Total score		

1.25 PERFORMING VENIPUNCTURE AND BLOOD SAMPLE COLLECTION

Neha Jain

Objective

One should be able to perform safe, clean and effective blood sample collection.

Equipment and Supplies

- Sterile gloves
- 24/26 G needle
- Swab and cotton balls soaked in chlorhexidine
- Prelabeled blood collection tubes and lab forms.

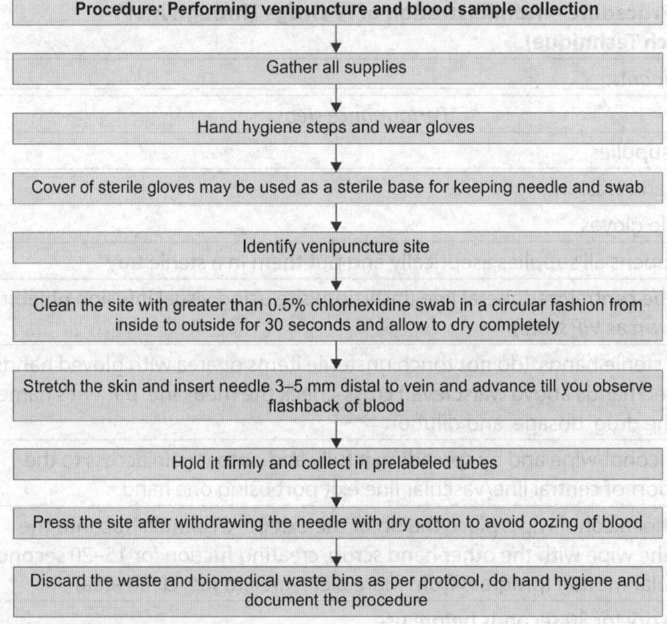

Key Points to Remember

What else can be done?

- Use nonpharmacological measures and developmentally supportive care.
- Fresh disposable needles and syringes are to be used always.

What to be avoided?

- Do not palpate the area of puncture after site preparation.
- Continue monitoring of site for bleeding, hematoma, and signs of infection.

1.26 INTRAMUSCULAR INJECTION

Neha Jain

Objective

One should be able to administer medication through intramuscular injection

Indication

To administer Inj. vitamin K, vaccines, and antibiotics.

Site

Quadriceps group of muscles of upper, outer thigh.

Equipment and Supplies

- Sterile 1 inch needle of smallest size (22–24 gauze)
- Sterile syringe of smallest size available that has adequate markings for proper dose (1–3 mL)
- Dry cotton wool ball.

Pain Management

- Ensure pain management with breastfeeds/assisted feeds with EBM or 10%D/swaddling.
- Using sharp of smallest diameter (22–24 gauze) using minimal volume injection (e.g., 2 mL or less)
- Avoid rapid injection of drug/vaccine using alternative injection site for subsequent injections.

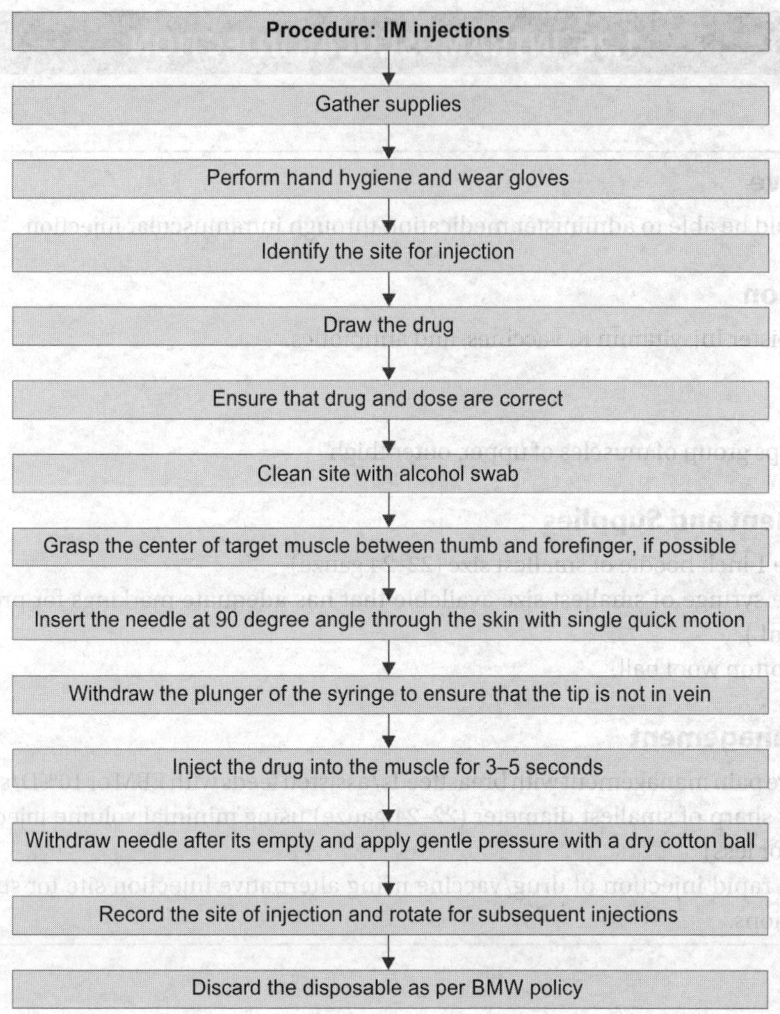

Key Points to Remember

If the needle is in a vein:

- Withdraw the needle without injecting the drug.
- Apply gentle pressure to the site with a dry cotton-wool ball to prevent bruising.
- Place a new, sterile needle on the syringe.
- Choose a new site for injection.
- Repeat the procedure described above.

If the needle is in the muscle:

If the needle is in the muscle, inject the material with steady pressure for 3–5 seconds.

- Upon completion of the injection, withdraw the needle and apply gentle pressure with a dry cotton wool ball.
- Record the site of the injection and rotate the site of subsequent injections.

Complications:

- Inadvertent intra-arterial or IV injection
- Infection from contaminated injection material
- Neural injury
- Local tissue damage due to injection of irritants

Complications can be avoided by following methods:

- Selecting the safest agents for injection.
- Choosing the proper injection site.
- Establishing anatomic landmarks.
- Cleansing the skin thoroughly.
- Alternating sites for subsequent injections.
- Aspirating before injecting the drug/vaccine.
- Avoiding tracking the drug into superficial tissues.
- Using a needle of adequate length to reach the intended injection site.

OSCE/Checklist: Procedure—Insertion of IM

*Name of the participants:*____

S. No.	*Performance steps*	Yes	No
1.	Collects all items needed		
2.	Perform hand washing		
3.	Wear sterile gloves		
4.	Assistant opens all supplies aseptically and put them in a sterile tray		
5.	Prepare the skin with spirit swab for 30 seconds		
6.	Locate the site of injection		
7.	Insert the needle at 90° angle		
8.	Withdraws the plunger to ensure that needle is not in the vein		
9.	Inject the medication		
10.	Withdraws the needle and apply gentle pressure with dry cotton		
11.	Dispose all the disposable as per BMW protocol		
12.	Document in the record		
	Total score		

Equipment

*Manish Diwedi, Swati Upadhyay, Mrinal Sinha, Swati Jangra, Anantika Garg,
Boby Varghese, Arun Gautam, Neha Jain, Jubilant James, Garima Saxena*

2.1 RADIANT WARMER/OPEN CARE SYSTEM

Manish Diwedi

About the Equipment

- Radiant warmers are open care systems used to provide warmth to babies.
- They provide intense source of radiant heat energy and reduce the conductive losses by providing a warm microenvironment surrounding the baby.

Principles of Working

- The overhead quartz/ceramic heating element produces heat, which is reflected by the parabolic reflector onto the baby on the bassinet.
- There are two modes—*servocontrol mode* and *manual mode* in radiant warmers.
- In servo mode, the heater output is determined automatically based on skin temperature sensed by the temperature probe applied on baby. Servosystem is the preferred method of running the open care system.
- In manual mode, the heater output from the heating rod can be increased or decreased manually by the heater output control knobs.

Parts (Fig. 1)

1. *Bassinet:* For placing the neonate.
2. *Heating element (quartz/ceramic rod/silicon quartz):* Provides radiant heat.
3. Parabolic reflectors
4. *Control panel:* It has a collection of display and control features/knobs.
5. *Mode selector:* Selects manual or servo mode.
6. *Heater output control knobs:* For increasing or decreasing the heater output manually
7. *Heater output display:* Indicates how much is the heater output.
8. *Temperature selection key/knob:* To set desired skin temperature.
9. *Temperature display:* Display temperature of the baby's skin (via skin probe) and the set temperature.
10. Alarm display for power failure, system failure, skin probe failure, skin temperature high/low, and heater failure.
11. Skin probe

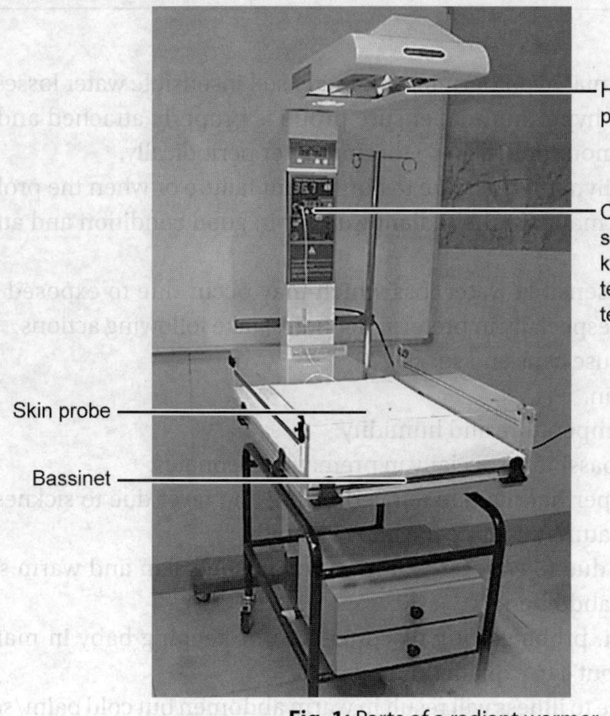

Fig. 1: Parts of a radiant warmer.

Setting up a radiant warmer
↓
Connect the unit to mains and switch on
↓
Select the manual mode and keep heater output to 100% for 15–20 minutes for prewarming the bassinet and linen
↓
Select servo mode and set the desired skin temperature as 36.5°C. Heater output adjusts automatically to keep the baby at set temperature
↓
Place baby on the bassinet. Cover head with cap, feet with socks, and hands with mittens
↓
Connect skin probe to baby's abdomen with a skin friendly tape
↓
For keeping a baby on manual mode, select the desired heater output. In manual mode, record baby's axillary temperature at 30 minutes and then 2 hourly
↓
Respond to alarms immediately. Identify the fault and rectify it
↓
Never leave baby unmonitored, when being cared for, under a warmer

Adverse Effects

- To watch out for hyperthermia, hypothermia, and increased insensible water losses
  - To prevent inadvertent hyperthermia, ensure probe is properly attached and the temperature of baby is monitored using a thermometer periodically.
  - To prevent inadvertent hypothermia due to equipment failure or when the probe is malfunctioning, always maintain the radiant warmer in good condition and attend to alarms immediately.
  - To reduce increased insensible water loss which may occur due to exposed skin surface to radiant heat, especially in preterm neonates, take following actions:
    - Clothe the baby and use caps and socks.
    - Coconut oil to the skin.
    - Maintain ambient temperature and humidity.
    - Use cling wrap over bassinet especially in premature neonates.
- Differentiating between hyperthermia due to overheating and fever due to sickness: If baby is having high temperature, examine the baby carefully.
- A baby who is overheated due to warmer will have red flushed skin and warm sole/palms in addition to warm abdomen.
- Malfunction of equipment, probe getting disconnected or keeping baby in manual mode with high heater output can explain this situation.
- On the other hand, fever due to illness will result in warm abdomen but cold palm/soles.
- In addition, clinical examination will reveal features that point toward sepsis in the baby.

■ TROUBLESHOOTING

Problem	Action
Machine does not switch on	Check power supply, check the plug and check fuse, if all the above okay, call engineer
Power on but heater not working	Call engineer
No skin temperature display	Faulty skin sensor (replace sensor/call engineer)
Display temperature and baby temperature variation >1°C	Calibration required. Call engineer
Sudden overheating on servo control mode	Check attachment of the probe—if correct probe failure—call engineer

Cleaning and Disinfection

- When bassinet is occupied—use only mild soap and water wipes daily. Do not use spirit or other chemicals to clean the plastic/acrylic parts.
- When bassinet is unoccupied—clean using disinfectant, like 2% bacillocid or glutaraldehyde, when the bassinet is unoccupied or weekly (move the baby while using disinfectant).

- Every seventh day, after shifting the baby to another cot, the warmer should be cleaned thoroughly, first by light detergent solution and then by antiseptic solution. All detachable assemblies are to be treated similarly.
- *Probe:* Clean the probe using isopropyl alcohol swab before and after each use.

Maintenance

- Calibration should be done every 4–6 months as per manufacturer's manual.
- At the time of purchase, take comprehensive warranty for 5 years and annual maintenance contract (AMC) to be done thereafter.

Key Points to Remember

- Maintaining euthermia is essential to ensure optimal growth.
- Energy expenditure and oxygen consumption is minimal in thermoneutral range.
- *Application of skin probes:*
  - Prepare the skin using an alcohol/spirit swab to ensure good adhesion to the skin.
  - Use skin friendly adhesive tape to secure the probe in place. Do not place probe on bony structures.
  - Apply probe over the right hypochondrium area in the supine position and over the flank in prone position.
  - Check sensor probe regularly to ensure that it is in place. In the event of displaced probe from baby's abdominal skin, overheating of the baby will occur because the skin probe depicts air temperature and heater output keeps on increasing till probe temperature matches control temperature.
  - Cover probe with a reflective cover pad, if available (foil covered foam adhesive pad).
  - *Do not* apply probe to bruised skin.
  - *Do not* reuse disposable probes.
- Do not use the warmer in a very cold room. It works best when the environmental temperature is above 20°C.
- Avoid air currents in vicinity as this reduces the warmer efficiency.
- Check temperature manually, at least once per shift.
- Always respond to alarms promptly and take corrective measures.
- *Manual mode:* Manual mode is used only for following situations—
  - When you are anticipating a new baby to be brought under warmer care. Keep warmer on with 100% heater output and once the baby arrives, shift to servo mode.
  - While rapid warming of a hypothermic baby.
  - Make sure that baby is never left unattended while using manual mode.

■ FURTHER READING

1. Facility Based Newborn Care (FBNC). Ministry of Health and Family Welfare (MoHFW); Government of India; 2022.
2. Rennie JM. Rennie & Roberton's Textbook of Neonatology, 5th edition. United Kingdom: Churchill Livingstone; 2012. .

2.2 INCUBATOR (CLOSED CARE SYSTEM)

Manish Diwedi

About the Equipment

- Maintaining euthermia is essential to ensure optimal growth.
- When temperature is maintained in thermoneutral range, caloric expenditure, and oxygen consumption is minimal.
- Incubators are closed care systems used to provide warmth and humidity to babies.

Indications

- Caring for neonates born <32 weeks or <1,800 g.
- For humidification, especially for ELBW babies.
- For isolating an infected baby to achieve barrier nursing.
- For providing oxygen. Depending on oxygen flow rate, ambient oxygen concentration can be maintained.
- For transporting babies (using transport incubator).
- For use at extremely low ambient temperatures.

Principles of Working

- Incubators work on the principle of forced convection.
- Air or an air-oxygen mixture is sucked in through a microfilter, streamed over the heating element, and the humidifier using a fan. The warm humidified air is then circulated through the hood to attain a uniform temperature within.
- Incubators reduce convective and radiation heat losses by reducing exposure to air currents and by providing a warm environment.
- Evaporative losses are minimized by maintaining high humidity in the incubator.
- Radiation losses are curtailed by the hood or canopy on the baby or by using double-walled incubators.

Temperature control modes in incubator: Two modes—air mode and servo mode.

- *In the air mode,* desired temperature around the baby is set and the heater output adjusts itself to maintain this. The appropriate set temperature is decided by using thermoneutral temperature charts **(Table 1)** as applicable to an individual baby based on gestation and postnatal age.
- The air temperature sensing probe should be placed near the baby and care should be taken that it is not displaced or covered.
- Air mode should be used whenever a procedure is being done and the hood or canopy is expected to stay open for a long time.

TABLE 1: Neutral range of environmental temperature (°C) for low-birth-weight babies.

Age	BW <1,200 g	1,200–1,500 g	1,501–22,500 g
1st day	35.0 ± 0.5	34.3 ± 0.5	33.4 ± 1.0
2nd day	34.5 ± 0.5	33.7 ± 0.5	32.7 ± 1.0
3rd day	34.0 ± 0.5	33.5 ± 0.5	33.0 ± 1.0
≥4th day	33.5 ± 0.5	32.8 ± 0.5	32.2 ± 1.0

Source: Adapted from Standards and Recommendations for Hospital Care of Newborn Infants, 5th edition. Evanston, Illinois: American Academy of Pediatrics; 1971.

- *In the servo-controlled mode* or the skin temperature-controlled mode, the desired skin temperature is set to 36.5°C.
- The baby's temperature is monitored by a skin probe, fixed firmly using a tape on the abdominal wall. The feedback system modifies heater output to keep the baby temperature constant.

Humidification protocol: Incubators reduce insensible water losses.

- It is done by filling the humidification tray with 1 liter of sterile water. In some incubators, water-soaked sponges are used.
- Protocol for setting humidity is as follows:
  - *For babies <28 weeks:* Commence 80% incubator humidity. After 7 days, wean by 5% each day. Cease incubator humidity when 40% is reached.
  - *For babies 28 weeks and above:* Commence 80% incubator humidity. After 1 day, wean humidity by 5% each day. Cease incubator humidity when 40% is reached.
- Commence humidity as soon after admission as possible. Do not delay unless necessary (e.g., an urgent procedure). Extremely preterm babies (<25 weeks) may require humidification for longer if there are problems with dehydration/hypernatremia.
- Water must be changed daily. Use sterile water only, to prevent colonization by bacteria.
- Check water levels regularly especially on high humidity. Incubator will alarm if water levels are low. Empty the water tank when the humidity is turned off.
- Minimize the opening of doors so that humidity inside incubator remains constant.
- Incubator temperature may need to be increased when the humidity is decreased to ensure thermal stability for the baby.
- There are concerns that prolonged humidification may increase the risks of sepsis, so prolonged humidification should not be routine and should be reviewed regularly.
- Change incubators weekly.

Parts of an Incubator (Fig. 1)

- *Hood or canopy:* Single or double walled. Made of acrylic/plexiglass/fiberglass.
- *Iris ports:* Access ports which are meant to be elbow operated
- Under deck area and conditioning chamber
- Air inlet, filter, fan, or blower system

- Humidity chamber
- Baby tray with the mattress
- An inlet for oxygen and IV tubings
- Skin and air temperature probes
- Display panel with temperature and humidity control knobs
- *Additional optional features:* Intravenous stand, weighing scale, timer, tilt facility, battery backup, oxygen analyzer, resuscitator, vital signs monitor, phototherapy unit, oxygen flow meter, suction, and ventilator.

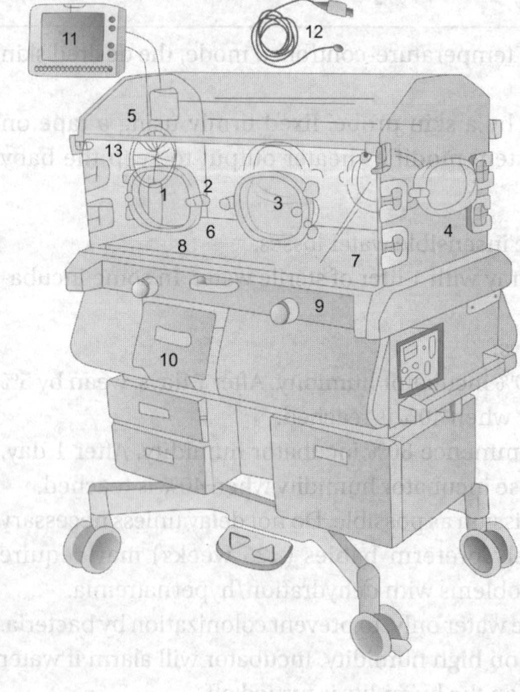

Fig. 1: *Parts of incubator:* 1—Porthole (external); 2—porthole lock; 3—porthole (internal); 4—small wall; 5—small wall; 6—superior face of the mattress (head); 7—superior face of the mattress (buttock/feet); 8—platform in contact with inferior face of the mattress (head); 9—air conditioning chamber; 10—humidity chambers; 11—control panel; 12—probe/sensor for skin temperature; and 13—access port cover.

Cleaning and Disinfection

- When the equipment is in use, all approachable internal and external surfaces should be cleaned daily with soap water or antiseptic. Spirit or other organic solvents must not be used to clean the incubator hood or panel.
- Every 7th day, after shifting the baby to another clean incubator, the used equipment should be cleaned thoroughly, first by light detergent solution and then by antiseptic solution. All detachable assemblies, especially from the under-deck area, are to be treated similarly. After drying, the parts are reassembled and sterilized using a vaporizing agent and/or fumigation. Adding 50 mL of formalin to 50 mL of distilled water in humidity tank and plugging it for 4 hours leads to fumigation of the incubator. After fumigation it should be thoroughly aired.
- The sleeves of the access windows must preferably be changed daily and cleaned.

Maintenance

- The hospital biomedical engineer must regularly check equipment. Authorized company engineer must be called for preventive checks and major breakdowns.
- Air filters generally require change every 3 months or if they are visibly dirty. A clogged filter reduces the oxygen entry and promotes carbon dioxide build up in incubator.
- The control and power units should be calibrated every 4–6 months and thorough servicing should be done annually.
- Temperature calibration should ensure sensitivity to ±0.5° of the set value.

Key Points to Remember

- Double-walled incubators or dome shields may be used if environmental temperatures are low. Room temperature between 21° and 28°C is ideal.
- Double-walled incubators are better than single walled as they reduce the radiant heat losses by 29%.
- Positioning the incubator parallel to the wall should be avoided because it hampers air circulation.
- Baby can be clothed while inside an incubator.
- The choice of an incubator should be made according to the level of neonatal care for which it will be used—minimum care, subintensive care, intensive care, or superintensive care.

■ FURTHER READING

1. Rennie JM. Rennie & Roberton's Textbook of Neonatology, 5th edition. United Kingdom: Churchill Livingstone; 2012.

2.3 PULSE OXIMETER

Swati Upadhyay

Indications

- Pulse oximeter used for monitoring of oxygenation in a continuous and noninvasive manner.
- While resuscitating a neonate, use pulse oximetry as an adjunct for assessing response to resuscitation when PPV is required, to confirm perception of persistent central cyanosis in delivery room and as a guide to titrate oxygen therapy to maintain baby's SpO_2 in target range.
- Monitoring of sick babies in NICU and titrating their oxygen therapy.
- Detection of apnea (bradycardia and desaturation) in neonates.
- Monitoring of babies while transport.
- It may be useful in addition to Allen's test to detect ulnar artery patency.
- As a screening tool for detection of critical congenital heart disease in all neonates after 24 hours of life.

Principles and Mechanism of Action

- The concept of pulse oximetry is based on the Beer-Lambert law, which states that the concentration of an unknown solute in a solvent can be determined by amount of light absorbed by the solute.
- *Pulse oximetry utilizes following two principles:*
  - Difference in peak absorption spectra of oxyhemoglobin (HbO) and reduced hemoglobin (HbH) at wavelengths of 660 nm (red) and 940 nm (infrared): Reduced hemoglobin absorbs more red light than infrared light and oxygenated hemoglobin absorbs more infrared than red **(Fig. 1)**.

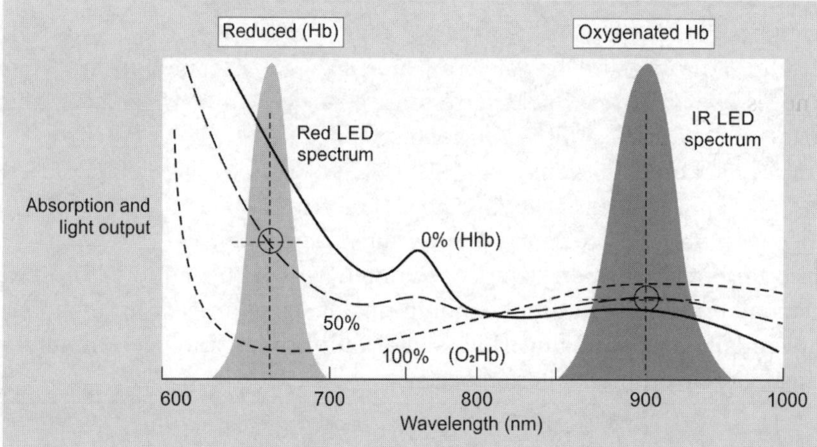

Fig. 1: The absorption spectra of oxyhemoglobin and reduced hemoglobin across the red (660 nm) and infrared (940 nm) spectra with middle-dashed line depicting spectra of 50% saturated hemoglobin.

- *Presence of a pulsatile signal generated by the arterial blood flow:* Only the pulsatile change in light transmission through living tissue is measured to calculate arterial saturation. The absorption of light by venous blood, skin pigments, tissue, and bone is eliminated from consideration.

How does pulse oximeter work?

- Probe of pulse oximeter consists of two diodes which emit equal intensities of red and infrared light in sequence into pulsatile tissue bed.
- One light-emitting diode emits light in the red spectrum, at a wavelength of 660 nm, at which the light absorption of deoxyhemoglobin is greater than that of oxyhemoglobin.
- The other diode emits light in the infrared spectrum, at a wavelength of 940 nm, at which oxyhemoglobin absorbs more light than deoxyhemoglobin.
- A photodetector placed on the opposite side senses the ratio of red and infrared light based on which the proportion of oxygenated and reduced hemoglobin is estimated by an in-built microprocessor and digitally displayed **(Fig. 2)**.

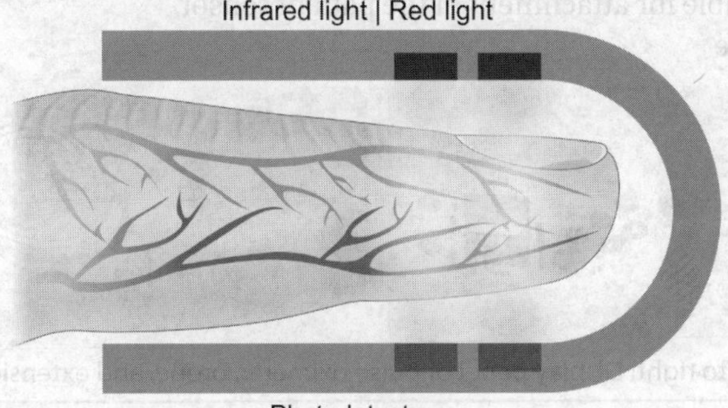

Fig. 2: Light emitting diodes and photodetector in pulse oximeter probe.

Masimo SET versus Conventional Pulse Oximetry

- Conventional pulse oximetry assumes that arterial blood is the only blood moving (pulsating) at the measurement site. However, during patient motion, the venous blood also moves, which causes conventional pulse oximetry to under-read because it cannot distinguish between the arterial and venous blood.
- Masimo signal extraction technology (SET) identifies the venous blood signal, isolates it and using adaptive filters, cancels the noise, and extracts the arterial signal only. It then reports the true arterial oxygen saturation and pulse rate.
- Masimo SET pulse oximetry works accurately where conventional pulse oximetry tends to fail or provide inaccurate monitoring or signal dropout as in patient motion or movement, low perfusion (low signal amplitude), intense ambient light, or electrosurgical instrument interference.

Masimo Rainbow SET Technology

- It is a noninvasive monitoring platform enabling the assessment of multiple blood constituents and physiologic parameters that previously required invasive or complicated procedures.
- In this technology, adaptive filters along with seven different algorithms are used to noninvasively measure blood constituents and fluid status using pulse oximeters.
- It can measure total hemoglobin (Sp Hb), respiratory rate (RRa), pleth variability index (PVI), oxygen content, and levels of carboxyhemoglobin (SpCO) and methemoglobin (Sp Met).

Parts

- Display panel—numeric and graphic display
- A patient sensor/probe which is to be connected to the extension cable. Probes may be disposable or reusable.
- An extension cable for attachment of the patient sensor.
- An electric cable

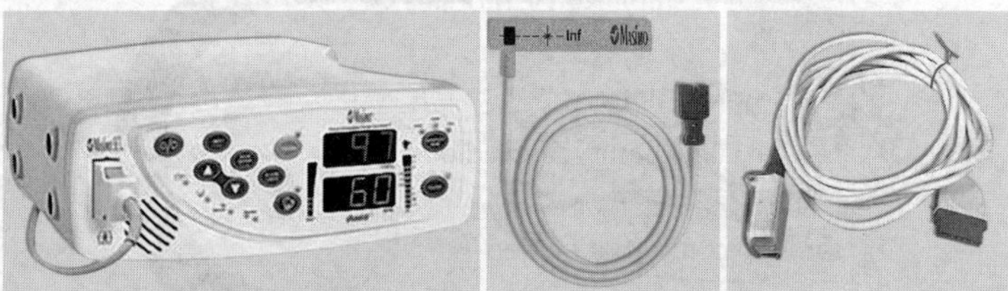

From left to right: Display panel of pulse oximeter, probe, and extension cable.

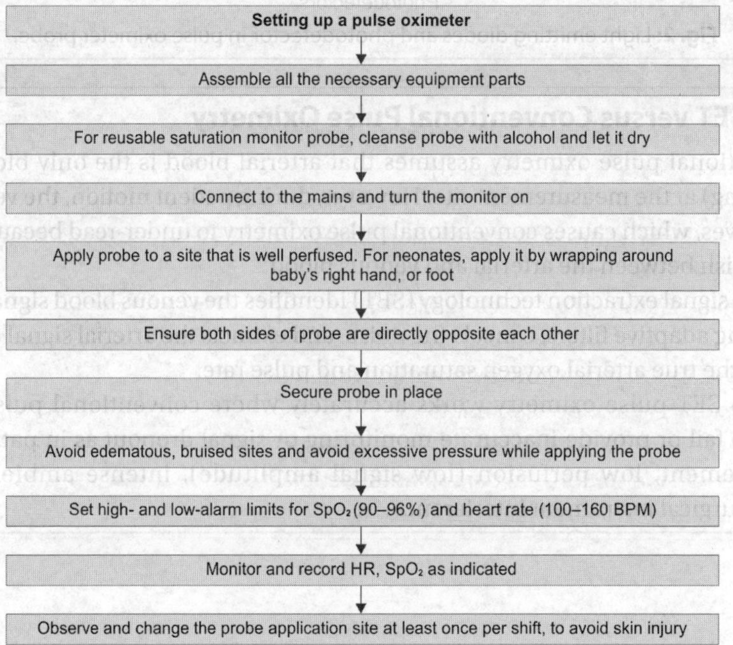

Cleaning and Disinfection

- Clean display panel with a moist soft cloth.
- Clean body with soft cloth dampened with soap water followed by moist soft cloth.
- Clean reusable sensors with spirit after each patient use.
- Do not autoclave.
- Carefully connect and disconnect probes and plugs to avoid damage. Grip the hub and not the cable.

Troubleshooting		
Alarm/display message	**Possible cause**	**Corrective action**
Check sensor	Motion, low perfusion, wrong position	Reposition, relocate
Check probe	Probe not connected properly or faulty probe	Check probe condition and connection. Connect probe correctly
Pulse search	Low perfusion, edema, movement	Change sensor site
Interference detected	Electric signal with electromagnetic waves in vicinity like TV, mobile phone	Remove interference
Low battery	Low internal battery	Connect to AC power
Sensor failure	Broken cable, faulty photodiode, sensor damage	Replace sensor
System failure	Internal component failed	Unit needs service/change
Ambient light	Excessive light on sensor like phototherapy lights	Relocate/cover with opaque paper or cloth/aluminum foil

Key Points to Remember

- Inspect sensor site every 2–4 hours for any erythema or discoloration.
- Change sensor site every 4–6 hourly.
- Pulse oximeter may be less accurate in the following situations:
    - Hypovolemic states or low perfusion states
    - Severe hypothermia/cold extremities
    - Dyshemoglobinemias—COHb, Meth Hb
    - Dyes and pigments including nail polish, methylene blue
    - Optical interference from external light sources (phototherapy unit, fluorescent light, and sunlight) and optical shunts.
    - Excess movement artifacts
    - Excess pigmentation—in dark skinned people it may be less accurate.
    - Electrosurgical instrument interference

- Pulse oximeters are accurate mainly when the oxygen saturation is between 80 and 95%. The accuracy of pulse oximetry is about ±4–5% at or above 80% saturation. Accuracy declines below a saturation of 80%.
- Pulse oximeter cannot detect hyperoxia.
- Pulse oximetry does not take clinical impact of anemia into account; hence it may be less accurate in severe anemia.
- Conventional pulse oximeters may not distinguish different types of hemoglobins. Hence, in the presence of COHb (carboxyhemoglobin) and Meth Hb (methemoglobin), the saturation readings may be falsely and significantly elevated, thus masking the presence of hypoxemia.
- Pulse oximetry reflects state of oxygenation and has no value in assessing adequacy of ventilation.
- Always check the baby and the plethysmograph before interpreting the SpO_2 and heart rate value. It is mandatory to have a sharp, well-defined pulsatile waveform tracing with dicrotic notch, for the saturation and heart rate readings to be accurate.
- Values are reliable when the plethysmography waveform or bar signal is good and when the display is constant and not blinking or repeatedly changing.
- Too much tightly attached probe can cause false reading, pressure injury and limb ischemia. Inspect sensor site every 2–4 hours for any erythema or discoloration.
- Change sensor site every 4–6 hourly. Do not apply sensor too tightly. Do not apply probe to edematous or bruised sites.
- *Cross-talk phenomenon:* If probe does not fit properly, the light can be shunted from the LEDs directly to photodetector affecting the accuracy of the measurement.
- *Lag monitor phenomenon:* Often a fall in partial pressure of oxygen precedes, the fall in oxygen saturations by several minutes and there may be a delay in picking up hypoxemia episode.
- *Response delay:* Although it is used for continuous real-time monitoring of oxygen saturations, there is often a delay of 5–20 seconds due to signal averaging. Hence, actual drop in saturations usually precedes the displayed drop in SpO_2.
- Pulse oximeter software varies between different manufactures. Hence one manufacturer's sensor may give false results if used by another manufacturer's monitors (e.g., Nellcor sensor for Philips monitor).
- Avoid edematous, bruised sites, and avoid excessive pressure while applying the probe.
- Avoid excess ambient light shining on the probe. If so, cover with opaque material.
- Do not tie BP cuff proximal to the limb where probe is fixed to avoid poor perfusion.
- Keep the pulse oximeter battery fully charged but do not run the oximeter on battery alone if power is available.

OSCE/Checklist: Procedure—SpO$_2$ Measurement by Using Pulse Oximeter			
Name of the participants: ____			
S. No.	Performance steps	Yes	No
1.	Perform hand hygiene and identify neonate with indications		
2.	Cleans SpO$_2$ probe with 70% alcohol		
3.	Connects the power cord, turns on the power switch		
4.	Checks/sets the alarm limits		
5.	Applies the probe properly to right hand (preductal)		
6.	Wait for stable plethysmography tracings and pulse rate		
7.	Documents the SpO$_2$ reading and the pulse rate		
		Total score	

■ FURTHER READING

1. Facility Based Newborn Care (FBNC). Ministry of Health and Family Welfare (MoHFW); Government of India; 2022.
2. Rennie JM. Rennie & Roberton's Textbook of Neonatology, 5th edition. United Kingdom: Churchill Livingstone; 2012.

2.4 INFUSION PUMPS

Swati Upadhyay

About the Equipment

- Accurate fluid and drug infusion are critical for the optimum management of sick neonates.
- Infusion pumps assure continuous, precise, and accurate delivery of prescribed fluid and drug volumes over a specified time.
- They are especially important while administering drugs with short half-lives, to maintain a desirable constant serum concentration and in situations when constant infusion of glucose is needed.

Principles of Working

- Gravity controlled pumps rely solely on gravity to regulate the rate of flow. Infusion rate is dependent on pressure difference across the valve.
- Drip rate controllers rely on gravity to provide the infusion pressure also. Positive displacement pumps provide a positive displacement of fluid with the help of a motor.
- Positive displacement pumps have either a peristaltic or a piston mechanism.

Parts

- Syringe barrel clamp
- Pusher and push guard/flange guard
- Handle assembly bolt
- Swing lock clamp
- On/off
- Screen
- Silence alarm
- Bolus or prime
- Value selection
- Prealarm and alarm warning
- Stop—infusion stop
- Menu

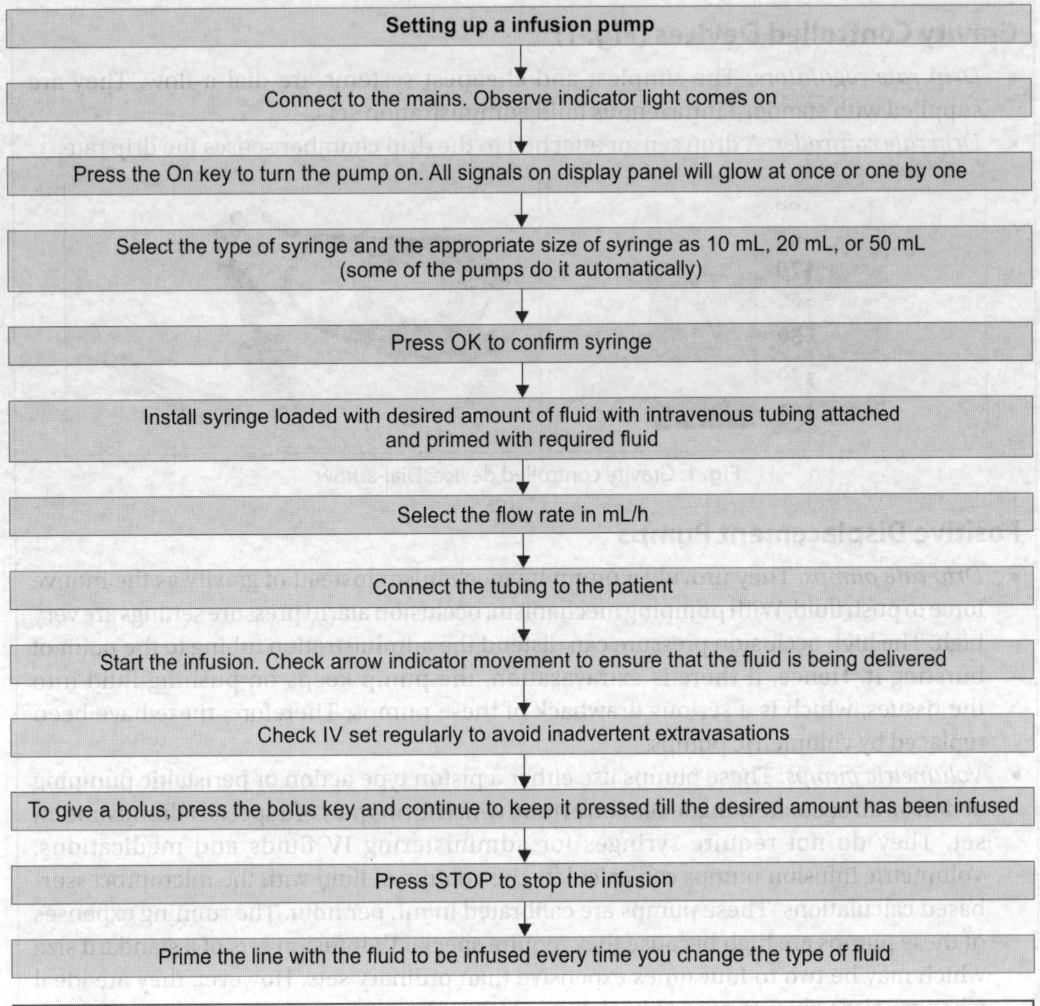

Types

- *Gravity controlled:*
  - Drip rate regulators
  - Drip rate controllers
- *Positive displacement pumps:*
  - Drip rate pumps
  - Volumetric pumps
  - Syringe pumps
  - Multichannel pumps
  - Characteristic features of different infusion pumps

Gravity Controlled Devices (Fig. 1)

- *Drip rate regulators:* The simplest and cheapest systems are dial-a-flow. They are supplied with standard intravenous fluid administration sets.
- *Drip rate controller:* A drop sensor attached to the drip chamber senses the drip rate.

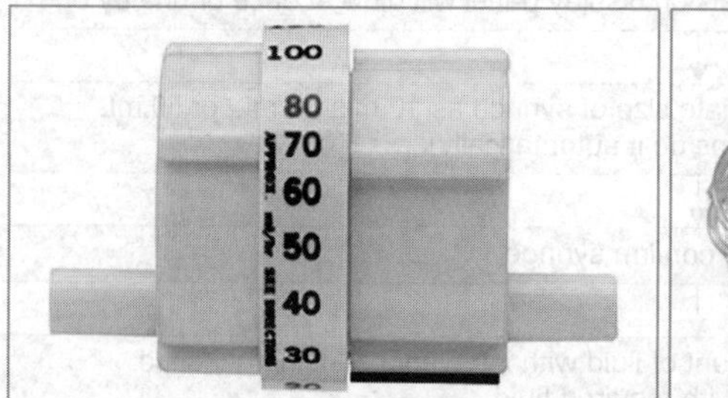
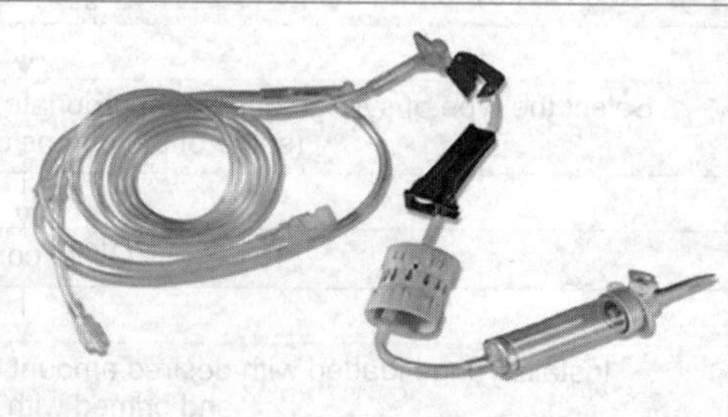

Fig. 1: Gravity controlled device: Dial-a-flow.

Positive Displacement Pumps

- *Drip rate pumps:* They provide a pumping mechanism instead of gravity as the motive force to push fluid. With pumping mechanism, occlusion alarm pressure settings are very high. The high occlusion pressure can distend the administration tubing to the point of bursting it. Hence, if there is extravasation, the pump keeps on pushing fluid into the tissues, which is a serious drawback of these pumps. Therefore, these have been replaced by volumetric pumps.
- *Volumetric pumps:* These pumps use either a piston type action or peristaltic pumping action on an accurately made section of tube which forms part of a special administration set. They do not require syringes for administering IV fluids and medications. Volumetric infusion pumps can calculate the volume of fluid with the microprocessor-based calculations. These pumps are calibrated in mL per hour. The running expenses of these pumps are high because they require special IV infusion sets of a standard size which may be two to four times expensive than ordinary sets. However, they are ideal when precise volumes need to be delivered **(Fig. 2)**.

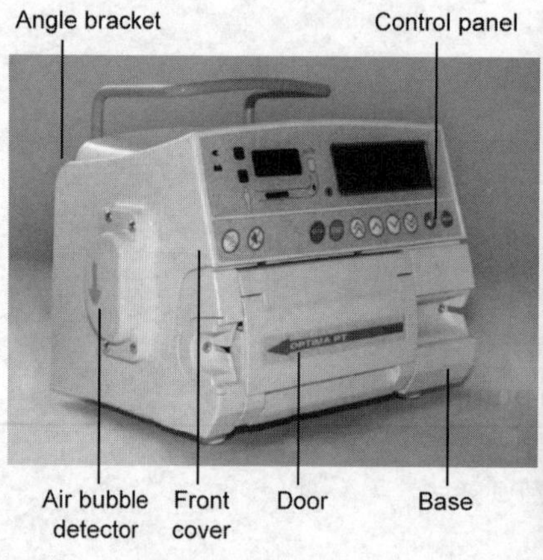

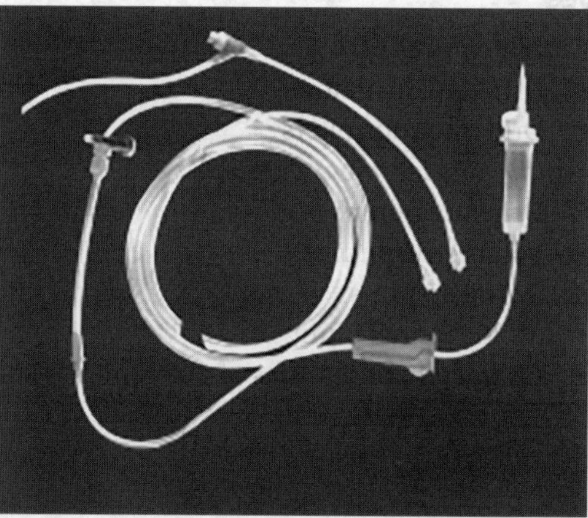

Fig. 2: Volumetric infusion pump along with special IV administration set.

- *Syringe pumps (**Fig. 3**):* The most used pumps for the administration of intravenous drugs are positive displacement syringe pumps that utilize a gear reduction mechanism and lead screw. They do not require specialized IV administration sets. They can accept all syringe sizes from 10 to 100 mL and have two independent microprocessors to monitor and control infusion processes for consistent delivery.

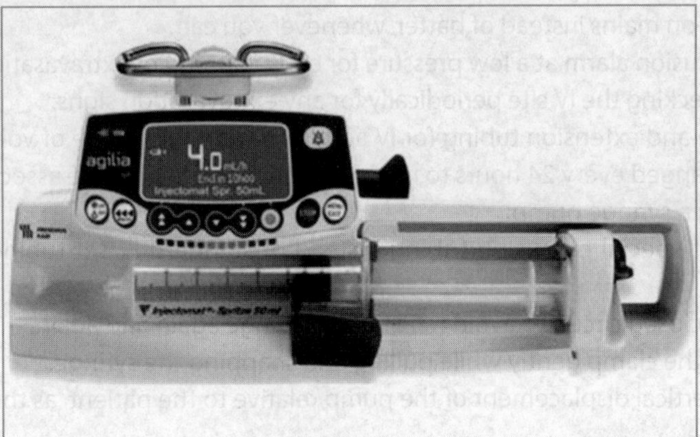

Fig. 3: Syringe pump.

- *Multichannel pumps:* There are now several multichannel pumps available, which permit simultaneous administration of two or three infusions. However, one potential problem with such a system is the possibility of incompatible mixing.
- *Ambulatory pumps:* These are pocket size pumps, which use linear peristaltic mechanism and have a fluid container in the form of a small floppy bag or cassette. The pumps are designed for users who need to wear them for long periods, and they have good alarm and display systems.
- *"Smart" infusion pumps:* These are new generation infusion pumps that incorporate a software that includes a "drug library" wherein hospital-defined drug infusion parameters, such as acceptable concentrations, infusion rates, dosing units, maximum and minimum loading, and maintenance dose bolus limits for 60 or more medications can be preprogrammed. With rapid advancements in computer technology, these pumps are likely to be used in future along with computerized prescriber order entry (CPOE) and automatic medication dispensing systems.

Troubleshooting

Problem	Action
No power on the switching on the instrument	Check power supply, fuse, plug If all above are okay, call engineer
Alarms	Check syringe position and clamps
Occlusion alarm with no block in line (easy fluid infusion when manually pushed)	Call engineer

Key Points to Remember

- Crosscheck the flow rate to assure no inadvertent medication/fluid administration errors (e.g., 5 mL/h instead of 0.5 mL/h).
- Label the syringe with the drug/fluid name.
- Respond to alarms and take corrective action immediately.
- Always run-on mains instead of batter, whenever you can.
- Set the occlusion alarm at a low pressure for early warning of extravasation or block.
- Keep on checking the IV site periodically for any extravasation signs.
- The syringe and extension tubing (or IV administration set in case of volumetric pumps) must be changed every 24 hours to minimize the risk of healthcare associated infections.
- While using a syringe pump:
    - Connect special extension tubing instead of standard IV set tubing to the loaded syringe.
    - Make a closed circuit to avoid refilling the syringe again and again.
    - Handle the clamp gently while pulling and snapping the syringe.
- Minimize vertical displacement of the pump relative to the patient, as this may influence the flow rate.
- Minimize total compliance of the IV administration set by making use of tubing, add-on devices, and filters that are low compliant and have a low volume.
- Choose a low-compliant syringe (i.e., rigid wall and a close fit of the plunger to the plunger head) with the smallest size and diameter that matches the preprogrammed flow rate while preventing the need for frequent replacing of the syringe.
- Use valves to prevent backflow and/or siphonage, but make sure that the opening pressure of the valves is low.
- Always prime the IV administration set.
- Side effects—inadvertent IV extravasation, if IV cannula is displaced.
- **Cleaning and disinfection:** Use damp cloth soaked in soap-water (detergent) for cleansing the panel daily.

■ FURTHER READING

1. Facility Based Newborn Care (FBNC). Ministry of Health and Family Welfare (MoHFW); Government of India; 2022.
2. Rennie JM. Rennie & Roberton's Textbook of Neonatology, 5th edition. United Kingdom: Churchill Livingstone; 2012.

2.5 MEASUREMENT OF SERUM BILIRUBIN BY TRANSCUTANEOUS BILIRUBINOMETER

Swati Upadhyay

About the Equipment

- Proper assessment and appropriate management of hyperbilirubinemia are very important to prevent acute and chronic bilirubin encephalopathy.
- Serum bilirubin [transcutaneous bilirubinometer (TCB)] measurement in clinical laboratory is an objective method, but it is expensive, invasive and there is significant interlaboratory and intralaboratory variability.
- Blood sampling is painful and repeated pricks carry a risk of infection. Visual assessment of bilirubin is observer-dependent and therefore less reliable. This is where TCB comes into play.
- The use of a TCB meter for screening has several advantages, including being a point-of-care, noninvasive method for estimating bilirubin levels and providing nearly instantaneous results.
- In multiple studies, TCB measurements have been shown to provide reasonably accurate estimates of total serum bilirubin (TSB) levels with few exceptions.

Indication

Screening for hyperbilirubinemia in term and late preterm infants (>35 weeks gestation) who have not received phototherapy or exchange transfusion.

Commonly Used Devices

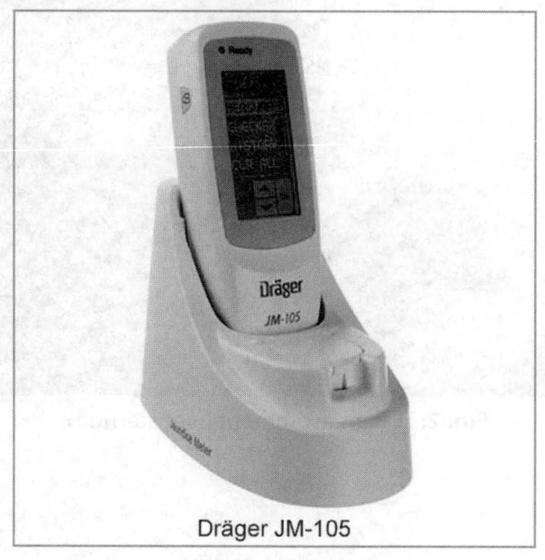

Dräger JM-105

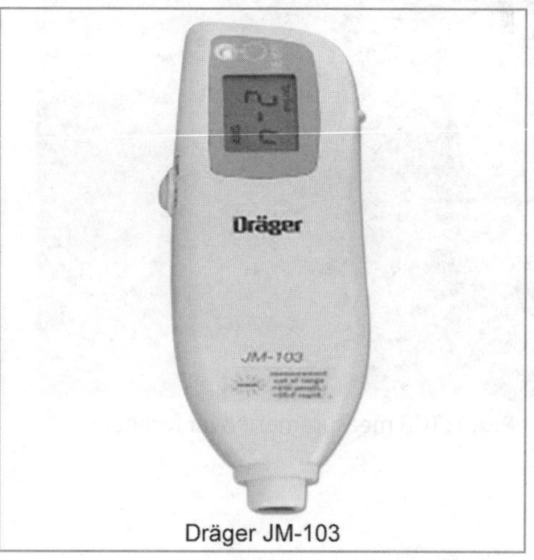

Dräger JM-103

Note: Dräger JM-105 is indicated for use in neonatal patients born ≥24 weeks gestation who have not undergone exchange transfusion. The device is indicated for use before, during, and after phototherapy treatment.

Principles of Working

- There is high degree of correlation between cutaneous bilirubin and TCB is the basis of transcutaneous bilirubinometry.
- Transcutaneous bilirubinometer is based on principle of reflectance photospectrometry. TSBs measure yellowness of the skin by analysis of spectrum of optical signal (including dual or multiple wavelengths) reflected by the baby's skin.
- These optical signals are converted to electrical signals by a photocell. These are analyzed by a microprocessor to generate a serum bilirubin value.

How to Use

- Perform hand hygiene
- Set the number of average measurements needed. Averaging 3 or more readings (computed automatically by the TCB meter when the desired number of measurements is set) provide more precise TCB measurements than using a single measurement.
- Ensure that "ready" lamp is illuminated.
- *Site of measurement:* The recommended sites are the forehead and the upper end of sternum **(Figs. 1 and 2)**.
- Place the optic head of the meter against the forehead or sternum of the neonate and press gently.
- The first measurement is complete when the measuring probe is pressed against the patient and the unit clicks. The probe must be lifted from the patient and reapplied for total number of measurements selected. At the end, TCB machine will automatically display the averaged reading.

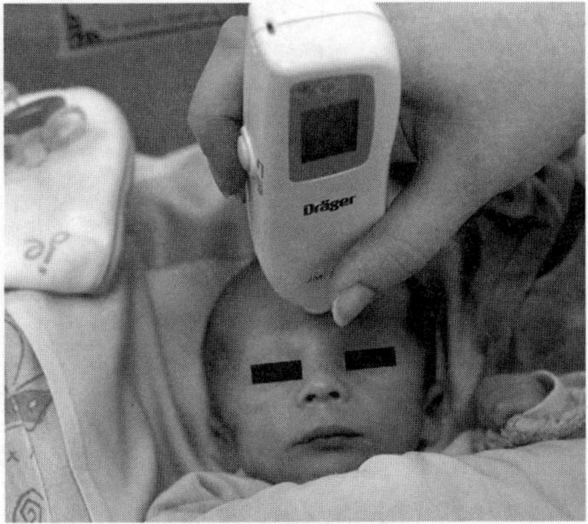

Fig. 1: TCB measurement over forehead.

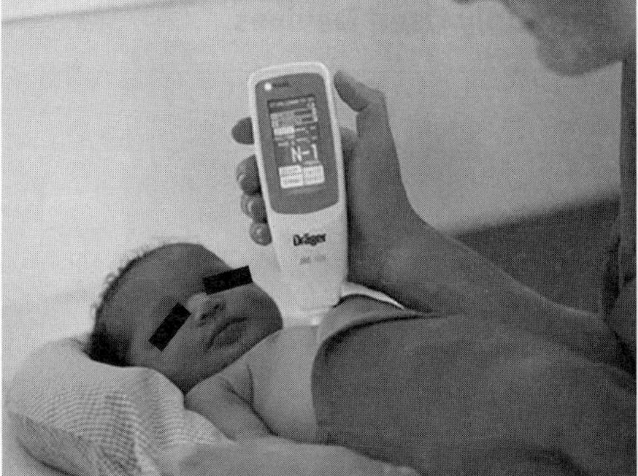

Fig. 2: TCB measurement over sternum.

CONTRAINDICATIONS AND LIMITATIONS

- TCB is not intended as a diagnostic device. It is a screening device for the detection of neonatal hyperbilirubinemia in the early stage and should be used in conjunction with other clinical symptoms and laboratory measurements for diagnosis and therapy decisions.
- Do not use this device on infants with hemolytic jaundice or pathologic jaundice because of an incompatible blood type. In such babies, total serum bilirubin should be measured.
- Do not use this device on patients with hydrops fetalis major, congenital malformations, diseases or skin conditions or thickness that would preclude or interfere with the use of the TCB meter (e.g., skin infections, purpura, etc.)
- Hyperemia at the test site may affect the results. Measurements against bruises, birthmarks, and subcutaneous hematoma should be avoided.
- Use only in babies up to 14 days old.
- In following cases, TCB measurements may not be reliable and decisions for treatment should be made based on TSB alone:
  - Babies less than completed 35 weeks of gestation
  - Jaundice in first 24 hours of life
  - Babies >14 days old
  - TCB measurements >15 mg/dL
  - Babies under phototherapy or postphototherapy
  - TCB measurement within 3 mg/dL of TSB phototherapy cut off. For example, if TSB cut off for phototherapy is 15 mg/dL and TCB measurement is 12 mg/dL or above, then TSB should be measured. In other words, if "TCB + 3" would change the management, then TSB should be obtained.
  - Babies where conjugated hyperbilirubinemia is suspected.

Cleaning and Disinfection

- *Cleaning:* Wipe off obvious soiling with a disposable cloth soaked in surface disinfectant.
- *Surface disinfection:*
  - Wipe cleaned surfaces again to visibly wet all surfaces to be disinfected with surface disinfectant. Wait for the surface disinfectant contact time.
  - At the end of the contact time, moisten a new uncontaminated and lint-free cloth with water (at least drinking water quality). Wipe all surfaces with this cloth until no remains of the surface disinfectant visible. Wait until the surfaces are dry.
  - Clean the measuring probe with alcohol before and after taking a measurement on the next patient. Wipe with a dry cloth.

> ### Key Points to Remember
>
> - Transcutaneous bilirubin measurement may be used to screen for hyperbilirubinemia in term and preterm neonates.
> - If TCB values fall within 2.9 mg/dL (~50 µmol/L) below or above the age appropriate phototherapy threshold, total serum bilirubin (TSB) should be measured to decide on the need for phototherapy or exchange transfusion.

◼ MEASUREMENT OF SERUM BILIRUBIN BY MICROCENTRIFUGE

OSCE/Checklist: Procedure		
Name of the participants: ______________________________		
S. No. — *Performance steps*	*Yes*	*No*
1. Wash hands with soap and water		
2. Wear sterile gloves		
3. Disinfect the area of skin to be pricked in alcohol-betadine-alcohol sequence		
4. Use a 24/26G needle and collect capillary or venous blood in 2–3 heparinized capillaries		
5. Seal the capillary base with clay and then soap		
6. Place the capillaries in microcentrifuge diagonally opposite to one another with sealed end facing outward		
7. Close the microcentrifuge cover and lid		
8. Turn on the microcentrifuge @10,000 rpm for 4–5 minutes		
9. Let the machine come to a stop by itself		
10. Switch on the spectrophotometer and calibrate with a blank capillary		
11. Place the centrifuged capillary in the slit		
12. Measure and document serum bilirubin		
Total score		

◼ FURTHER READING

1. Facility Based Newborn Care (FBNC). Ministry of Health and Family Welfare (MoHFW); Government of India; 2022.
2. Rennie JM. Rennie & Roberton's Textbook of Neonatology, 5th edition. United Kingdom: Churchill Livingstone; 2012.

2.6 PHOTOTHERAPY UNIT

Mrinal Sinha, Swati Jangra

About the Equipment

- *Indication:* Provide phototherapy to a newborn presented with neonatal hyperbilirubinemia.
- *Types of unit:*
  - Fluorescent lights (conventional phototherapy):
    - Fluorescent 6–8 white light OR a combination of two special blue and four to six white fluorescent lights with a plexiglass shield.
    - Tube life is 1,000 hours/6 months whichever is earlier
    - *Irradiance:* White light 6–8 $\mu w/cm^2/nm$), blue + white light 8–12 $\mu w/cm^2/nm$.
  - Compact fluorescent lights (CFL)
    - Compact high intensity bulbs (4 blue and 2 white) enclosed in the unit with reflecting grills
    - Irradiance: 12–18 $\mu w/cm^2/nm$
    - Lamp life is 2,000–3,000 hours
  - Light emitting diode (LED)
    - Multiple high intensity LED bulb in a panel
    - *Irradiance:* 20–40 $\mu w/cm^2/nm$
    - Bulb life is 20,000–30,000 hours.
- *Other parts:* Radiator fan and hour meter (counts total working hours)

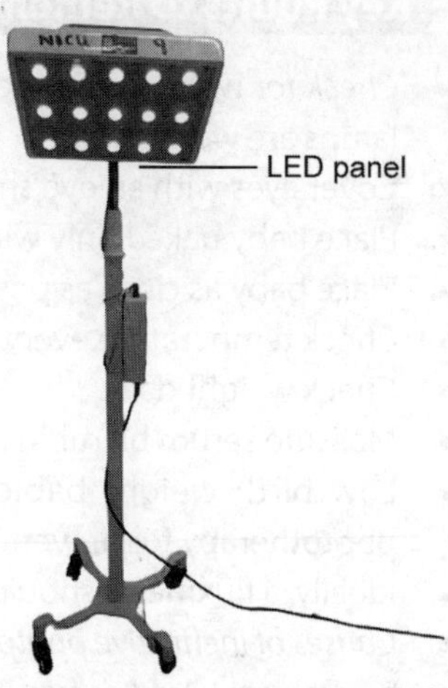

Principle of Working

All phototherapy units have a light source to provide irradiance ranging from 6 to 40 $\mu w/cm^2/nm$ in the wavelength of 420–460 nm.

Maintenance

- LED bulb has longer life approximately 30,000 hours or every 6 years whichever is earlier.
- Use a flux meter to monitor the irradiance of the unit once a week.
- Change the tube light if irradiance is below <15 $\mu w/cm^2/nm$.
- Do not place anything on the phototherapy unit.
- Cleaning:
  - Soap/detergent once daily
  - Clean with disinfectant once a week
  - Keep the lamps, the covering shield and the grill clean

Troubleshooting

S. No.	Problem	Probable reason	Action
1.	Insufficient irradiance	Light or reflector covered with dust or life of bulb is over	Clean the dust/change the tube light
2.	Bulb flickering or end of tube blackened	Starter problem or life of tube is over	Change starter/tube
3.	Noisy machine or baby getting overheated	Fan not working or faulty choke	Call engineer—get the fan or choke repaired
4.	Timer not working	Need to change	Call engineer

Key Points to Remember

- *Check for working:* Connect to mains and switch on the unit and check that all tubes/lamps are working.
- Cover eyes with an eye shield.
- Place baby naked only with the nappy to cover genitalia.
- Place baby as close as possible to light source avoiding hyperthermia.
- Check temperature every 4 hourly to monitor for hypo/hyperthermia.
- Check weight daily.
- Measure serum bilirubin as clinically indicated.
- Low birth weight babies can have their socks, caps and mittens on while under phototherapy for preventing hypothermia.
- Ideally, a fluxmeter should be used to check for and ensure optimal irradiance.
- *Causes of ineffective phototherapy:*
  - Baby covered or frequently removed from phototherapy.
  - Low irradiance (tubes old, flickering, black ends, and bulbs covered with dust or reflectors dirty).
  - Distance between phototherapy lights and baby is more than recommended.
  - Hemolytic conditions can cause bilirubin to rise (>0.5 mg/dL/h) in spite of phototherapy.
- *Side effects and dangers:*
  - Transient maculopapular rash on the trunk
  - Hyperthermia/hypothermia
  - Increased insensible water loss and dehydration
  - Loose stools
  - Bronzing of the skin in the presence of direct hyperbilirubinemia

OSCE/Checklist: Procedure—Managing the Baby Under Phototherapy			
Name of the participants: ____			
S. No.	*Performance steps*	*Yes*	*No*
1.	Switch on the phototherapy unit and check if all the LED/lamps are working		
2.	Undress the baby. Cover the external genitalia with a diaper		
3.	Cover the eyes with eye shades		
4.	Place the baby in the bassinet and lower the unit as close to the baby as possible (If using LED phototherapy)		
5.	Turn the baby to expose all the body surface		
6.	Encourage the mother to breast feed every two hours		
7.	Monitor temperature 4 hourly		
8.	Monitor urine output and weight daily		
9.	Monitor S. bilirubin—Clinical and TcB assessment may not be reliable under phototherapy		
	Total score		

◼ FURTHER READING

1. Facility Based Newborn Care (FBNC). Ministry of Health and Family Welfare (MoHFW); Government of India; 2022.
2. Rennie JM. Rennie & Roberton's Textbook of Neonatology, 5th edition. United Kingdom: Churchill Livingstone; 2012.

2.7 SUCTION EQUIPMENT

Anantika Garg, Boby Varghese

SUCTION MACHINE

About the Equipment

Parts:
- Suction tubing
- Suction bottles
- Pressure gauze

Types:
- Electrical
- Mechanical foot operated
- Wall suction

Working

Electrical:
- Connect to the mains
- Switch on the unit and occlude distal end with your thumb to check the suction pressure. Ensure it does not exceed 100 mm Hg.
- Use disposable suction catheters.
- Connect the desired size disposable suction catheter to suction tubing.
- Perform suction gently and intermittently.
- Switch off the suction machine.

Foot operated:
- Pedal to build the desired level of suction pressure.
- Connect the desired size disposable suction catheter to suction tubing.
- Perform suction gently and intermittently.
- Switch off the suction machine.

Wall suction:
- Turn knob to ON position.
- Check and adjust the pressure gauze.
- Connect the desired size disposable suction catheter to suction tubing.
- Perform suction gently and intermittently.
- Switch off the suction machine.

Cleaning and Disinfection

- Wash suction bottle and tubing's with soap and water daily.
- After cleaning soak, the tubing's and the bottle in 2% glutaraldehyde solution for 20 minutes daily.
- Take out from glutaraldehyde solution and wash under running water.
- Connect to the machine after placing disinfectant solution (3% phenol or 5% lysol) in the bottle.
- Flush the suction tubing by suctioning with clean water after each use.

Troubleshooting

Problem	Possible cause	Action
Machine not working	Check power supply, fuse and cord, plug, and socket	Ensure power supply change fuse, cord plug, or socket if needed
No suction pressure	Check for leakages in the bottle, tubing and manifold room for malfunctioning wall suction	• Replace tubes/bottles, ensure airtight connections • Rectify malfunctioning in manifold room

MUCUS EXTRACTOR

Steps of Mucous Extraction

Using mucous extractor:
- Remove the mucous extractor aseptically from its packet.
- During suction, the proximal portion is kept in the resuscitator's mouth.
- Use the distal end to clear secretions from mouths then nose.
- Keep the mucus extractor in upright position.
- The mucus trapped in the drip chamber.

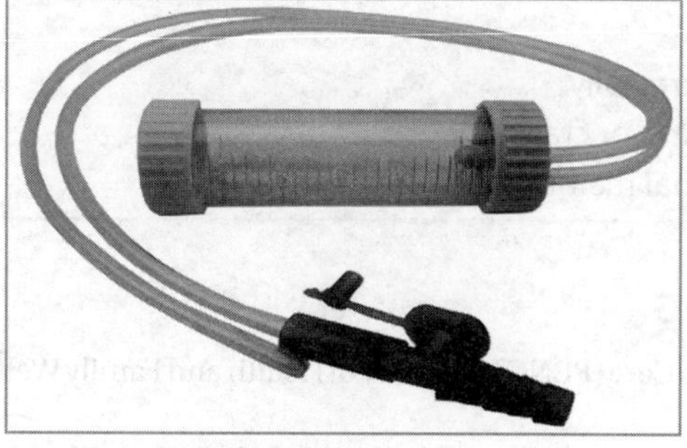

Using the bulb syringe:
- Squeeze the air out from the bulb, keep squeezing the bulb.
- Insert the tip of the squeezed bulb into one nostril gently and release.
- Repeat the same process if needed.
- If the mucus is too thick to suction, use saline to irrigate.

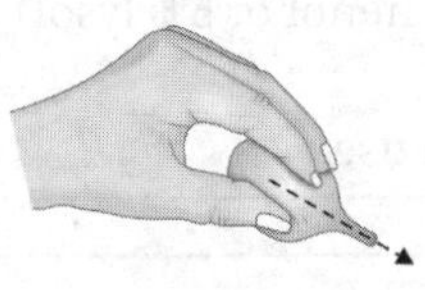

Squeeze the bulb

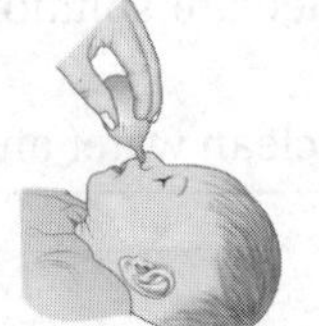

Place bulb in nostril

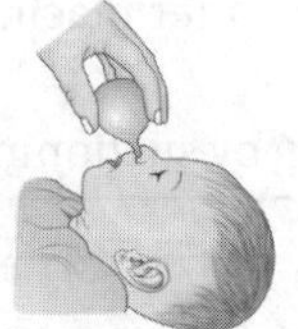

Mucus will be drawn
out of the nose

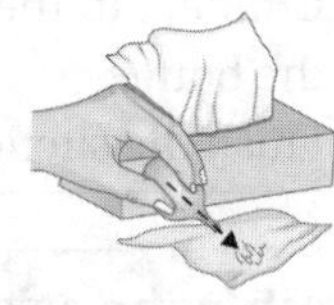

Squeeze the mucus
on to tissue

Key Points to Remember

- The first few minutes of an infant's life are critical to prevent birth asphyxia.
- As the initial steps of the resuscitation at birth, establish an open airway following the ABCs of resuscitation.
- By using bulb syringes, mucus traps, or electric suction, secretions are removed from the mouth and nose first.
- Suction gently and intermittently.
- Do not perform vigorous and deep suction.
- Use only disposable suction catheters and discard them after single use.
- Check adequacy of suction pressure prior to use.

Side effects and dangers of suctioning:
- Local trauma
- Bradycardia
- Apnea
- Infection
- Check suction pressure daily
- Change tubing for leaks or cracks
- Comprehensive/annual maintenance contract

■ FURTHER READING

1. Facility Based Newborn Care (FBNC). Ministry of Health and Family Welfare (MoHFW); Government of India; 2022.
2. Rennie JM. Rennie & Roberton's Textbook of Neonatology, 5th edition. United Kingdom: Churchill Livingstone; 2012.

2.8 SELF-INFLATING BAG

Arun Gautam

About the Equipment

- The self-inflating bag (SIB) remains inflates automatically without a compressed gas source, hence portable.
- Also known as AMBU—artificial manual breathing unit
- *Parts:*
  - Air inlet—air is drawn into the bag through a one-way valve during re-expansion after compression
  - Oxygen inlet—a small projection to which oxygen tubing can be attached when oxygen is needed.
  - Patient outlet—air exits from the bag to the infant and is where the mask or endotracheal tube connector can be attached.
  - Fish mouth valve—located at patient outlet, allowing one way movement of air from bag to patient and prevent exhaled air movement in to bag.
  - Reservoir port—attachment port provided for oxygen reservoir bag.
  - Pop off valve (pressure releasing valve)—safety measure to prevent excessive pressure. 30–40 cmH$_2$O is limit.
  - PEEP valve—additional attachment to provide PEEP.
- *Oxygen delivery:*
  - Only bag—21% oxygen
  - Bag with oxygen, no reservoir—40–50%
  - Bag with oxygen and reservoir bag—90–95%.

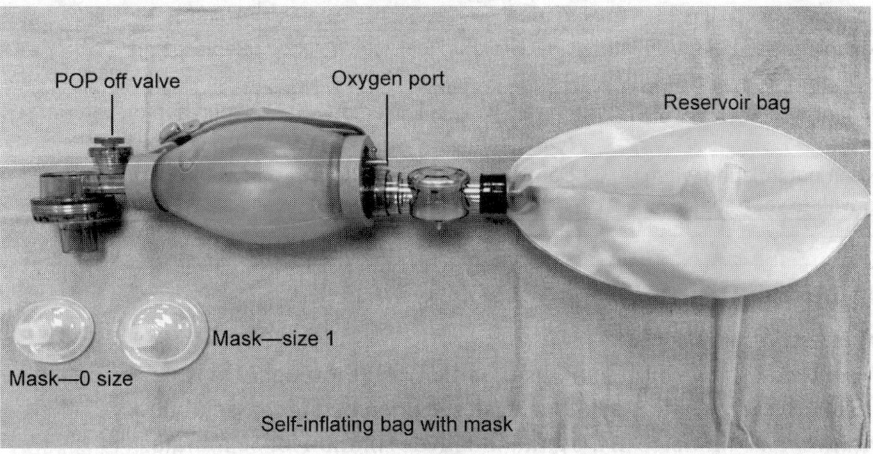

Self-inflating bag with mask

Indication

To provide positive pressure ventilation with mask or endotracheal tube.

Contraindication

Congenital diaphragmatic hernia.

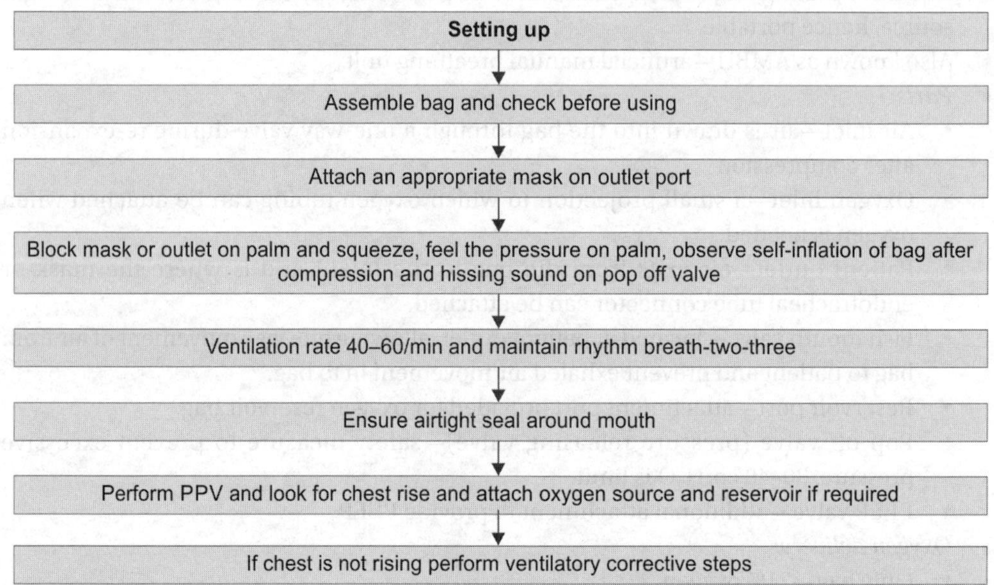

Troubleshooting

Problem	Reason	Action
Bag unable to self-inflate/deflate without pressure on squeezing	Check for bag leak (cut/hole in bag)	Replace bag
No hissing sound on pop off valve	Pop off valve is locked or nonworking	Open pop off valve or replace bag
Reservoir not inflating when using with oxygen source	Damaged reservoir bag	Replace reservoir bag

Cleaning and Disinfection

- *Disinfect daily and sterile weekly*
- *Decontamination*—disassemble all parts. Wash thoroughly in water using a detergent, rinse with clean water, and dry with sterile linen before reassembling.
- *Disinfection*—immerse in 2% glutaraldehyde solution for 30 minutes.
- *Sterilization*—immerse in 2% glutaraldehyde solution for 6 hours.
- After removing from glutaraldehyde rinse with clean water, dry with sterile cloth and reassemble.
- Clean mask with spirit between patient use.

> **Key Points to Remember**
>
> - Check bag prior to use.
> - Look for adequate chest rise.
> - Ensure proper seal around mouth.
> - Free flow oxygen cannot be delivered.
> - Do not place/leave it under radiant warmer.
> - PIP is controlled by how hard the bag is squeezed.
> - PEEP may be administered if an additional valve is attached to the bag.

FURTHER READING

1. Facility Based Newborn Care (FBNC). Ministry of Health and Family Welfare (MoHFW); Government of India; 2022.
2. Rennie JM. Rennie & Roberton's Textbook of Neonatology, 5th edition. United Kingdom: Churchill Livingstone; 2012.

2.9 T-PIECE RESUSCITATORS

Swati Upadhyay

About the Equipment

- T-piece resuscitator is a device which can be used to deliver peak inspiratory pressure (PIP), positive end-expiratory pressure (PEEP) as well as free-flow oxygen during neonatal resuscitation.
- It is easy to use and delivers more accurate and consistent PIP and PEEP than other PPV devices, resulting in more stable tidal volume delivery.

Parts

There are nine parts of a T-piece resuscitator. The position and function of control dials on the T-piece resuscitator can vary by manufacturer.

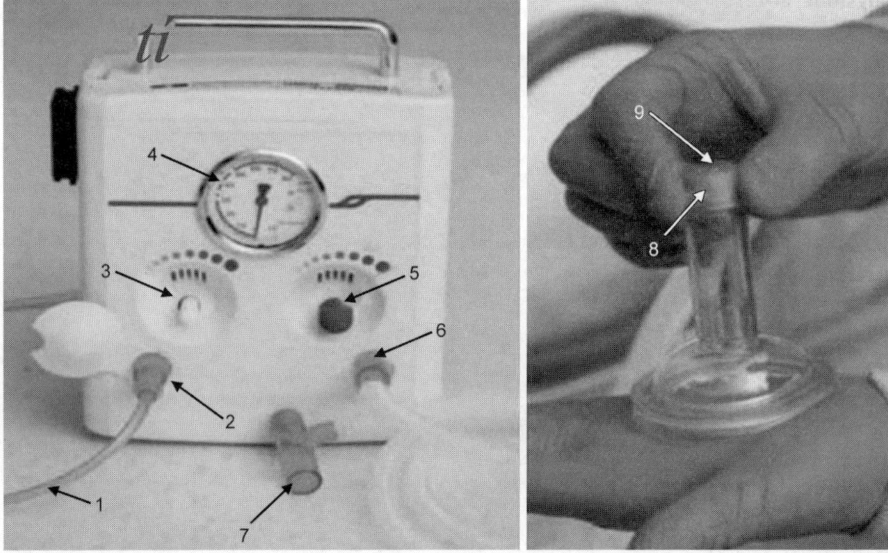

Parts of a T-piece resuscitator—1. Gas tubing, 2. Gas inlet, 3. Maximum pressure-relief control, 4. Manometer, 5. Inflation pressure control, 6. Gas outlet (proximal), 7. T-piece gas outlet (patient), 8. T-piece PEEP adjustment dial, and 9. Opening on T-piece cap.

Mechanism of Working

- Gas from a compressed source enters the T-piece resuscitator through gas tubing at the gas inlet.
- Gas exits the control box from the gas outlet (proximal) and travels through corrugated tubing to the T-piece gas outlet (patient), where a face mask, laryngeal mask, or endotracheal tube attaches.
- When the opening on the T-piece cap is occluded by the operator, the preset peak inflation pressure is delivered to the patient for as long as the T-piece opening is occluded.
- PEEP is adjusted using a dial on the T-piece cap.

| **Setting up a T-piece resuscitator** |
| Assemble the parts of the T-piece resuscitator as instructed by the manufacturer |
| Occlude the patient outlet (using a test lung, outlet-occluding cap, or palm) |
| Connect the device to the compressed gas source using gas tubing. Adjust the pressure settings as follows |
| Adjust the gas flow rate to 10–15 L/min |
| Set the desired peak inspiratory pressure (PIP) by occluding the T-piece cap with your finger (20–25 cmH$_2$O) **(Fig. 1)** |
| Set the PEEP, adjusting the dial on the cap to the desired setting (5 cmH$_2$O) **(Fig. 2)** |
| Apply mask or endotracheal tube to adapter to T-piece gas outlet |
| Administer a breath by alternately covering and releasing the opening on the T-piece cap |
| The *inflation time* is controlled by how long your finger covers the opening |
| The *ventilation rate* is determined by how often you occlude the opening on the cap |
| The concentration of oxygen delivered by the T-piece resuscitator is controlled by the oxygen blender |

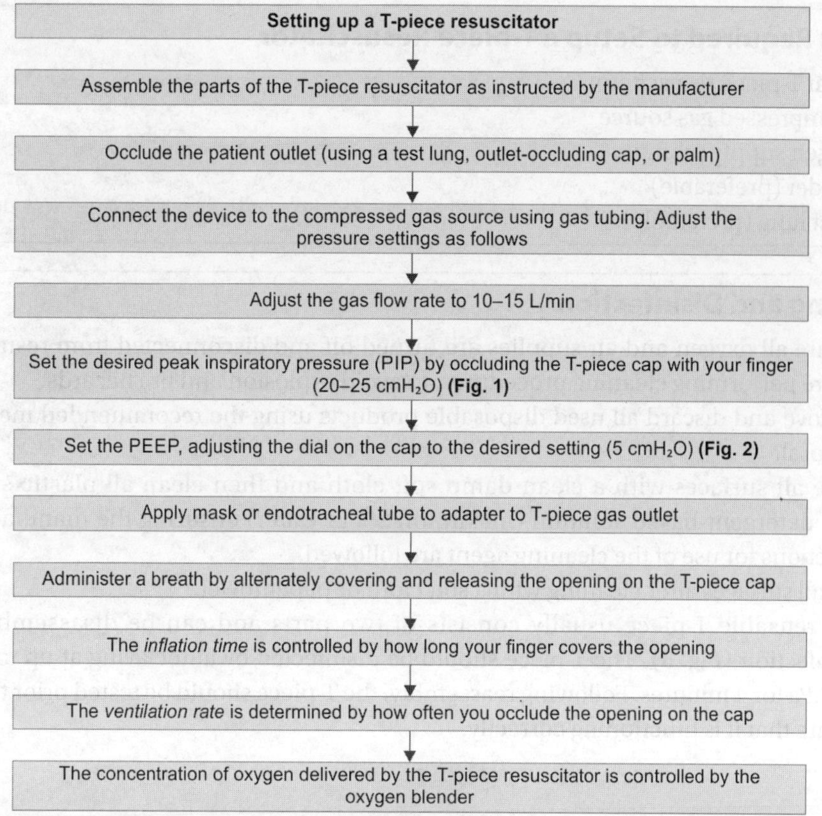

Fig. 1: Adjusting PIP.

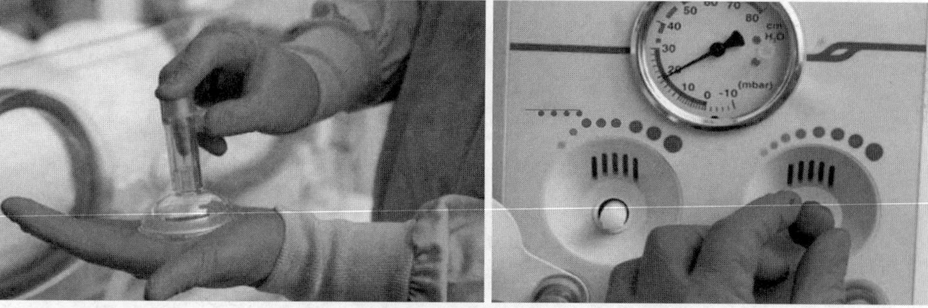

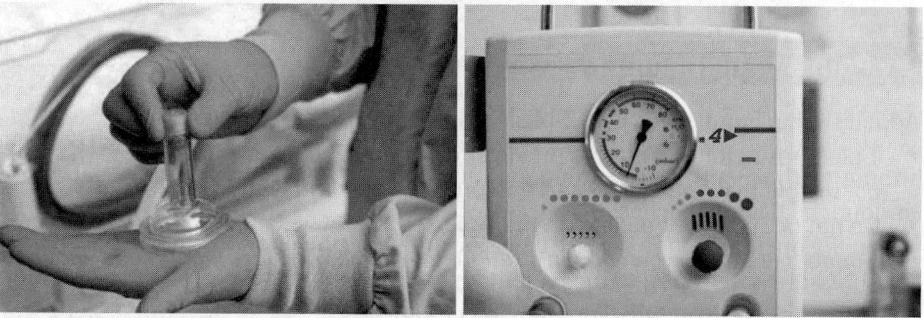

Fig. 2: Adjusting PEEP.

Things Required to Setup a T-piece Resuscitator

- Infant T-piece resuscitator
- A compressed gas source
- Oxygen supply tubing
- Blender (preferable)
- A test lung (preferable).

Cleaning and Disinfection

- Ensure all oxygen and air supplies are turned off and disconnected from resuscitator before performing cleaning procedures, to avoid explosion and fire hazards.
- Remove and discard all used disposable products using the recommended method of disposal.
- Wipe all surfaces with a clean damp soft cloth and then clean all plastic surfaces with detergent-based solution (maximum 2% in water) ensuring the manufacturer's directions for use of the cleaning agent are followed.
- Dry all surfaces after cleaning with a soft cloth or paper towel.
- The reusable T-piece usually consists of two parts and can be disassembled for disinfection **(Fig. 3)**. The T-piece should be disinfected by autoclaving at up to 136°C, 220 kPa for 4 minutes. Following reassembly, the T-piece should be tested prior to use to ensure that it is functioning correctly.

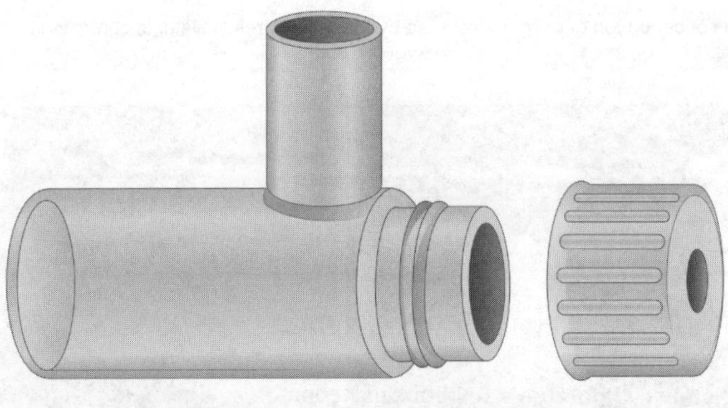

Fig. 3: Disassembling T-piece for disinfection.

Key Points to Remember

- Administering free-flow O_2 with T-piece resuscitator
  - T-piece resuscitator is used to provide free-flow O_2, hold the mask close to the face but *not so tight* that you make a seal and pressure builds up within the mask.
  - Do not occlude the opening on the T-piece cap.
  - *During free-flow oxygen administration, the T-piece pressure manometer should read zero.*

- Testing a T-piece resuscitator
  - Block the mask or T-piece gas outlet without occluding the opening on the T-piece cap. The manometer should display PEEP of 5 cmH$_2$O (or whatever is set).
  - Occlude the opening on the T-piece cap. The manometer should read peak pressure of 20–25 cmH$_2$O.
  - While using on a baby, look for following signs:
    - Listen for a soft whistle of gas through the PEEP cap.
    - Manometer readings should be according to set PIP and PEEP.
    - Increase in the heart rate >100/min if used for resuscitation.
    - A slight rise of the chest and upper abdomen with each inflation.
    - An improvement in oxygenation.
- *Troubleshooting when baby does not improve, or desired peak pressure not achieved:*
  - *Check the seal of mask:* Is the T-piece gas outlet sealed?
  - *Check the flow rate:* Is the gas flow set at 10 L/min?
  - Is the gas tubing connected to the gas inlet?
  - Is the gas outlet (proximal) disconnected?
  - Check if the maximum circuit pressure, PIP, or PEEP may be incorrectly set.
- Advantages and disadvantages of T-piece resuscitator.
  Advantages:
  - Provides consistent pressure
  - Reliable control of PIP and PEEP
  - No operator fatigue from bagging

  Disadvantages:
  - Always requires compressed gas supply for working.
  - Changing inflation pressures during resuscitation may be difficult.
  - 100% oxygen delivery may be harmful in preterm infants if blender is not available.

◼ FURTHER READING

1. Facility Based Newborn Care (FBNC). Ministry of Health and Family Welfare (MoHFW); Government of India; 2022.
2. Rennie JM. Rennie & Roberton's Textbook of Neonatology, 5th edition. United Kingdom: Churchill Livingstone; 2012.

2.10 LARYNGOSCOPE

Arun Gautam

About the Equipment

- It is used for endotracheal intubation.
- *Parts:*
  - Handle—(contains batteries)
  - Blade—straight (Miller), curved (Macintosh)
  - Neonates and infants—prefer straight blade
  - Sizes—00 (extreme preterm), 0 (preterm), 1 (term newborn).

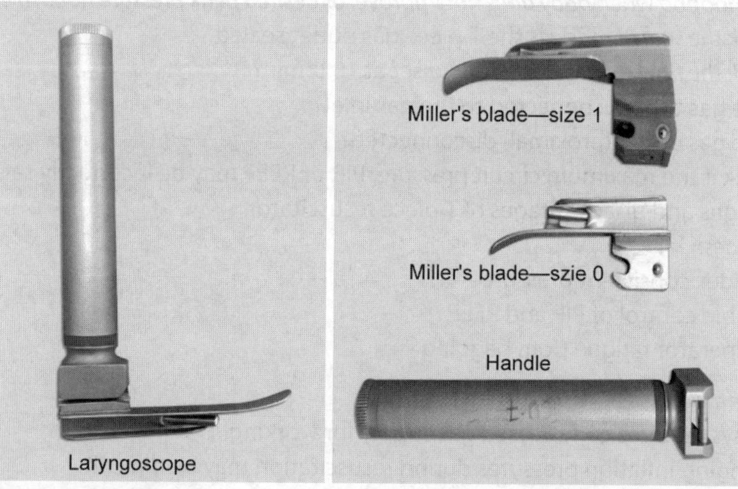

Indications

- *Therapeutic:*
  - Endotracheal intubation for invasive ventilation
  - Surfactant administration through ET or catheter
- Diagnostic
- Laryngeal inspection for edema or foreign body.

Contraindication

If cervical spinal injury is present then use of laryngoscope is contraindicated.

Setting up

↓

Always hold laryngoscope in left hand

↓

Put blade in hinge over handle and open in upward direction, blade will fix in handle with a click sound and bulb will light up

↓

Now laryngoscope is ready to use for intubation

Troubleshooting	
Problem	Action
Flickering of light in bulb	Check or replace bulb
No light in bulb	Check or replace battery, check bulb also

Disinfection

- Wash blade with running water and soap for visible soiling.
- Sterilization—ETO preferred. Boiling and autoclave can also be used but after removing bulb from blade.

■ FURTHER READING

1. Facility Based Newborn Care (FBNC). Ministry of Health and Family Welfare (MoHFW); Government of India; 2022.
2. Rennie JM. Rennie & Roberton's Textbook of Neonatology, 5th edition. United Kingdom: Churchill Livingstone; 2012.

2.11 OXYGEN CONCENTRATOR

Arun Gautam

About the Equipment

An oxygen concentrator is a self-contained, electrically powered medical device designed to concentrate oxygen from ambient air.

Types

- *Stationary:*
  - Weigh <27 kg
  - Can provide oxygen flow rates up to 10 litres per minute (LPM).
  - Generally used in health facilities.
- *Portable:*
  - Have lower output capacity (3 LPM or less)
  - Ideal for individual patients as ambulatory oxygen systems.
  - Pulsed-dose or intermittent flow allows oxygen delivery only during inspiration.
  - Pulse-dosed concentrator is not suitable for infants and young children may not generate enough negative pressure during inspiration to reliably trigger oxygen flow.

Indications

- As an alternative to oxygen cylinder or central oxygen distribution system in a small hospital
- For home-based therapy in patient with chronic lung disease (BPD).

Principles of Working

- Operate on *pressure swing adsorption* method.
- Produces up to 95.5% concentrated oxygen.
- *Components:* Compressor, solenoid valves, sieve beds, mixing tank (reservoir), and flow meter
- Zeolite preferentially adsorbs nitrogen gas (N_2) at high pressures.

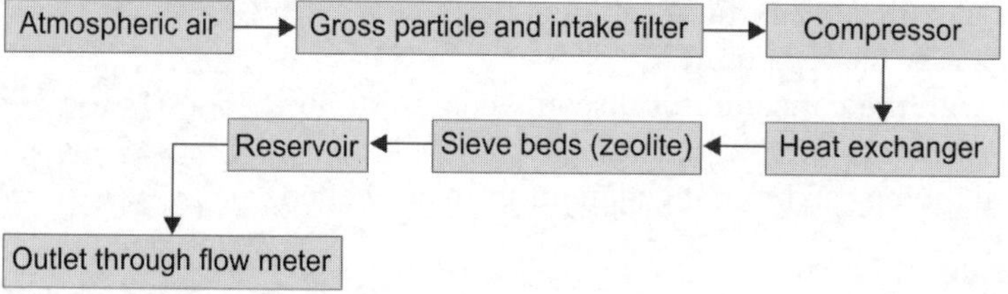

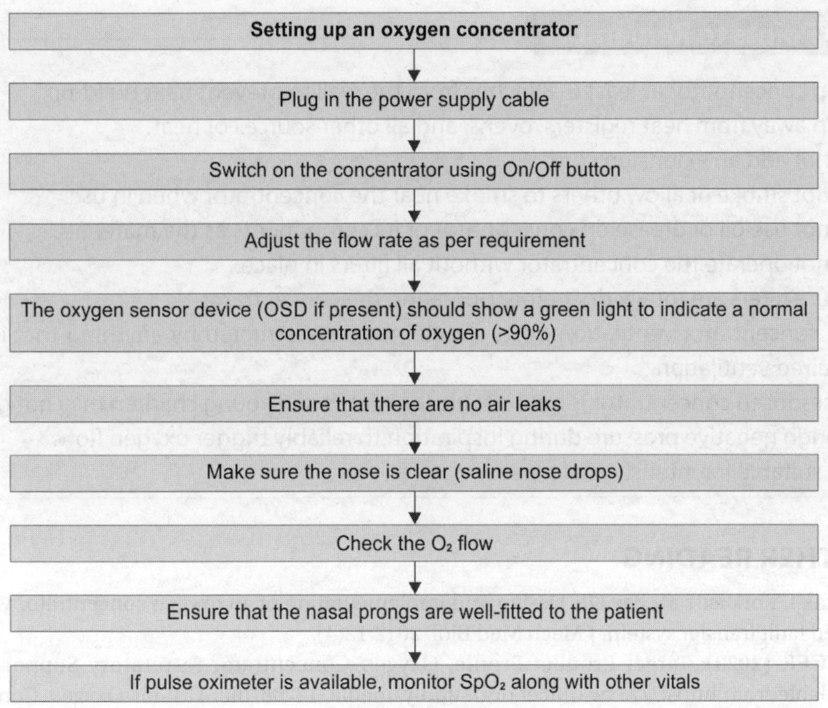

Troubleshooting	
Problem	*Action*
No power	Check power supply
No flow	Check for leaks
Machine is too noisy	Coarse filter may be blocked—was filter daily
Room/machine gets heated	Keep away from the walls to get free circulation of air
Yellow light is On	Flow rate is too high—decrease flow rate
Compressor gets heats up	Malfunctioning of compressor—call service center

Disinfection

- Routine preventive maintenance by medical supplier.
- Weekly, clean the concentrator cabinet filter(s) in a mild detergent solution.
- Weekly, change nasal cannulas.
- Monthly, with the concentrator disconnected from power source, wipe the outside of the concentrator cabinet with a damp cloth and mild detergent.
- Additional tubing can be changed monthly or as needed.

Maintenance

- *Coarse filter*—ensure it is dust free, wash daily
- *Zeolite granules*—change every 20,000 hours
- *Bacteria filter*—change every year

> ### Key Points to Remember
>
> - Keep concentrator at least 6–8 inches from the wall to prevent heat build-up.
> - Keep away from heat registers, ovens, and all other sources of heat.
> - Do not add an extension cord.
> - Do not smoke or allow others to smoke near the concentrator when in use.
> - Do not use oil or grease on concentrator or its components as the materials.
> - Do not operate the concentrator without all filters in place.
> - Ensure filters are totally dry before operating the concentrator.
> - The concentrator ventilation ports should not be obstructed by anything that impedes required ventilation.
> - Pulse-dosed concentrator is not suitable for infants and young children may not generate enough negative pressure during inspiration to reliably trigger oxygen flow.
> - Not suitable for intensive care areas.

◼ FURTHER READING

1. Atacak İ, Korkusuz M, Bay OF. Design and implementation of an oxygen concentrator with GPRS-based fault transfer system. J Mech Med Biol. 2012;12(4).
2. UNICEF. (2020). Target Product Profile, Oxygen Concentrator-respiratory Support. [online] Available from https://www.unicef.org/supply/media/12706/file/TPP-for-Oxygen-Concentrator-March-2020.pdf [Last accessed October, 2022].
3. WHO. (2015). Technical specifications for oxygen concentrators. [online] Available from https://apps.who.int/iris/handle/10665/199326 [Last accessed October, 2022].

2.12 USE OF NEBULIZER
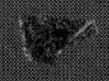

Neha Jain

Objective

One should be able to provide safe and effective nebulization use in neonates.

Indication

Nebulization and delivery for medication

Equipment and Supplies

- Two pairs of sterile gloves
- Nebulizing chamber and mouthpiece or mask
- Tubing to attach the gas inlet in the chamber to either an air or oxygen supply
- Oxygen hood
- Medications with appropriate dilution and quantity

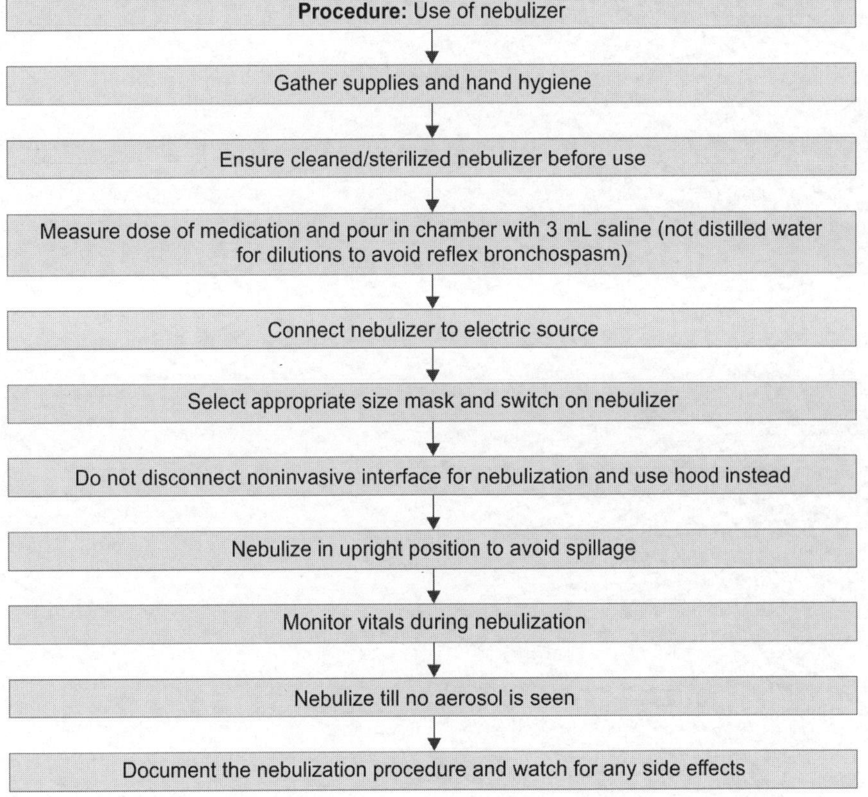

What else can be done?

- Ensure parts of nebulizer are clean before use.
- Use saline, not distilled water for dilutions to avoid reflex bronchospasm.
- Discard the residual solutions since it can get contaminated from environment.
- Monitor vitals and do clean the filter.

What is to be avoided?

- Chlorhexidine solutions to be avoided.
- Do not use chamber if it is discolored/stickiness/crack.
- Do not disconnect noninvasive interface for nebulization and use hood.

FURTHER READING

1. Facility Based Newborn Care (FBNC). Ministry of Health and Family Welfare (MoHFW); Government of India; 2022.
2. Rennie JM. Rennie & Roberton's Textbook of Neonatology, 5th edition. United Kingdom: Churchill Livingstone; 2012.

2.13 INFANTOMETER

Manish Diwedi

About the Equipment

- The stature or height of an individual is an inherent characteristic that defines as the measurement of an individual from head to foot, taking into consideration the standard landmarks.
- In scenarios of clinical significance ranging from estimating the body mass index (BMI) to diagnosing certain physical growth disorders and assessment of nutritional status.
- *Dimensions:* Length range from 0 to 1,000 mm.
- *Scale:* The graduation is given in mm/cm/inch.
- Foot piece that can be locked.

Indications

- The World Health Organization (WHO) standards for monitoring growth standards are used to analyze the physical growth and development of infants.
- It usually estimates the percentile and z-scores for length/height for age, weight for age, weight for length, weight for height, and BMI for age.
- The aforesaid parameters included in the growth chart are used to diagnose growth abnormalities, the nutritional needs of children and type of feeding.

Various Modes of Measurement

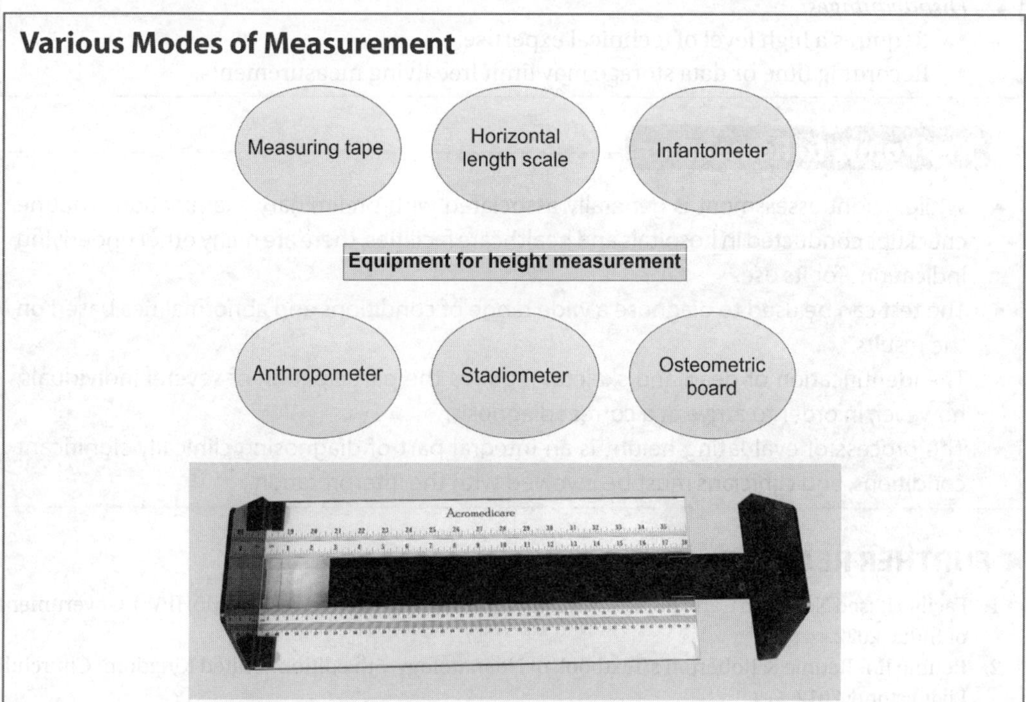

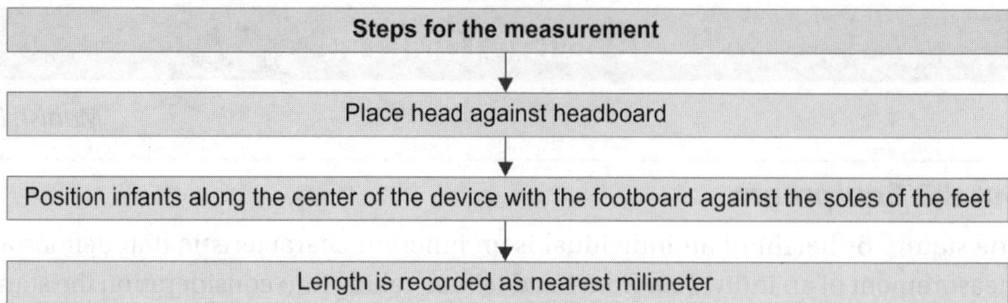

Clinical Significance

- Clinically, height is necessary for maintaining physical growth records. This is especially significant when it comes to monitoring the growth patterns of infants.
- Height assessment and the growth patterns linked to it, either directly or indirectly, point toward the socioeconomic status of an individual, amongst other things.
- Growth indicators such as the height of the individual and hence the BMI can help diagnose conditions such as marasmus and kwashiorkor in children.
- *Advantages:*
  - Frequently measuring an infant's length is crucial to determining growth velocity and ensuring infant is developing normally.
  - The technique would allow for frequent measurement of infant length and tracking of growth rate. Based on height and weight, BMI is calculated.
  - It measures the healthy weight compared with the unhealthy weight.
  - The results can also be used to monitor a child's growth.
- *Disadvantages:*
  - Requires a high level of technical expertise.
  - Recording time or data storage may limit free living measurements.

Key Points to Remember

- While height assessment is generally associated with preliminary examinations/routine checkups conducted in hospitals and healthcare facilities, there are many other underlying indications for its use.
- The test can be used to diagnose a wide range of conditions and abnormalities based on the results.
- The identification of dead and skeletal requires the participation of several individuals, however, in order to arrive at a correct diagnosis.
- The process of evaluating height is an integral part of diagnosing clinically significant conditions, and clinicians must be involved with the interpretation.

■ FURTHER READING

1. Facility Based Newborn Care (FBNC). Ministry of Health and Family Welfare (MoHFW); Government of India; 2022.
2. Rennie JM. Rennie & Roberton's Textbook of Neonatology, 5th edition. United Kingdom: Churchill Livingstone; 2012.

2.14 WEIGHING SCALE

Manish Diwedi

About the Equipment

- Scales are instruments that measure a material's weight (mass) accurately and precisely. The fact that they can measure as much as 50 kg as well as little as 10 µg makes them very common.
- Monitoring nutrition and fluid balance with a weight record are essential.
- For all neonatal units and delivery rooms that provide special care, an accurate weighing scale is a must.
- Very low birth weight (VLBW) babies must have their weight recorded throughout their lives. Neonatal mortality and morbidity are strongly influenced by weight at birth.
- *Unit of measurement:*
  The unit of weight is the *Newton,* the force with which gravity exerts on a kg mass.
  $$Weight = Mass \times Gravity\ constant$$
- A weight-sensitive device is attached below the baby pan in scales with a conventional spring balance and an electronic sensor in scales with an electronic balance.
- *Types of scale:*
  - Spring balance
  - Beam balance
  - Electronic weighing scale.

Indications

Weighing scales help in predicting the following points:
- All babies at birth
- All LBW babies on follow-up.
- Sick newborn once or twice a day
- VLBW (<1,500 g) babies once or twice daily to monitor fluid therapy.
- Measuring urine output by preweighed napkins.

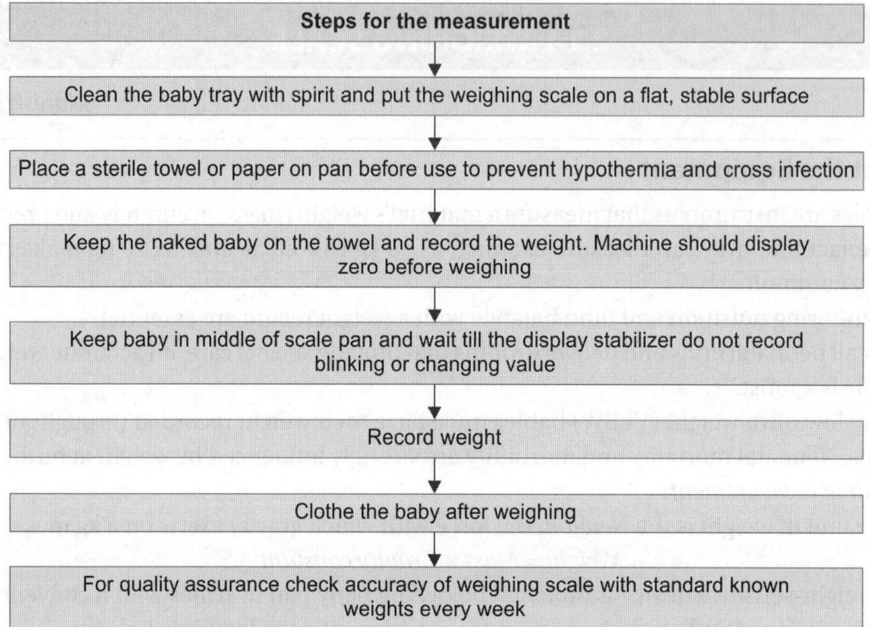

Cleaning and Disinfection

- Clean with soap and water daily.
- Wipe with sprit swab before each patient use.
- Calibration of the scales once weekly or as required.

Key Points to Remember

- Always look for ZERO and adjust zero error by pressing "TARE" key.
- Weigh the baby naked.
- Machine should be placed on flat surface when in use.
- Do not place anything on weighing pan when not in use.
- Calibration of the scales by using a known weight once weekly or as required.

■ FURTHER READING

1. Facility Based Newborn Care (FBNC). Ministry of Health and Family Welfare (MoHFW); Government of India; 2022.
2. Rennie JM. Rennie & Roberton's Textbook of Neonatology, 5th edition. United Kingdom: Churchill Livingstone; 2012.

2.15 OXYGEN TUBE

Boby Varghese

About the Equipment

- Oxygen tube is connecting device to supply oxygen from source to delivery device at patient end.
- Ends are fitted with soft funnel shaped connectors for easy attachments to ports.
- Usually come as accessory in oxygen mask, self-inflating bag, or nebulizer mask.

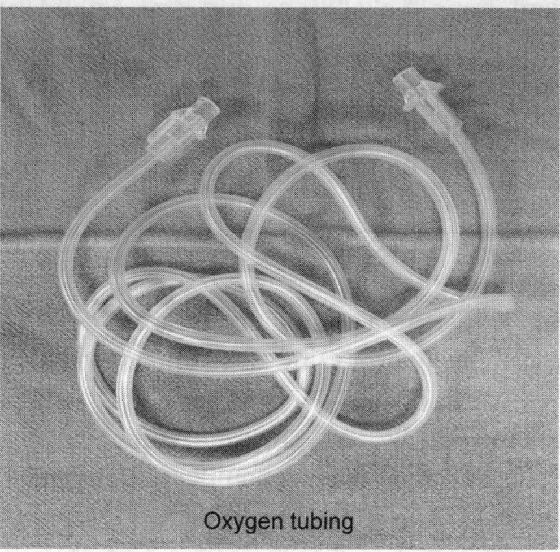

Oxygen tubing

Indications

- It can be used in both high-flow (oxygen hood) and low-flow oxygen devices (oxygen mask).
- As part in nebulizer mask

Troubleshooting

If oxygen flow is not there at delivery end, look for any leak/damage in tube.

Cleaning and Disinfection

- **Disinfection:** Immerse in 2% glutaraldehyde solution for 30 minutes.
- **Sterilization:** Immerse in 2% glutaraldehyde solution for 6 hours.
- Rinse with clean water, dry with sterile cloth after removing from glutaraldehyde solution.

2.16 MICRODRIP SET

Jubilant James

About the Equipment

- It is used for delivering small amounts of intravenous solutions in pediatric patients at specific flow rate.
- The rate of flow (drops per minute) is controlled by dial attached on tube.
- 1 macro drop = 4 micro drop
- 1 mL of fluid = 60 micro drops (No. of drops/min = mL of fluid/h)
- *Parts:*
  - *Volume chamber:* Available in 110 or 150 mL. Measured graduation on wall for accurate measurement of fluid.
  - *Chamber vent:* Allows air to enter chamber and prevent vacuum inside and maintain continuous flow out of chamber.
- *Inlet tube with spike and thumb lock:* Required amount of fluid filled in chamber from a larger fluid bottle/bag through inlet tube.
  - *Murphy's chamber:* Transit area between volume chamber and outlet tube. It allows holding area and visibility of drops flow rate. A fluid level must be maintained in this chamber.
  - *Regulator:* Control flow rate by adjusting tube diameter.
  - *Outlet tube:* Connecting part between chamber to fluid recipient.

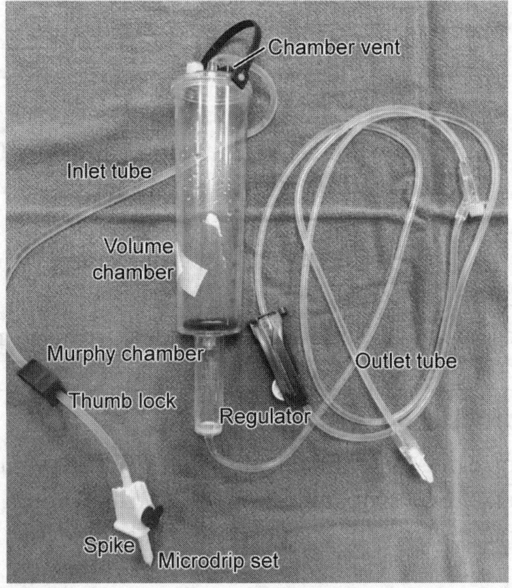

Indications

- Intravenous fluid administration
- Drug administration
- Parenteral nutrition
- Measured fluid in peritoneal dialysis in infants

Disinfection

Discard after 24 hours of use on a single patient.

◼ FURTHER READING

1. Facility Based Newborn Care (FBNC). Ministry of Health and Family Welfare (MoHFW); Government of India; 2022.
2. Rennie JM. Rennie & Roberton's Textbook of Neonatology, 5th edition. United Kingdom: Churchill Livingstone; 2012.

Medication

Richa Malik

COMMON NEONATAL MEDICATIONS IN DAY-TO-DAY PRACTICE

Acetaminophen

Indications	Dosing and administration	Adverse effects
• Closure of PDA in preterm infants • Fever reduction • Treatment of mild to moderate pain	• 10–15 mg/kg/dose IV over 15 minutes or orally 6–8 hourly • *Rectal dose:* 30 mg/kg rectally, then 12–18 mg/kg/dose 6–8 hourly or as needed	• Injection site events • Vomiting • Hepatotoxicity occurs with excessive dose

Acetylcysteine

Indications	Dosing and administration	Adverse effects
Antidote for acetaminophen overdose to prevent hepatic injury	• *Oral-loading dose:* 140 mg/kg, maintenance dose: 70 mg/kg orally every 4 hours for 17 doses starting 4 hours after loading dose • *IV-loading dose:* 150 mg/kg for those weighing >5 kg administered over 1 hour, maintenance dose: 50 mg/kg orally for two doses	Hypernatremia

Acyclovir

Indications	Dosing and administration	Adverse effects
• Treatment of neonatal HSV infection, known or suspected, also its chronic suppressive therapy • *Varicella-zoster* virus infection with CNS and pulmonary involvement	• For herpes simplex virus infection: 20 mg/kg/dose every 8 hours as IV infusion over 1 hour • Treat skin, eye, mouth disease for 14 days; CNS or disseminated infection for 21 days • *For chronic suppression:* 300 mg/m^2/dose orally three times a day when disease is severe and recurrent • For *Varicella-zoster* virus infection: 10–15 mg/kg/dose IV every 8 hours	• Nausea, vomiting • Rash • Cardiovascular events: Hypotension • Elevated hepatic transaminases • Leukopenia, thrombocytopenia • Phlebitis at injection site

Adenosine

Indications	Dosing and administration	Adverse effects
Acute treatment of sustained paroxysmal supraventricular tachycardia (PSVT)	• *Starting dose:* 50 µg/kg rapid IV push over 1–2 seconds into a vein as close to heart as possible followed by rapid saline flush of 5–10 mL after each bolus • Increase the dose by 50 µg/kg every 2 minutes until return of sinus rhythm • *Maximum dose:* 250 µg/kg	• Flushing, dyspnea, irritability • Transient arrhythmia • Recurrence of PSVT

Adrenaline

Indications	Dosing and administration	Adverse effects
• Neonatal resuscitation • Fluid refractory shock	• *Resuscitation:* 1:10,000 solution—IV rapid push 0.1–0.3 mL/kg, ET 0.5–1 mL/kg • *Continuous IV infusion:* 0.01–0.1 µg/kg/min, maximum recommended dose: 1 µg/kg/min • *Nebulization:* 1:1,000 solution, 0.5 mL/kg + 2–3 mL NS	• Tachycardia, arrhythmia • Hypertension • Injection site events—pallor, gangrene • Hypokalemia, lactic acidosis

Albumin (Human)

Indications	Dosing and administration	Adverse effects
• Cardiopulmonary bypass • Hemolytic disease of newborn • Hypotension • Septic shock • Nephrotic syndrome	0.5–1 g/kg of 25% albumin given IV over 1 hour (for hemolytic disease) or over 20–30 minutes (for hypotension)	• Flushing, urticaria, fever, chills, vomiting, tachycardia, hypotension • Lid edema

Alprostadil

Indications	Dosing and administration	Adverse effects
To promote dilatation of ductus arteriosus in cases of duct dependent congenital heart	• *Initial dose:* 0.05–0.1 µg/kg/min as continuous IV infusion via a large vein. Titrate to infant's oxygenation • *Maintenance dose:* As low as 0.01 µg/kg/min	• Apnea, hypotension • Fever, leukocytosis, flushing, bradycardia • Hypokalemia, reversible cortical proliferation of long bones, gastric outlet obstruction with long-term therapy

Amikacin

Indications	Dosing and administration	Adverse effects
• Infections caused by gram-negative bacilli that are resistant to other aminoglycosides • Generally used in combination with a beta-lactam antibiotic for neonatal sepsis	• Based on postnatal age: Postmenstrual (*see* Table below) • Amikacin is administered as IV infusion over 20–30 minutes in neonates	• Transient and reversible renal tubular dysfunction • Vestibular and auditory ototoxicity • Neuromuscular weakness when used with neuromuscular blocking agents/in patients with hypermagnesemia • *C. difficile*-associated diarrhea

Postmenstrual age (PMA)	Postnatal age	Dosage (mg/kg/dose)	Frequency
29 weeks or less	• 0–7 days • 8–28 days • 29 days or older	• 14 • 12 • 12	• Every 48 hours • Every 36 hours • Every 24 hours
30–34 weeks	• 0–7 days • 8 days or older	• 12 • 12	• Every 36 hours • Every 24 hours
35 weeks or more	• All	• 12	• Every 24 hours

Hughes, 2017

Aminophylline

Indications	Dosing and administration	Adverse effects
• Treatment of neonatal apnea including postextubation, postanesthesia • As bronchodilator	• *Loading dose:* 8 mg/kg IV infusion over 20–30 minutes or orally • *Maintenance dose:* 1.5–3 mg/kg/dose IV or oral every 8–12 hourly (start 8–12 hours after loading dose)	• GI irritation • Hyperglycemia • CNS irritability • *Signs of toxicity:* Tachycardia, vomiting, jitteriness, failure to gain weight, seizures, hyperreflexia

Amiodarone

Indications	Dosing and administration	Adverse effects
Treatment of drug-resistant SVT, ventricular tachyarrhythmia, junctional ectopic tachycardia	• *Loading dose:* 5 mg/kg IV infusion over 20–60 minutes preferably in a central vein • *Maintenance dose:* 7–15 µg/kg/min IV infusion. Switch to oral therapy within 24–48 hours • *Oral dose:* 5–10 mg/kg/dose every 12 hours	• Bradycardia, hypotension • AV block • Cardiac failure • *Long-term toxicity:* Hyper or hypothyroidism, hepatitis

Amphotericin B deoxycholate (conventional)

Indications	Dosing and administration	Adverse effects
Treatment of systemic fungal infection and severe superficial mycoses	• 1–1.5 mg/kg every 24 hours as IV infusion over 2 hours. *Do not mix with saline solution as precipitation will occur* • Duration of therapy for candidemia is 2 weeks after documented clearance of Candida from bloodstream • For CNS infections, continue until all signs and CSF abnormalities resolved	• *Hypokalemia:* More common with amphotericin liposome • *Infusion-related reactions:* Rash, fever, chills, tachycardia—more common in pediatric patients, not seen in infants <90 days • Pain at injection site with/without phlebitis • Renal function abnormalities

Amphotericin B lipid complex

Indications	Dosing and administration	Adverse effects
Treatment of systemic fungal infection resistant to conventional amphotericin B or in patients with renal or hepatic dysfunction	• 2.5–5 mg/kg/dose every 24 hours as IV infusion over 2–6 hours • Do not mix it with saline solution as precipitation will occur	• Anemia, thrombocytopenia • Hypokalemia • Nausea, vomiting • Fever/chills

Amphotericin B liposome

Indications	Dosing and administration	Adverse effects
Treatment of systemic fungal infection resistant to conventional amphotericin B or in patients with renal or hepatic dysfunction	• 2.5–7 mg/kg/dose every 24 hours as IV infusion over 60–120 minutes • Do not mix it with saline solution as precipitation will occur	• Safety not established in patients <1 month • Hypokalemia, chills, vomiting, hypertension are reported more than deoxycholate form • *Infusion-related reactions:* Reported less in pediatric patients • Hepatotoxicity • Nephrotoxicity more than deoxycholate form

Ampicillin

Indications	Dosing and administration	Adverse effects
• Broad spectrum antibiotic useful against gram-positive organisms (*Streptococcus* species, penicillin G susceptible staphylococci, *Listeria*) • Also gram-negative sepsis caused by *E. coli* • Addition of an aminoglycoside enhances its effectiveness	• *Usual dose:* 50 mg/kg/dose administered IV slowly over 3–5 minutes. For high doses (>1 g) administer over 10–15 minutes • Dosing interval depends on postnatal age and PMA (*see* Table below)	• Very large doses may cause CNS excitation or seizure activity • Moderate prolongation of bleeding time has been reported after three to four doses • Hypersensitivity reactions are rare in neonates

Dosing interval chart		
PMA (weeks)	**Postnatal age (days)**	**Interval (hours)**
29 or less	• 0–28 • >28	• 12 • 8
30–36	• 0–14 • >14	• 12 • 8
37–44	• 0–7 • >7	• 12 • 8
>44	All	• 6

Atropine

Indications	*Dosing and administration*	*Adverse effects*
Reversal of severe sinus bradycardia, prevention of bradycardia during endotracheal intubation	• *IV:* 0.01–0.03 mg/kg/dose over 1 minute or IM. Dose can be repeated every 10–15 minutes • *ET dose:* 0.01–0.03 mg/kg/dose followed by 1 mL NS	• Cardiac arrhythmia • Abdominal distension, esophageal reflux • Mydriasis, cycloplegia • Post-op respiratory acidosis

Azithromycin

Indications	*Dosing and administration*	*Adverse effects*
• Bordetella pertussis treatment and postexposure prophylaxis • Treatment of ophthalmia neonatorum caused by Chlamydia trachomatis	• 10 mg/kg/dose IV or oral every 24 hours for 5 days • Oral suspension can be given with or without feeding	• *GI symptoms:* Vomiting, diarrhea, feed intolerance, abdominal tenderness • Association with infantile hypertrophic pyloric stenosis (highest risk in infants exposed at 0–14 days of age)

Budesonide

Indications	*Dosing and administration*	*Adverse effects*
Prevention of chronic lung disease, recurrent wheezing	*Nebulization:* 0.25–0.5 mg + 3 mL NS every 12 hours	Risk of oral candidiasis, viral infection

Caffeine citrate

Indications	*Dosing and administration*	*Adverse effects*
• Treatment of apnea of prematurity • Prevention of BPD in extremely preterm neonates • Weaning from ventilator	• *Loading dose:* 20 mg/kg of caffeine citrate IV over 30 minutes or orally • *Maintenance dose:* 5–10 mg/kg/dose IV over 10–15 minutes or oral every 24 hours • High doses (40 mg/kg loading, 20 mg/kg/day maintenance dose) have been used in some trials	• Restlessness, vomiting • Tachycardia • Slow weight gain • Hyperglycemia

Calcium gluconate 10%

Indications	Dosing and administration	Adverse effects
Acute treatment of neonatal symptomatic hypocalcemia	• *Hypocalcemia:* 100–200 mg/kg/dose (1–2 mL/kg/dose) as IV infusion in 1:1 dilution over 10–30 minutes while monitoring heart rate • *Maintenance treatment:* 200–800 mg/kg/day (2–8 mL/kg/day), treat for 3–5 days	• Vasodilatation, hypotension, bradycardia, cardiac arrest with rapid infusion • Precipitation in infusion line and crystalline deposits in lungs and kidney reported if coadministered with IV ceftriaxone • Thrombophlebitis at injection site

Calcium, oral

Indications	Dosing and administration	Adverse effects
• Nonacute hypocalcemia • Treatment of osteopenia of prematurity	• 150–220 mg/kg/day orally for preterm neonates • Calcium gluconate 10% IV formulation can be given orally as 2–8 mL/kg/day	• Gastric irritation • Diarrhea

Caspofungin

Indications	Dosing and administration	Adverse effects
• Treatment of refractory candidemia, intra-abdominal abscess, peritonitis, pleural space infections • Refractory invasive aspergillosis and those intolerant to amphotericin B	• 25 mg/m^2/ dose every 24 hours as IV infusion over 60 minutes • Do not dilute in dextrose containing solutions • Duration of therapy for candidemia without metastatic complications, is 2 weeks after documented clearance of Candida from bloodstream and resolution of symptoms	• Thrombophlebitis • Hypercalcemia, hypokalemia • Elevated liver enzymes • Isolated direct hyperbilirubinemia

Cefotaxime

Indications	Dosing and administration	Adverse effects
• Neonatal sepsis, lower respiratory tract infections, UTI, skin infection, intra-abdominal or bone and joint infections caused by susceptible gram-negative organisms (e.g., *E. coli, H. influenzae, Klebsiella*) • Empirical agent for treatment of neonatal meningitis. Reassess therapy based on culture-sensitivity results	• Dosing based on postnatal age and PMA (*see* Table below) • *Meningitis:* 0–7 days of age 100–150 mg/kg/day IV divided every 8–12 hours. *8 days or older:* 150–200 mg/kg/day IV divided every 6–8 hours • Administered as slow IV push over 3–5 minutes or intermittent IV infusion over 10–30 minutes or by IM injection	• *Rarely:* Rash, phlebitis, leukopenia, granulocytopenia, eosiophilia, diarrhea • C. difficile-associated diarrhea • Drug-resistant bacteria may develop if used in the absence of bacterial infection • Early use in ELBW neonates associated with high risk of candidiasis

PMA (weeks)	Postnatal age (days)	Dosage (mg/kg/dose)	Frequency
All weeks	<7	50	Every 12 hours
<32	7 or older	50	Every 8 hours
32 or more	7 or older	50	Every 6 hours
Leroux, 2016			

Ceftazidime

Indications	Dosing and administration	Adverse effects
• Neonatal sepsis and meningitis caused by susceptible gram-negative organisms (e.g., *P. aeruginosa*, *E. coli*, *H. influenzae*, *Neisseria*, *Klebsiella*, and *Proteus* species) • Empirical agent for treatment of neonatal meningitis. Reassess therapy based on culture and sensitivity results	• 30 mg/kg/dose administered as IV infusion over 30 minutes or deep IM injection or less serious infections • Dosing interval depends on postnatal age and PMA (*see* Table below) • *Meningitis:* 0–7 days of age 100–150 mg/kg/day IV divided every 8–12 hours • *8 days or older:* 150 mg/kg/day IV divided every 8 hours	• *Rarely:* Rash, diarrhea, elevated hepatic enzymes, eosinophilia, positive Coombs test • Early use in ELBW neonates associated with high risk of candidiasis (prospective cohort study)

Dosing interval chart		
PMA (weeks)	**Postnatal age (days)**	**Interval (hours)**
29 or less	• 0–28 • >28	• 12 • 8
30–36	• 0–14 • >14	• 12 • 8
37–44	• 0–7 • >7	• 12 • 8
>44	All	• 8

Ceftriaxone

Indications	Dosing and administration	Adverse effects
• Neonatal sepsis and meningitis caused by susceptible gram-negative organisms (e.g., *E. coli*, *H. influenzae*, *Pseudomonas*, *Klebsiella*) • It is contraindicated due to high risk of kernicterus in neonates	• *Sepsis:* 50 mg/kg/dose IV every 24 hours administered as IV infusion over 60 minutes • Do not mix with calcium containing solutions in the same IV line due to risk of precipitation • *Meningitis:* 100 mg/kg/day IV loading dose, then 80 mg/kg IV every 24 hours	• Hypersensitivity reactions • Methemoglobinemia • Hemolytic anemia • Prothrombin time alteration in patients with low vitamin K stores • Eosinophilia, thrombocytosis, leukopenia • *C. difficile*-associated diarrhea • Raised BUN and serum creatinine • Elevated liver enzymes

Chloramphenicol

Indications	Dosing and administration	Adverse effects
• Wide spectrum bacteriostatic agent • May be bactericidal to *H. influenzae* and *Neisseria meningitidis*	• 0–7 days age, <2 kg–25 mg/kg/day every 24 hours as intermittent IV infusion over 15–60 minutes • 8–28 days age, >2 kg–12.5 mg/kg/dose every 6 hours or 25 mg/kg/dose IV every 12 hours	• Reversible bone marrow suppression • Irreversible aplastic anemia • Gray-baby syndrome • Fungal overgrowth

Ciprofloxacin

Indications	Dosing and administration	Adverse effects
Wide spectrum bactericidal agent for treating systemic infection and meningitis caused by multiple resistant organisms	• *0–28 days age:* 10 mg/kg/dose every 12 hours as IV infusion over 30–60 minutes • Higher dose 20 mg/kg/dose for treating *Pseudomonas* infection • *>28 days age:* 10 mg/kg/dose every 8 hours as IV infusion	• More frequent in pediatric age group than neonates • Abnormal liver function test • Change in WBC counts • Nausea, vomiting • Osteoarticular problems, joint deformities, growth impairment are not reported on long-term follow-up of preterm or term infants treated with this drug

Clindamycin

Indications	Dosing and administration	Adverse effects
• Bacteriostatic agent for treatment of systemic infection, pulmonary and deep tissue infections caused by anaerobic bacteria and few gram-positive cocci • Not to be used in treating meningitis due to poor CSF penetration	• 5–7.5 mg/kg/dose as IV infusion over 60 minutes or orally • Dosing interval depends on postnatal age and PMA (*see* Table below)	• Hypersensitivity reactions • Jaundice and abnormal liver function test • Concomitant use with oral or topical erythromycin is contraindicated

Dosing interval chart		
PMA (weeks)	**Postnatal age (days)**	**Interval (hours)**
29 or less	• 0–28 • >28	• 12 • 8
30–36	• 0–14 • >14	• 12 • 8
37–44	• 0–7 • >7	• 12 • 8
>44	All	• 6

Colistin

Indications	Dosing and administration	Adverse effects
Used in combination with at least one other antibiotic for treating gram-negative multidrug-resistant infection, mostly *Acinetobacter baumannii* and *Klebsiella pneumoniae*	• 2.5–5 mg/kg/day or 50,000–75,000 IU/kg/day of colistin base IV or IM in two to four divided doses (1 million unit = 80 mg) • Administered as intermittent IV infusion over 5–30 minutes or by deep IM injection	• Gastrointestinal upset • Dizziness, slurred speech, tingling of extremities or tongue, rash, fever, urticaria • Respiratory distress, apnea • Nephrotoxicity

Co-trimoxazole (trimethoprim + sulfamethoxazole)

Indications	Dosing and administration	Adverse effects
• Despite the safety label warning for its use in neonates <2 months age, it is still used in home-based neonatal care in developing countries • Also used for prophylaxis of UTI in at risk patients	*TMP:* 4–6 mg/kg/dose IV over 60–90 minutes or orally every 12 hours	• Contraindicated in G6PD deficiency • Not recommended in infants at risk of jaundice • Bone marrow suppression • *Allergic reactions:* Fever, rash, nausea, vomiting • Megaloblastic anemia, methemoglobinemia • Hyperkalemia (cautious use with potassium sparing diuretics)

Dexamethasone

Indications	Dosing and administration	Adverse effects
• To facilitate extubation • To improve lung function in preterm neonates with risk of BPD	• *DART trial protocol:* 0.075 mg/kg/dose every 12 hours for 3 days, 0.05 mg/kg/dose every 12 hours for 3 days, 0.025 mg/kg/dose every 12 hours for 2 days, and 0.01 mg/kg/dose every 12 hours for 2 days; given as slow push IV or orally (total 10 days) • *Extubation protocol:* 0.25 mg/kg/dose every 8 hours for up to three doses. Commence 4 hours prior to extubation	• Routine use of dexamethasone is discouraged. If required for BPD risk reduction, start treatment only after 7 days • Increased risk of cerebral palsy if used in first week of life • Hypertension • Hyperglycemia, glycosuria • GI perforation and hemorrhage • Cardiac effects • Sodium and water retention • Hypokalemia, hypocalcemia, hypertriglyceridemia • Increased risk of sepsis • Osteopenia, inhibition of growth • Adrenal insufficiency secondary to pituitary suppression

Dextrose

Indications	Dosing and administration	Adverse effects
• To treat hypoglycemia • Hyperkalemia along with insulin • As nutritional supplement in PN solutions	• *Hypoglycemia:* 2 mL/kg of 10% D IV bolus followed by continuous IV infusion of 5–10% D • *Parenteral nutrition (PN):* Start at dextrose infusion rate of 6–8 mg/kg/min, advanced up to 10–12 mg/kg/min • *Hyperkalemia:* Continuous IV infusion of 0.5 g/kg/h dextrose along with insulin	• Excessive glucose can cause fat deposition, liver impairment, and steatosis • Impaired protein metabolism

Diazoxide

Indications	Dosing and administration	Adverse effects
• To treat hypoglycemia due to hyperinsulinemia • Concurrent treatment with thiazide diuretic is recommended to prevent fluid retention	• *Initial dose:* 10 mg/kg/day orally divided every 8 hours • *Maintenance dose:* 8–15 mg/kg/day orally divided every 8–12 hours	• Hirsutism, hypertrichosis • Fluid retention causing CHF • Hypotension, thrombocytopenia, leukopenia—rare

Dobutamine

Indications	Dosing and administration	Adverse effects
Hypotension and hypoperfusion related to myocardial dysfunction, septic shock	2–25 µg/kg/min as continuous IV infusion into a large vein	• May cause hypotension if patient is hypovolemic • Tachycardia, arrhythmia, hypertension • Cutaneous vasodilation • Tissue ischemia occurs with infiltration

Domperidone

Indications	Dosing and administration	Adverse effects
• Symptomatic management of GI motility disorders • Enhances gastric emptying and intestinal motility	0.25–0.3 mg/kg/dose orally every 6–8 hours	• Drowsiness, dry mouth, malaise • QT interval prolongation, sudden cardiac death • Extrapyramidal disorder

Dopamine

Indications	Dosing and administration	Adverse effects
• Hypotension • Severe sepsis and septic shock	2–20 µg/kg/min as continuous IV infusion into a large vein	• Tachycardia, arrhythmia • Increase in pulmonary artery pressure at high doses • Reversible suppression of prolactin and thyrotropin secretion

Erythromycin

Indications	Dosing and administration	Adverse effects
• Infection by chlamydia, mycoplasma, and ureaplasma • Gonococcal ophthalmia neonatarum prophylaxis • Feed intolerance due to dysmotility	• *Treatment of pneumonitis, conjunctivitis due to Chlamydia trachomatis:* 12.5 mg/kg/dose orally every 6 hours for 14 days • *Prokinetic:* 10 mg/kg/dose orally every 6 hours for 2 days followed by 4 mg/kg/dose orally every 6 hours for 5 days	• Hypertrophic pyloric stenosis • QT interval prolongation

Erythropoietin

Indications	Dosing and administration	Adverse effects
Prevention of blood transfusion in the treatment of anemia of prematurity in preterm <34 weeks	200–400 IU/kg/dose IV/SC three times a week	• Iron deficiency • Neutropenia • Thrombocytopenia, thrombocytosis

Fentanyl

Indications	Dosing and administration	Adverse effects
• For sedation and analgesia • Naloxone should be available to reverse adverse effects	• *Single/intermittent dose:* 0.5–3 µg/kg/dose slow IV push. Repeat as required (every 2–4 hours) • *Continuous infusion:* 1–5 µg/kg/h. Tolerance may develop rapidly with constant infusion	• Respiratory depression • Chest wall rigidity • Laryngospasm • Urinary retention • Withdrawal symptoms occur with continuous infusion for 5 days or longer

Flecainide

Indications	Dosing and administration	Adverse effects
• Treatment of supraventricular arrhythmias not responding to conventional therapy • Contraindicated in patients with structural heart defects	• Begin at 2 mg/kg/dose every 12 hours orally, maximum dose: 4 mg/kg/dose • Time to achieve optimal effect is 2–3 days • Correct preexisting hyper/hypokalemia if any	• *Newer arrhythmia:* AV block, bradycardia, ventricular tachycardia, torsade de pointes • Negative ionotropic effect • Dizziness, blurred vision

Fluconazole

Indications	Dosing and administration	Adverse effects
• Treatment of systemic fungal infection caused by Candida species and for prophylaxis of invasive candidiasis • Resistance reported with *C. glabrata* and *C. krusei*	• 12–25 mg/kg loading dose, then 12 mg/kg/dose as IV infusion over 60–120 minutes or orally • *Prophylaxis (for neonates <1 kg):* 3–6 mg/kg/dose twice weekly IV or oral for 6 weeks in NICU with high incidence rate of Candida infections • *Duration of therapy for candidemia:* 2 weeks after documented clearance of Candida from bloodstream and resolution of symptoms	• Vomiting, pain abdomen, diarrhea • Elevated liver enzymes • Conjugated hyperbilirubinemia in ELBW babies

Invasive candidiasis dosing interval chart

PMA (weeks)	Postnatal age (days)	Interval (hours)
29 or less	• 0–14 • >14	• 48 • 24
30 or older	• 0–7 • >7	• 48 • 24

Furosemide

Indications	Dosing and administration	Adverse effects
• Adjunct therapy for BPD • Heart failure	*Bolus dose:* 0.5–2 mg/kg/dose IV or orally every 24 hours (for premature infants), or 12 hourly (term neonates) or 6–8 hourly (infants >1 month)	• Hyponatremia • Ototoxicity • Nephrocalcinosis, nephrolithiasis • Hypercalciuria, bone demineralization

Ganciclovir

Indications	Dosing and administration	Adverse effects
Prevention of progressive hearing loss and lessening of developmental delay in babies with symptomatic congenital CMV infection involving CNS	• 6 mg/kg/dose IV every 12 hours over 1 hour • Treat for minimum 6 weeks. Reduce dose by half for neutropenia (<500 cells/mm^3) • *Chronic oral suppression:* 30–40 mg/kg/dose orally every 8 hours	• Significant neutropenia • Use with caution in cases with impaired renal function

Gentamicin

Indications	*Dosing and administration*	*Adverse effects*
• Infections caused by aerobic gram-negative bacilli • Usually used in combination with a beta-lactam antibiotic	• Based on postnatal age and PMA (*see* Table below) • Administered as IV infusion over 30–120 minutes • IM route has variable absorption	• Transient and reversible renal tubular dysfunction • Vestibular and auditory ototoxicity • Neuromuscular weakness may occur when used with neuromuscular blocking agents/in patients with hypermagnesemia

Postmenstrual age (PMA)	*Postnatal age*	*Dosage (mg/kg/dose)*	*Frequency*
29 weeks or less	• 0–7 days • 8–28 days • 29 days or older	• 5 • 4 • 4	• Every 48 hours • Every 36 hours • Every 24 hours
30–34 weeks	• 0–7 days • 8 days or older	• 4.5 • 4	• Every 36 hours • Every 24 hours
35 weeks or more	All	• 4	• Every 24 hours

Glucagon

Indications	*Dosing and administration*	*Adverse effects*
Treatment of hypoglycemia refractory to IV dextrose infusion, or in cases of documented glucagon deficiency	• *Refractory hypoglycemia:* 200 µg/kg/dose IV push, IM or subQ • *Continuous infusion:* Start with 10–20 µg/kg/h	• Tachycardia • Nausea, vomiting • Ileus • Hyponatremia, thrombocytopenia

Heparin

Indications	*Dosing and administration*	*Adverse effects*
• Maintenance of peripheral arterial and central venous catheter patency • Treating thrombosis	• To maintain patency of IV catheters: 0.5–1 IU/mL of IV fluid • *Thrombosis:* 75 IU/kg IV over 10 minutes followed by 28 IU/kg/h continuous infusion. Measure aPTT after 4 hours and adjust the dose. Treatment is limited to 10–14 days	• Contraindicated in case of intracranial or GI bleeding or thrombocytopenia ($<50,000/mm^3$) • Heparin-induced thrombocytopenia • *Long-term use:* Osteoporosis

Hydrochlorothiazide

Indications	*Dosing and administration*	*Adverse effects*
• BPD • Edema and hypertension • Pulmonary hypertension with right-sided heart failure	1–2 mg/kg/dose orally every 12 hours. Administer with food (improves absorption)	• Hypokalemia • Hyperglycemia • Hyperuricemia

Hydrocortisone

Indications	Dosing and administration	Adverse effects
• Prevention of BPD in ELBW neonates • Treatment of cortisol deficiency • Treatment of pressor-resistant hypotension • Adjunctive therapy for persistent hypoglycemia	1 mg/kg/dose IV over 30 seconds every 8 hours	• Hyperglycemia • Hypertension • Salt and water retention • Risk of GI perforation • Risk of disseminated *Candida* infection • Prolonged course associated with fine motor and language delay by 20 months corrected age

Ibuprofen

Indications	Dosing and administration	Adverse effects
Closure of PDA	• *Closure of patent ductus arteriosus (PDA):* 10 mg/kg orally or IV infusion over 15 minutes, followed by 5 mg/kg/dose at 24 and 48 hours • Two courses can be given	• GI bleeding • Spontaneous intestinal perforation • Acute kidney injury

Imipenem

Indications	Dosing and administration	Adverse effects
• Lower respiratory tract infections, intra-abdominal infections, skin and soft tissue infections, septicemia caused by susceptible drug-resistant organisms • Not recommended in meningitis as safety and efficacy have not been established	• *Body weight <2 kg:* 0–7 days—20 mg/kg/dose IV infusion over 20–30 minutes every 12 hours • *8 days or older:* 25 mg/kg/dose IV every 12 hours • *Body weight 2 kg or more:* <7 days—25 mg/kg/dose IV every 12 hours • *7 days or older:* 25 mg/kg/dose IV every 8 hours	• Seizures can occur in patients with meningitis, preexisting CNS pathology • Local reactions at injection site • Increased platelet count • Elevated liver transaminases

Indomethacin

Indications	Dosing and administration	Adverse effects
Closure of PDA	• Usually three IV doses per course (*see* Table below) • Give at 12–24 hour interval • IV dose is administered over 20–30 minutes • Two courses can be given • *Longer treatment course:* 0.2 mg/kg every 24 hours for total 5–7 days	• Hypoglycemia • Platelet dysfunction • Rapid infusion can cause reduction in organ blood flow • GI perforation, NEC • *Renal effects:* Oliguria, rise in serum creatinine

PDA closure dose (mg/kg)			
Age at first dose	*First dose*	*Second dose*	*Third dose*
<48 hours	0.2	0.1	0.1
2–7 days	0.2	0.2	0.2
>7 days	0.2	0.25	0.25

Insulin human regular

Indications	Dosing and administration	Adverse effects
• Hyperglycemia in critically ill neonates • Hyperkalemia	• *For hyperglycemia-intermittent dose:* 0.1–0.2 unit/kg subQ every 6–12 hours • *Continuous IV infusion:* 0.01–0.1 unit/kg/h • *For hyperkalemia:* Regular insulin 0.1–0.2 unit/kg along with 0.5 g/kg/h dextrose as continuous IV infusion • Saturate the plastic tubing binding sites by filling the IV tubing with insulin solution and wait for 20 minutes	• Hyperglycemia • Insulin resistance

Ipratropium bromide

Indications	Dosing and administration	Adverse effects
• Treatment of chronic obstructive pulmonary diseases • Acute bronchospasm	• Used as nebulization 0.25 mg + 3 mL NS every 6–8 hours • Optimal dose in neonates has yet to be determined	• Blurring of vision • Precipitation of narrow angle glaucoma

Iron—oral

Indications	Dosing and administration	Adverse effects
Treatment and prophylaxis of anemia of prematurity	2–3 mg/kg/dose orally every 12 hours	• Vomiting • Constipation

IVIG (human immune globulin)

Indications	Dosing and administration	Adverse effects
• Treatment of isoimmune hemolytic disease refractory to phototherapy • NAIT • Measles exposure	• 0.5–1 g/kg/dose IV over 4–5 hours, may repeat in 12 hours for isoimmune hemolytic disease • *For neonatal alloimmune thrombocytopenia (NAIT):* 1 g/kg/dose IV every day for two doses	• Transient tachycardia • Hypotension • Risk of NEC • Infusion reactions • Aseptic meningitis • Risk of infection—rare

Kayexelate (K bind)

Indications	Dosing and administration	Adverse effects
Correction of hyperkalemia	1–2 g/kg/dose per rectally every 4–6 hours	• Rectal pain • Constipation, diarrhea • Nausea, vomiting

Levetiracetam

Indications	Dosing and administration	Adverse effects
Treatment of seizures	• *Loading dose:* 20 g/kg IV over 15 minutes, maximum total loading dose up to 150 mg/kg • *Maintenance dose:* 20–65 mg/kg/day divided every 12 hours IV or orally	• Anaphylactic reactions • Behavioral disorders with long-term use

Levothyroxine

Indications	Dosing and administration	Adverse effects
Replacement therapy for congenital or acquired hypothyroidism (primary/secondary/tertiary)	*Initial dose:* 10–15 µg/kg/day orally. Begin at a lower starting dose and adjust the dose every 4–6 weeks based on clinical and laboratory response	Prolonged over treatment can cause premature craniosynostosis and acceleration of bone age

Lidocaine—antiarrhythmic

Indications	Dosing and administration	Adverse effects
Short-term control of ventricular arrhythmias and arrhythmia due to digitalis intoxication	• 0.5–1 mg/kg IV push over 5 minutes. Repeat every 10 minutes as necessary to control arrhythmia • *Maintenance IV infusion:* 10–50 µg/kg/min	• *CNS toxicity:* Drowsiness, agitation, vomiting, muscle twitching • Seizures, respiratory depression, apnea may occur • High dose can lead to cardiac toxicity

Linezolid

Indications	Dosing and administration	Adverse effects
• Infections caused by gram-positive organisms (methicillin resistant *S. aureus*, penicillin-resistant *Streptococcus pneumoniae*, vancomycin-resistant *Enterococcus faecium*) refractory to vancomycin and other antibiotics • Do not use as empirical therapy or for infections by gram-negative bacteria	• 10 mg/kg/dose every 8 hours as IV infusion over 30–120 minutes or orally • *Preterm neonates (<34 weeks) <1 week age:* 10 mg/kg/dose IV or orally every 12 hours	• Elevated liver transaminases • Diarrhea • Anemia, thrombocytopenia • *Severe cutaneous reactions:* Toxic epidermal necrolysis, Stevens-Johnson syndrome • Sideroblastic anemia

Magnesium sulfate

Indications	Dosing and administration	Adverse effects
• Treatment of torsades de pointes • Treatment and prevention of hypomagnesemia	• 25–50 mg/kg/dose rapid IV infusion over 10–20 minutes for torsades with pulses, over 30–60 minutes for hypomagnesemia • *Daily maintenance dose (parenteral nutrition):* 0.25–0.5 mEq/kg/day IV	• Flushing, sweating, hypothermia, stupor • Osteopenia or fractures may occur in developing fetus with prolonged use (5–7 days) in pregnant mothers for stopping preterm labor

Meropenem

Indications	Dosing and administration	Adverse effects
Serious/complicated infections caused by susceptible gram-negative organisms that are resistant to other antibiotics	• Based on postnatal age and PMA (*see* Table below) • *For meningitis:* 40 mg/kg/dose at age-specific dose interval • Administered as IV infusion over 30 minutes, prolonged infusion (over 4 hours) for resistant organisms may be more effective • Consider concomitant use of an aminoglycoside	• Diarrhea, vomiting • Rash • Inflammation at injection site • Use of carbapenems can result in development of cephalosporin resistance in many organisms • Increased risk of pseudo-membranous colitis and fungal infections

Postmenstrual age (PMA)	Postnatal age	Dosage (mg/kg/dose)	Frequency
<32 weeks	• <14 days • 14 days or older	• 20 • 20	• Every 12 hours • Every 8 hours
32 weeks or older	• <14 days • 14 days or older	• 20 • 30	• Every 8 hours • Every 8 hours

Metoclopramide

Indications	Dosing and administration	Adverse effects
• To facilitate gastric emptying and gastrointestinal motility • May improve feed intolerance	0.033–0.1 mg/kg/dose oral or IV over 10–15 minutes every 8 hours	Dystonic reactions and extrapyramidal symptoms seen at higher doses

Metronidazole

Indications	Dosing and administration	Adverse effects
Anerobic bacteremia and CNS infections caused by susceptible organisms	• Dosing based on PMA (*see* Table below) • *Surgical prophylaxis:* <1.2 kg—single dose of 7.5 mg/kg IV 60 minutes before incision. For 1.2 kg or more—single dose of 15 mg/kg IV 60 minutes before incision • Administered as IV infusion over 30–60 minutes	• *Gastrointestinal symptoms:* Nausea, vomiting, diarrhea, abdominal cramps • Hepatic impairment

PMA (weeks)	Loading dose IV or oral (mg/kg)	Maintenance dose IV or oral (mg/kg)	Interval
24–25	15	7.5	Every 24 hours
26–27	15	10	Every 24 hours
28–33	15	7.5	Every 12 hours
34–40	15	7.5	Every 8 hours
>40	15	7.5	Every 6 hours

Midazolam

Indications	Dosing and administration	Adverse effects
For anesthesia induction, sedation, refractory seizures	• *Sedation-IV:* 0.05–0.15 mg/kg over 10 minutes • *Continuous IV infusion:* 10–60 µg/kg/h, may be increased after few days due to tolerance • *Intranasal:* 0.2–0.3 mg/kg/dose • *Sublingual:* 0.2 mg/kg/dose mixed with a flavored syrup • *Anticonvulsant:* Load@ 0.15 mg/kg IV followed by maintenance infusion of 20–150 µg/kg/h	• Respiratory depression, hypotension • Seizure-like myoclonus • *Nasal route:* Burning sensation

Milrinone

Indications	Dosing and administration	Adverse effects
• For low-cardiac output postcardiac surgery prophylaxis • Severe PPHN with left ventricular dysfunction • Septic shock with poor LV function and normal BP	• *Low-cardiac output, postcardiac surgery:* Loading dose 50 µg/kg IV over 15 minutes followed by maintenance dose—0.25–0.75 µg/kg/min for 35 hours	• *Hypotension:* Ensure adequate vascular volume prior to initiating therapy • Tachycardia • Thrombocytopenia

Morphine

Indications	Dosing and administration	Adverse effects
• Analgesia • NAS • Sedation • Opioid dependence	• 0.05–0.2 mg/kg/dose IV, IM, or subQ • *Continuous infusion for pain:* Load with 100 µg/kg IV followed by 10–20 µg/kg/h • *Neonatal abstinence syndrome (NAS):* 0.03–0.1 mg/kg/dose orally every 3–4 hours. Wean dose by 10–20% every 2–3 days based on scoring	• Naloxone should be readily available to reverse adverse effects • Marked respiratory depression • Hypotension, bradycardia • Transient hypertonia • Ileus, delayed gastric emptying • Urine retention • Tolerance

Netilmicin

Indications	Dosing and administration	Adverse effects
• Infections by aerobic gram-negative bacilli (*Pseudomonas, E. coli, Klebsiella*) • Usually used in combination with a beta lactam antibiotic	• Based on postnatal age and postmenstrual age (*see* Table below) • Administered as IV infusion over 30 minutes	• Transient and reversible renal tubular dysfunction • Vestibular and auditory ototoxicity • Neuromuscular weakness may occur when used with neuromuscular blocking agents/in patients with hypermagnesemia

Postmenstrual age (PMA)	Postnatal age	Dosage	Frequency
29 weeks or less	• 0–7 days • 8–28 days	• 5 mg/kg/dose • 4 mg/kg/dose	• Every 48 hours • Every 36 hours
	• 29 days or older	• 4 mg/kg/dose	• Every 24 hours
30–34 weeks	• 0–7 days • 8 days or older	• 4.5 mg/kg/dose • 4 mg/kg/dose	• Every 36 hours • Every 24 hours
35 weeks or more	All	• 4 mg/kg/dose	• Every 24 hours

Nevirapine

Indications	Dosing and administration	Adverse effects
• Prevention of maternal–fetal HIV transmission • Treatment of HIV 1 infection	• *Perinatal HIV transmission, prophylaxis:* Birth weight—1.5–2 kg– 8 mg/dose orally for three doses • Birth weight >2 kg—12 mg/dose orally for three doses • Give first dose within 48 hours of birth, preferably within 6–12 hours, second dose 48 hours after first dose and third dose 96 hours after second dose. It must be given with zidovudine	• Granulocytopenia, anemia • *Hepatotoxicity:* Less severe in pediatric patients

Noradrenaline

Indications	Dosing and administration	Adverse effects
• Septic shock • PPHN with circulatory failure	0.2–2 µg/kg/min by continuous IV infusion into a large peripheral vein or central vein	Extravasation events

Octreotide

Indications	Dosing and administration	Adverse effects
• Refractory hyperinsulinemic hypoglycemia • Congenital and postoperative chylothorax	• *Hyperinsulinemic hypoglycemia:* 1 µg/kg/dose subQ or IV every 6 hours, maximum: 10 µg/kg/dose every 6 hours • *Chylothorax:* Begin at 1 µg/kg/h IV continuous infusion, maximum dose: 10 µg/kg/h	• Vomiting, diarrhea, abdominal distension, steatorrhea • Hyperglycemia • Pulmonary hypertension • NEC

Omeprazole

Indications	Dosing and administration	Adverse effects
• Crying and irritability • Gastroesophageal reflux in preterm, GERD	0.5–1 mg/kg/dose orally once daily	• Hypergastrinemia • Mild transaminase elevation

Pantoprazole

Indications	Dosing and administration	Adverse effects
• Crying and irritability • Gastroesophageal reflux in preterm, GERD • Stress ulcer prophylaxis, upper GI bleeding	1–1.5 mg/kg/dose IV over 15–30 minutes every 24 hours	• Anemia • Constipation • Contact dermatitis • Vomiting

Phenobarbitone

Indications	Dosing and administration	Adverse effects
• Anticonvulsant • Cholestasis • NAS	• *Loading dose:* 20 mg/kg IV over 15–30 minutes. Give additional doses of 10 mg/kg maximum up to 40 mg/kg • *Maintenance:* 3–5 mg/kg/day IV in one to two divided doses started 12 hours after loading dose • VLBW (<1,500 g) babies require loading dose of <15 mg/kg IV followed by single dose of <3 mg/kg/day 24 hours later • *NAS:* 16 mg/kg orally on day 1 followed by 1–4 mg/kg/dose orally every 12 hours	• Vomiting, diarrhea, abdominal distension, steatorrhea • Hyperglycemia • Pulmonary hypertension • NEC

Phenytoin

Indications	Dosing and administration	Adverse effects
As anticonvulsant to treat seizures refractory to phenobarbital	1–1.5 mg/kg/dose IV over 15–30 minutes every 24 hours	• Extravasation events • Hypotension, cardiac arrhythmia • Nystagmus • Movement disorders • *Long-term effects:* Gingival hyperplasia, coarse facies, hirsutism, hyperglycemia, hypoinsulinemia • Cutaneous side effects

Phytonadione (Vitamin K$_1$)

Indications	Dosing and administration	Adverse effect
• Vitamin K deficiency bleeding • Prophylaxis for early and late bleeding	• *Prophylaxis at birth:* Infants <1.5 kg–0.5 mg IM; Infants >1.5 kg–1 mg IM to be given within 6 hours of birth • *Vitamin K deficiency bleeding:* 1 mg by subcutaneous route is preferred. Avoid IM route in coagulopathy	• Pain, swelling at IM injection site • Anaphylaxis—rare

Piperacillin/Tazobactam

Indications	Dosing and administration	Adverse effects
• Infections by beta lactamase producing isolates of *S. aureus* and gram-negative organisms (e.g., *E. coli, H. influenzae, Pseudomonas, Klebsiella, Citrobacter, Enterobacter*) • It has poor CSF penetration	• Based on postnatal age and PMA (*see* Table below) • Administered as IV infusion over at least 30 minutes	• Diarrhea or constipation, nausea • Cautious use in patients with renal failure

PMA (weeks)	Postnatal age (days)	Dose IV* (mg/kg/dose)	Interval (hours)
29 or less	• 0–28 • >28	100	• 12 • 8
30–36	• 0–14 • >14	100	• 12 • 8
37–44	• 0–7 • >7	100	• 12 • 8
>44	All	100	• 8

*Dose for piperacillin component

Ranitidine

Indications	Dosing and administration	Adverse effects
• Treatment of GER • Postoperative prophylaxis in tracheoesophageal fistula, GI bleeding • To reduce stress ulcers	1 mg/kg/dose IV over 5 minutes every 12 hours	• Increase in risk of NEC • Increase in risk of late onset sepsis in NICU • Risk of *C. difficile* infection • Reversible changes in liver function test

Sildenafil

Indications	Dosing and administration	Adverse effects
Adjunct therapy in PPHN	• *IV:* Loading dose of 0.4 mg/kg over 3 hours followed by continuous infusion of 1.6 mg/kg/day • *Oral:* 0.5–1 mg/kg/dose three to four times a day	• Worsening of oxygenation • Systemic hypotension • May increase risk of retinopathy of prematurity if used in extremely preterm neonates

Sodium bicarbonate

Indications	Dosing and administration	Adverse effects
Treatment of normal anion gap metabolic acidosis	• *Metabolic acidosis:* Slow IV push • HCO_3 needed = HCO_3 deficit (mEq/L) × 0.3 × body weight (kg) • Administer half of calculated dose, then reassess need for remainder	• Rapid infusion associated with intracranial hemorrhage • Extravasation injuries • Fluid overload, hypocalcemia, hypernatremia, hypokalemia • Metabolic alkalosis

Sodium chloride (normal saline)

Indications	Dosing and administration	Adverse effects
In neonatal resuscitation	• 10 mL/kg of 0.9% sodium chloride IV over 15–20 minutes • Consider second dose if no improvement after first dose	Large volume can cause fluid overload or intracranial hemorrhage in preterm neonates

Spironolactone

Indications	Dosing and administration	Adverse effects
Used in combination with other diuretics in case of BPD, heart failure	1–3 mg/kg/dose orally every 24 hours	• Rashes, vomiting, diarrhea, paresthesia • Hyponatremia, hypovolemia • Androgenic effect in females and gynecomastia in males • Drowsiness

Sucrose 24%

Indications	Dosing and administration	Adverse effects
Mild analgesia and behavioral comforting prior to painful procedure (vaccination, heel prick) in infants	• *Preterm infants:* 0.5–1 mL orally • *Term infants:* 2 mL orally • Administer sucrose solution directly to tongue 2 minutes prior to painful procedure	• Osmolarity of 24% sucrose is 1,000 mOsm/L • Adverse effects of repeated doses in preterm are not known

Teicoplanin

Indications	Dosing and administration	Adverse effects
Narrow spectrum antibiotic active only against gram-positive organisms (both methicillin sensitive and resistant *S. aureus*, enterococci), *Listeria*, *Clostridium* spp., anaerobic gram-positive cocci	• *Loading dose:* 16 mg/kg as IV infusion over 30–60 minutes • *After 24 hours:* 8 mg/kg/day IV every 24 hours	• Skin rash • *Nephrotoxicity and ototoxicity:* Less than vancomycin • Hypersensitivity reactions, eosinophilia, bronchospasm • Transient decrease in white cell count

Tigecycline

Indications	Dosing and administration	Adverse effects
Rarely used in neonatal sepsis caused by extensively drug-resistant gram-negative organisms (e.g., *Klebsiella*, *Acinetobacter*) associated with nosocomial infection	• *Loading dose:* 2–3 mg/kg as IV infusion over 30–60 minutes • *Maintenance dose:* 1–1.5 mg/kg/dose IV infusion over 30–60 minutes every 12 hours	• Nausea, vomiting, diarrhea • *Long-term side effects:* Teeth discoloration, delay in ossification

Tropicamide 0.5% (ophthalmic)

Indications	Dosing and administration	Adverse effects
Induction of mydriasis and cycloplegia for ophthalmic procedures	• One drop instilled in each eye 10 minutes prior to fundus examination • Feeding should be withheld for 4 hours following procedure	*Systemic effects:* Fever, tachycardia, vasodilatation, dry mouth, restlessness, decreased GI motility, urine retention

Ursodiol

Indications	Dosing and administration	Adverse effects
Treatment of cholestasis associated with parenteral nutrition, biliary atresia	10–15 mg/kg/dose orally every 12 hours	• Nausea, vomiting • Abdominal pain • Constipation, flatulence

Vancomycin

Indications	Dosing and administration	Adverse effects
Gram-positive organisms (both methicillin sensitive and resistant strains), CLABSI, ventricular device-associated infections, Clostridium difficile-associated diarrhea	• 10–15 mg/kg/dose IV every 6–18 hours • Higher dose is used in cases of meningitis • Administered as IV infusion over 60–120 minutes • Dosing interval based on PMA and postnatal age (*see* Table below)	• Nephrotoxicity and ototoxicity • Rash and hypotension (red-man syndrome) • Neutropenia • *Phlebitis:* Minimized by slow infusion and dilution of the drug

Dosing interval chart		
PMA (weeks)	**Postnatal age (days)**	**Interval (hours)**
29 or less	• 0–14 • >14	• 18 • 12
30–36	• 0–14 • >14	• 12 • 8
37–44	• 0–7 • >7	• 12 • 8
>44	All	• 6

Vasopressin

Indications	Dosing and administration	Adverse effects
• Catecholamine-resistant shock • Hypotension from ventricular outflow tract obstruction • Postcardiopulmonary bypass • PPHN	0.01–0.05 IU/kg/h as continuous IV infusion	• Atrial fibrillation, bradycardia, right heart failure • Hyponatremia • Decrease in platelet count • Renal insufficiency

Vecuronium

Indications	Dosing and administration	Adverse effects
Skeletal muscle paralysis/relaxation in infants requiring mechanical ventilation	0.1 mg/kg (0.03–0.15 mg/kg) IV push, as needed for paralysis at interval of 1–2 hours	• Hypoxemia • Bradycardia • Hypotension

Vitamin A

Indications	Dosing and administration	Adverse effects
To reduce the risk of BPD in high-risk preterm infants, to reduce the incidence of ROP	*Vitamin A deficiency:* VLBW and ELBW neonates: 5,000 units three times weekly for 4 weeks administered IM using an insulin syringe	• *Signs of toxicity:* Full fontanel, lethargy, irritability, hepatomegaly, edema, bony tenderness • Avoid concomitant use with glucocorticoids

Vitamin D$_3$

Indications	Dosing and administration	Adverse effects
Prevention and treatment of vitamin D deficiency, rickets	• *Routine supplementation for neonates:* 400–800 IU/day orally • *For vitamin D deficiency:* 1,000–2,000 IU/day orally. *Target 25:* Hydroxyvitamin D concentration >20 ng/mL (50 nmol/L)	*Signs of toxicity (at concentration >250 nmol/L):* Hypercalcemia, azotemia, vomiting, nephrocalcinosis

Vitamin E

Indications	Dosing and administration	Adverse effects
Prevention of vitamin E deficiency, may be indicated in babies receiving erythropoietin and high-iron dosages	5–25 units/day orally with feeds, do not administer simultaneously with iron	• Feed intolerance • NEC due to hyperosmolarity of preparation • Increased rate of sepsis

Zidovudine

Indications	Dosing and administration	Adverse effects
• Prevention of maternal–fetal HIV transmission • Treatment of HIV 1 infection	Perinatal HIV transmission, prophylaxis (*see* Table below)	• Anemia, neutropenia • Transient lactic academia

Dosing

PMA (weeks)	Postnatal age	Dose	Interval
35 or older	Birth to 4 weeks	4 mg/kg/dose orally	Every 12 hours
30 to <35	Birth to 2 weeks	2 mg/kg/dose orally	Every 12 hours
	2 up to 4–6 weeks	3 mg/kg/dose orally	Every 12 hours
<30	Birth to 4–6 weeks	2 mg/kg/dose orally	Every 12 hours

Key Points to Remember

Decreasing Medication Errors in NICU

Definition: Any error in the medication-use process such as prescribing, transcribing, dispensing, administering, and monitoring of medications.

Neonates are more prone to medication errors due to:

- Increased need for calculations, dilutions, and manipulations of medications.
- Many medications are used off-label in neonatal setting, resulting in prescribing, and administration challenges.
- Relative physiological immaturity (renal/hepatic)

- Limited dosing protocols and evidence-based information regarding efficacy, safety, dosing, pharmacokinetic, and clinical use of medications in neonates.
- Dosing-based on postnatal age and postmenstrual age.

Interventions for Reducing Medication Errors in Neonatal Care

Intervention type	Examples
Personnel	• Personalized feedback of medication prescribing errors • Report errors, mistakes, and adverse events without fear • Committed leadership • Policies for reduction of workplace stress • Family involvement and patient-centered approach • Training programs for staff
Technology	• Introduction of a computerized physician order entry system • Electronic tool to verify parenteral nutrition orders (online parenteral nutrition calculator) • Implementation of a barcode medication administration system • Use of automated infusion/dispensing devices • Implementation of electronic health records (EHRs)
Organizational	• Development of preformatted medication order sheets • Preparation of prediluted medications for administration • Transcription of paper-based orders to electronic orders by nursing staff
Communication (written)	• Medication order in legible handwriting and in capital letters • Use standardized notation (doses given in mg, mcg, g) • Leading zeros to be used for values <1 (e.g., 0.2 mg instead of .2 mg) • No trailing zeros (e.g., 2 mg instead of 2.0 mg) • Avoid < or >(use "less than" or "greater than")
Communication (verbal)	• Prompt warnings for drug interactions, allergy, or overdose • Avoid oral orders or use of telephone in emergency situations • Confirm identity of patients before administering medications • For lookalike and soundalike drug names, establish a policy
Quality improvement tools	• Use of failure modes, effects, and criticality analyses to redesign care processes • Automated detection of medication errors

■ FURTHER READING

1. Micromedix Neofax Essentials 2020: Thomas Reuters; 2020.

Common Laboratory Reference Value

Sachin Garg

LABORATORY REFERENCE RANGE VALUES

Cerebrospinal Fluid

Component	Preterm newborn	Full-term 1–7 days	Full-term 8–30 days
Color	Clear or xanthochromic	Clear or xanthochromic	Clear or xanthochromic
WBCs (µL)	21–28	<30	<12
Protein (mg/dL)	65–150	79 (23)	68 (20)
Glucose (mg/dL)	24–63 (1.3–3.5 mmol/L)	>50 (>2.8 mmol/L)	≥38 (2.1 mmol/L), >50% in serum
CSF glucose/blood glucose	0.55–1.05	>0.6	>0.6
Polymorphonuclear cells	19–60%	37–60%	<10%

Clinical chemistry	Age	Valves
Alanine aminotransferase (ALT) (U/L)	1–<13 y	9–25
Aspartate aminotransferase (AST) (U/L)	15 d–<1 y	20–67
Alkaline phosphatase (ALP) (U/L)	1 d–6 m	104–455
Bilirubin (conjugated) (mg/dL)	Neonates	<0.4
Bilirubin (total) (mg/dL)	• 0–24 h • 1–2 d • 3–5 d	• <5.1 • <7.2 • <10.3
Ammonia (µmol/L)	30 d	<51
Calcium (total) (mg/dL)	0–<1 y	8.5–11.0
Magnesium (mg/dL)	• 0–14 d • 15 d–<1 y	• 1.99–3.94 • 1.97–3.09

Contd...

Contd...

Clinical chemistry	Age	Valves
Sodium (mEq/L)	• 0–<7 d • 7–31 d	• 131–144 • 132–142
Chloride (mmol/L)	1–<18 y	102–112
Potassium (mEq/L)	• 0–<1 wk • 1 wk–<1 mo	• 3.2–5.7 • 3.4–6.2
Lipase (U/L)	0–<19 y	4.0–39.0
Amylase (U/L)	• 0–14 d • 15 d–<13 wk • 13 wk–<1 y	• 3–10 • 2–22 • 3–50
Lipids (mg/dL)	Cholesterol	• *Optimal:* <170 • *Borderline:* 170–199 • *High:* >200

Triglycerides (mg/dL)	Age	Male	Female
	• 0–7 d • 8–30 d	• 19–174 • 37–279	• 26–159 • 33–270

Clinical chemistry	Age	Valves
C-reactive protein (mg/L)	Newborn	0.01–0.44
Creatinine (enzymatic) (mg/dL)	• 0–14 d • 15 d–<2 y	• 0.33–0.93 • 0.10–0.36
Iron (mcg/dL)	0–<14 y	16–128
Lactate (serum) (mmol/L)	0–2 mo	1.0–3.5
Lactate dehydrogenase (LDH) (U/L)	1–14 d 15 d–<1 y	• 309–1,222 • 163–452
Methemoglobin (% of hemoglobin)	All	0.04–1.50
Osmolality (serum or plasma) (mOsm/kg)	• Neonates • All	• 266–295 • 275–295
Phosphate (mg/dL)	• 0–14 d • 15 d–<1 y	• 5.6–10.5 • 4.8–8.4
Urea nitrogen (BUN) (mg/dL)	• 0–4 d • 5 d–2 y	• 3–19 • 6–17
Uric acid (mg/dL)	• 0–14 d • 15 d–<1 y	• 2.8–12.7 • 1.6–6.3
Vitamin D (total) (25-hydroxyvitamin D) (ng/mL)	• Sufficiency • Insufficiency • Deficiency	• ≥20 • 12–<20 • <12
Zinc (mcg/dL)	All	70–120
Troponin I (ng/L)	5–<15 d	<968

(d: days; h: hours; mo: months; wk: weeks; y: years)

For Newborns ABG Values

Analyte	Cord blood	2–4-hour venous blood
pH	7.25–7.45	7.28–7.44
pCO_2 (mm Hg)	28–52	29–57
Hct (%)	38–58	47–67
Hb (g/L)	1.33–1.97	1.46–2.34
Sodium (mmol/L)	132–144	131–143
Potassium (mmol/L)	2.7–7.9	4.2–6.2
Chloride (mmol/L)	99–115	101–121
Calcium (ionized) (mmol/L)	0.4–1.85	0.97–1.29

Thyroid Function Tests

TSH, Total T_3, Total T_4, and free T_4 values of children:

Function	Age	Values	
Thyroid-stimulating hormone (TSH) (mIU/L)	4 d–<1 y	0.73–4.77	
Triiodothyronine (total) (T_3) (ng/dL)	4 d–<1 y	84.64–234.38	
Thyroxine (total) (T_4) (mcg/dL)	7 d–<1 y	5.87–13.67	
Thyroxine (free) (T_4) (ng/dL)	• 5–<15 d • 15–<30 d • 30 d–<1 y	• 1.05–3.21 • 0.68–2.53 • 0.89–1.7	
17-Hydroxyprogesterone (ng/dL)	• 0–<6 mo • 6 mo–<6 y	• 25–248 • Girl: 3–107	Boy: 7–100
Cortisol (mcg/dL)	• Age • 0–24 mo	• 5:00–11:00 AM • 1.0–34.0	• 5:00–11:00 PM • 1.0–30.0

(d: days; mo: months; y: years)

Hematology Values

Age	Hemoglobin (g)	Hematocrit (%)	Mean corpuscular volume (fL)	Mean corpuscular hemoglobin concentration (g/dL per RBC)	Reticulocytes (%)	White blood cells ($\times 10^3/\mu L$)	Platelets ($\times 10^3/\mu L$)	Red blood cells ($\times 10^{12}/L$)
1–3 days	M: 12.5–16.6 F: 12.7–16.4	M: 36.4–47.4 F: 36.5–47.7	M: 94.0–106.3 F: 89.7–105.4	M: 32.8–36.4 F: 31.7–36.3	M: 2.2–4.8 F: 2.1–3.7	M: 7.69–13.12 F: 7.51–15.83	M: 140–238 F: 133–255	M: 3.69–4.75 F: 3.79–4.76
4–7 days	M: 12.5–16.3 F: 12.6–15.3	M: 35.9–46.6 F: 36.1–44.0	M: 87.1–96.5 F: 86.5–93.8	M: 30.9–33.4 F: 30.6–32.3	M: 0.4–2.7 F: 0.4–2.0	M: 6.54–12.32 F: 5.86–12.23	M: 129–271 F: 95–230	M: 3.98–5.08 F: 4.05–4.83
8–14 days	M: 11.9–15.7 F: 12.7–14.9	M: 34.4–45.4 F: 36.6–43.2	M: 87.1–94.8 F: 87.4–92.2	M: 30.4–33.0 F: 30.5–31.9	M: 0.4–2.7 F: 0.4–2.0	M: 7.66–14.05 F: 7.46–14.55	M: 120–297 F: 106–294	M: 3.75–4.93 F: 4.01–4.73
2 weeks–<1 month	M: 11.6–14.2 F: 11.6–14.3	M: 33.6–41.0 F: 34.1–41.8	M: 88.0–95.2 F: 88.4–93.3	M: 30.6–32.6 F: 30.5–32.0	M: 0.4–2.7 F: 0.4–2.0	M: 8.90–16.69 F: 8.55–15.72	M: 157–406 F: 114–364	M: 3.61–4.46 F: 3.70–4.59

Age-specific Coagulation Values—Healthy, Full-term Infants

Common coagulation tests	Day 1 after birth	Day 5 after birth	Day 30 after birth
PT (s)	13.00 (1.43)	12.40 (1.46)	11.80 (1.25)
aPTT (s)	42.90 (5.80)	42.60 (8.62)	40.40 (7.42)
Thrombin time (s)	23.50 (2.38)	23.10 (3.07)	24.30 (2.44)
Plasminogen (U/mL)	1.95 (0.35)	2.17 (0.38)	1.98 (0.36)

Biostatistics

Ramji Bhardwaj, Amit Yadav, Aparna Prasad

■ STUDY DESIGN

Research Questions

A research study should always be designed to answer a particular research question. The question usually relates to a specific population.

For example:
Is low birth weight associated with hypertension in later life?
A well-built clinical foreground question should have four components.

The *PICO model* is a helpful tool that assists you in organizing and focusing your foreground question into a searchable query:

- *P = Patient, population*
  - How would you describe a group of patients similar to you?
  - What are the most important characteristics of the patient?
- I = Intervention, prognostic factor, exposure
  - What main intervention are you considering?
  - What do you want to do with this patient?
- *C = Comparison (can be none or placebo)*
  - What is the main alternative to compare with the intervention?
  - Are you trying to decide between two drugs, a drug and no medication or placebo, or two diagnostic tests?
- *O = Outcome*
  - What are you trying to accomplish, measure, improve, or affect?
  - Outcomes may be disease-oriented or patient-oriented

For example:
P = newborns; I = low birthweight; C = normal birthweight; O = hypertension

Confounding

Confounding may be an important source of error.

- A confounding factor is a background variable (i.e., something not of direct interest) which:
  - Is different between the groups being compared, and
  - Affects the outcome being studied

In the comparison of hypertension rates between LBW and not LBW, social class could be a confounder if:

- The LBW babies are more likely to have lower social class.
- Social class is associated with the risk of hypertension.

Confounding may be avoided by matching individuals in the groups according to potential confounders

For example, we could recruit individuals of low and normal birth weight from similar social classes.

Different Types of Studies

- *Descriptive studies:*
  - Case reports
  - Case-series
  - Surveys studies
  - Qualitative studies
- *Observational studies:*
  - Case-control study
  - Cross-sectional study
  - Cohort study
  - Ecological study
- *Experimental studies:*
  - Randomized control trials
    - Double blind study
    - Single blind study
    - Unblinded study
  - Crossover study

Observational Studies

When an observational study compares two groups; it may be categorized as being either:

1. Case control study—consider differences between the groups in the *past*
2. Cross-sectional study—consider differences between the groups at the *present time*
3. Cohort study—consider differences between the groups in the *future*

Case control study:

- It is a *retrospective* study. This means that you begin at the end (with the disease), and then work backward, to hunt for possible causes.
- It usually *compare diseased and healthy groups*, and look back in time to see what they have done differently in the past that may have led to disease.
- These studies are concerned with *etiology* rather than treatment. They are more suitable for *rare diseases*.
- These studies can't calculate incidence, prevalence, or relative risk (RR). Results are expressed as *odds ratios (ORs)*.
- Case control studies are less reliable than either randomized controlled trials (RCTs) or cohort studies.

For example, a study in which colon cancer patients are asked what kinds of food they have eaten in the past and the answers are compared with a selected healthy control group.

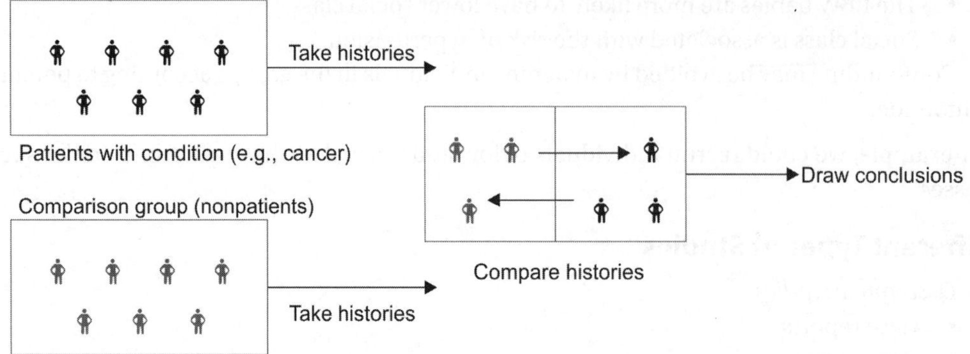

- *Cross-sectional study (transversal study and prevalence study):*
  - A study that examines the relationship between diseases (or other health-related characteristics) and other variables of interest as they exist in a defined population at a specified time (i.e., exposure and outcomes are both measured at the same time).
  - It is usually used for quantifying:
    - The prevalence of a disease or risk factor
    - The accuracy of a diagnostic test
  - These studies allow determination of prevalence and RR; but *not the incidence*
  - It cannot evaluate hypotheses about causation, as it does not take into account how the timing of exposure to a risk factor relates to the development of disease
  - *For example*—what is the current prevalence of cystic fibrosis in a population of adolescents?
  - *Another example*—Is there an association between diabetes and overweight?
- *Cohort study (longitudinal study):*
  - Two or more groups of subjects are selected on the basis of their exposure or lack of exposure to a particular risk factor or agent (e.g., drinking alcohol or not, smoking or not, eating a high-fat diet or not), and follow the groups forward in time to see how many in each group develop a particular disease.
  - Cohort studies are used to evaluate association between a factor and the outcome/impact of treatment, when randomized controlled clinical trials are not possible (more suitable for *common diseases*).

Cohort studies may be either:
- Prospective—exposure factors are identified at the beginning of a study and a defined population is followed into the future.
- Retrospective—past medical records for the defined population are used to identify exposure factors:
  - Prospective cohort studies are *more reliable* than retrospective cohort studies
  - Cohort studies allow determination of incidence and RR; but *not the prevalence*
  - Disadvantages include the large numbers required for rare outcomes, problems of *drop-out bias,* and changes in practice during long follow-up periods

- Cohort studies are used for determining the outcome of infants born prematurely.

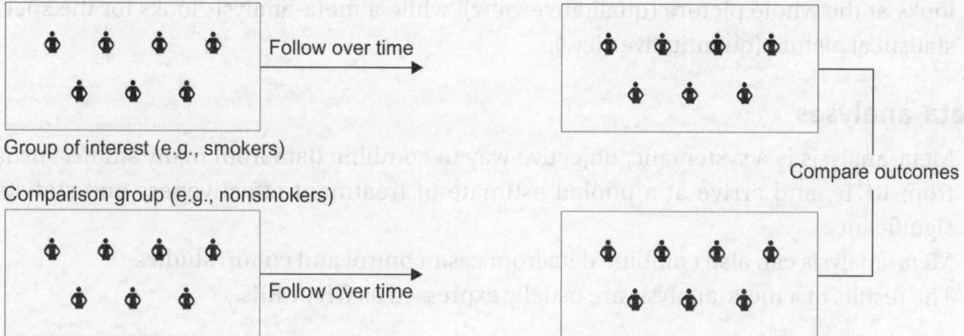

Randomized Controlled Trial (Randomized Clinical Trial)

- It is the mainstay of *experimental* medical studies, normally used in testing new drugs and treatments.
- *In randomized controlled studies,* there are two groups, one treatment group and one control group. The treatment group receives the treatment under investigation, and the control group receives either no treatment (placebo) or standard treatment. Patients are *randomly* assigned to all groups.
- *Placebo* is a pharmacologically inert dummy, identical in appearance to the treatment(s), should normally be used for the control group.
- Having a control group allows for a comparison of treatments (e.g., treatment A produced favorable results 56% of the time versus treatment B in which only 25% of patients had favorable results)
- *Randomization* means that each patient has the same chance of being assigned to either of the groups, regardless of their personal characteristics. Note that random does not mean haphazard or systematic.
- Randomization helps to avoid the *selection bias* in the assignment process. It also increases the probability that differences between groups can be attributed to the treatment(s) under study.
- *Allocation concealment* means that the allocation (to treatment or control) is unknown before the individual is entered into the study.

Systematic Review

- It is a comprehensive survey of a topic that takes great care to find all relevant studies (both published and unpublished)—assess each study—synthesize the findings from individual studies in an unbiased, explicit and reproducible way, and present a balanced and impartial summary of the findings with due consideration of any flaws in the evidence.
- In this way, it can be used for the evaluation of either existing or new technologies and practices.
- A systematic review is more rigorous than a traditional literature review and attempts to reduce influence of bias.

- The difference between a systematic review and a meta-analysis is that a systematic review looks at the whole picture (qualitative view), while a meta-analysis looks for the specific statistical picture (quantitative view).

Meta-analyses

- Meta-analysis is a systematic, objective way to combine data from many studies, usually from RCTs, and arrive at a pooled estimate of treatment effectiveness and statistical significance.
- Meta-analysis can also combine data from case-control and cohort studies.
- The results of a meta-analysis are usually expressed as OR or RRs.

Bias

- *Sampling bias*—volunteer subjects in a study may not be representative of the population being studied; as a consequence, the results of the study may not be generalizable to the entire population.
- *Selection bias*—occurs when there is a systematic difference in the way study groups are chosen. One method of decreasing this bias is *randomization.*
- *Recall bias*—patients who experience an adverse outcome have a different likelihood of recalling an exposure than do patients who do not have an adverse outcome, independent of the true extent of the exposure
- *Expectancy bias*—occurs when a physician knows which patients are in treatment versus placebo group, causing the physician to draw conclusions supporting the expected outcome. One method of decreasing this bias is a *double-blind design.*
- *Late-look bias*—results from information being gathered too late to draw conclusions about the disease or exposure of interest from the entire study population. For instance, more severe cases may have already died.

Quantifying Risk

Risk

It is the probability that an event will happen.

Absolute Risk

- It is the probability that a person will have a medical event.
- It is the ratio of the number of people who have an event divided by all of the people who could have the event.
- Absolute risk is expressed as a percentage.
- *Absolute risk is equal to the incidence rate.*

Relative Risk (RR)

- It compares the incidence rate of an outcome among individuals exposed to a risk factor (e.g., lung cancer among smokers) with the incidence rate of the *same* outcome among individuals *not* exposed to risk factor.

- Relative risk is the incidence rate of the *exposed* (or treated) group (i.e., experimental event rate = EER) divided by the incidence rate of the *unexposed* (or untreated) group (i.e., control event rate = CER)

$$RR = EER \div CER$$

Attributable Risk

- Attributable risk is useful for determining what would happen in a study population if the risk factor were removed (e.g., determining how common lung cancer would be in a study if people did not smoke).
- Attributable risk is the incidence rate of the unexposed group *subtracted* from the incidence rate of the exposed group

$$Attributable\ risk = EER - CER$$

Odds Ratios

- An OR is a measure of association between an exposure and an outcome.
- An OR is a relative measure of effect, which allows the comparison of the intervention group of a study relative to the comparison or placebo group.
- Since incidence data are not available in a case-control study, the OR (i.e., odds risk ratio) can be used as an estimate of RR in such studies.
- They are calculated by dividing odds of having been exposed to a risk factor by odds in a control group.
- An OR of 1—the likelihood of exposure to the risk factor is *identical* for both cases and controls.
- An OR of >1—the likelihood of exposure to the risk factor is *greater* for cases than for controls.
- An OR of <1—the likelihood of exposure to the risk factor is *lower* for cases than for controls.
- Relative risk as well as ORs should always be presented with their (95%) confidence intervals (CIs).
  - If CI includes 1, the relationship between risk exposure and disease occurrence is not statistically significant.
  - If CI does not include 1, the relationship between risk exposure and disease occurrence is statistically significant.
  - The width of the interval estimates the precision of the OR.
  - A small CI—indicates a higher level of precision of the OR.
  - A large CI—indicates a lower level of precision of the OR.

Number Needed to Treat

- Number needed to treat (NNT) is the number of persons who need to take a treatment for one additional person to benefit from the new treatment.
- It is the reciprocal of absolute risk reduction (ARR), and is more meaningful than the relative risk reduction (RRR) for assessing the efficacy of a treatment.

- RRR is constant regardless of risk in reference group, whereas NNT is likely to be higher if risk of having the outcome is low in reference group.
- NNT is 1 divided by the ARR *(NNT = 1 ÷ ARR)*.

Number Needed to Harm

- Number needed to harm (NNH) is the number of persons who need to be exposed to a risk factor for one person to be harmed who would otherwise not be harmed.
- NNH is 1 divided by the attributable risk *(NNH = 1 ÷ attributable risk)*.

Screening tests:

Screening test result	Diseased	Disease-free	Total
Positive (indicating possible disease	a (true +ve)	b (false +ve)	a + b
Negative	c (false –ve)	d (true –ve)	c + d
Totals	a + c	b + d	a + b + c + d

- *Sensitivity* is the proportion of true positives correctly identified by the test proportion of true positive screening test in diseased individuals [a ÷ (a + c)] × 100.
- *Specificity* is the proportion of true negatives correctly identified by the test proportion of true negative screening test in healthy individuals [d ÷ (b + d)] × 100.
- *Positive predictive value* describes the chance of a patient having the disease if the test is positive proportion of true positive screening test in all positive individuals [a ÷ (a + b)] × 100.
- *Negative predictive value* describes the chance of a patient being disease free if the test is negative proportion of true negative screening test in all negative individuals [d ÷ (c + d)] × 100.

■ DISTRIBUTIONS

Types of Data

Data may be either qualitative (categoric) or quantitative (numeric):

- Qualitative data can be nominal or ordinal
- Quantitative data can be discrete or continuous
- *Qualitative (categoric) data:*
  - Deals with descriptions
  - Data can be observed but not measured. For example:
    - Color of eyes—blue, green, brown, etc.
    - Socioeconomic status—low, middle, or high
  - *Qualitative data are classified as either:*
    - Nominal—if there is no natural order between the categories (e.g., eye color).
    - Ordinal—if there is a natural order between the categories (e.g., disease severity: mild, moderate, severe, and socioeconomic status: lower, middle, and upper)
  - If there are only two categories, then the variable is *binary*

- *Quantitative (numeric) data:*
  - Deals with numbers
  - Data can be measured (e.g., length, height, area, volume, weight, speed, time, temperature, and humidity)
  - *Quantitative data are classified as either:*
- Discrete—if the measurements are integers (i.e., a whole number such as 3 or 4, but not 3.5) (e.g., number of people in a household, number of cigarettes smoked per day, and number of antibiotic courses)
- Continuous—if the measurements can take on any value, usually within some range (BW, HR, BP)
  - Quantities such as sex and weight are called *variables*, because the value of these quantities vary from one observation to another
  - Numbers calculated to describe important features of the data are called *statistics*.

Measures of Central Tendency

- *Mean (= average):*
  - The sum of the values of the observations divided by the numbers of observations
  - Use the mean to describe the middle of a set of data that *does not* have an outlier, i.e., data has Gaussian distribution.
- *Median (= middle):*
  - The central value of data series when the values are lined up in order of magnitude (50th percentile value).
  - Use the median to describe the *middle* of a set of data that does have an *outlier.*
  - To get the median—you first put your numbers in an ascending or descending order.
  - If you have an odd number of numbers—the median is the center number (e.g., 3 is the median for the numbers 1, 1, 3, 4, and 9).
  - If you have an even number of numbers—the median is the average of the two innermost numbers (e.g., 2.5 is the median for the numbers 1, 2, 3, and 7).
- *Mode = (most frequent):*
  - The most frequently.

Normal Distribution (Gaussian or Bell-shaped Distribution)

- The normal distribution is symmetrical and bell-shaped, with one side the mirror image of the other.
- If distribution is normal:
  - The *mean* and standard deviation are preferable as a summary of the data.
  - The mean, median, and mode are *equal.*
- About *68%* of the observations fall within 1 standard deviation of the mean.
- About *95%* of the observations fall within 2 standard deviations of the mean.
- About *99.7%* of the observations fall within 3 standard deviations of the mean occurring value in a set of observations.

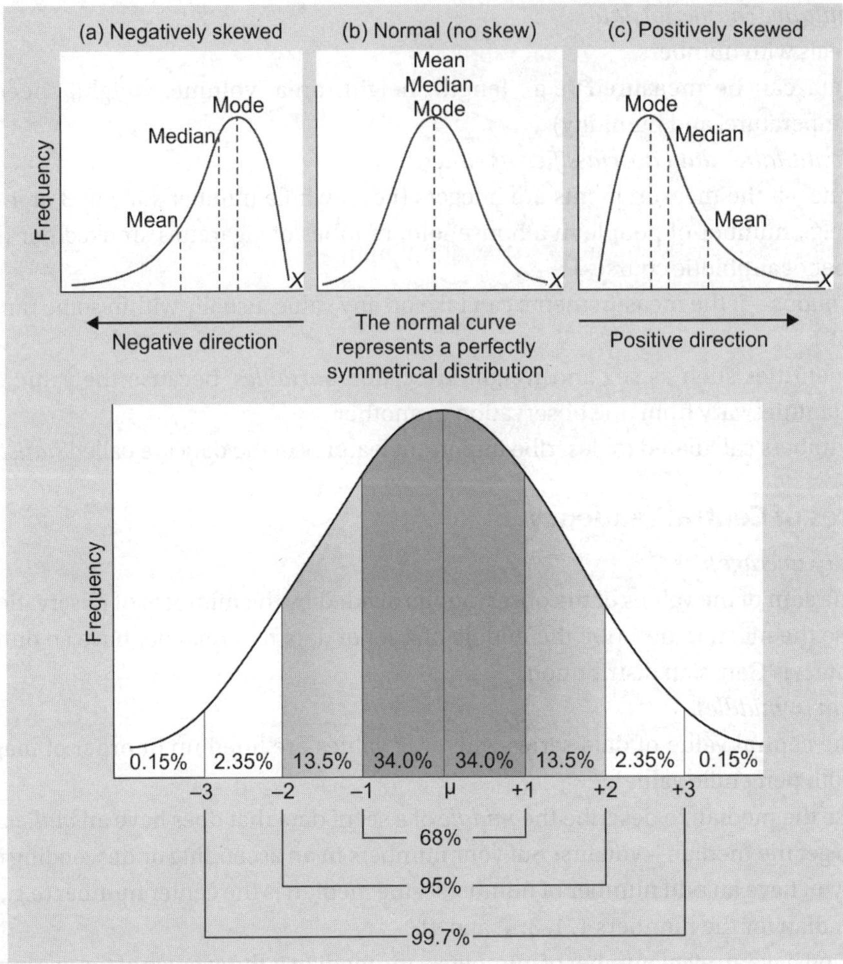

▌ MEASURES OF VARIABILITY

- Measures of variability tell you how "spread out" or how much variability is present in a set of numbers.
- Measures of variability should be reported along with measures of central tendency because they provide very different but complementary and important information.
- An easy way to get the idea of variability is to look at two sets of data, one that is highly variable and one that is not very variable.
- For example, which of these two sets of numbers appears to be the most spread out, Set A or Set B?
  - Set A → 93, 96, 98, 99, 99, 99, 100
  - Set B → 10, 29, 52, 69, 87, 92, 100
    - If you said set B is more spread out, then you are right! The numbers in set B are more "spread out"; that is, they are more variability.
    - Measures of variability include the range, the variance, and the standard deviation.

- *Range:*
  - ◆ *It is the difference between the largest and smallest value.*
  - ◆ For example, the range in set A shown above is 7, and the range in set B shown above is 90
- *Variance (σ^2):*
  - *It is the average of the squared differences between each value and the mean.*
  - It measures how far a set of numbers is spread out.
  - It tells you (exactly) the average deviation from the mean, in "squared units".
  - A small variance indicates that the data points tend to be very close to the mean and hence to each other, while a high variance indicates that the data points are very spread out from the mean and from each other.
  - *A variance of zero* indicates that all the values are identical (e.g., for the data 3, 3, 3, 3, 3, 3, the variance, and standard deviation will equal zero).
  - For example, how to calculate the variance for the following data 3, 4, 4, 5, 6, and 8.
    - ◆ Firstly, calculate the mean $\rightarrow (3 + 4 + 4 + 5 + 6 + 8) \div 6 = 5$
    - ◆ Then for each number; subtract the mean and square the result $\rightarrow [(3\text{-}5)2 + (4\text{-}5)2 + (4\text{-}5)2 + (5\text{-}5)2 + (6\text{-}5)2 + (8\text{-}5)2] = 4 + 1 + 1 + 0 + 1 + 9 = 16$
    - ◆ Finally, calculate the average of those squared differences $\rightarrow 16 \div 6 = 2.7$
- Standard deviation (σ):
  - *It is the square root of the variance.*
  - The standard deviation tells you (approximately) how far the numbers tend to vary from the mean.
  - *SD should only be used when the data has a normal distribution.*
  - It is important to distinguish between the standard deviation of a population and the standard deviation of a sample. They have different notation, and they are computed differently.
  - The standard deviation of a population is denoted by σ, and the standard deviation of a sample, by *s*.
    - ◆ Percentile or centile—the value below which a certain percentage of values fall. The value at the 50th percentile means that half the data is above and half below that value.
    - ◆ Interquartile range $\rightarrow$ usually describes the data which fall between the 25th and 75th percentile.

Confidence Interval

- It is a range of values in which we are fairly confident the true population value lies.
- It gives an estimated range (interval) of values which is likely to include an unknown population parameter.
- Confidence interval is usually reported as 95% CI (i.e., we can be 95% confident that the population value lies within those limits).
- CI = mean $\pm$ (z × SE)
- The CI is equal to the mean of the sample (X) plus or minus the z score multiplied by the SE.
  - For the 95% CI $\rightarrow$ a z score of 2 is used
  - For the 99% CI $\rightarrow$ a z score of 2.5 is used
  - For the 99.7% CI $\rightarrow$ a z score of 3 is used

- *Confidence interval is affected by two main factors:*
  - Variation in the population
  - Sample size—the larger the sample size, the smaller the CI.

■ SIGNIFICANCE TESTS

- Statistical significance tests, or hypothesis tests, use the sample data to assess how likely some specified null hypothesis is to be correct.
- The measure of "how likely" is given by a probability known as the *p*-value.
- Usually, the null hypothesis is that there is "no difference" between the groups.

Null Hypotheses

- The *null hypothesis (Ho)* underlies all statistical tests.
- Null hypothesis says that the findings are the result of chance or random factors.
- If you want to show that a drug works, the null hypothesis will be that the drug does not work.
- *Example of the null hypothesis:*
  - A group of 20 patients who have similar systolic blood pressures at the beginning of a study (Time 1) is divided into two groups of 10 patients each. One group is given daily doses of an experimental drug meant to lower blood pressure (experimental group); the other group is given daily doses of a placebo (placebo group). Blood pressure in all 20 patients is measured 2 weeks later (Time 2).
  - The null hypothesis assumes that there are no significant differences in blood pressure between the two groups at Time 2.
  - If, at Time 2, patients in the experimental group show systolic blood pressures similar to those in the placebo group—the null hypothesis is not rejected.
  - If, at Time 2, patients in the experimental group have significantly lower or higher blood pressures than those in the placebo group → the null hypothesis is rejected.

Critical Level (*p*-value)

- *p*-value is the probability of the null hypothesis to be true.
- *p*-value is a measure of the strength of the evidence against the null hypothesis.
- Since the *p*-value is a probability, it takes values between 0 and 1.
- The *p*-value *never* is actually zero, so we never totally disprove the null hypothesis.
- The smaller the value (nearer to 0), the less likely the null hypothesis is to be true, suggesting that there is likely to be a difference between groups.
- A *p*-value equal to or <0.05 is generally considered to be statistically significant.
- If $p \leq 0.05$—reject the null hypothesis.
- If $p > 0.05$—do not reject the null hypothesis.
- $p = 0.05$—means that the difference will only have happened by chance 1 in 20 or 5%. This is considered to be "statistically significant".
- $p = 0.01$—means that the difference will only have happened by chance 1 in 100 or 1%. This is considered to be "highly significant".

- $p = 0.001$—means that the difference will have happened by chance 1 in 1,000 times. This is considered to be "very highly significant".

Meaning of the *p*-value

- Provides criterion for making decisions about the null hypothesis
- Quantifies the chances that a decision to reject the null hypothesis will be wrong
- Tells statistical significance, not clinical significance or likelihood of benefit
- Limits to the *p*-value —the *p*-value does not tell us:
  - The chance that an individual patient will benefit.
  - The percentage of patients who will benefit.
  - The degree of benefit expected for a given patient.

Types of Error

- *Type 1 error (false positive)*
  - Rejection of the null hypothesis when it is really true (i.e., assuming that there is a difference between data sets when in fact there is not) (e.g., asserting that the drug works when it doesn't).
  - The chance of type I error is given by the *p*-value.
  - If $p = 0.05$—the chance of a type I error is 5 in 100, or 1 in 20.
  - The probability of a type I error is designated by the Greek letter alpha (α), and is called type I error rate or significance level.
- *Type 2 error (false negative):*
  - Failing to reject the null hypothesis when it is really false (i.e., assuming that there is no difference when there is one) (e.g., asserting the drug does not work when it really does)
  - The chance of a type II error cannot be directly estimated from the *p*-value
  - The probability of a type II error is designated by the Greek letter beta (β), and is called type II error rate.
  - One minus the type II error ($1-\beta$) is the *power* of the test
  - Type I error (error of commission) is generally considered worse than type II error (error of omission). For the same reason, acceptable cut off for type 1 error is 0.05 and type II error is 0.2.
  - If the null hypothesis is not rejected → there is no chance of a type I error.
- If the null hypothesis is rejected, there is no chance of a type II error.

■ TYPES OF SIGNIFICANCE TESTS

- Statistical tests are used to analyze data from medical studies.
- The results of statistical tests indicate whether to reject or not reject the null hypothesis.
- Statistical tests can be parametric or nonparametric.

Parametric Tests

- Parametric tests use population parameters (e.g., mean scores) and are usually used to identify the presence of statistically significant differences between groups when:

- Data is *normally* distributed.
  - The sample size is large.
- *Commonly used parametric statistical tests include:*
  - t-test (sometimes called "Student's t-test" or "Student's paired t-test")
  - Analysis of variance (ANOVA)
  - Pearson's coefficient of linear correlation
- *Student's t-test:*
  - It is a statistic that checks if two means (averages) are reliably different from each other.
  - It is used for comparing a single *small* sample with a population or to compare the difference in means between two *small* samples.
  - Use Student's t-test when you have one *nominal* variable and one *measurement* variable, and you want to compare the mean values of the measurement variable. The nominal variable must have only *two* values, such as "male" and "female" or "treated" and "untreated".
  - It is inappropriate if more than two means are compared.
  - The larger the t-value—the larger the difference between the two means—the smaller the p-value—the stronger the evidence that the null hypothesis is untrue
  - *t-value* = variance between groups ÷ variance within groups
  - The t-test may be paired or unpaired.
    - *Unpaired (independent) t-test*—used to compare the average (means) of two groups of numerical.
    - Data, provided the values are approximately *normally* distributed and the samples are *not* small.
    - *Paired (dependent) t-test*—compares the means of two small *paired* observations of numerical data, either on the same individual or on *matched* individuals.
  - If the two-sample *t*-test is invalid (non-normality and/or small samples) → Mann-Whitney *U* test is used.
- Analysis of variance (ANOVA):
  - This is a set of techniques used to compare the means of *more than two samples.*
  - They can also allow for independent variables which may affect the outcome.

■ NONPARAMETRIC TESTS

They are usually used to identify the presence of statistically significant differences between groups when:

- Data is *not* normally distributed
- The sample size is small
- *Commonly used nonparametric statistical tests include:*
  - Chi-square (χ^2) test
  - Wilcoxon signed rank test—used for matched or paired data
  - Wilcoxon rank sum test → used for unpaired data

- Mann-Whitney U test gives equivalent results to the Wilcoxon rank sum test
- *Kruskal-Wallis test:* It is used to compare non-normally distributed quantitative data, with more than 2 groups

- *Chi-square (χ^2) test:*
  - It is used to compare *proportions* between two groups, provided the samples are *large* enough and the proportions in each group *not extreme*
  - If only small samples are available and/or the proportions are extreme → Fisher's exact test is used
  - If proportions are paired—McNemar's test should be used.
    - Nonparametric tests are less powerful than parametric tests
    - *t*-tests are appropriate for continuous numeric outcomes
    - The t-test is used to compare the differences between 2 means
  - If the samples are large and the proportions are not extreme—χ^2 test
  - If the samples are small and the proportions are extreme—Fisher's exact test
    - χ^2 is *not* applicable for extreme percentages (e.g., 10% and 0.5%). Therefore, in order to compare 10% with 0.5% seen in two different groups, Fisher's exact test should be used.
    - The χ^2 test ranges from –1.0 to +1.0
    - The larger the χ^2 value—the lower the *p*-value—the more statistically significant difference.
    - The Fisher exact test is used only for categorical measures.
    - 95% CIs are calculated as 1.96 times standard deviation.
    - The most appropriate statistical test for a non-normally distributed continuous measure when the groups are independent is the Mann-Whiney U-test.

Forest Plots

- Forest plot is graphical manner of presenting means and CI of studies, so that they can be easily reviewed and compared.
- It is convenient and easily understandable manner of presenting study results in a systematic review/meta-analysis.
- It is used mainly to present results of individual study in a systematic review/ meta-analysis as well as the systematic review/meta-analysis itself.
- It shows effect size of all studies and results of meta-analysis.

Parts of a Forest Plot

- *Left side:* It enumerates the names of various studies which have been included in the meta-analysis in a chronological order.
- *Right side:* It represents the measure of effect of the studies included.
- The square in diagram is a measure of effect of the study (example: mean, OR, and RR) and the horizontal line represents the 95% CI of the study.

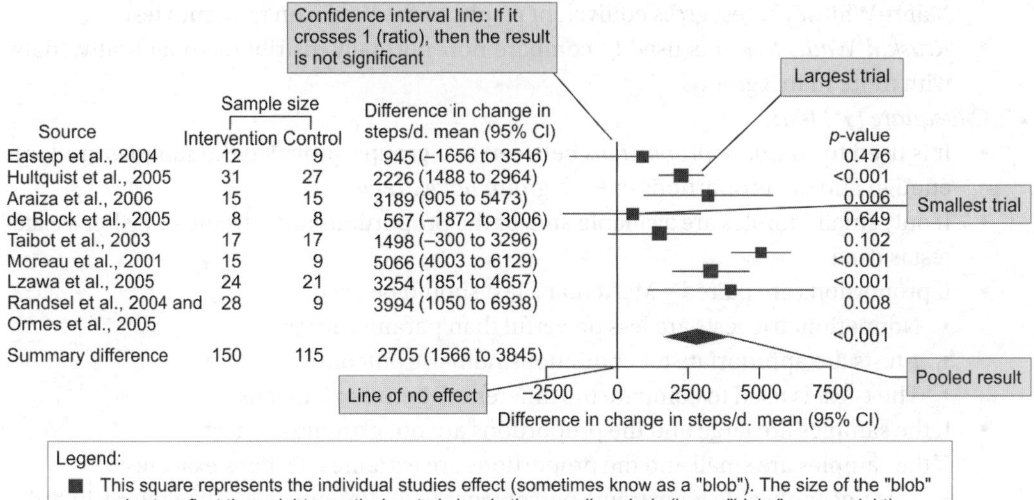

- Size of each square or the area of a square is proportional to the weight of the study in the meta-analysis.
- The diamond in the plot represents the overall measure of effect of the meta-analysis. The vertical line represents the line of no effect/ null hypothesis.

Receiver Operating Characteristic Curve

- Receiver operating characteristic (ROC) is a plot of sensitivity vs 1—specificity or plot of true positive rate against the false positive rate, for the different possible cut offs (threshold values) of a diagnostic test.
- It shows the relationship between sensitivity and specificity (any increase in sensitivity is accompanied by a decrease in specificity).
- ROC curve gives an idea of accuracy of a test (efficiency of the test to discriminate between true positive and true negative).
- The area under the curve gives the measure of test accuracy.
- Area of ROC curves is calculated by complex mathematical models but can be obtained easily by various computer programs.

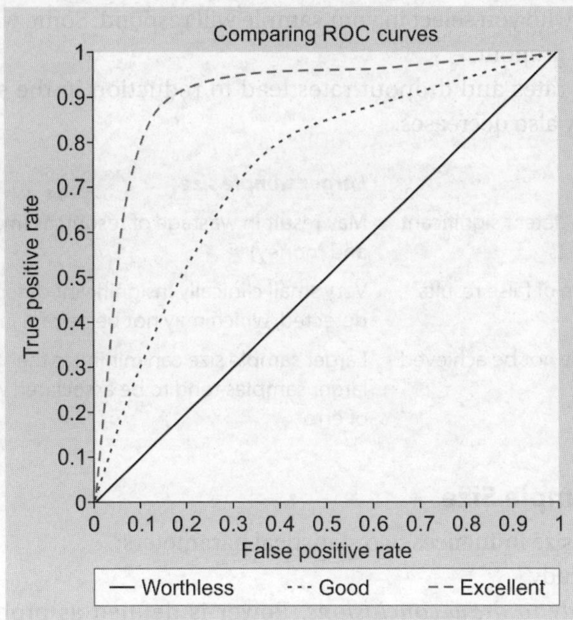

Sample Size

- Sample size is defined as the number of subjects that are included in a given research study.
- It is impossible to study whole population, so a sample is selected from the population in a random manner.
- The sample size should be just large enough to be able to detect a difference if it exists.
- This number is usually represented by the term "n".
- Importance of sample size:
  - Calculation of sample size helps in planning study.
  - Calculation of sample size helps to estimate the resources that would be required, that is: manpower, money, material and time that would be required to complete the research.
  - Sample size calculation helps to ensure scientific and ethical integrity of the research study.
- Factors to consider while calculating sample size:
  - Type of study?
  - What is the primary outcome variable of the study?
  - What is estimated value of primary outcome variable and acceptable precision?
  - What is acceptable Type 1 and 2 error for hypothesis testing?
  - What is the desired effect size?
- *Factors affecting sample size:*
  - *Feasibility:* It refers to what is possible or what one can do, depending upon the resources available to you.
  - Nonresponse rates and dropout rates

- Not everyone who you select in your sample will respond. Some will be nonresponders and some will dropout.
- Nonresponse rates and dropout rates lead to reduction in the sample size studied. Power of study also decreases.

Small sample size	*Larger sample size*
May not be possible to detect significant difference even if it exists	May result in wastage of resources (manpower, time, effort, and money)
May result in estimation of false results	Very small clinically insignificant differences may be detected, which may not be helpful in clinical practice
Objectives of study may not be achieved	Larger sample size can minimize the sampling error. That is, larger samples tend to be associated with smaller margin of error

Calculation of Sample Size

Significance: Sample size influences two statistical parameters:

1. Precision of the study
2. *Power of the study to draw conclusions:* Power is defined as probability of finding a statistically significant result.

Key Points to Remember

- *Incidence*—the number of *new* cases within a defined population at a specified time.
- *Prevalence*—the total number of cases within a defined population at a specified time.
- *Stillbirth rate*—number of stillbirths (i.e., babies born with no signs of life after 24 weeks' gestation) per 1,000 total births.
- *Perinatal mortality rate*—number of stillbirths and deaths within the first week of life per 1,000 total births
- *Neonatal mortality rate*—number of deaths of live born babies aged up to 1 month per 1,000 live births.

Hierarchy of evidence:

Study type	*Level of evidence*	*Strength of recommendation*
• Systematic reviews and meta-analyses of randomized controlled trials • Randomized controlled trials	Ia Ib	A
• Nonrandomized controlled trials • Cohort studies	2a 2b	B
Case-control studies	3	C
Case studies, expert opinions	4	D
Diagnostic studies	–	–

Reporting formats:

- *PRISMA (http://www.prisma-statement.org/:*
  - PRISMA (Preferred Reporting Items for Systematic Reviews and Meta-analyses) is developed for the reporting of systematic reviews and meta-analyses.
  - The PRISMA statement consists of a checklist of 27 items, which are divided into the following categories: Title, abstract, introduction, methods, results, discussion, and funding.
  - The PRISMA statement also endorses the use of a flow diagram. The aim of this statement is to increase transparency and to improve the reporting of systematic reviews and meta-analyses.
- *CONSORT (http://www.consort-statement.org/):*
  - CONSORT (Consolidated Standards of Reporting Trials) is a guideline for reporting RCTs.
  - The CONSORT consists of a 25-item checklist and is divided into subcategories: title and abstract, introduction, methods, results, discussion, and other information. This structure is intended to promote complete reporting and transparent research.
- *STROBE (http://www.strobe-statement.org/).* STROBE (STrengthening the Reporting of OBservational studies in Epidemiology):
  - It is used as a guideline for reporting observational studies, specifically cohort, case-control, and cross-sectional studies.
  - The STROBE statement consists of a 22-item checklist under the following headings: title and abstract, introduction, methods, results, discussion, and other information.
- *MOOSE (http://www.consort-statement.org/downloads):*
  - MOOSE (Meta-analysis Of Observational Studies in Epidemiology) is a guideline used for reporting meta-analyses of observational studies.
  - The result was a 35-item checklist with the following headings: background, search strategy, methods, results, discussion, and conclusion.
- *STARD (http://www.stard-statement.org/):*
  - STARD (STAndards for the Reporting of Diagnostic accuracy studies) is intended for reporting studies of diagnostic or prognostic accuracy.
  - The checklist concluded on 25 items under the following headlines: title/abstract/keywords, introduction, methods, results, and discussion.
  - A flow diagram adds to the checklist bringing information about the method used for patient recruitment and information about in which order the tests had been carried out.

Another way of securing adherence to reporting guidelines is the instruction of the Committee on Publication Ethics (COPE) Ethical Guidelines for Peer Reviewers.

Guideline	Study type	Sections	Number of items	Flow diagram
PRISMA	Systematic reviews and meta-analyses	Title; abstract; introduction; methods; results; discussion; funding	27	Yes
CONSORT	Parallel group randomized controlled trials	Title and abstract; introduction; methods; results; discussion; other information	25	Yes
STROBE	Observational studies in epidemiology	Title and abstract; introduction; methods; results; discussion; other information	22	No
MOOSE	Meta-analyses of observation studies in epidemiology	Background; search strategy; methods; results; discussion; conclusion	35	No
STARD	Studies of diagnostic accuracy	Title/abstract/keywords; introduction; methods; results; discussion	25	Yes
SPIRIT	Standard protocol items for clinical trials	Administrative information; introduction; methods; ethics and dissemination; appendices	33	No

Suggested checklist submission any article to the Journal	Yes	No
Submitted by: Email/post/both		
Covering letter and submission		
• Covering letter (in original)		
• Copyright transfer form (in original)		
• Illustrations (in original)		
• Manuscript (Email/original)		
• Category for which submitted		
• Number of authors restricted as per instructions		
• Word count restricted as per instructions.		
Presentations and formats		
• Printed on A4 paper with 1st margins on all sides in double space		
• Abstract, text, acknowledgment, what is already known and what this study adds, references, legends, and tables starting on a new page		

• *Title page contains the following:*
  – Full title of the paper
  – Short running title in 40 characters
  – Initials, surname, and highest degree of authors, affiliations
  – Name of Departments/Institution
  – Details of corresponding authors including email
  – Contributor's credit
  – Source of funding
  – Competing interests
  – Word count of the text		

Contd...

Contd...

• Abstract and key words provided (for research papers, Short communications, Perspective, Case reports, Research letters and reviews)		
• "What is already known" and "What this study adds" boxes (only for research papers and short communications)		
• References cited in parenthesis according to journals instructions.		
• Pages numbered consecutively		
• Language and grammar		
• Uniform American English		
• Abbreviations spelt out in full for first time		
• Text arranged as per IMRAD format		
• Follows style of writing in Indian pediatrics		
• Conventional units used throughout manuscript		
Tables and figures		
• No repetition of data in table/graphs and in text		
• Figures are black and white (except images), good quality; with labels on back		
• Able numbers in roman numerals and Figure numbers in Arabic numerals		
• Correct symbols used for footnotes to tables		
• Figure legends provided		
• Patient Privacy maintained		

OSCE

Swati Upadhyay, Sidharth Nayyar, Naveen Prakash Gupta

OSCE

1. **A 24-year-old G2A1 mother with "O negative" blood group has been following up in your associated antenatal clinic. Husband's blood group is "B positive". There is history of one spontaneous abortion 2 years back. Maternal ICT at 12 weeks of pregnancy was negative. Now she is 24 weeks gestation and ICT has become positive with anti-D titers 1:64.**
   a. What is the anticipated risk to baby?
   b. What is the next step in management?
   c. Would you administer anti-D to this mother?
   d. What would be the indication for cordocentesis in this case?
   e. What are the criteria for intrauterine transfusion in such cases? What are the methods for intrauterine transfusion?
   f. What investigations would you perform on the baby postnatal?
   g. This mother comes to you in next pregnancy again and anti-D titers are 1:1,028 at 18 weeks of pregnancy. How would you proceed?

2. **A 38-week male infant weighing 3,200 g was born after an uncomplicated pregnancy. The mother is a 35-year-old primipara with type A Rh-positive blood group. The baby's course in the hospital was uneventful and baby was roomed-in with mother. Although the mother needed significant help in establishing effective breastfeeding, baby was exclusively breastfed at discharge and thereafter. Prior to discharge, jaundice was noted at the age of 48 hours. The total serum bilirubin level was 10.5 mg/dL.**
   a. What are the major risk factors for development of severe hyperbilirubinemia in infants >35 weeks of gestation?
   b. What are the risk factors for neurotoxicity in babies with hyperbilirubinemia?
   c. What chart would you use predischarge to designate the risk of subsequent severe hyperbilirubinemia?
   d. What is the risk of developing subsequent severe hyperbilirubinemia in this baby? What would be your follow-up recommendation based on that?
   e. The baby was discharged at the age of 48 hours and comes to you 2 days later with marked jaundice and icterus up to soles. The results of his physical examination are

otherwise normal, but his weight is now 2,800 g. Mother reports nipple crack and breast engorgement. His total serum bilirubin level is 19.5 mg/dL and his conjugated (direct) bilirubin level 0.6 mg/dL. There is no pallor or splenomegaly. The complete blood count and peripheral with blood smear are normal. The infant has type A Rh-positive blood. What would be your next line of management?

f. What score would you use to assess the neurological status of this baby? What are its components? How do you interpret the score?

g. What is the possible reason for hyperbilirubinemia in this baby?

3. **You have started intensive phototherapy for the above-mentioned baby in room with mother. You repeat a serum bilirubin after 6 hours, but it has not dropped and is same. You visit the room and find that the baby is lying on bed and phototherapy unit is placed high above and is fixed at maximum possible distance.**

a. What corrective action would you take in this baby?

b. What is the mechanism of action of phototherapy?

c. What factors affect the dose and efficacy of phototherapy?

d. What are the criteria for defining intensive phototherapy?

e. What is the irradiance footprint of phototherapy?

f. What are the advantages of LED phototherapy over conventional phototherapy?

g. How frequently would you monitor serum bilirubin values in a baby receiving phototherapy?

h. What are the criteria for stopping phototherapy and checking rebound serum bilirubin values?

4. **A 5-day-old male newborn is admitted with severe jaundice. He is a first-born child, via cesarean delivery at a gestational age of 39^{+6} weeks, with APGAR scores of 9 at 1 and 5 minutes after birth. The blood types of both the baby and the mother are B positive. Maternal ICT was negative. Total serum bilirubin (TSB) is reported as 24.5 mg/dL. There is no cephalhematoma, bruise, or subgaleal bleed. There is no encephalopathy. Baby is otherwise well to examine. There is no significant weight loss. The glucose-6-phosphate dehydrogenase deficiency screen and direct Coombs test are negative. Blood examination shows hemoglobin level is 12.2 g/dL with a reticulocyte of 10%. There is family history of recurrent blood transfusion and gallstones in father and paternal uncle. You have started intensive phototherapy for this baby while preparing for exchange transfusion.**

a. What would be your differential diagnosis in this baby?

b. What are the diagnostic criteria for hereditary spherocytosis?

c. What is the spectrum of clinical features of HS in neonatal period?

d. What investigation would you advise to confirm the diagnosis of HS?

e. What is the most common genetic defect involved in HS?

f. What are the short- and long-term complications associated with HS?

g. What are the treatment modalities for HS? What is the definitive treatment and when should it be offered?

5. **You are following up a 3-day-old baby in your OPD. The baby was born at 38 weeks with birth weight of 2.9 kg. Mother is O positive and baby A positive. There was no jaundice in first 24 hours. Baby is exclusively breastfed and was discharged at 40 hours of life with transcutaneous bilirubin (TCB) of 6.5 mg/dL. TCB in your OPD at follow-up at 72 hours is 15.5 mg/dL. Baby is otherwise well to examine without any significant weight loss.**
   a. What would be your next step?
   b. What is the principle behind TCB?
   c. What are few pitfalls of TCB and in which conditions would you avoid using TCB?
   d. What are the indications for doing serum bilirubin while monitoring a baby with TCB?
   e. Up to what age can you do TCB in neonates?
   f. What are the common devices available?
   g. What is the latest upgrade in TCB machine and how is it different from previous version in terms of intended use?
   h. Name one more method for noninvasive measurement of bilirubin in neonates.

6. **A 28-day-old boy baby presents to you in OPD with history of high-colored urine. On enquiring, mother clearly gives history of pigmented stools. Baby is exclusively breastfed and thriving well. You note icterus and request for total and direct bilirubin. Total serum bilirubin is 15 mg/dL and direct bilirubin is 13 mg/dL. You plan to evaluate the baby for neonatal cholestasis.**
   a. What investigations would you plan for this baby?
   b. USG abdomen reveals normal gallbladder morphology and contractility and no evidence of choledochal cyst. LFT shows moderately elevated ALT and *normal GGT*. What would be your differential diagnoses?
   c. What would be your next step in managing this baby? What is the current consensus on role of HIDA scan in evaluation of neonatal cholestasis?
   d. You plan liver biopsy for this baby. Liver histology shows cholestasis, giant cell hepatitis, hepatocellular necrosis, and portal fibrosis. Biopsy specimen is subjected to immunohistochemistry which shows absent canalicular staining with BSEP antibodies. Electron microscopy showed amorphous bile. What is the most probable diagnosis?
   e. What are the medical and surgical treatment options available for this condition?
   f. What is the expected course of disease and what are the anticipated long-term complications?

7. **You have been called to attend delivery of a term baby with suspected Rh isoimmunization. Mother is A negative with positive ICT (anti-D titers 1:64) since 24 weeks of pregnancy. The baby is born and has pallor and splenomegaly. Cord bilirubin is 8 mg/dL and Hb is 7.5 g/dL. Retic count is 8%. Baby's DCT is +++. You had immediately shifted the baby to NICU and started intensive phototherapy while preparing for exchange transfusion.**
   a. What are the indications of exchange transfusion for hyperbilirubinemia in neonates?
   b. What percentage of circulating RBCs are removed by double volume exchange transfusion? How much drop in bilirubin levels is expected by DVET?
   c. Baby's blood group is B positive. What type of blood would you use for exchange transfusion in this baby?

d. Baby's weight is 3 kg. How would you calculate the amount of blood needed for double volume exchange transfusion?

e. What are the complications associated with exchange transfusion?

f. You have requested the blood bank for desired blood product and type, but it is not available anywhere at present. What would you do?

g. What are the indications of IV immunoglobulin in neonatal jaundice?

8. **A 19-day-old term born 3.2 kg birth weight baby boy has been brought to you with complain of yellowish discoloration of body. The baby was born by cesarean section. You note that baby is icteric till soles. The baby had already received phototherapy twice after birth for serum bilirubin of 18 and 22 mg/dL on days 4 and 9 of life. The baby is thriving well. There is no pallor, no hepatosplenomegaly. There is no cephalhematoma, bruising, or any evidence of concealed bleed. Baby has been on breastfeeds as well as formula feeds. Baby's vitals are stable. There is no setting of blood group incompatibility. Baby's DCT is negative, and CBC is WNL. You request for a total serum bilirubin, and it is 22 mg/dL again with direct bilirubin only 0.5 mg/dL.**

a. What additional investigations would you carry out?

b. What are the probable causes of marked prolonged unconjugated hyperbilirubinemia in neonates?

c. G-6-P-D levels for this baby are very low. What advice would you give to the family?

d. How is the neonatal presentation of G-6-P-D deficiency different from classical presentation later?

e. What are the congenital nonhemolytic unconjugated hyperbilirubinemia clinical syndromes? Which of these has most severe presentation and what is the definitive treatment for same?

9. **A term 38-week gestation, boy baby with birth weight 2,920 g was born to a 28-year-old primigravida mother by cesarean section for fetal distress. It was a booked pregnancy with regular antenatal visits and normal antenatal ultrasounds. Breastfeeding was initiated at 3 hours of life and continued thereafter. Baby passed urine and stools on the first day of life. Baby was noted to have icterus till soles on day 3 of life. The baby was admitted in NICU, and phototherapy was started. Investigations showed TSB of 26.2 mg/dL with direct fraction of 1.2 mg/dL at 72 hours of life. Baby had pallor and splenomegaly of 2 cm below LCM. There was no encephalopathy, no cephalhematoma or bruise. The blood group of the baby and both the parents was type A Rh (+). Direct Coombs test of the baby was positive (++++). Hemoglobin was 12 g/dL. Glucose-6-phosphate dehydrogenase enzyme levels were normal. Peripheral smear showed evidence of hemolysis with reticulocyte count of 8.5%. Maternal ICT was positive.**

a. What would be your most probable diagnosis?

b. What investigations would you plan in this baby to confirm the diagnosis?

c. What are the current recommendations for routine antibody screening during pregnancy?

d. You did exchange transfusion in this baby along with intensive phototherapy. Now the baby is ready for discharge after 1 week of hospital stay. How would you plan the long-term follow-up for this baby?

10. **A 28-day-old well thriving neonate has come to you for routine follow-up visit. Mother does not have any medical concerns. However, as a routine practice, you ask the color of stool and mother says it is "white". She takes out the diaper and you find pale unpigmented stool. You plan to evaluate the baby. Laboratory tests reveal conjugated hyperbilirubinemia and a raised GGT. Next you plan an USG abdomen.**
    a. What USG findings would suggest biliary atresia?
    b. What are the clinical forms of biliary atresia?
    c. What are the characteristic histologic features in biliary atresia?
    d. What is the initial surgical management? Before what age should it be preferably done to achieve best outcomes?
    e. How would you medically support this baby?
    f. What are the ways to reduce the risk of ascending cholangitis after surgery? What are its clinical implications?
    g. When will you refer this baby for liver transplantation?
    h. What screening method may be utilized in office practice for early detection of biliary atresia?

11. **A neonate is admitted with complain of poor feeding, lethargy, and fast breathing on day 21 of life. On examination, baby has tachycardia, tachypnea, CFT 2 seconds, and normal BP. The ECG of this baby is as shown in Figure 1.**
    a. What is the diagnosis?
    b. What is the drug of choice? What is its serum half-life?
    c. Write the dose and technique by which this drug is administered.
    d. The baby did not respond to this drug and developed cold peripheries and hypotension. How will you manage this baby now?
    e. What are the indications for long-term medical treatment of this condition? Which drugs are used for chronic medical treatment?

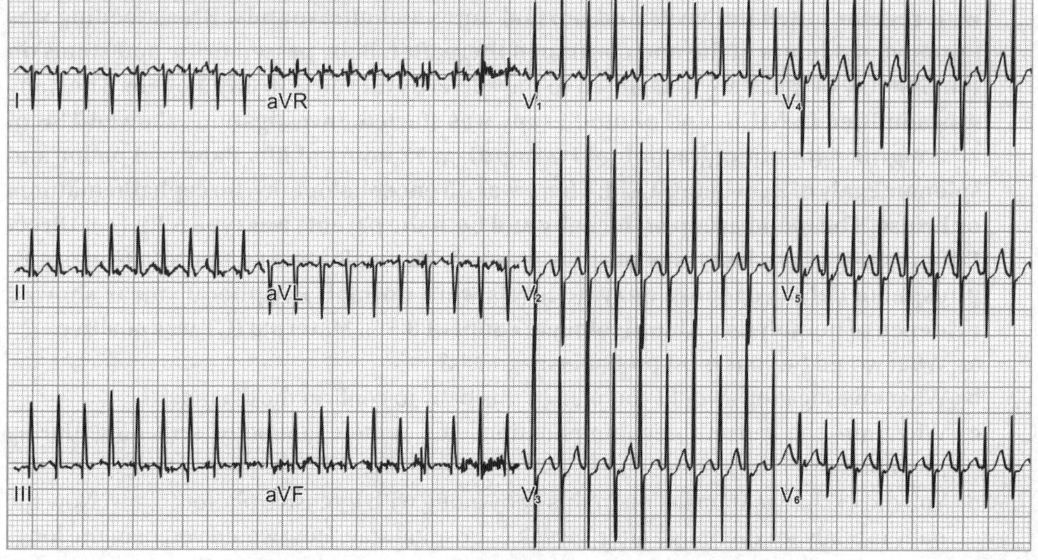

Fig. 1

12. **A 10-day-old neonate is admitted in ER with fine rash over periorbital area. On systemic examination, baby is noted to have irregular heart rhythm. ECG of this baby is as shown in Figure 2. Laboratory evaluation shows raised transaminases.**

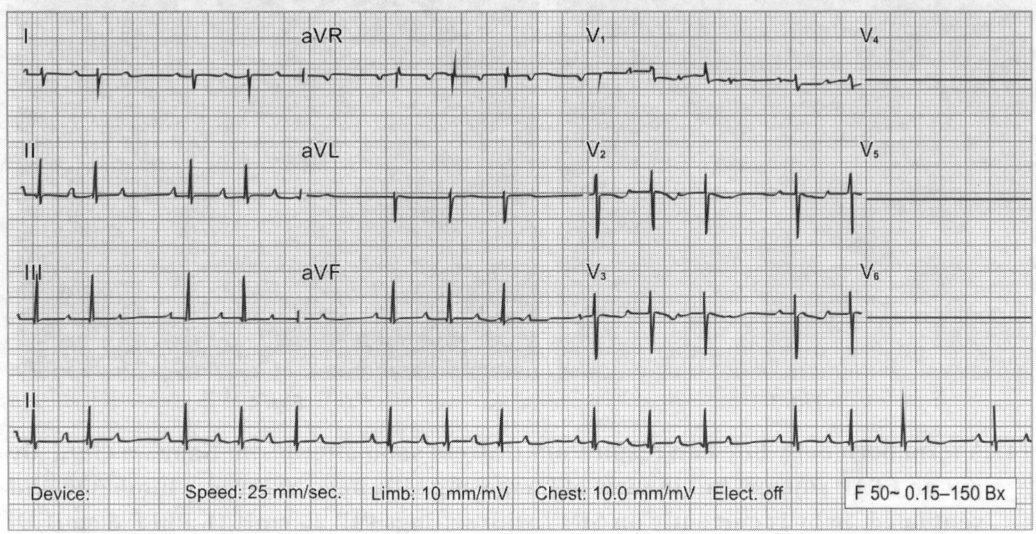

Fig. 2

   a. Interpret the ECG.
   b. What is the probable diagnosis? What investigation would you do to confirm the diagnosis?
   c. What is the underlying pathogenesis of the disease?
   d. What are the indications for permanent pacemaker implantation in neonates?

13. **A 27-week 980 g preterm baby on SIMV ventilation has worsening clinical condition on day 3 of life. Baby has increasing FiO_2, and pressure requirements and pinkish secretions are noted in ET tube. Heart rate is 170/min. Baby has low diastolic pressure and dorsalis pedis is well felt. Sepsis screen is negative.**

   a. What is your probable clinical diagnosis?
   b. 2D ECHO is planned and images are as shown below. Identify the view in **Figure 3**. What are the ECHO findings suggestive of?
   c. Identify the view and structures labeled in **Figure 4**. Which important parameter related to above clinical condition is measured in this view and how is it measured? What is the clinical utility of this parameter?
   d. What neonatal complications may be associated with this condition?
   e. What drugs are used for medical management of this condition? What are the side effects associated with these drugs?

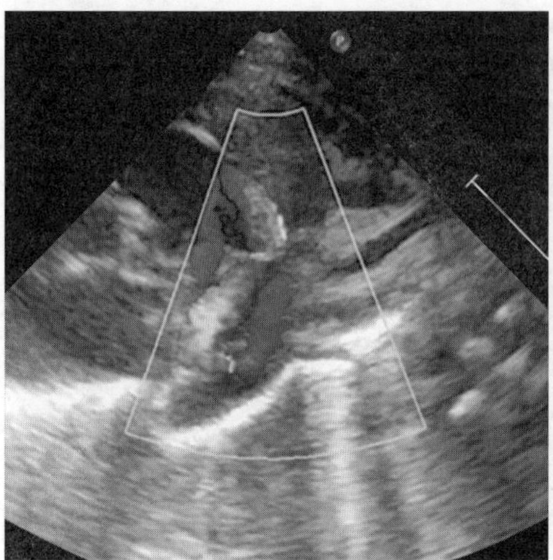
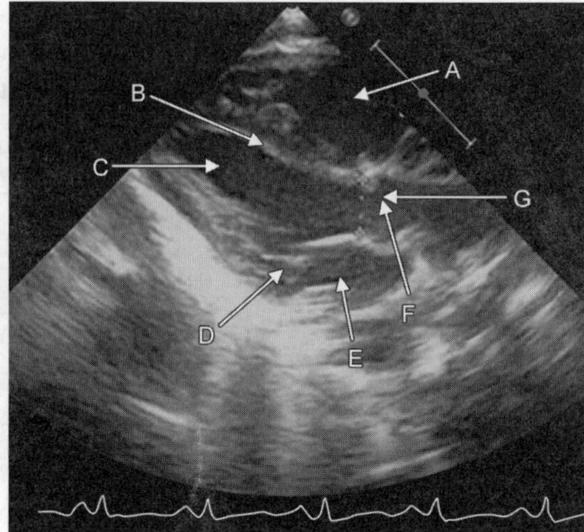

Fig. 3   Fig. 4

14. **A term born baby boy had respiratory distress soon after birth. Baby was initially put on CPAP support but in view of increasing FiO_2 need, baby was intubated and ventilated. Baby is currently on SIMV with settings PIP 25 cmH_2O, PEEP 6 cmH_2O, MAP 12 cmH_2O FiO_2 100%, rate 60 bpm. SpO_2 is between 80 and 85%, pulses are well felt, CFT <3 seconds and mean BP 55 mm Hg. C-X-ray showed appropriately placed ET with bilateral eight posterior intercostal spaces, no collapse, and no pneumothorax. Blood gas revealed pH 7.3, PaO_2 50 mm Hg, pCO_2 45 mm Hg, HCO_3 17. A 2D ECHO is planned. Based on echocardiographic assessment of ductal and atrial shunts, what would be your differential diagnoses and treatment considerations in scenarios a, b, and c mentioned below?**

    a. Right-to-left shunt at the ductal and atrial level.

    b. Right-to-left shunt at the ductal level but a left-to-right shunt at the atrial level.

    c. Left-to-right shunt at ductal level but a right-to-left shunt at the atrial level.

15. **The above-mentioned baby had labile hypoxemia and right-to-left shunt at both ductal and atrial level. 2D ECHO is as shown in Figure 5.**

    a. Identify the view and abnormality. What is your diagnosis?

    b. TR jet velocity is 3.99 m/s. Calculate the pulmonary artery systolic pressure in this baby.

    c. Calculate OI in this baby based on above parameters.

    d. What would be your line of management in this baby based on OI?

    e. What parameter for assessment of RV systolic function is being measured in view shown in **Figure 6**? What value is considered normal in term neonates and what value indicates severe pulmonary hypertension?

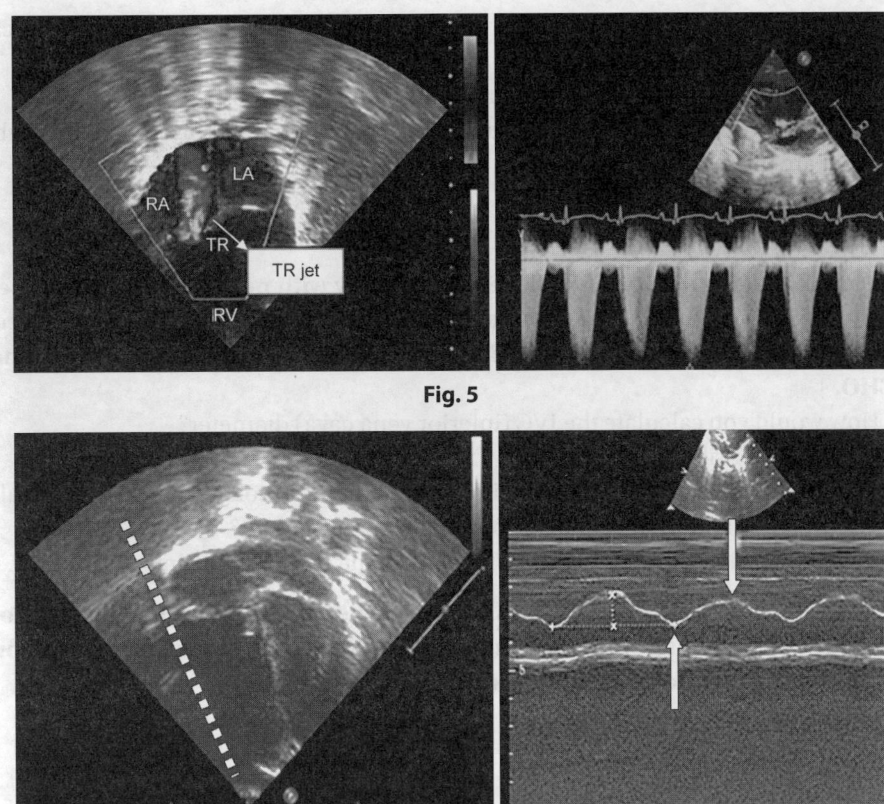

Fig. 5

Fig. 6

16. **A 3-kg baby boy, term born, developed cyanosis within first few hours of life. SpO$_2$ is 70% and hypoxia is unresponsive to oxygen. Auscultation revealed loud single S2. Chest X-ray revealed narrow mediastinum with slight predominance of right ventricle. 2D ECHO is done and PLAX view is as shown in Figure 7. The vessel arising from LV is traced and Figure 8 demonstrates its bifurcation.**

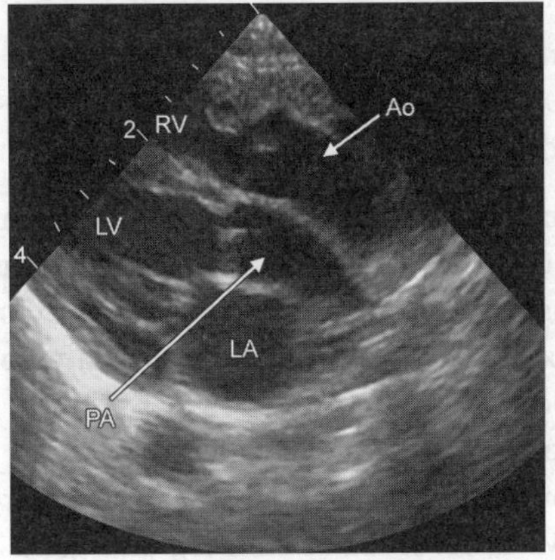

Fig. 7

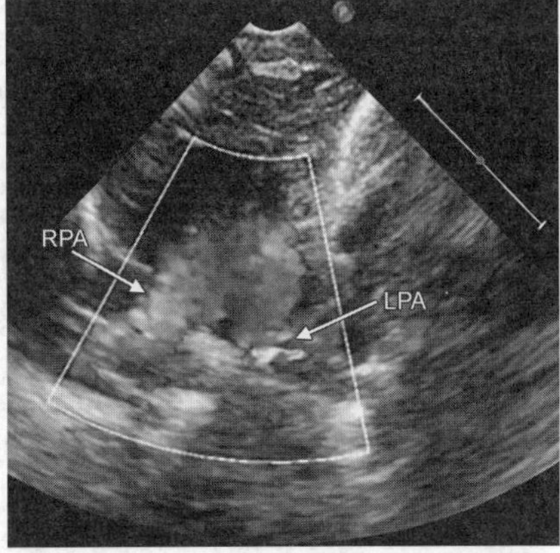

Fig. 8

a. What is the diagnosis? What percentage of these babies may have extracardiac malformations?
b. What will be the initial management in this baby?
c. Write the dose and adverse effects of drug used for initial stabilization in this baby.
d. What are the indications of balloon atrial septostomy?
e. What is the definitive treatment?
f. What is the ideal timing of surgery in lesions with intact ventricular septum?

17. **You are managing a critically sick ventilated baby with perinatal asphyxia. The baby has borderline perfusion. You want to assess the intravascular fluid status for deciding total fluid intake in this baby and decide to perform point of care ultrasound and ECHO.**
    a. How would you calculate the IVC (inferior vena cava) diameter?
    b. What is distensibility index of IVC?
    c. The diameter of IVC in this baby is 7 mm with >50% collapsibility. How would you interpret this and what would be your line of management?
    d. What are the key findings in favor of hypovolemia on 2D ECHO imaging?

18. **Given below are few drugs used for managing cardiopulmonary conditions in neonates. Write in one word, their mechanism of action/name of the receptor they act upon. Also mention important side effect of each drug.**
    a. Sildenafil
    b. Levosimendan
    c. Bosentan
    d. Digoxin

19. **A sick neonate is being ventilated postoperatively after cardiac surgery. The baby has signs of poor perfusion and is receiving dopamine and dobutamine 10 µg/kg/min, but there is no significant improvement. Baby still has cold peripheries, CFT 4 seconds but mean BP is 60 mm Hg. Bedside ECHO is suggestive of LV dysfunction and a low-cardiac output state. You decide to start milrinone based on clinical and ECHO findings.**
    a. What is the mechanism of action of milrinone?
    b. What is the half-life of this drug?
    c. What is the immediate and most common side effect of milrinone?
    d. What are the indications for using milrinone in neonates?
    e. What is the primary route of excretion of this drug?

20. **A 2-hour-old term neonate with meconium aspiration syndrome is being ventilated. Currently baby is on SIMV PIP 22 cmH$_2$O, PEEP 6 cmH$_2$O rate 50 bpm, and FiO$_2$ 100%. Baby has labile oxygen saturations, ranging from 80 to 90%. X-ray of chest shows bilateral diffuse patchy opacities, six posterior intercostal spaces and low-lung volume. Currently, baby's perfusion is good.**
    a. What is the first step you will take to manage hypoxia in this baby?
    b. Baby stabilizes after your intervention but after 6 hours, baby again has very labile oxygen saturations. 2D echo is suggestive of RVSP of 48 mm Hg and good cardiac function. Clinically, baby also has signs of poor perfusion and low blood pressure

(mean BP 34 mm Hg). X-ray chest shows adequate lung expansion. What will be your line of management now?

c. What are the indications of ECMO in a neonate with persistent hypoxemia?

21. **A 3-week-old baby girl was admitted in NICU with respiratory distress of 4 days duration. She was born at term and birth weight was 3.2 kg. She had passed her CCHD pulse oximetry screen and metabolic screen and was discharged on day 3 of life. Her current weight is 2.8 kg. There is no history of fever, cough, cold, vomiting, and diarrhea. Mother reveals that baby has severe forehead sweating during feeding and there is history of suck-rest-suck cycle. On examination, she looks pale but alert. Her heart rate is 176 beats/min, oxygen saturation 88% on room air and 96% with 25% FiO_2. RR 80 breaths/min, with subcostal and intercostal retractions, pulse volume is good, and blood pressure—72/45 (52) mm Hg. There is a loud pansystolic murmur in the tricuspid region with loud S2, and ejection systolic murmur in pulmonary area. There is hepatomegaly of 4 cm below the right costal margin.**

a. What is your clinical diagnosis?

b. What would be your immediate line of management in this baby?

c. 2D ECHO revealed a 4 mm VSD and 3 mm ostium secundum ASD. How would you follow-up this baby?

d. What are the indications for ASD closure? What are the techniques available for ASD closure?

e. What are the indications for VSD closure and what is the preferred modality?

22. **A 14-day-old neonate is brought to the ER with irritability for last 3 hours. On evaluation temperature is normal, there is marked tachycardia, CFT 3 seconds, and pulses are well palpable. SpO_2 is 95% on room air. The infant is on exclusive breastfeeds. ECG is as shown in Figure 9.**

a. Interpret the ECG. What is your diagnosis?

b. What medical conditions can precipitate this in neonates?

c. What are the differential diagnoses of wide QRS complex tachycardia in neonates?

d. What drugs are used for managing this condition?

e. This baby did not respond to medical therapy and developed hypotension after 4 hours. What would be the treatment of choice now?

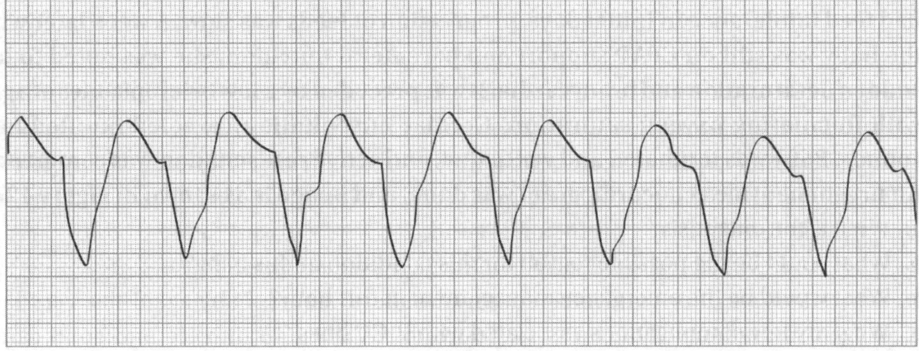

Fig. 9

23. A term neonate, AGA, presented with tachypnea and cyanosis 6 hours after birth. Baby had cried soon after birth, no history of meconium aspiration and no antenatal risk factors for sepsis. SpO_2 was 85% on room air, HR 168/min, RR 68/min, mean BP 50 mm Hg, and there is hepatomegaly 3 cm below RCM. Chest X-ray was suggestive of massive cardiomegaly as shown in Figure 10. 2D ECHO is done and apical four chamber view is as shown in Figure 11.

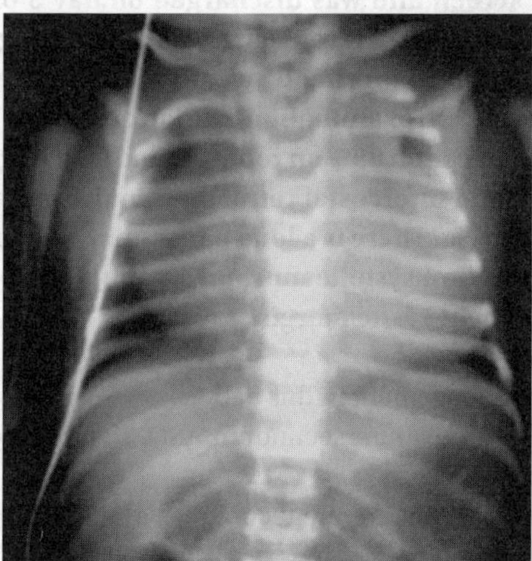
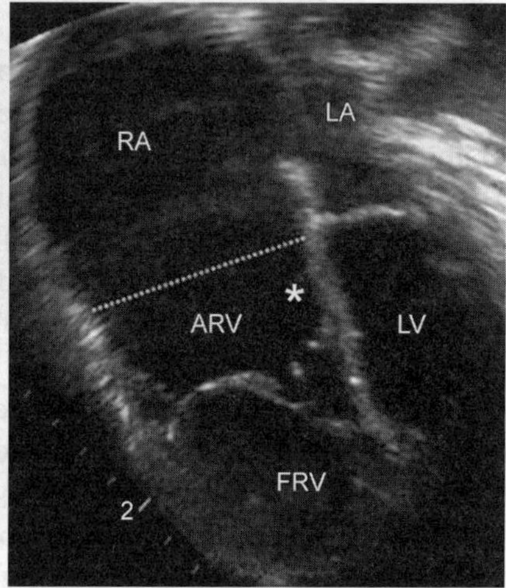

Fig. 10   Fig. 11

a. What are the ECHO findings in **Figure 11** and what is the most probable diagnosis?
b. What is GOSE score and what is its clinical utility?
c. What drugs are used for medical management of these babies?
d. This baby had worsening clinical condition after starting prostaglandin infusion. What could be the possible reason?
e. What are the indications for surgical intervention in neonates?
f. What other cardiac problems would you monitor these babies for?

24. A preterm neonate, 29 weeks, 1.1 kg, was being cared for in NICU. She had severe RDS requiring two doses of surfactant and mechanical ventilation for 2 days, followed by CPAP support. She was started on minimal enteral nutrition and was receiving parenteral nutrition through a PICC line inserted via right antecubital fossa. As she had feed intolerance in initial days, progression of feeds was slow. A week later whilst the baby was still on CPAP support and parenteral nutrition, she was noted to have sudden desaturation and bradycardia. It was preceded by a few brief episodes of apnea with fluctuating oxygen saturation. Cardiac auscultation revealed muffled heart sounds. Baby was intubated and ventilated, and active resuscitation was commenced. An urgent bedside echocardiogram was done, and image is as shown in Figure 12.
a. What is the diagnosis?
b. What could be the possible reason for this condition in this baby?
c. What would be the emergency management in this baby?
d. What are few complications associated with PICC lines?

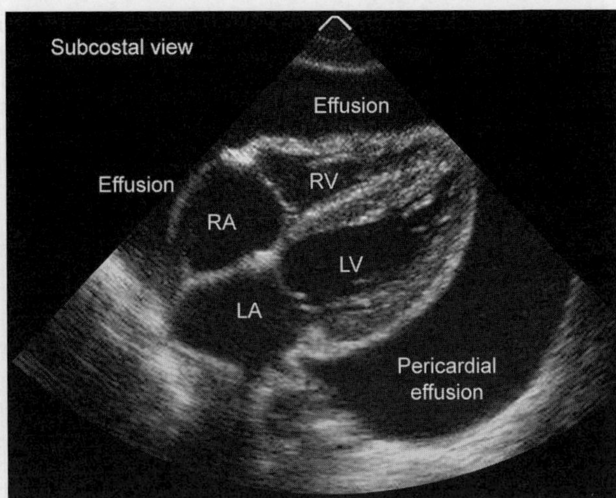

Fig. 12

25. A 1-month-old neonate was admitted with feeding difficulties and respiratory distress. Hypotonia and generalized areflexia were observed during examination. Laboratory evaluation showed elevated creatine kinase levels. Chest X-ray, ECG, and 2D ECHO are as shown in Figures 13 to 15, respectively.
    a. What are the findings in chest X-ray, ECG, and ECHO?
    b. What is the probable diagnosis?
    c. How would you confirm the diagnosis?
    d. What is the definitive treatment for this condition?

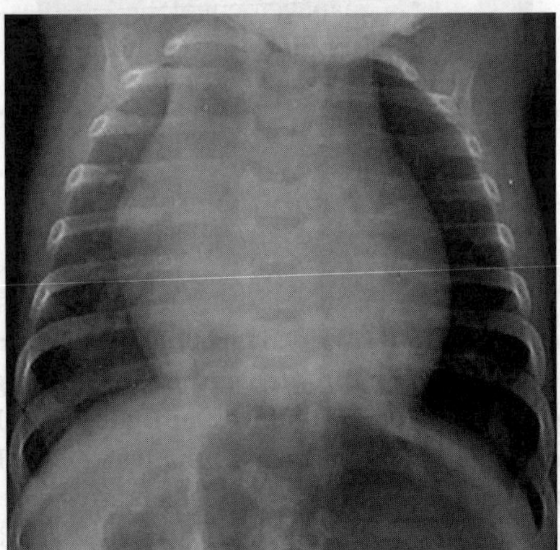

Fig. 13

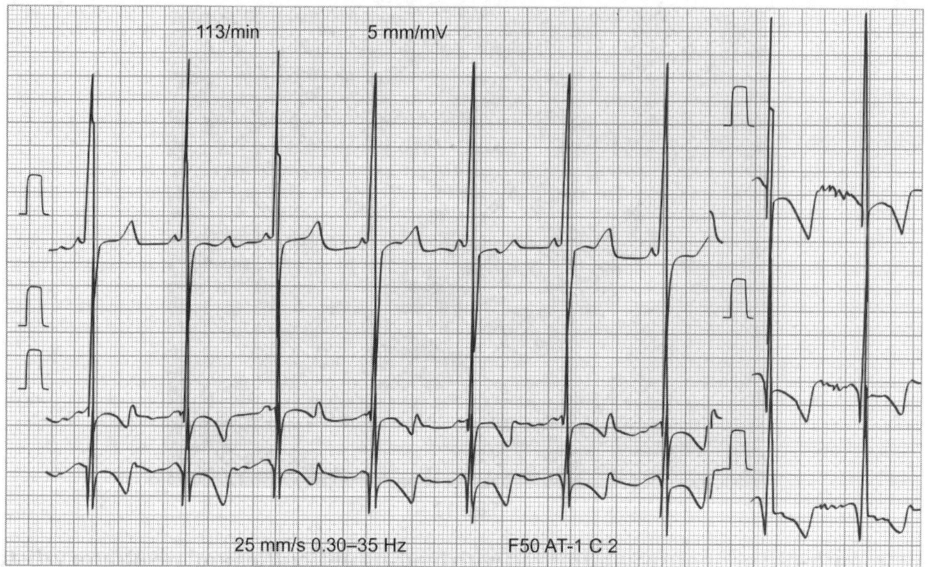

Fig. 14

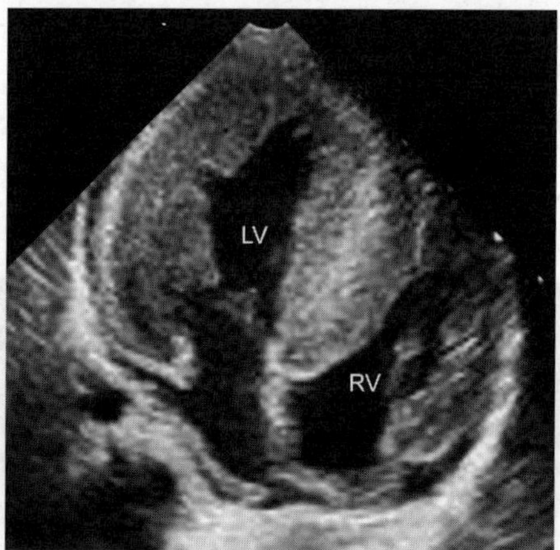

Fig. 15

26. **You are called by nursing staff to review a term born, 36-hour-old well baby. Baby is feeding well and has passed urine and meconium. The nursing staff performed pulse oximetry screening and reported SpO$_2$ of 97% in right upper limb and 92% in lower limb. You examined the baby and performed the test again. The findings are same. Baby's vitals are otherwise stable.**

   a. How would you interpret this pulse oximetry screening result? What would be your next step?

   b. Name five congenital heart defects which can be diagnosed or strongly suspected on basis of pulse oximetry screening results.

   c. What law is pulse oximetry based upon?

   d. What are the advantages of signal extraction technology in pulse oximetry?

e. At what SpO_2 range is pulse oximetry most reliable?

f. Name two conditions with reversal of differential cyanosis (preductal SpO_2 less than postductal SpO_2).

27. **Below is the drug prescribed to a 20-day-old neonate (Figure 16).**

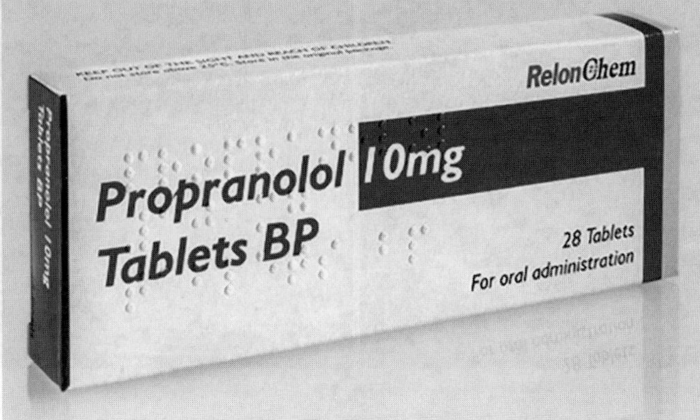

Fig. 16

a. What is the mechanism of action of this drug?

b. Which class of antiarrhythmic is propranolol, according to Voughan William classification?

c. What are the indications for use of propranolol in neonates?

d. What is the dose of propranolol in neonates?

e. What would you monitor after starting propranolol therapy in a neonate?

28. **A 27-day-old neonate presented with tachypnea, poor feeding, cold peripheries, and lethargy. On evaluation, baby was critically sick. RR 80/min, HR 176/min, SpO_2 75% on room air, CFT 3 seconds, peripheries cold, pulses feeble, mean BP 40 mm Hg. Baby had hepatomegaly 4 cm below RCM. Baby was intubated and mechanically ventilated and initiated on antiheart failure treatment. Chest X-ray revealed cardiomegaly. 2D ECHO ruled out structural heart defect and was suggestive of marked left ventricular (LV) dilatation with global hypokinesia. LV fractional shortening was 15% and LV ejection fraction (LVEF) 25%. LA dilated, and the mitral valve leaflets showed sluggish movement. The baby was discharged after 25 days with furosemide and ACE inhibitors. During the follow-up period, the baby had two episodes of decompensated heart failure again and had failure to thrive.**

a. What is the diagnosis?

b. What are the probable causes of this condition in neonates?

c. How would you evaluate such babies?

d. What is the long-term prognosis in these babies?

e. What are the indications for cardiac transplantation in these infants?

29. **A term 3.2-kg boy baby was brought to the ER on day 10 of life with a history of poor feeding and lethargy. On examination, he was mottled with poor peripheral pulses. An ejection systolic murmur was appreciated. Bilateral femoral pulses were not**

palpable, and he was hypotensive. 2D ECHO was done after primary stabilization and arch view is as shown in Figure 17.

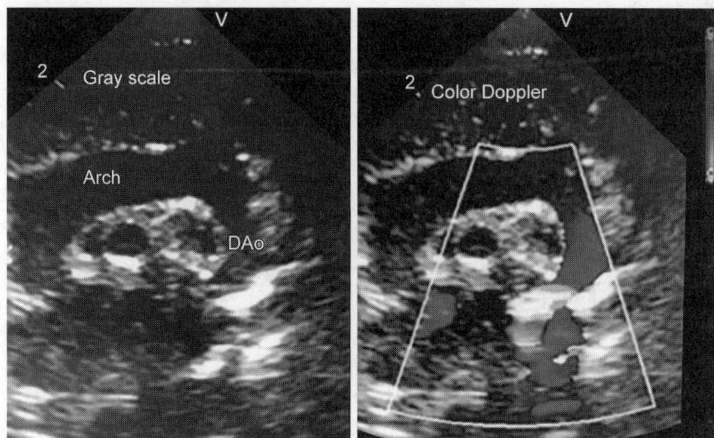

Fig. 17

a. Describe the ECHO finding.

b. What is the diagnosis?

c. What drug will you immediately start to improve the systemic circulation in this baby?

d. What would be the definitive treatment of choice in this condition?

e. What are the risks associated with balloon angioplasty of native coarctation in early infancy?

f. What percentage of babies will have recurrence of this condition? How is it managed later?

30. What are the most common cardiac defects found in chromosomal anomalies and syndromes mentioned below?

a. Trisomy 18

b. Trisomy 21

c. Turner's syndrome

d. Noonan's syndrome

e. DiGeorge's syndrome (deletion 22q11)

f. CHARGE syndrome

31. a. Identify the abnormality in this waveform (Figure 18).

b. What complications can occur due to this abnormality?

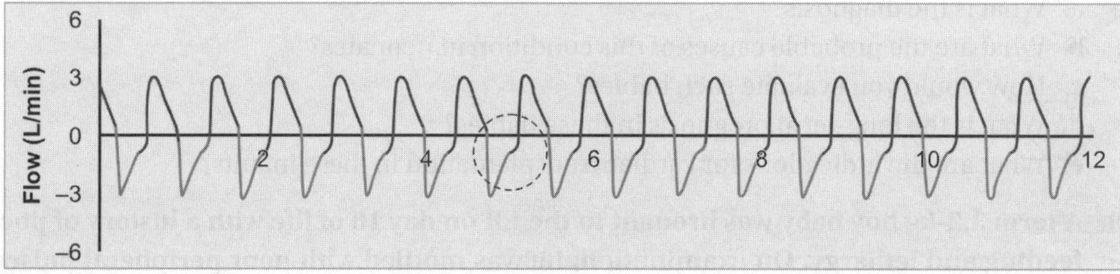

Fig. 18

32. **A term born baby girl is noted to have progressive respiratory distress after birth (Fig. 19).**
    a. What is the diagnosis here?
    b. What investigation will you do to confirm the diagnosis?
    c. What is the definitive management for this condition?
    d. During anesthesia induction, the infant is noted to be blue. What could be the possible reason?

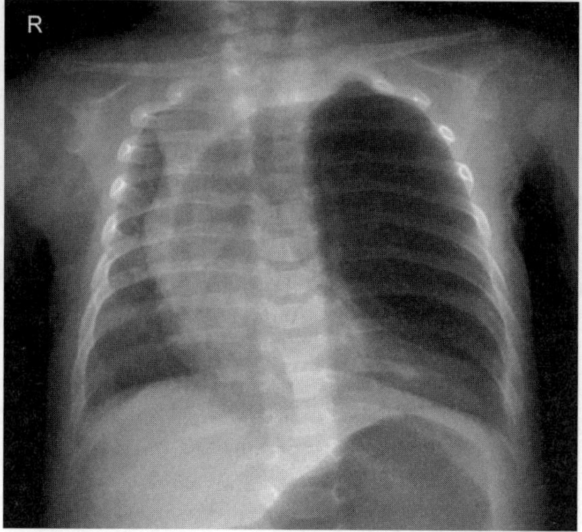

Fig. 19

33. **Below are shown two graphs.**
    a. Identify the graphs below **(Figs. 20 and 21)** and mention their use in ventilated babies.
    b. Identify phases of respiration shown in A and B in **Figure 20**.
    c. Name two possible events that occurred between arrows 1 and 2 **(Fig. 21)** in a ventilated baby.

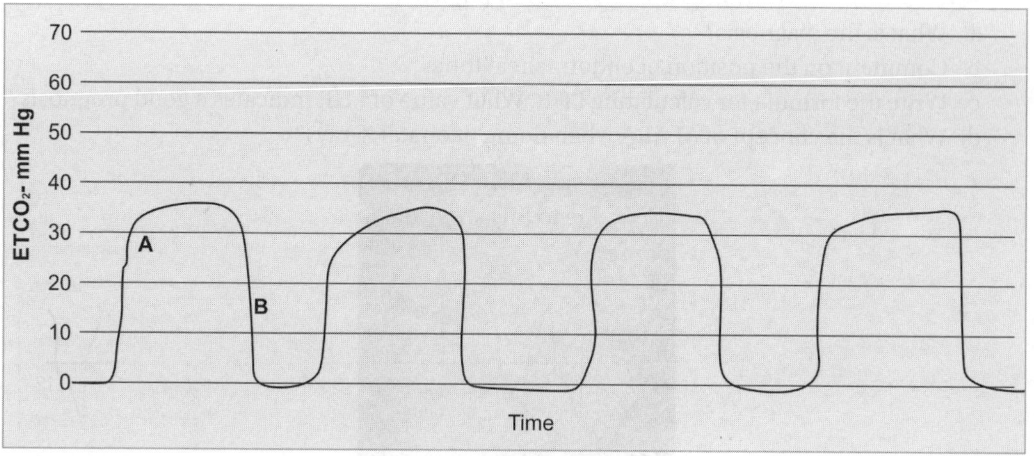

Fig. 20

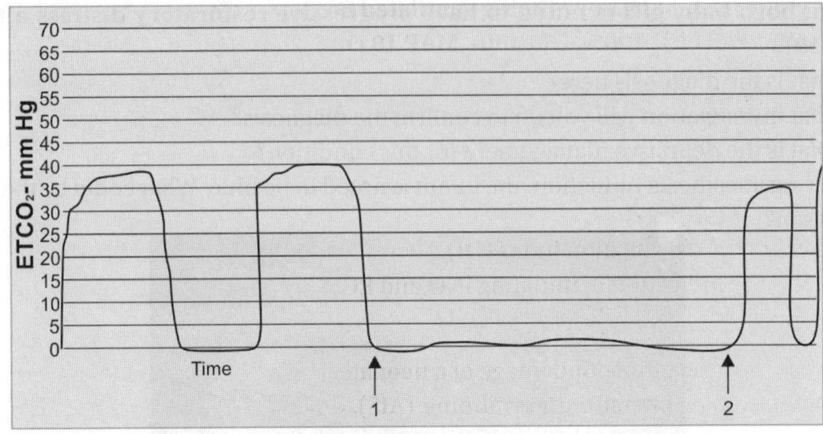

Fig. 21

34. **Consider the following two ABG analyses of two ventilated term babies:**

Baby A	Baby B
pH 7.40	pH 7.30
pCO_2 35 mm Hg	pCO_2 74 mm Hg
pO_2 75 mm Hg	pO_2 50 mm Hg
SaO_2 92%	SaO_2 80%
Hb 6 g%	Hb 13 g%

   a. How do you calculate arterial oxygen content?

   b. Which of the above two babies is more hypoxic and why?

   c. What is the normal value of arterial oxygen content?

35. **A term born baby boy 3.2 kg, is born floppy and gets intubated in labor room. Baby is ventilated and put on SIMV mode of ventilation with PIP 17, PEEP 6, FiO_2 40%, and rate 40/min. Chest radiograph is shown in Figure 22.**

   a. What is the diagnosis?

   b. Comment on the position of endotracheal tube.

   c. Write the formula for calculating LHR. What value of LHR indicates a good prognosis?

   d. What is the concept of ALARA when doing neonatal X-rays?

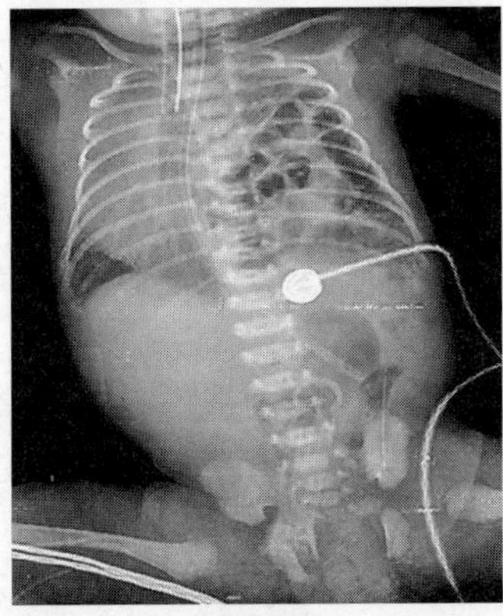

Fig. 22

36. A 2-day-old-term baby boy is being ventilated for MAS with PPHN on SIMV mode with PIP 28, PEEP 6, FiO_2 100%, f 50/min, MAP 18 cmH_2O. ABG is as given below.

    pH 7.21

    pCO_2 54 mm Hg

    pO_2 44 mm Hg

    HCO_3 13 mmol/L

    a. Interpret this ABG.
    b. Calculate the oxygenation index (OI).
    c. What is the indication of initiating iNO and ECMO based on OI?

37.

    a. Here is the lung ultrasound image of a neonate. Identify A, B, and C (**Fig. 23**).
    b. Define alveolar interstitium syndrome (AIS), white lung and comet tail sign seen in neonatal lung ultrasound.

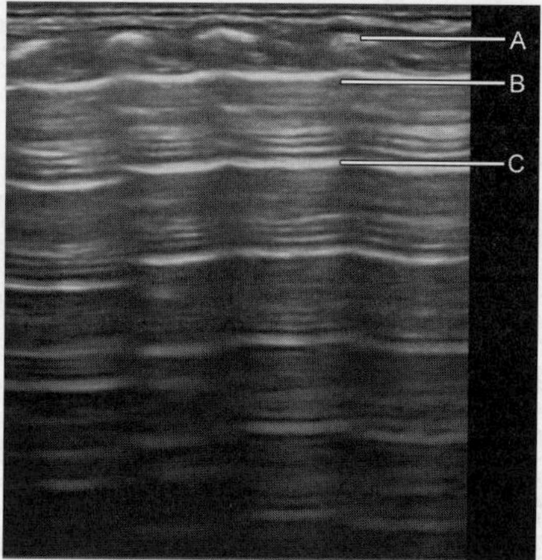

Fig. 23

38.

    a. Identify the loops shown in **Figures 24 and 25**.
    b. Identify A and B in **Figure 25**.
    c. What abnormality is seen in **Figure 25**?
    d. What could be the possible reasons for this abnormality?

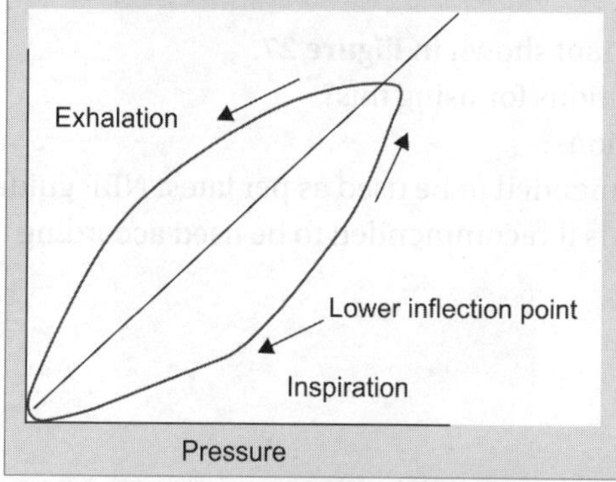

Fig. 24

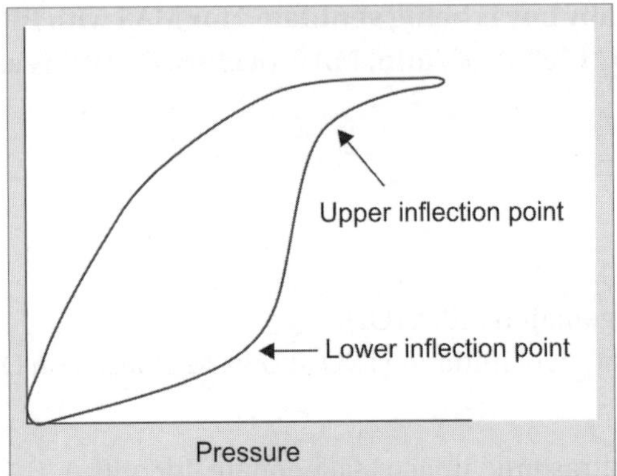

Fig. 25

39. **A late preterm baby 2.5 kg had respiratory distress soon after birth. Baby was noted to have frothy secretions. Chest radiograph is shown in Figure 26.**
   a. Identify the condition.
   b. What is the Spitz classification for prognostication in these babies?
   c. What two findings in antenatal ultrasound would raise the suspicion of this condition?

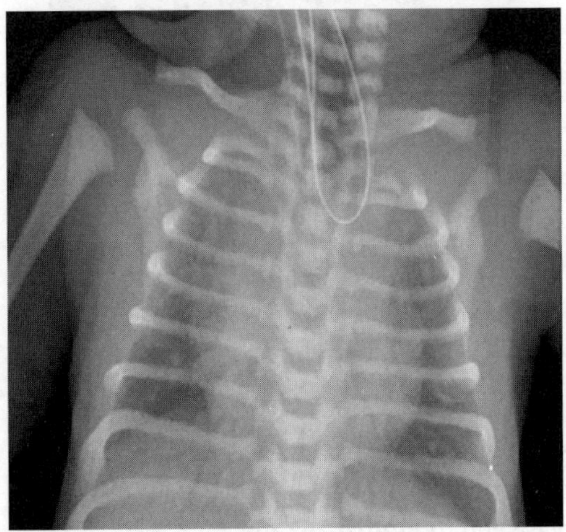

Fig. 26

40.
   a. Identify the equipment shown in **Figure 27**.
   b. What are the indications for using this?
   c. What are its limitations?
   d. What size is recommended to be used as per latest NRP guidelines?
   e. Above what weight is it recommended to be used according to latest NRP guidelines?

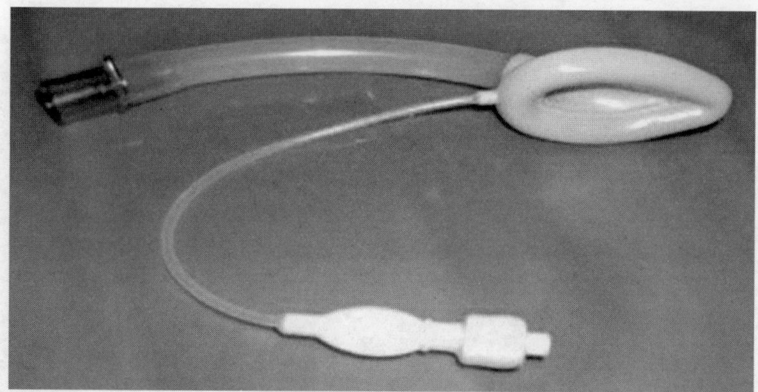

Fig. 27

41. **You have been called to attend delivery of a term baby. Baby is born limp. You have provided warmth, dried, stimulated, positioned the head and neck, and cleared the airway of secretions. It is now 60 seconds after birth and the baby is still apneic and limp.**
    a. What is your next action?
    b. What concentration of oxygen will you use to start positive-pressure ventilation in this baby?
    c. What ventilation rate should be used during positive pressure ventilation?
    d. How much pressure should be used to start positive pressure ventilation?
    e. How do you evaluate the baby's response to positive pressure ventilation?

42. **You have been called to attend delivery of 35-year-old mother with some ultrasonographic abnormalities. The baby is born limp and does not improve after initial steps. You have started positive-pressure ventilation in this baby. After 15 seconds, the heart rate is 40 beats per minute and is not improving. Your assistant does not see chest movement.**
    a. What will be your next step?
    b. The baby required prolonged bag and mask ventilation and you decide to insert OG tube to deflate the stomach. How would you measure the length to be inserted?
    c. You decide to intubate this baby and capnography is available at your center. What change in color of CO_2 detector would suggest inflation and aeration of the lungs appropriately?
    d. The baby had micrognathia and intubation attempts are unsuccessful. You decide to insert a laryngeal mask airway. Up to what landmark would you insert the laryngeal mask into the baby's mouth?

43. **Follow the figure.**
    a. Identify the equipment shown in **Figure 28**.
    b. Identify the parts labeled in **Figure 28**.

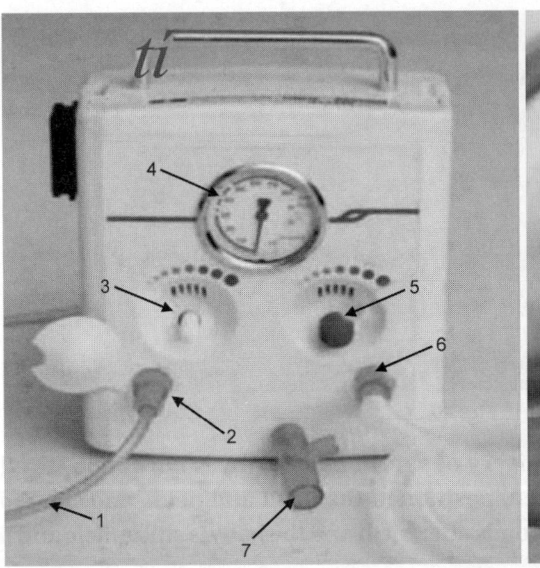
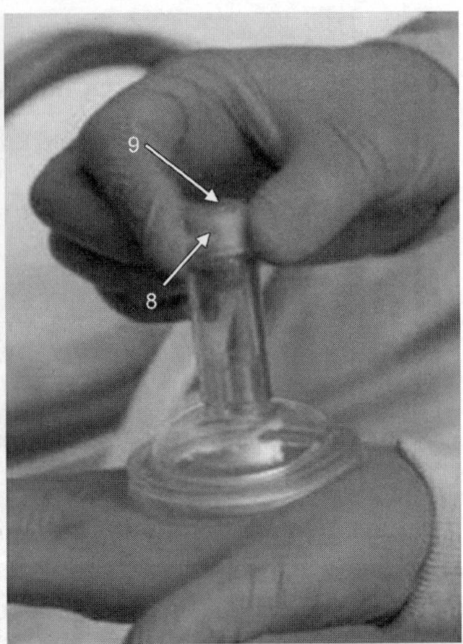

Fig. 28

44. **Your team is called to attend the birth for a woman at 36 weeks' gestation whose pregnancy and labor is complicated by preeclampsia, intrauterine growth restriction, and a category II fetal heart rate pattern. The amniotic fluid is clear. After birth, the obstetrician dries and stimulates the baby, but the baby remains limp and apneic. The umbilical cord is clamped and cut, and the baby is moved to the radiant warmer. You finish drying the baby, provide brief additional stimulation, and position and clear secretions from the airway, but the baby is still not breathing. Within 1 minute of birth, you start positive-pressure ventilation (PPV) with 21% oxygen. After 15 seconds, the heart rate is not increasing, and chest is not moving. You initiate the ventilation corrective steps, but baby is not improving, and you decide to intubate the baby. Baby's weight is around 2.2 kg.**

   a. Identify the important anatomic landmarks in the neonatal airway as shown in **Figure 29**.
   b. What are the indications for endotracheal intubation other than being an alternative airway?
   c. What endotracheal size tube would you use in this baby and how would you estimate the depth of insertion?
   d. Within how much time should you complete the endotracheal intubation procedure?
   e. Baby's condition worsens after endotracheal intubation. What could be the four possible causes?
   f. You have inserted a laryngoscope and are attempting intubation. You see the view depicted in **Figure 30**. What action would you take to visualize the glottis?

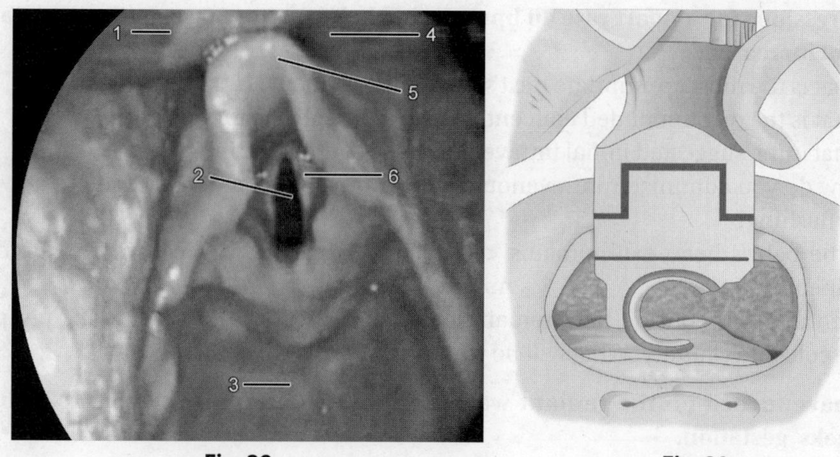

Fig. 29   **Fig. 30**

45. **A newborn is apneic at birth. The baby does not improve with the initial steps and positive-pressure ventilation. An endotracheal tube is inserted, and chest is moving well. After 30 seconds of effective PPV, the heart rate is remaining 40 beats per minute.**
    a. What will be your next step?
    b. Mark the area on the baby shown in **Figure 31**, where you would apply chest compressions.
    c. What is the correct depth of chest compressions?
    d. What important things should you consider when starting chest compressions?
    e. After how much time would you assess the baby's heart rate response once you have started chest compressions?

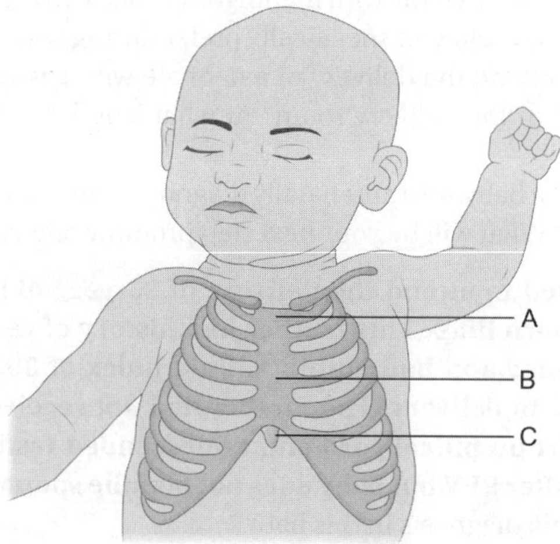

Fig. 31

46. **You are called to attend delivery of a term baby with maternal history of abruptio placentae. Baby is born limp and pale. During resuscitation, you have established adequate ventilation with an endotracheal tube and your colleague has begun chest**

compressions for a heart rate 40 bpm. Nevertheless, after 60 seconds, the heart rate has not increased.

a. What is the most appropriate next step in management?
b. What is the recommended concentration of epinephrine for newborns?
c. What is the suggested initial intravenous dose of epinephrine?
d. How do you administer intravenous epinephrine? What amount of saline do you use for flushing?
e. If the baby's heart rate remains <60 beats per minute, you can repeat the dose of epinephrine every ____________ minutes.
f. Even after epinephrine, baby remains pale, heart rate is not improving, and peripheries are cold and clammy. What will be your next step?

47. **You have turned on the radiant warmer in anticipation of the birth of a baby at 27 weeks' gestation.**
    a. List four additional steps that will help maintain this baby's temperature.
    b. After initial steps, baby needs positive pressure ventilation. What is preferred device to provide positive pressure ventilation in this baby?
    c. What FiO_2 will you use to initiate PPV?
    d. What should be the position of baby's leg as compared to head to decrease neurologic injury in a premature newborn during and after resuscitation?

48. **Miscellaneous scenarios:**
    a. A newborn has respiratory distress after birth. The baby has small jaw, glossoptosis, and cleft palate. What will you do in the delivery room to manage respiratory distress in this baby?
    b. How would you position a baby with meningomyelocele in the delivery room and later? What type of gloves would you specifically prefer during resuscitation of this baby?
    c. You have gone to attend the delivery of a neonate with gastroschisis. How would you position this baby in the delivery room? At what length would you cut the umbilical cord in this baby?
    d. You attend birth of a baby with antenatally diagnosed congenital diaphragmatic hernia. Baby is born limp. What will be your next step promptly after birth?

49. **You have been called to attend the delivery of 33-year-old primi mother at term gestation. Baby is born limp. This mother had history of reduced fetal movements throughout pregnancy and had amniotic fluid index of 35. There is no history of sentinel event prior to delivery. The mother had not received any opiates. Baby is born limp, has short umbilical cord and undescended testis. Heart rate and SpO_2 promptly improve after PPV but baby does not breathe spontaneously.**
    a. What is the possible diagnosis in this baby?
    b. What are the other possible causes of poor respiratory drive in neonates at birth, when there is no history of sentinel event?
    c. What will be your priority management in a baby if mother had received opiate shortly before birth?
    d. What is the current state of evidence regarding use of naloxone in such babies and what are few complications reported with use of naloxone?

50. **A woman is admitted to the hospital at 23-week gestation with contractions, fever, fetal tachycardia, and ruptured membranes leaking purulent amniotic fluid.**
    a. What important points you would include while counseling the parents in this case?
    b. What role should parents play in decisions about resuscitation?
    c. What ethical principles apply to neonatal resuscitation?

51. **A 4 hours old term small for gestational age (SGA) baby boy born with a birth weight of 1800 g to 27-year-old primigravida mother was admitted with poor feeding and lethargy. Blood sugar was 25 mg/dL. Dextrose 10% bolus was given, followed by continuous infusion with glucose infusion rate (GIR) of 6 mg/kg/min. His blood sugars remained less than 40 mg/dL and GIR was increased in stepwise manner to 12 mg/kg/min. Hydrocortisone was added. There was no history of perinatal asphyxia and no risk factors for early onset neonatal sepsis. Mother was not receiving any drugs apart from routine supplementation. There were no visible external malformations and no organomegaly. The family history was unremarkable.**
    d. What do you think is underlying cause of hypoglycemia in this case and how would you investigate this baby further?
    e. Enumerate diagnostic criteria for hyperinsulinemic hypoglycemia?
    f. Baby had elevated insulin levels (sample was taken at time when RBS was 32 mg/dL). His free fatty acid and ketone levels were low. His GIR needs were 15 mg/kg/min to maintain blood sugars in normal range. Lactate and ammonia were within acceptable range; urine ketones and sepsis workup were negative.
        i.   What will be your drug of choice in this scenario?
        ii. What is its mechanism of action?
        iii. What is the recommended dose?
        iv. What are the adverse effects of this drug?
    g. In spite of diazoxide hypoglycemia persisted. What other drugs would you consider in this baby?
    h. What genetic work up would you plan for this baby?

52. **A 29-year-old primigravida mother delivered a term female baby at 38 weeks gestation with weight 3.2 kg. Routine cord blood TSH screening showed TSH levels of 90 mIU/L.**
    a. How will you proceed?
    b. Repeat venous sampling was done at 72 hours of life. Repeat TSH was 100 mIU/L and free T4 was low (0.2 ng/dL). Suspecting congenital hypothyroidism, what additional tests will you perform?
    c. What is the time frame within which ultrasound and radionuclide scan can be done in babies with congenital hypothyroidism?
    d. USG of thyroid gland showed small gland in this baby and thyroid scan showed absent uptake. What is the most probable diagnosis?
    e. How would you initiate and titrate treatment in this baby? When would you repeat thyroid function tests after starting treatment?
    f. How would you plan long-term follow-up for this baby?

g. What are the current criteria for initiation of levothyroxine therapy in term newborns based on confirmatory venous sample results after newborn screening?

h. When should screening for congenital hypothyroidism (CH) be done in preterm babies?

53. **A preterm 26-week male baby boy with birth weight 700 g is admitted in your NICU. Baby is now 4-week-old and is still on HHHFNC support (25% FiO$_2$ and 4 L/min flow). He had a stormy initial course, required invasive ventilation for 2 weeks and had suspect NEC warranting parenteral nutrition for 15 days. Calcium and vitamin D was added in milk once baby reached full feeds. He also received a course of postnatal steroids and diuretics for evolving bronchopulmonary dysplasia (BPD).**

a. When would you start evaluating this baby for metabolic bone disease? What lab tests would you use for screening and what are the cut-off values for diagnosing metabolic bone disease (MBD)?

b. What risk factors in this baby put him at a higher risk for developing the metabolic bone disease?

c. This baby had a serum phosphorus level of 3 mg/dL and alkaline phosphatase (ALP) of 1200 IU/L, despite optimal Ca and P supplementation. How would you investigate this baby further?

d. On further evaluation, the baby had serum parathormone (PTH) of 150 pg/mL and TRP of 70%. Vitamin D levels were low. What would be your interpretation and how would your management change?

e. What is the current recommendation for calcium, phosphate and vitamin D supplementation in preterm VLBW babies? Up to what age is fortification indicated?

54. **A multigravida mother with gestational diabetes mellitus (GDM), with poor glycemic control during pregnancy delivered a male baby with weight 4.5 kg. There was no history of perinatal asphyxia and no risk factors for early-onset neonatal sepsis. The baby was started on feeds. On screening, blood sugars were with in normal range. He has an episode of multifocal clonic seizure at 24 hours of life. RBS was 64 mg/dL. Baby was shifted to NICU and stabilized. Baby remained hemodynamically stable.**

a. Enumerate possible reasons for seizure in this baby?

b. This baby had a calcium level of 6 mg/dL. How would you manage the baby?

c. Despite adequate treatment with IV calcium, the baby had another seizure on 3rd day of life. You repeated calcium levels and they were still 6.1 mg/dL. What will be your next step in managing this baby?

d. What other systemic and metabolic complications can occur in this baby? What are the long-term complications which can occur in infants of diabetic mothers?

e. What are the current recommendations on the timing of delivery in pregnant women with GDM?

f. This mother is concerned regarding her own follow-up and risk of developing diabetes. What are the current ACOG recommendations for follow-up of women with GDM?

55. **A 30-day-old baby boy is admitted with complaints of poor feeding, vomiting and lethargy. On examination, the baby is dehydrated, dull and has hypotonia. There is no history of diarrhea. The mother reported that she had been giving supplements as advised to the baby. His HR is 160/min, RR is 58/min, and SpO$_2$ is 100% on room air. RBS is 80 mg/dL. IV fluids and antibiotics are started, and investigations are sent. The lab tests are as follows: Hb 15 g/dL, TLC 6000, platelet count 4 lakh, CRP negative, sodium 140 mEq/L, potassium 4.5 mmol/L, pH 7.38, calcium 17 mg/dL.**
    a. What is your diagnosis?
    b. What are the common causes of this condition in neonates?
    c. What medication history would you particularly ask from mother?
    d. How would you evaluate this baby further?
    e. Upon checking the medications, you find that child has been receiving 0.5 mL/day of a cholecalciferol preparation containing 60,000 IU/5 mL, instead of standard formulation. The baby had suppressed PTH levels and vitamin D level >100 ng/mL. What is your diagnosis? What would be your line of management?

56. **A girl child is delivered at 38 weeks of gestation to 27-year-old primigravida mother with Graves' disease. She was diagnosed to have Graves' disease at 24 years of age and had received treatment in form of oral medications, followed by radioactive ablation of thyroid gland. Subsequently, she received thyroxine and had remained euthyroid throughout pregnancy.**
    a. How would you evaluate the baby? Is this baby at risk of developing hyperthyroidism despite maternal thyroid gland ablation and adequate treatment? If yes, then why?
    b. On day 4 of life, the baby was noticed to have tachycardia and irritability. Baby's free T4 was 7 ng/dL and TSH was 0.1 mIU/mL. What drugs would you use for managing this baby? What doses would you use?
    c. What are the current recommendations for antenatal evaluation of mothers with history of Graves' disease?
    d. Which drugs are used for antenatal treatment of maternal and fetal hyperthyroidism? What are the potential adverse effects of these drugs?
    e. Which drug is preferred for treatment of hyperthyroidism in lactating women?

57. **A term born SGA baby boy, presented on day 26 of life with weight loss, vomiting and dehydration. He was admitted and IV fluids and antibiotics were started. Blood sugar levels on admission were 400 mg/dL and remained high even on subsequent readings.**
    a. How do you define neonatal hyperglycemia? What are the common causes of neonatal hyperglycemia?
    b. What treatment would you initiate for hyperglycemia? What are the current suggested operational thresholds at which treatment for hyperglycemia should be initiated?
    c. How would you diagnose neonatal diabetes mellitus (NDM)?
    d. What is the etiology of NDM? What treatment options are available for NDM?
    e. This baby required insulin during the hospital stay and blood sugars normalized. Insulin was gradually stopped. Postdischarge, this baby had recurrent infections, dermatitis, persistent diarrhea and required re-initiation of insulin for hyperglycemia. Which syndrome would you suspect? What genetic defect is involved in this syndrome?

58. **A 12-day-old neonate is admitted with complaints of lethargy, vomiting and poor feeding. The baby was born at 38 weeks and had a birth weight of 3 kg. On examination, the baby was dehydrated, had feeble pulses with prolonged CFT and mean BP of 35 mm Hg. Head-to-toe examination revealed findings as shown in Figure 32. There was hyperpigmentation in the umbilical and genital regions. Palpation of genitals revealed "empty scrotum". RBS was 40 mg/dL. Blood gas revealed metabolic acidosis. Sodium levels were 120 mEq/L and potassium levels were 7.8 mEq/L.**

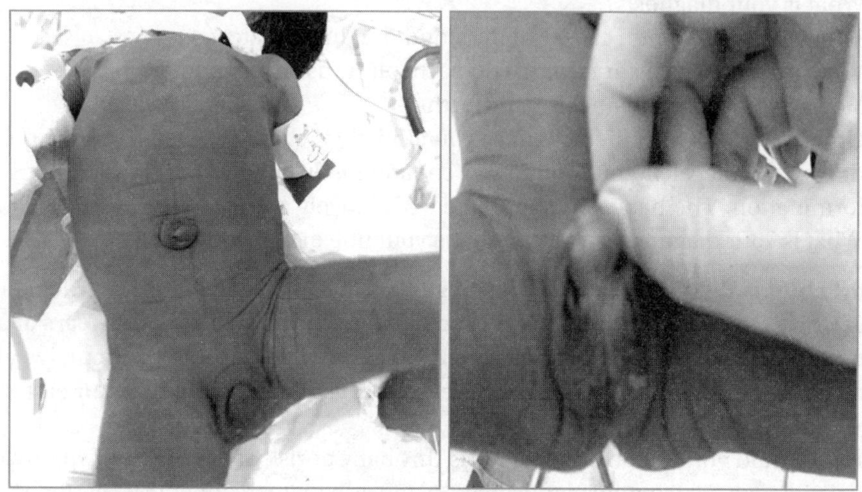

Fig. 32: Empty scrotum and hyperpigmented genitals and umbilical regions.

   a. What would be your provisional diagnosis?
   b. How would you investigate this baby?
   c. This baby had markedly elevated 17-OHP levels and low cortisol levels. Other adrenocortical hormones were within range. USG pelvis showed Müllerian structures. FISH analysis suggested 46,XX pattern. What would be your final diagnosis and how would you manage this baby immediately and thereafter?
   d. What factors would you consider while assigning sex of rearing in this baby?
   e. How would you plan follow-up for this baby and what instructions would you give to parents for intercurrent illnesses?
   f. What is the current consensus on the timing of genital surgery in these babies?
   g. What is the current consensus on prenatal dexamethasone administration to pregnant women with a prior CAH-affected child?

59. **A 3-week-old baby boy is referred to you with a history of recurrent hypoglycemia and persistent jaundice. The child was born full term and had birth weight of 2 kg. The antenatal period was uneventful, except for the absent cavum septum pellucidum in antenatal scans. Family history was unremarkable and there was no history of consanguinity. On examination, the baby was hemodynamically stable. He had a midline cleft lip, hypospadias, micropenis and icterus till legs.**

   a. What would you suspect? What hormonal deficiencies are the baby expected to have?

b. On lab evaluation, the baby had conjugated hyperbilirubinemia, mildly raised transaminases, low stimulated cortisol levels, low free T4 levels and TSH levels. Other pituitary hormones were normal. How would you manage this baby?

c. What associated CNS anomalies you may find in the MRI brain of this baby?

d. How would you diagnose neonatal growth hormone deficiency? Is there any role of GH stimulation test in newborns?

e. What is the ideal time to evaluate this baby for central hypogonadism associated with hypopituitarism?

60. **A baby is delivered at 39 weeks of gestation to a primigravida mother. The baby has small phallus with separation of the scrotal sac, penoscrotal hypospadias and single palpable testis. The antenatal period was uneventful.**

a. In which babies would you suspect DSD?

b. What is the external masculinization score?

c. What important points would you elicit in antenatal and family history?

d. Which disorder of sex development is this baby likely to have?

e. What are the causes of 46,XY DSD?

f. Parents were apprehensive and therefore FISH was sent while karyotype results were awaited. FISH detected Y chromosome material. How would you further evaluate the baby? At what age would you do biochemical and hormonal evaluation?

61. **A full term 3.2 kg baby boy delivered by elective LSCS to a primi mother, was admitted with complaints of poor feeding, lethargy, fast breathing, and unresponsiveness on day 3 of life. There were no maternal risk factors for early onset sepsis. Ultrasound scans in antenatal period were normal. Baby had cried soon after birth and had not required any resuscitation. He was being nursed with mother before the illness. On examination at the time of admission, baby was encephalopathic. Baby's respiratory rate was 70/min and baby had fast deep breathing. Heart rate was 158/min. Pulse volume was good and CFT was 2 seconds. Temperature was normal. RBS was 74 mg/dL.**

a. What are your differential diagnoses? How would you like to evaluate this baby?

b. What preliminary basic investigations would you do when suspecting inborn error of metabolism?

c. This baby's counts were normal, CRP was negative and blood culture was sterile. CSF analysis revealed no meningitis. USG cranium was normal. RBS was 74 mg/dL. Serum electrolytes (sodium, potassium, calcium, magnesium) were normal. Blood gas revealed pH 7.47, pCO_2 24, BE-1. Lactate was 4 mmol/L and serum ammonia 1000 mmol/L (1785 µg/dL). Urine ketones were negative. What is the interpretation? What is the probable diagnosis?

d. How would you confirm the diagnosis? How would you manage this baby?

e. TMS showed high glutamine and decreased levels of citrulline. Urine GCMS showed increased orotic acid. What is the probable diagnosis?

f. What is the long-term therapy for this condition?

62. **A term born 3 kg baby girl was admitted on day 5 of life with history of difficulty in feeding, lethargy, abnormal movements, and fast breathing. Her temperature was 37°C, heart rate 180/min, respiratory rate 80/min, mean BP 68 mm Hg. Pulses were well felt. She had hepatomegaly (3 cm below right costal margin). RBS was 90 mg/dL. Treatment for congestive cardiac failure and probable sepsis was initiated while awaiting evaluation. Chest X-ray revealed cardiomegaly. 2D ECHO showed normal cardiac morphology. CRP was negative and blood culture sterile. Electrolytes (sodium and calcium) were normal. USG brain and MRI were done, and images are as shown in Figures 33 and 34.**

    a. What is the probable diagnosis?

    b. What are the potential complications associated with this condition?

    c. What is the pathophysiology of cardiac failure in this condition?

    d. What is the treatment modality?

    e. What are few complications that can happen after treatment?

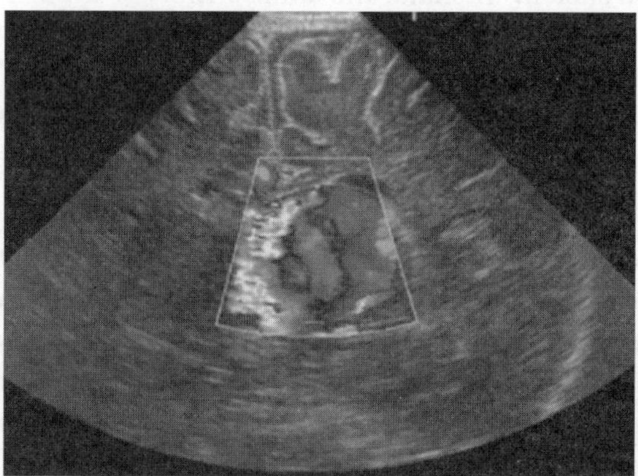

Fig. 33: USG brain Doppler.   Fig. 34: MRI brain.

63. **A 5-day-old term born neonate was admitted with history of abnormal movements in form of multiple, successive, unilateral, clonic movements affecting the face and the limbs. It was a full term normal vaginal delivery and immediate perinatal period was uneventful. Apgar scores were 8, 9, 9 at 1, 5 and 10 minutes respectively. Baby was discharged to home at 48 hours. There were no risk factors for sepsis and baby was being exclusively breastfed.**

    a. How would you evaluate this baby?

    b. After admission, RBS was 90 mg/dL. Electrolytes (sodium, calcium, magnesium) were normal. Sepsis workup was negative. Basic metabolic work was negative. Phenobarbitone and phenytoin were administered for repetitive seizures. USG brain and MRI brain were normal. EEG was done and is as shown in **Figure 35**. It showed "theta pointu alternant pattern". What would be the probable diagnosis?

    c. How would you differentiate between familial and nonfamilial variant of this disease?

    d. What is the long-term prognosis of this condition?

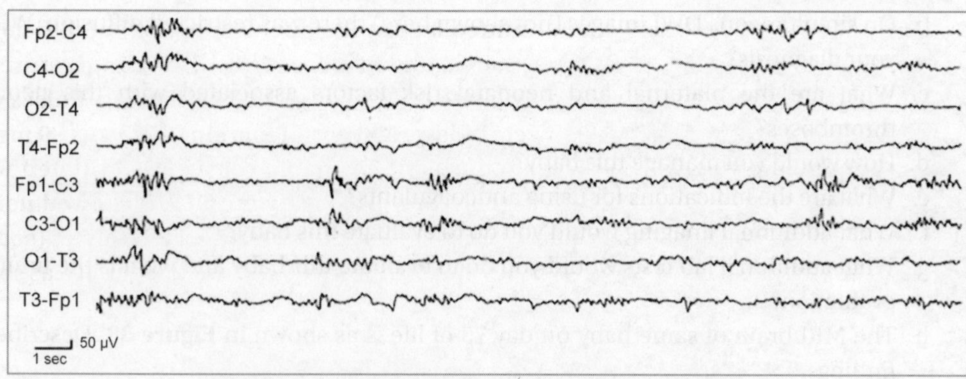

Fig. 35: EEG showing theta pointu alternant pattern.

64. **A full term 2.9 kg baby boy developed marked hypotonia and refractory seizures requiring multiple antiepileptic drugs on day 3 of life, after an uneventful normal vaginal delivery. It was an un-booked pregnancy and antenatal scans were not available. Baby had not required any resuscitation at birth. RBS, electrolytes were normal, and sepsis workup was negative. MRI brain is as shown in Figure 36.**
   a. What is the diagnosis?
   b. Name few conditions with which it is associated?
   c. At what gestational age during pregnancy is this brain malformation likely to occur?
   d. What are the other disorders of neuronal migration?

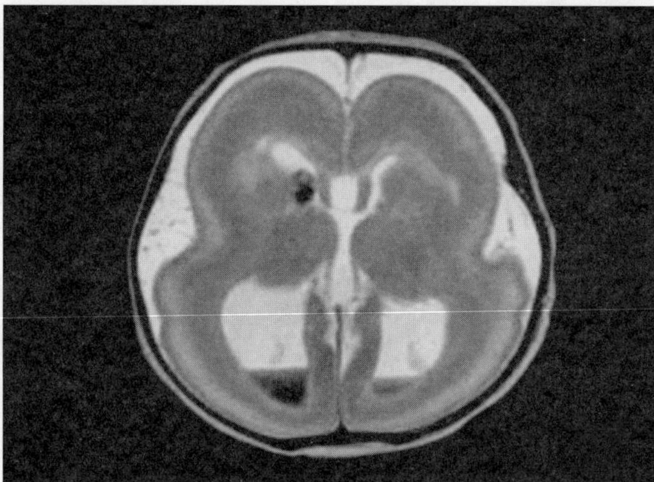

Fig. 36: MRI brain.

65. **A full term 3.1 kg baby girl developed feeding difficulty and increased sleepiness on day 2 of life, followed by refractory seizures requiring multiple antiepileptic drugs within next 12 hours. It was an uneventful normal vaginal delivery. Baby had not required any resuscitation at birth. RBS, electrolytes were normal, and sepsis workup was negative. MRI brain on day 3 of life is as shown in Figure 37.**
   a. Describe the MRI findings.

b. On simultaneous DWI images (not shown here) there was restricted diffusion. What is your diagnosis?

c. What are the maternal and neonatal risk factors associated with this neonatal thromboses?

d. How would you manage this baby?

e. What are the indications for using anticoagulants?

f. What additional imaging would you do to evaluate this baby?

g. What additional lab tests would you do to evaluate this baby and what is the timing of evaluation?

h. The MRI brain of same baby on day 75 of life is as shown in **Figure 38**. Describe the findings.

i. What are the long-term problems expected in this baby?

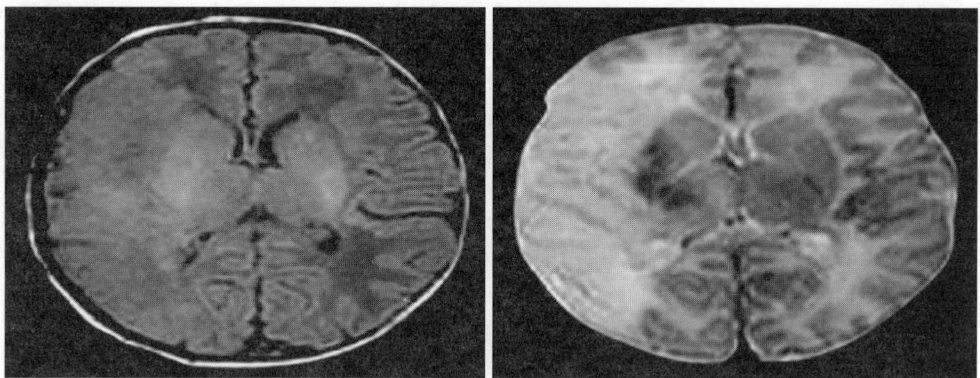

Fig. 37: MRI brain on day 3 of life.

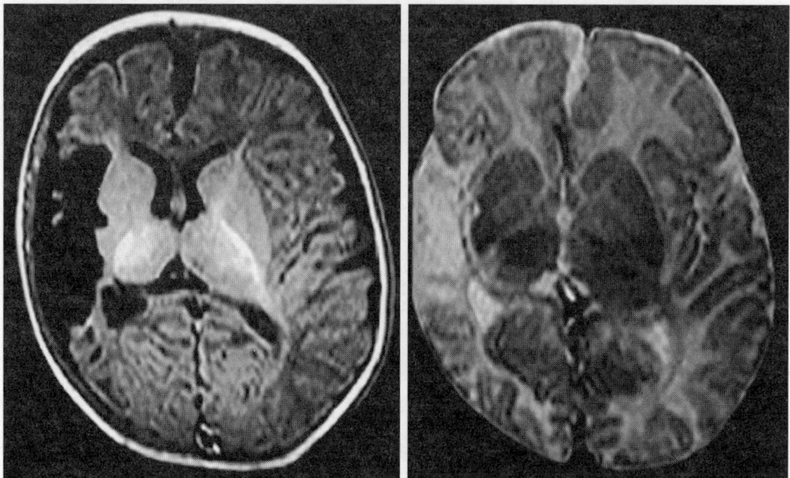

Fig. 38: MRI brain on day 75.

66. **A 25-day-old neonate with culture positive sepsis (*Acinetobacter*), was referred to you due to worsening sensorium and clinical condition. At the time of admission, baby had temperature of 38.5°C and poor sensorium. Perfusion was stable. RBS was 82**

mg/dL. The baby is stabilized, and antibiotics are administered as per blood culture sensitivity report. You decide to perform lumbar puncture. CSF analysis showed 60 cells with 10% neutrophils, sugar 25 mg/dL and protein 170 g/dL. CSF culture also grew *Acinetobacter* and sensitive antibiotics were being given. After 3 days of antibiotic treatment, the baby became afebrile, and sensorium improved. However, during the second week of treatment, the baby developed bulging fontanelle and multiple episodes of seizures.

a. What are the possible complications of meningitis?
b. What is the utility of USG brain in evaluating meningitis and its complications?
c. How would you diagnose ventriculitis?
d. What is the recommended duration of treatment for ventriculitis?
e. Cranial ultrasound of this baby showed a large cystic mass with internal debris and shaggy wall in the parietal region of the right cerebral hemisphere. MRI brain is as shown in **Figure 39**. Describe the findings. What is your diagnosis?
f. How would you manage this baby further?

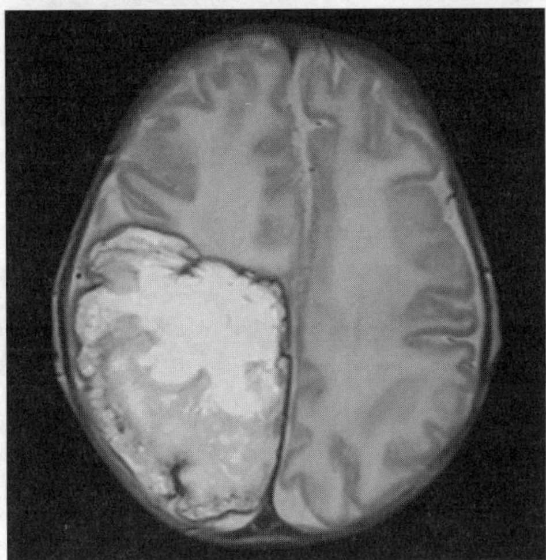

Fig. 39: MRI brain

67. A 2-month-old baby is brought to you with paucity of spontaneous movements and difficulty in feeding for last 2–3 weeks. Mother had noted looseness while handling the baby. Baby sucked intermittently for few minutes and mother was struggling with breast and bottle feeding. Baby otherwise looked around and was responsive. Antenatally, there was h/o reduced fetal movement compared to earlier pregnancy. There was polyhydramnios in 3rd trimester. No h/o any drug exposure in mother. No h/o fever, rash suggestive of intrauterine infection. Antenatal scans were normal. Baby was delivered in breech presentation with no perinatal complication. There was no history of NICU admission. There was no h/o consanguinity or similar condition in family. On examination, baby had normal sensorium, had an alert look, marked hypotonia with absent deep tendon reflexes. There is weakness and paucity of movements in upper as well as lower limbs. There was no dysmorphism,

no microcephaly, no neurocutaneous markers and no other external visible malformations.

a. How would you differentiate between central and peripheral hypotonia?
b. What are the possible sites of involvement and respective differential diagnoses in peripheral hypotonia?
c. What are the differential diagnoses for central hypotonia?
d. What is the probable diagnosis in this child?
e. What would be your approach in managing this baby?
f. Name two FDA approved drugs for use in infants with SMA.

68. **A term baby is admitted with seizures on day 1 of life. Mother had no antenatal check-ups. There was no history of perinatal asphyxia and need for resuscitation. Initial blood and lab investigations (RBS, blood gas, electrolytes, CRP, blood culture and CSF analysis) were all normal. MRI scan is as shown in Figure 40.**

a. What are the findings in this MRI scan?
b. What is the diagnosis?
c. What are the three characteristic features of this condition?
d. What are the associated abnormalities in this condition?
e. What are the differential diagnoses of posterior fossa abnormalities that may be associated with hydrocephalus?
f. How would you manage this baby?
g. What is the prognosis of this disease?

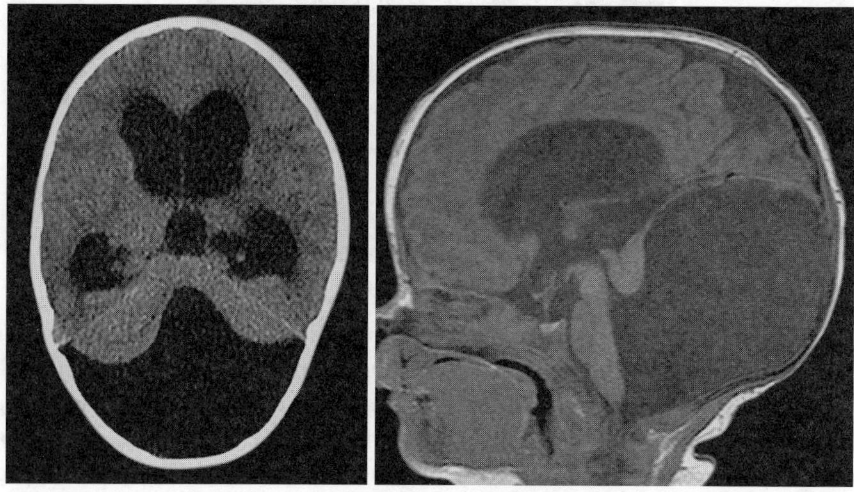

Fig. 40: MRI scan.

69. Identify the amplitude integrated EEG patterns as shown in Figures 41 to 44:

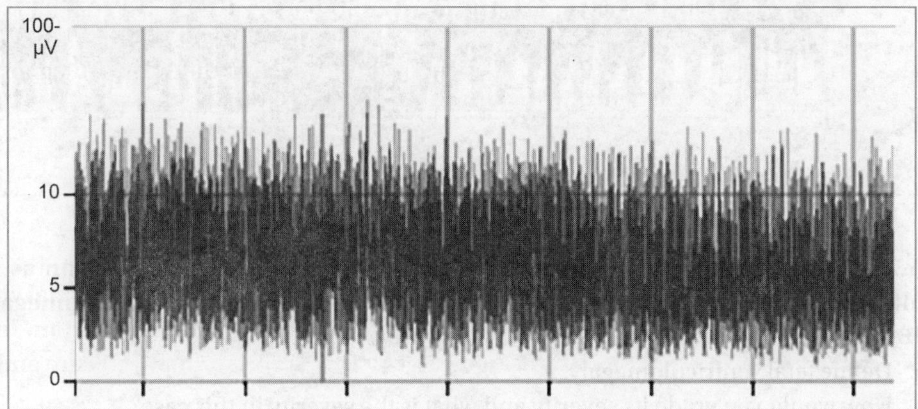

Fig. 41

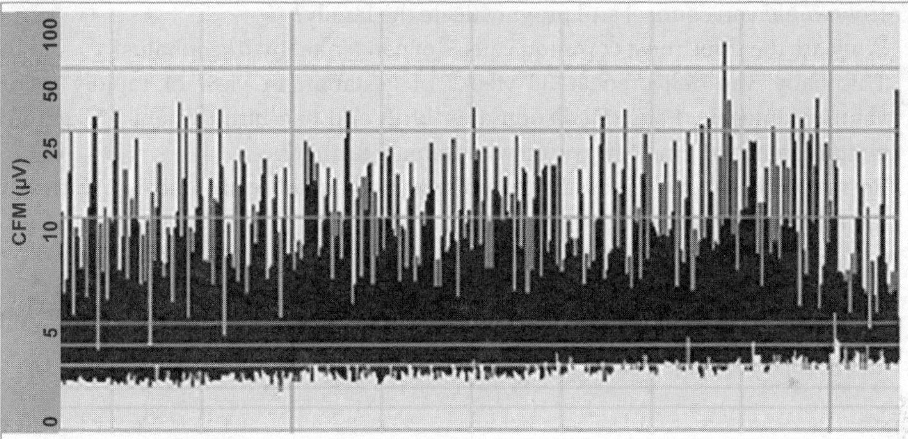

Fig. 42

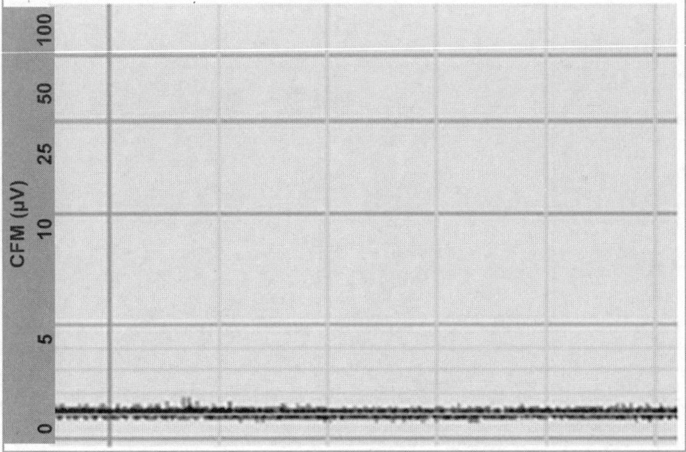

Fig. 43

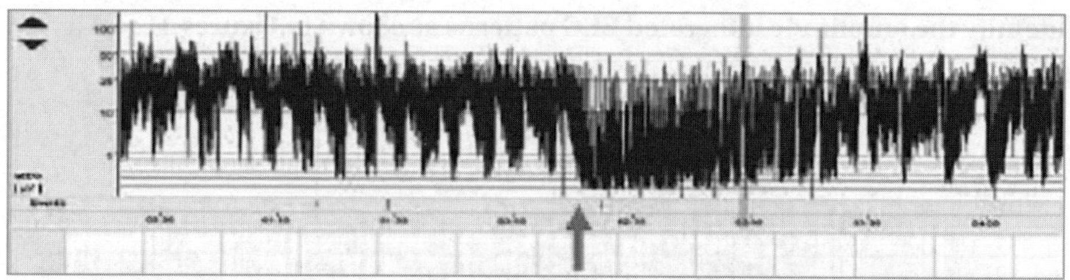

Fig. 44

70. **A 25-year-old primigravida is referred to you for antenatal consultation as fetal ultrasonography at 25 weeks of gestation is showing bilateral ventriculomegaly of 16 mm size.**
    a. Define fetal ventriculomegaly.
    b. How would you grade its severity and what is the severity in this case?
    c. What further evaluation would you plan in this mother?
    d. How would you counsel and prognosticate the family?
    e. What are the three most common causes of congenital hydrocephalus?
    f. This baby was delivered at 36 weeks of gestation in view of rapidly increasing ventriculomegaly. Baby cried soon after birth and had birth weight 3.2 kg and head circumference 41 cm. How would you evaluate further?
    g. Postnatal MRI showed gross hydrocephalus and aqueductal stenosis. What would be the mainstay of treatment?

ANSWERS

1. a. Rh isoimmunization. Hemolytic disease of fetus and newborn.
    b. MCA Doppler for MCA-PSV (middle cerebral artery-peak systolic velocity) at 1–2 weeks intervals to detect fetal anemia.
    c. No.
    d. MCA-PSV more than 1.5 times MoM.
    e. Fetal hemoglobin lower than 2 SD below the mean for gestational age or hematocrit <30% with gestation <35 weeks. Methods of IUT are intravascular and intraperitoneal.
    f. ABO Rh, CBC, DCT, reticulocyte count, peripheral smear for hemolysis, and serum bilirubin.
    g. Plasmapheresis and IVIg may be considered in mother. Start weekly MCA Dopplers and if MCA PSV is more than 1.5 MoM, check fetal hemoglobin by cordocentesis. Indications for IUT as mentioned above.

2. a. Predischarge TSB or TcB level in the high-risk zone of hour-specific normogram, jaundice observed in the first 24 hours, blood group incompatibility with positive direct antiglobulin test, other known hemolytic disease (e.g., G6PD deficiency), gestational age 35–36 weeks, previous sibling received phototherapy, cephalohematoma or significant bruising, feeding problems particularly if nursing is not going well and weight loss is excessive, East Asian race.
    b. Isoimmune hemolytic disease, G6PD deficiency, asphyxia, sepsis, acidosis, albumin <3.0 mg/dL, significant lethargy, and temperature instability.
    c. Bhutani's hour-specific nomogram.
    d. Low intermediate risk zone. Follow-up in 2 days.
    e. Start intensive phototherapy and correct hydration and feeding as baby has 12.5% weight loss.
    f. BIND score or BIND-M score.
        BIND score components: Mental status, muscle tone, and cry
        BIND-M: Mental status, muscle tone, cry, and altered gaze
        Interpretation:
        BIND Score Interpretation
        0: No indication of acute bilirubin encephalopathy (ABE).
        1–3: Subtle signs of mild acute bilirubin encephalopathy (ABE).
        4–6: Moderate acute bilirubin encephalopathy (ABE), urgent bilirubin reduction intervention is likely to reverse the acute damage.
        7–9: Advanced acute bilirubin encephalopathy (ABE), urgent bilirubin intervention is needed to prevent further brain damage and reduce the severity of sequelae.
        BIND-M Score Interpretation
        <3: No indication of diagnosis of acute bilirubin encephalopathy (ABE)
        ≥3: Positive diagnosis of acute bilirubin encephalopathy (ABE)
    g. Breastfeeding jaundice. Increased enterohepatic circulation due to decreased feeding.

3. a. Decrease the vertical distance between baby and phototherapy.

b. Structural isomerization, photoisomerization, and photooxidation.

c. Spectrum of light emitted, spectral irradiance, spectral power, cause of jaundice, and TSB level at the start of jaundice.

d. The American Academy of Pediatrics defines intensive phototherapy as a spectral irradiance of at least 30 μW/cm^2/nm over the same bandwidth delivered to as much of the infant's body-surface area as possible.

e. The area illuminated by the PT device with sufficient spectral irradiance. It is measured with the help of radiance meter.

f. *Advantages of LED phototherapy:* Less heat generation, less hyperthermia, lesser insensible losses, less power consumption, and more shelf life.

g. If TSB is close to exchange range and/or hemolytic jaundice is anticipated—repeat value within 2–3 hours

TSB >25—repeat in 2–3 hours

TSB 20-25–repeat in 3–4 hours

TSB <20—repeat in 4–6 hours

If continues to fall—repeat in 8–12 hours.

h. *For stopping:*

TSB <3 mg/dL below phototherapy range. 2 values for hemolytic jaundice. Single value otherwise. In readmission jaundice, stop phototherapy once TSB <14 mg/dL.

For Rebound testing, after 24 hours of stopping (particularly in hemolytic or early jaundice). In readmission jaundice, option of clinical review after 24 hours can be given.

4. a. Nonimmune-mediated hemolytic jaundice:

- Inherited RBC defects
- *Enzyme defects:* Glucose-6-phospate/pyruvate kinase deficiency
- *Membrane defects:* Hereditary spherocytosis/hereditary elliptocytosis
- *Hemoglobinopathies:* Severe forms of thalassemias/sickle cell disease

b. The diagnosis of hereditary spherocytosis (HS) in a newborn infant is generally made based on a positive family history, spherocytes on blood film and Coombs-negative hemolytic jaundice of variable severity with an elevated mean corpuscular hemoglobin concentration (MCHC) and a low mean corpuscular volume (MCV). If MCHC/MCV ratio >0.36, it is likely to be HS. Positive osmotic fragility test. Definitive diagnosis is by genetic testing.

c. During the perinatal period, the clinical manifestation of HS ranges from severe fetal anemia with hydrops fetalis to no clinical symptoms. In the neonatal period, jaundice is the most common manifestation.

d. EMA binding test, acidified glycerol lysis time test, genetic testing (next-generation DNA sequencing).

e. *ANK1*, located at 8p11.21, encodes erythroid ankyrin, and its mutations are the most common causes of HS1.

f. Anemia, hyperbilirubinemia, folate deficiency, cholelithiasis, and aplastic crisis.

g. Phototherapy/exchange transfusion for jaundice as and when indicated, management of anemia using blood transfusion, folate supplementation. Definitive treatment is splenectomy, and it is usually offered after 5 years of age.

5. a. We will do total serum bilirubin.

b. Multiwavelength reflectance photo spectrometry.

c. Babies less than completed 35 weeks of gestation
   - Jaundice in first 24 hours of life
   - Babies >14 days old
   - Babies under phototherapy or postphototherapy
   - Babies where conjugated hyperbilirubinemia is suspected.

d. TCB measurements >13 mg/dL. TCB >75th centile on Bhutani's hour-specific normogram/TCB is at 70% of TSB level recommended for phototherapy/TCB measurement within 3 mg/dL of TSB phototherapy cut off. In other words, if "TCB + 3" would change the management, then TSB should be obtained.

e. 14 days.

f. JM-105, JM-103, Bilicheck.

g. Dräger JM-105 is indicated for use in neonatal patients born ≥24 weeks gestation who have not undergone exchange transfusion. The device is indicated for use before, during, and after phototherapy treatment.

h. End-tidal carbon monoxide measurement.

6. a. Liver function tests, fasting ultrasound, sepsis screen, metabolic tests, genetic tests, and liver biopsy.

b. PFIC I and II

Inborn errors of bile acid metabolism.

c. We shall plan liver biopsy.

Hepatobiliary-iminodiacetic acid (HIDA) scan has limited role in evaluation of NC especially if the baby has clearly documented pale or pigmented stools. The time required (5–7 days) for priming before the scan, especially in patients who are referred late, is a limitation. The sensitivity of scintigraphy for biliary atresia is relatively high (83–100%); however, its specificity is very low (33–80%). A recent meta-analysis of 81 studies has shown a pooled sensitivity and specificity of 98.7 % and 70.4%, respectively. A nonexcreting scan may be seen both in biliary atresia as well as severe hepatocellular dysfunction. However, excretion of the tracer into the bowel despite of biliary atresia is extremely rare and thus an excreting scan may help in ruling out biliary atresia, but without providing any other diagnostic information. Good-quality HIDA scan may not be available everywhere in our country. Since HIDA scan is expensive, time-consuming, and poorly specific, many centers do not routinely use this test in the evaluation of cholestatic infants because it may delay the diagnostic evaluation without providing definitive diagnostic information. However, others think that it still has a role where the liver biopsy is ambiguous, in the evaluation of preterm infants and in the diagnosis of the uncommon causes like spontaneous perforation of the bile duct.

(*Reference:* Consensus Statement of the Pediatric Gastroenterology Chapter of Indian Academy of Pediatrics; Italian guidelines for the management and treatment of neonatal cholestasis by Task Force for Hyperbilirubinemia of the Italian Society of Neonatology)

d. Progressive Familial Intrahepatic Cholestasis Type II (PFIC II).

e. *Drugs:* UDCA, rifampicin, and cholestyramine.

Nutritional rehabilitation: Water soluble vitamins are given at 1–2 times of the age-appropriate RDA. The fat-soluble vitamins are usually supplemented in the following dosage in children: vitamin A—5,000–25,000 IU/day PO, vitamin D 400–800 IU/day PO, vitamin E 50–100 IU/day PO and vitamin K 2.5–5 mg/day PO or 2–5 mg intravenous every 3–4 weeks. Adequate sunlight exposure and dietary intake of calcium (800–2,000 mg/day PO) are also essential.

Surgical: Biliary diversion procedures and liver transplantation.

f. PFIC patients have a variable prognosis depending on the type of PFIC and severity of genetic defect within each type. Approximately 30% children respond to UDCA therapy and about 70–80% to partial biliary diversion, if offered early in course of disease, before development of cirrhosis. Patients with cirrhosis and end-stage liver disease require liver transplant.

Anticipated long-term complications: Cirrhosis, hepatocellular carcinoma, and cholangiocarcinoma.

7. a. *Indications for exchange transfusion*: Immediate exchange transfusion is indicated in any infant with acute bilirubin encephalopathy or if TSB is ≥5 mg/dL above the threshold for exchange transfusion in AAP chart. It should be considered when TSB reaches the exchange transfusion threshold and is not decreasing despite of intensive phototherapy.

b. 85% of circulating RBCs are replaced and bilirubin level decreases by about 50% by DVET.

c. B or O Rh negative PRBC suspended in AB positive plasma.

d. 160 mL/kg. For this baby, it will be 480 mL. For dead space loss in circuit, around 20–25 mL extra blood should be taken. Two-thirds of the total amount should be PRBC and rest one-third plasma.

e. Adverse effects associated with exchange transfusion: Infection, thrombocytopenia, electrolyte disturbances like hypocalcemia, hyperkalemia, hypo or hyperglycemia, fluid overload, cardiac arrhythmias, coagulopathies, graft-versus-host disease, necrotizing enterocolitis, portal vein thrombosis, and a mortality rate of approximately 0.5–2%.

f. Continue intensive phototherapy and give IV immunoglobulin 0.5–1 g/kg IV over 2 hours.

g. *Indications of IVIg*: In isoimmune hemolytic disease, administration of intravenous globulin (0.5–1 g/kg over 2 hours) is recommended if the TSB is rising despite intensive phototherapy, or the TSB level is within 2–3 mg/dL (34–51 mol/L) of the exchange level. If necessary, this dose can be repeated in 12 hours.

8. a. G6PD, TSH, and sepsis screen.

b. Breast milk jaundice, hypothyroidism, G6PD deficiency, pyloric stenosis, Crigler-Najjar syndrome, Gilbert syndrome, and extravasated blood.

c. G6PD deficiency is a genetic disorder. It happens when the body doesn't have enough of an enzyme called glucose-6-phosphate dehydrogenase (G6PD). G6PD helps red blood cells work. It also protects them from substances in the blood that could harm them. In people with G6PD deficiency, either the red blood cells do not make enough

G6PD or what they do make does not work as it should. Without enough G6PD to protect them, the red blood cells break apart. This can cause anemia and jaundice. Red blood cells that do not have enough G6PD are sensitive to some triggers which can be medicines, foods, and infections. Triggers of hemolysis in kids with G6PD deficiency include illness, such as bacterial and viral infections, some painkillers and fever-lowering drugs, some antibiotics (most often those with "sulf" in their names), some antimalarial drugs (most often those with "quine" in their names), fava beans (also called broad beans), naphthalene (a chemical found in mothballs and moth crystals). Treating G6PD deficiency symptoms is usually as simple as removing the trigger. Often, this means treating the infection or stopping the use of a drug. A child with severe anemia may need treatment in the hospital to get oxygen and fluids. Sometimes, a child also needs a transfusion of healthy blood cells. The best way to care for your child is to limit exposure to anything that triggers symptoms. We will give written instructions, and a list of medicines and other things that could be a problem for your child with G6PD deficiency.

   d. Neonates usually present with severe or prolonged unconjugated hyperbilirubinemia. They may not present with classical hemolytic anemia crisis.

   e. Crigler–Najjar syndrome-1, Crigler–Najjar syndrome-2, Gilbert syndrome. Crigler–Najjar-1 is the most severe of these. Liver transplantation is the definitive treatment of Crigler–Najjar syndrome type 1.

9. a. Minor blood group incompatibility.
   b. Blood group typing of parents and baby for Kell, C, c, E, and e. Antibody titers in mother against these antigens.
   c. ABO, Rh(D) blood group antigen typing and screening for RBC antibodies at the booking visit.
   d. Regular follow-up for anemia till 3 months. BERA at 3 months. Long-term neuro-development assessment for tone abnormalities/athetoid CP.

10. a. Abdominal ultrasonography findings described in BA include the triangular cord sign, abnormal gallbladder morphology (not visualized or length <1.9 cm or lack of smooth/complete echogenic mucosal lining with an indistinct wall or irregular/lobular contour), no contraction of the gallbladder after oral feeding and non-visualized common bile duct (CBD). A distended gall bladder, however, does not rule out a proximal BA with a distal patent bile duct and mucus filled gallbladder. It is recommended that ultrasound should be done after 4 hours of fasting.
    b. Biliary atresia can be grouped into three categories:
       1. BA without any anomalies or malformations
       2. BA in association with laterality malformations (BASM—biliary atresia splenic malformation)
       3. BA in association with other congenital malformations.
    c. The characteristic histopathology features of BA are bile duct proliferation, bile plugs in ducts, fibrosis, and lymphocytic infiltrates in the portal tracts.

d. The standard treatment of biliary atresia is the Kasai hepatic portoenterostomy with intraoperative cholangiogram to confirm the site of the obstruction before surgery. It should preferably be done before 60 days.

e. *Drugs:* UDCA

   Nutritional rehabilitation: Water soluble vitamins are given at 1–2 times of the age-appropriate RDA. The fat-soluble vitamins are usually supplemented in the following dosage in children: vitamin A—5,000–25,000 IU/day PO, vitamin D 400–800 IU/day PO, vitamin E 50–100 IU/day PO and vitamin K 2.5–5 mg/day PO or 2–5 mg intravenous every 3–4 weeks. Adequate sunlight exposure and dietary intake of calcium (800–2,000 mg/day PO) are also essential.

f. Long loop hepatic portoenterostomy and prophylactic antibiotics after Kasai procedure help in reducing risk of ascending cholangitis. Recurrent cholangitis can progressively worsen liver function.

g. Referral for liver transplantation: Any baby, who has had Kasai's PE and the bilirubin remains >6 mg/dL, 3 months after surgery, should be referred to a transplant center. Babies with BA who present with decompensated cirrhosis (low albumin, prolonged INR, and ascites) are not likely to improve with a Kasai PE and should be referred for liver transplantation.

h. Stool color card test.

11. a. Narrow complex supraventricular tachycardia

   b. Adenosine is the drug of choice. Serum half-life is 10–15 seconds

   c. Dose: 0.05 to 0.2 mg/kg

   Technique: Two-syringe technique. Rapid IV bolus followed by a saline flush.

   Two syringes are attached to a three way which is open to the patient. The horizontal syringe has the adenosine and the vertical one has the normal saline flush. With pressure being firm on the horizontal syringe, push adenosine as fast as possible and immediately follow with the flush.

   d. Synchronized DC cardioversion: 0.5–1 J/kg first dose. Repeat dose 2–4 J/kg.

   e. Chronic medical treatment is appropriate for neonates who have hemodynamically significant SVT, frequent SVT requiring medical management, preexcitation on ECG, or congenital cardiac defect. Propranolol, flecainide, and amiodarone may be used for chronic medical treatment, depending upon clinical response.

12. a. Congenital heart block—type II a.

   b. Neonatal lupus is the most probable diagnosis. Anti-Ro and Anti-La antibodies shall confirm the diagnosis. Maternal testing for SLE (ANA, Anti ds DNA).

   c. Fetal exposure to maternal autoantibodies (anti-Ro and anti-La) results in fibrosis of the AV nodal structures, leading to progressive destructive process.

   d. Indications for permanent pacemaker implantation:

   Congenital third-degree AV block with ventricular rate (VR) 55 bpm or with CHD and VR <70 bpm

   Congenital third-degree AV block with wide QRS escape rhythm, complex ventricular ectopy, or ventricular dysfunction

Congenital third-degree AV block beyond the first year of life with an average rate <50 bpm, abrupt pauses in VR that are two to three times the basic cycle length or are associated with symptoms due to chronotropic incompetence.

13. a. Patent ductus arteriosus (PDA).
   b. Suprasternal view. ECHO findings are suggestive of PDA.
   c. PLAX (Parasternal Long Axis View)
   Structures:
   A: Right ventricle cavity
   B: Interventricular septum
   C: LV cavity
   D: Mitral valve
   E: Left atrium
   F: Aorta
   G: AV valve
   LA:Ao ratio is measured in parasternal LAX using M-Mode. A cut is made in the left atrium at the level of the aortic valve, with the transducer placed perpendicular to it. The aortic valve is measured just before its opening, at the end of the diastole, whereas the left atrium is measured at its maximal volume during the systole.
   Clinical utility: The LA:Ao ratio should not exceed 1.5. LA:Ao ratio >1.5 is one of the markers for hemodynamically significant PDA.
   d. CCF, acute kidney injury, BPD, NEC, and IVH.
   e. Drugs and their side effects:
   Indomethacin: Renal impairment, GI toxicity (NEC, GI hemorrhage, and perforation), altered platelet function
   Ibuprofen: Renal toxicity, GI toxicity, and altered platelet function
   Paracetamol: Lower antiplatelet activity. Long-term follow-up studies lacking.

14. a. *Right to left shunt at both levels:* PPHN.
   Treatment considerations: Lung recruitment, inhaled pulmonary vasodilators like iNO and sildenafil.
   b. Right-to-left shunt at the ductal level but a left-to-right shunt at the atrial level: Left ventricular dysfunction, pulmonary venous hypertension, and ductal-dependent systemic circulation.
   Treatment considerations: Milrinone, PGE1. iNO is contraindicated and may worsen pulmonary venous hypertension and reduce systemic blood flow.
   c. Left-to-right shunt at ductal level but a right-to-left shunt at the atrial level:
   Duct-dependent pulmonary circulation: Tricuspid atresia, pulmonary atresia, and critical PS.
   Treatment considerations: PGE1.

15. a. Apical 4-chamber view showing TR jet.
   Diagnosis: PPHN
   b. TR jet velocity (v) is 3.99 m/s.
   Pressure gradient = $4v^2$ = 4 × 3.99 × 3.99 = 62 mm Hg

Hence, RVSP (right ventricular systolic pressure) = 62 + 5 = 67 mm Hg

Hence, PA systolic pressure = 67 mm Hg

c. $OI = MAP \times FiO_2 \times 100/PaO_2$

OI in this baby is 24

d. As lung recruitment has already been optimized, pulmonary vasodilator like iNO would be the treatment of choice.

e. Tricuspid annular plane systolic excursion (TAPSE): TAPSE is a measure of the RV systolic excursion or displacement of the lateral (or medial) tricuspid annulus toward apex along the longitudinal axis. This parameter is particularly useful in cases of PPHN to determine the RV systolic function. Greater the excursion of the annulus, better is the systolic function.

In term neonates, an excursion of >8 mm (range: 8–11 mm) is considered as normal. TAPSE measurement <4 mm indicates severe pulmonary hypertension.

16. a. Transposition of great arteries. 10% of these babies may have extracardiac malformations.

b. Start intravenous infusion of prostaglandin E1 (PGE1), soon after delivery, if oxygen saturation is lower than 75% and/or lactic acidosis is present.

c. Prostaglandin infusion (PGE1) 0.03–0.1 µg/kg/min

Adverse effects: Apnea, fever, flushing, tachycardia, and hypotension.

d. Indications of BAS include:

- Low saturations despite PGE1 infusion and ASD are restrictive.
- Those presenting with low saturation and a restrictive ASD beyond 3–4 weeks with a closed PDA where PGE1 is likely to be ineffective.
- Patient with restrictive ASD, not fit for immediate surgery (e.g., having sepsis or respiratory infection).
- Restrictive ASD in TGA patients with large VSD or PDA: to decrease left atrial pressure and pulmonary venous hypertension.

e. Definitive treatment: Arterial Switch Operation (ASO).

f. As early as possible. 7 days–3 weeks, earlier if baby is unstable or has associated persistent pulmonary hypertension of the newborn. Best done before 4 weeks.

17. Answer

a. IVC diameter is measured within 1–2 cm of RA-IVC junction in subcostal longitudinal view.

b. Distensibility Index of IVC = D_{max} (inspiration) – D_{min} (expiration)/D_{mean}.

c. CVP is low, and poor perfusion is likely to be fluid responsive. We will give a fluid bolus and increase the total fluid intake.

d. Key findings in favor of hypovolemia on 2D ECHO imaging:

- LV and RV of small dimensions and hyperkinetic
- Small LV end-systolic and end-diastolic areas
- Increased LV ejection fraction shortening (>70%)
- Small IVC diameter with wide respiratory variation.

18. a. *Sildenafil:*
   Phosphodiesterase-5 inhibitor
   Adverse effect: Systemic hypotension
   b. *Levosimendan:*
   Calcium sensitizer
   Adverse effect: Hypotension
   c. *Bosentan:*
   Endothelial receptor (And B) antagonist
   Adverse effect: Hepatotoxicity, hypotension, decreased hematocrit, flushing
   d. *Digoxin:*
   Sodium-potassium ATPase inhibitor
   Adverse effect: Arrhythmia and hyperkalemia.

19. a. Phosphodiesterase-3 (PDE-3) inhibitor
   b. Around 4 hours
   c. Hypotension
   d. Indications: PPHN with LV/RV dysfunction; low cardiac output states especially after cardiac surgery; Ebstein's anomaly to increase the antegrade pulmonary blood flow
   e. Renal.

20. a. Lung recruitment by increasing MAP/HFOV/surfactant.
   b. Here, priority will be management of shock. In the presence of systemic hypotension and good cardiac function, 1 or 2 fluid boluses (10 mL/kg of NS) followed by dopamine are recommended. Some centers prefer the use of norepinephrine or vasopressin because these agents are thought to be more selective systemic vasoconstrictors. If high doses of vasopressors and multiple vasopressors are needed, hydrocortisone should be considered.
   c. *ECMO indication:* Persistent hypoxemia (OI of >40 or alveolar-arterial gradient >600 despite aggressive medical management of PPHN with mechanical ventilation and iNO) and the presence of hemodynamic instability.

21. a. Acyanotic congenital heart disease with congestive cardiac failure
   b. Stabilize airway, breathing, and circulation.
   Respiratory support to provide adequate PEEP
   Fluid restriction
   Diuretics (furosemide 1–2 mg/kg/dose Q12 hours). Digoxin/ACE inhibitors if not controlled on diuretic alone
   Treatment of concomitant infection and anemia
   Optimizing nutrition.
   c. A follow-up of growth and development every month for first 3 months and every 3 monthly thereafter. Follow-up ECHO at 1 month, followed by ECHO every 3–6 months.
   d. *Indication for ASD closure:* ASD with left-to-right shunt associated with evidence of right ventricular volume overload without evidence of irreversible pulmonary vascular disease.

Techniques:
- Transcatheter nonsurgical closure (Amplatzer device)
- Surgical closure.

e. *Indications for VSD closure:* Growth failure refractory to medical management; pulmonary artery pressure >50% of systemic pressure; Qp/Qs >2:1.
Modality: Direct surgical closure of the defect.

22. a. Wide QRS complex tachycardia.
    Diagnosis: Ventricular tachycardia
    b. Severe medical illness like shock, hypoxia, electrolyte disturbances, and SVT with aberrancy
    c. D/d of wide QRS complex tachycardia: VT, VF, Torsades de pointes, and SVT with aberrancy
    d. Lidocaine, amiodarone, and procainamide
    e. Synchronized cardioversion.

23. a. *ECHO findings:* Caudal displacement of the tricuspid valve with low implantation of posterior leaflet, moderate dilatation of the right ventricle and significant dilatation of the right atrium.
    Diagnosis: Ebstein anomaly.
    b. GOSE (Great Ormond Street Echocardiography score) or Celermajer score is defined as ratio of area of right atrium and arterialized right ventricle to the combined area of the functional RV, LA, and LV.
    GOSE score of 3 or more with mild cyanosis in a neonate is an indication for surgery in neonatal period.
    Also, GOSE score is helpful in grading Ebstein anomaly predicting mortality as follows:

Grade	GOSE score/ratio	Mortality
1	<0.5	8%
2	0.5–0.99	9%
3 (acyanotic)	1–1.49	• 10% (neonatal) • 45% (later)
3 (cyanotic)	1–1.49	100%
4	>1.5	100%

c. Drugs used for medical management of these babies: PGE1, iNO, and milrinone.
d. Pulmonary valve regurgitation. In this case, initiation of PGE1 may lead to creation of circular shunt resulting in low systemic output.
e. Indications for surgical intervention in neonates:
   - Severe persistent cyanosis
   - GOSE score 3 or more with mild cyanosis
   - Cardiothoracic ratio >80%
   - Severe TR with persistent right heart failure.
f. These babies should be monitored for arrhythmias.

24. a. Massive pericardial effusion with cardiac tamponade

b. PICC line migration and malposition of PICC tip in pericardial cavity

c. Emergency pericardiocentesis by substernal approach

d. PICC line complications: Catheter migration, malposition, catheter rupture, bloodstream infections, occlusions, thrombophlebitis, and pericardial or pleural effusion.

25. a. *Chest X-ray:* Cardiomegaly

ECG: Signs of left ventricular hypertrophy (large amplitude QRS complexes) and a short PR interval in precordial leads

2D *ECHO:* Severe generalized left ventricular hypertrophy, thick IVS, and right ventricle hypertrophy. Findings suggestive of hypertrophic cardiomyopathy.

b. Pompe disease.

c. *Diagnosis:* Absent or markedly reduced acid alpha glucosidase (GAA) enzyme activity in dried blood spots or cultured skin fibroblasts. Genetic testing by exome sequencing to demonstrate homozygous mutation in GAA coding gene.

d. *Enzyme replacement therapy:* Recombinant human acid alpha-glucosidase (GAA).

26. a. CCHD screen is positive. We would request for cardiac evaluation and echocardiography

b. Transposition of great arteries

- Truncus arteriosus
- Pulmonary atresia
- Hypoplastic left heart syndrome
- Obstructed TAPVC
- Tetralogy of Fallot

c. Beer Lambert Law

d. Decreases low perfusion artifact and motion artifact

e. 80–95%

f. TGA with coarctation of aorta; TGA with severe PPHN.

27. a. Nonselective beta blocker

b. First generation class II

c. Indications for use of propranolol in neonates:

- SVT and other tachyarrhythmias
- Hypertension
- Large hemangioma
- For management of cyanotic spells in TOF
- Thyrotoxicosis

d. Dose:

Oral: 0.5–1 mg/kg/dose BD

IV: 0.01–0.02 mg/kg/dose BD

e. Monitor for hypotension (BP) and hypoglycemia (RBS).

28. a. Dilated cardiomyopathy
  b. Probable causes of neonatal cardiomyopathy:
- Prenatal infections (CMV, HIV, and parvovirus)
- Familial or genetic causes
- Maternal autoimmune disease with anti-Ro and anti-La antibodies
- Prenatal drug exposure
- Arrhythmia-induced cardiomyopathy
- Twin-twin transfusion
- Storage and metabolic disorders.

  c. Evaluation should include detailed sequential assessment to rule out disorders mentioned above.
  d. Approximately one-third of patients with DCM die, one-third have chronic heart failure, and one-third experience improvement in their condition.
  e. Indications for heart transplantation include failure of medical therapy, severe failure to thrive, intractable arrhythmias, and severe limitations to activity.

29. a. *ECHO:* Gray scale and color Doppler demonstrating the narrowing of the isthmus and obstructed antegrade flow through the descending aorta (DAo)
  b. Coarctation of aorta
  c. PGE1
  d. *Surgical:* Resection of coarctation segment and end-to-end anastomosis
  e. Risks associated with balloon angioplasty of native coarct: Aneurysm, recoarctation, vascular injury at the site of access
  f. 10–15% of babies will have recoarctation. It is managed with balloon angioplasty.

30. a. *Trisomy 18:* VSD
  b. *Trisomy 21:* Complete AV canal defect and VSD
  c. *Turner's syndrome:* Coarctation and bicuspid aortic valve
  d. *Noonan's syndrome:* Pulmonary valve stenosis
  e. *DiGeorge's syndrome (deletion 22q11):* Interrupted aortic arch and conotruncal malformations
  f. *CHARGE syndrome:* Conotruncal anomalies.

31. a. Air trapping as expiratory flow is less than the inspiratory flow, resulting in more gas entering than leaving the lung.
  b. Auto PEEP may lead to pneumothorax.

32. a. Congenital lobar emphysema
  b. CT thorax
  c. Lobectomy
  d. These babies may not tolerate PPV as it may lead to air trapping, air leak, and rarely cardiac arrest.

33. a. It is a capnograph. It is used for continuous monitoring of $PaCO_2$.

b. A = Expiration; B = Inspiration

c. Tube dislodgement (1) and subsequent reintubation into trachea (2) *OR* Cardiopulmonary arrest (1) followed by resumption of spontaneous circulation (2) *OR* Equipment failure and apnea (1) followed by resumption of respiration (2).

34. a. $CaO_2 = 1.34 \times Hb\% \times SpO_2 + 0.003 \times paO_2$

b. Baby A is more hypoxic as oxygen content of baby A is 7.62 mL O_2/dL and oxygen content of baby B is 14.1 mL O_2/dL

c. 16–22 mL O_2/dL.

35. a. Congenital diaphragmatic hernia

b. Between T3 and T4. Deep tube

c. LHR = Lung area/Head circumference

where, Lung area = Longest Diameter of contralateral lung × Perpendicular diameter of contralateral lung.

LFR >1.4 indicates good prognosis.

d. ALARA is " as low as is reasonably achievable" which means making every reasonable effort to maintain exposures to ionizing radiation as far below the dose limits as practical.

36. a. Mixed respiratory and metabolic acidosis with hypoxemia

b. 40.9

c. iNO OI >20; ECMO OI >40.

37. a. A: Rib; B: Pleural line; C: A-lines

b. AIS: The presence of more than three B-lines in an examined area.

White lung: Presence of compact B-lines in all the regions examined.

Comet tail sign: Short-path vertical reverberation artifact that weakens with each reverberation so that it does not reach the edge of the screen. Resembles the shape of a comet tail.

38. a. Pressure—volume loop

b. A: Upper inflection point; B: Lower inflection point

c. Beaking/bird's beak at end of inspiration due to overdistension of lung

d. Excessive PIP, excessive PEEP, and prolonged I time.

39. a. Tracheoesophageal fistula/esophageal atresia.

b. Spitz classification:

- *Class I:* Low-risk group of patients without cardiac defect and weight >2,000 g.
- *Class II:* Moderate risk/weight <2,000 g.
- *Class III:* Relative high risk/weight >2,000 g but with a major cardiac anomaly.
- *Class IV:* High risk/weight <2,000 g and major cardiac anomaly.
- Survival decreases from class I to class IV as follows: 100%, 82%, 72%, and 27%.

c. Two antenatal findings: Polyhydramnios and absent or small stomach.

40. a. Laryngeal mask airway

b. As a short-term alternative airway when attempts at face mask ventilation or intubation are unsuccessful

c. Difficult to administer high pressures as air may leak through seal between pharynx and the mask; difficult to administer medications; cannot be used in very small babies

d. Size 1

e. Above 2 kg.

41. a. Start PPV

b. 21%. For the initial resuscitation of newborns greater than or equal to 35 weeks' gestation, set the blender to 21% oxygen. For the initial resuscitation of newborns <35 weeks gestation, set the blender to 21–30% oxygen. Set the flow meter to 10 L/min

c. 40–60 breaths per minute

d. Start with a PIP of 20–25 cmH$_2$O. When PEEP is also being used, the suggested initial setting for PEEP is 5 cmH$_2$O

e. The most important indicator of successful PPV is a rising heart rate:
   - If the baby's heart rate is increasing after the first 15 seconds, continue PPV and check the response again after total 30 seconds of PPV.
   - If the baby's heart rate is not increasing after the first 15 seconds, ask the assistant if the chest is moving.
   - If the chest is moving, continue PPV while you monitor your ventilation technique. Check the baby's response again after 30 seconds of PPV.
   - If the chest is NOT moving, you may not be ventilating the baby's lungs. Perform the ventilation corrective steps until you achieve chest movement with PPV.

42. a. Start ventilation corrective steps—MR SOPA (mask readjustment, reposition airway, suction, open mouth, pressure increase, and alternative airway).

b. Measure the distance from the bridge of the nose to the earlobe and from the earlobe to a point halfway between the xiphoid process and the umbilicus.

c. CO$_2$ detector changes to yellow color.

d. A laryngeal mask is inserted into the baby's mouth and advanced into the throat until it makes a seal over the entrance to the baby's trachea.

43. a. T-piece resuscitator

b. *Parts:*
   1. Gas tubing
   2. Gas inlet
   3. Maximum pressure-relief control
   4. Manometer
   5. Inflation pressure control
   6. Gas outlet (proximal)
   7. T-piece gas outlet (patient)
   8. T-piece PEEP adjustment dial
   9. Opening on T-piece cap which is occluded for providing PIP.

44. a. Important anatomic landmarks in the neonatal airway
    1. Tongue
    2. Glottis
    3. Esophagus
    4. Vallecula
    5. Epiglottis
    6. Vocal cords
  b. Indications for endotracheal intubation:
    As an alternative airway; before starting chest compressions; diaphragmatic hernia; for administering medications
  c. 3.5 size ET in this baby. Depth of insertion: NTL (nasotragal length + 1 cm)
  d. 30 seconds
  e. Displacement, obstruction, pneumothorax, equipment failure
  f. Advance the laryngoscope forward to visualize the glottis.

45. a. Start chest compressions coordinated with PPV
  b. B
  c. One-third of AP diameter of chest
  d. Intubation has been done; 100% FiO_2; ECG leads placement if available and call for additional help
  e. 60 seconds.

46. a. Administer epinephrine.
  b. The recommended concentration of epinephrine for newborns is 0.1 mg/mL.
  c. The suggested initial intravenous dose of epinephrine is 0.02 mg/kg.
  d. Intravenous epinephrine should be administered as quickly as possible, followed by a 3-mL normal saline flush.
  e. If the baby's heart rate remains <60 beats per minute, you can repeat the dose of epinephrine every 3–5 minutes.
  f. Administer normal saline or O negative packed red blood cells if available. The initial dose is 10 mL/kg.

47. a. Increase the room temperature to 23°–25°C (74°–77°F), prepare a thermal mattress, prepare a polyethylene plastic bag or wrap, and prewarm a transport incubator if the baby will be moved after birth.
  b. T-piece resuscitator/a PPV device that can deliver both PIP and PEEP.
  c. 21–30%.
  d. Avoid placing baby's legs higher than the head.

48. a. Baby's respiratory distress may improve by inserting a small endotracheal tube in the nose, advancing it to the pharynx (nasopharyngeal airway), and placing the baby prone.
  b. Babies with MMC should be placed prone or side-lying. Latex free gloves as babies with NTDs may have latex allergy.

   c. Babies with gastroschisis should be positioned on their right side. The umbilical cord should be clamped and cut 10–20 cm from the baby because the cord may be used as a part of surgical repair.

   d. Intubate.

49. a. Neuromuscular disorder.

   b. *Other causes of poor respiratory drive in absence of sentinel event:* Opiate administration before birth, general anesthesia, medications like narcotics self-administered by mother, structural brain abnormality, severe sepsis/meningitis leading to hypoxia and acidosis.

   c. PPV.

   d. There is insufficient evidence to evaluate safety and efficacy of this drug. Very little is known about the pharmacology of naloxone in the newborn. Animal studies and case reports have raised concerns about complications from naloxone, including pulmonary edema, cardiac arrest, and seizures.

50. a. We would review and include current national and local data describing the anticipated short- and long-term outcomes at this extremely early gestation. The parents should be provided information and explained the treatment options. The parents should be informed that some parents might decide that attempting resuscitation and life-sustaining medical treatment is not in their baby's best interest in view of the high risk of mortality and morbidity and might, instead, choose palliative care focusing on the baby's comfort after birth, while others may support full life support. Shared decision making would be done.

   b. Generally, parents are the best surrogate decision makers for their own babies, and they should be involved in shared decision-making whenever possible.

   c. Ethical principles that apply to all medical care, including neonatal care, include respecting an individual's rights to make choices that affect their life *(autonomy),* acting to benefit others *(beneficence),* avoiding harm *(nonmaleficence),* and treating people truthfully and fairly *(justice).*

51. a. Blood should be taken at time of hypoglycemia (critical samples) and sent for plasma glucose, serum insulin, serum cortisol, serum free fatty acids (FFA), serum Beta-hydroxybutyrate (BOHB), serum HCO_3, lactate.

b. Diagnostic criteria for hyperinsulinemic hypoglycemia (Ferrara C, Patel P, Becker S, et al. Biomarkers of Insulin for the Diagnosis of Hyperinsulinemic Hypoglycemia in Infants and Children. J Pediatr 2016; 168:212):
- At time of hypoglycemia (RB <50 mg/dL):
  - Insulin level ≥2 mIU/mL (Normally insulin levels should be undetectable in blood at time of hypoglycemia, so any detectable level of insulin at time of hypoglycemia can be taken as abnormal also)
  - Beta-hydroxybutyrate <1.8 mmol/L
  - FFA <1.7 mmol/L
  - Glucose rise ≥30 mg/dL after glucagon administration
  - Insulin like growth factor binding protein (IGFBP) ≤110 ng/mL
  - Low ketone and low FFA levels suggest insulin-mediated hypoglycemia. Low ketones and increased FFA levels suggest fatty acid oxidation defects.
- If GIR need is more than 12 mg/kg/min in absence of sepsis, hyperinsulinemia is likely etiology of hypoglycemia

c. (i) Diazoxide
   (ii) Binds to SUR1 subunit. It is a potassium channel opener.
   (iii) 5–20 mg/kg/day in 3 divided doses orally
   (iv) Fluid retention, hyponatremia, hypertrichosis, cardiac toxicity, rarely eosinophilia, leukopenia, hypotension

d. Octreotide, Nifedipine, and Sirolimus are other drugs which can be used in hyperinsulinemic hypoglycemia if there is no response to Diazoxide.

e. Genetic studies for mutational analysis of *ABCC8/KCNJ11* genes

52. a. Infants with TSH values above certain levels on the initial newborn screen, usually >30 mIU/L in serum units (equivalent to >15 mIU/L in whole blood units), are recalled for clinical evaluation and serum testing **(Flowchart 1)**, which occurs around 1 week of age. If a second test is done, the results should be interpreted using a lower TSH cutoff (typically >10 mIU/L after 1 week of age).

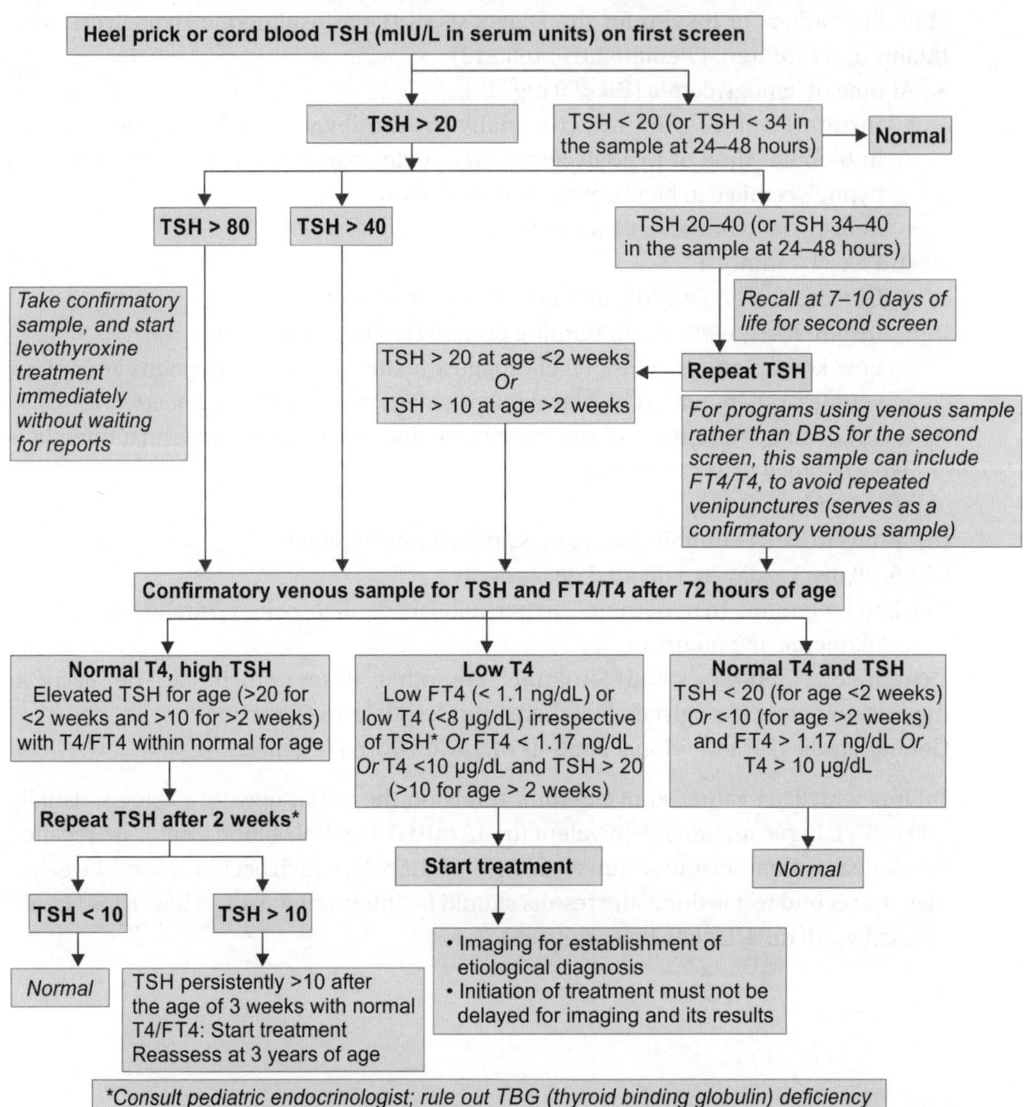

Flowchart 1: Screening and diagnosis of congenital hypothyroidism.

b. Thyroid ultrasound and radionuclide uptake and scan. Either 99m-pertechnetate or iodine-123 can be used. The 99m-pertechnetate scan is more readily available and allows a good scan picture, but because it is not organified, there is no measure of uptake. Iodine-123 must be especially ordered due to its short half-life, but it will provide both a scan and a measure of uptake. Iodine–123 scan is less readily available.

c. Ultrasound of thyroid gland should be done once congenital hypothyroidism (CH) is biochemically confirmed. Scintigraphy can be done either before or within 7 days of starting levothyroxine (till time TSH is elevated).

Please note that imaging should never be the reason to delay the initiation of therapy in CH.

d. Thyroid hypoplasia.

Interpretation of scan—A large gland in a normal location typically is seen with one of the enzymatic defects. A positive perchlorate discharge test is compatible with an organification defect. Decreased uptake on scan associated with a normally located thyroid gland on ultrasound suggests the possibility of a loss-of-function TSH receptor gene mutation or maternally transmitted TSH receptor-blocking antibodies.

e. The initial levothyroxine dose is 10–15 µg/kg, given as a single dose, as a crushed tablet in expressed breastmilk. The first follow-up including thyroid function tests (FT4/T4) should be done 2 weeks after starting treatment by which time normalization of FT4/T4 is expected. If the levels are low for age, a slight increase in the dose is required. On the other hand, the dose should not be decreased if a single value of T4 is found above the normal range. The next test, after 1 month, should include both T4/FT4 and TSH; normalization of TSH is expected by this time. The sample for thyroid function is taken before (or minimum 4 hours after) ingestion of LT4.

f. Follow-up is done every 2 months in early infancy till 6 months of age, every 3 months during age 6 months to 3 years and every 3–6 months thereafter, till growth and pubertal development is completed. Any dose change is followed by a biochemical evaluation after 4 weeks. Hearing test and clinical evaluation for other congenital malformations must be performed for all babies with CH. Babies with the possibility of transient CH should be re-evaluated at the age of 3 years, for permanence of CH and the need for lifelong therapy.

g. Criteria for initiating treatment
- Low T4 (<100 nmol/L or 8 µg/dL) or low FT4 (<12 pmol/L or <1.1 ng/dL) irrespective of TSH
- Mild low T4 (<128 nmol/L or 10 µg/dL) or low FT4 (<15 pmol/L or 1.17 ng/dL) in the presence of elevated venous TSH >20 mIU/L if age is <2 weeks and >10 mIU/L if age is >2 weeks
- Normal T4/FT4 with persistently elevated TSH >10 mIU/L at age >3 weeks

h. For preterm babies, screening for CH may be done at 2, 6 and 10 weeks of age using TSH and Free T4. This is because these babies will often have delayed rise of TSH due to immaturity of HPT axis.

53. a. We shall start screening for MBD at 4 weeks of age, using serum calcium, phosphorus and alkaline phosphatase (ALP). Combination of deceased serum phosphate levels <5.6 mg/dL (<1.8 mmol/L) and increased ALP levels >900 IU in preterm infants <33 weeks indicates low bone mineral density and has a sensitivity of 100% and specificity of 70% for diagnosing MBD.

b. Risk factors for MBD in this baby (apart from extreme prematurity and ELBW):
- Delayed initiation of enteral feeds
- Suspect NEC
- Bone active medications—diuretics and steroids

c. PTH, TRP (tubular reabsorption of phosphate), vitamin D levels, serum calcium levels, X-ray needed.

d. High PTH with low pO_4, high ALP and low TRP (normal TRP 85–95%) suggest primarily calcium deficient state. In this primarily calcium deficient state, mainstay of treatment will be calcium supplementation (40 to 100 mg/kg/day) in 2 to 4 divided doses. This would normalize elevated PTH, thus reversing resultant bone resorption and hypophosphatemia. Along with this, we would supplement vitamin D 800–1000 IU/day. Phosphate supplementation in this condition will result in binding to ionized calcium, therefore causing a further increase in PTH and in fact exacerbation of MBDP.

e. Current recommendations (ESPGHAN 2010):
   - Calcium 120–140 mg/kg/day
   - Phosphorus 60–90 mg/kg/day
   - Vitamin D 800–1000 IU/day

   Calcium phosphorus supplementation/fortification is continued until 40 weeks postmenstrual age. Vitamin D is continued till 1 year of age. Babies with MBD would need fortification for a longer duration, till phosphate normalizes and ALP touches baseline.

54. a. Hypocalcemia, hypomagnesemia

b. We will give a bolus dose of 2 mL/kg 10% calcium gluconate diluted 1:1 with 5% dextrose over 10 minutes under cardiac monitoring. This is followed by maintenance calcium at 80 mg/kg/day of elemental calcium (8 mL/kg/day of 10% calcium gluconate; 1 mL = 9.4 mg of elemental calcium) for 48 hours. This may be tapered to 50% dose if calcium levels normalize for another 24 hours and then discontinued.

c. Magnesium levels to be done. Magnesium level <1.5 mg/dL is suggestive of hypomagnesemia.

   Correction of associated hypomagnesemia: Give 50% magnesium sulfate solution (500 mg/mL or 4 mEq/mL)—50 mg/kg or 0.1 mL/kg/per dose every 12 hours, through IM or IV route. IV dose should be preferable in NICU and given over 2 hours.

d. Other complications:

   Systemic: Macrosomia, birth trauma, RDS, renal vein thrombosis, small left colon syndrome, asymmetric septal hypertrophy, poor feeding

   Metabolic: Hypoglycemia, hypocalcemia, hypomagnesemia, polycythemia, hyperbilirubinemia

   Long-term: Metabolic syndrome, obesity, diabetes

e. *Timing of delivery (ACOG):* For women with GDM that is controlled with diet and exercise, delivery should not be before 39 weeks of gestation, unless indicated otherwise. In such women, expectant management up to $40^{6/7}$ weeks is generally appropriate. For women with GDM that is well controlled by medications, delivery is recommended at $39^{0/7}$ to $39^{6/7}$ weeks of gestation.

f. Screening at 4–12 weeks postpartum is recommended for all women who had GDM to identify women with diabetes, impaired fasting glucose levels, or impaired glucose tolerance. They should be referred for preventive or medical therapy. The ADA and ACOG recommend repeat testing every 1–3 years for women who had a pregnancy affected by GDM and normal postpartum screening test results.

55. a. Hypercalcemia

b. Causes:
- Iatrogenic/improper medications/imbalance of calcium intake
- Hypervitaminosis D/vitamin D intoxication
- Hyperparathyroidism
- Familial hypocalciuric hypercalcemia
- Williams syndrome
- Subcutaneous fat necrosis

c. Vitamin D and calcium supplementation (if being given)—we should check the dose and preparation.

d. PTH levels, serum phosphorus, ALP, vitamin D levels
- Renal function tests
- USG KUB to look for nephrocalcinosis

e. Baby has hypervitaminosis D/vitamin D intoxication due to inappropriately high vitamin D ingestion over 1 month.

Treatment: Saline bolus (10–20 mL/kg), Furosemide (1 mg/kg/dose 8th hourly), glucocorticoids (Hydrocortisone/Methylprednisolone (4 mg/kg/day) followed by oral prednisolone (1 mg/kg/day). Calcitonin (8 IU/kg/day) and Pamidronate (0.5 mg/kg/day infusion) may be given in refractory hypercalcemia.

56. a. We will do following tests in the baby:
- Cord blood TRAb (TSH receptor antibody)
- Free T4 and TSH between day 3 and 5

Yes, this baby is still at risk of developing hyperthyroidism. Mothers with Graves' disease (GD) have TRAb. The treatment of Graves' disease consists of antithyroid drugs, radioactive iodine ablation or surgical thyroidectomy. None of these treatments target TRAb. Hence, even if the mother has been adequately treated for hyperthyroidism in the past, she may still have TRAb, which may persist lifelong though the risk decreases with time. The TRAb are of two types. They can inhibit the production of thyroxine or stimulate the production of thyroxine. The TRAb belong to the immunoglobulin G (IgG) and can easily cross the placenta and produce hyperthyroidism in the fetus and the neonate.

b. Baby has hyperthyroidism. Drugs for treatment:
- Methimazole (0.2–0.5 mg/kg/day in 2 divided doses)
- Propranolol (2 mg/kg/day in 2–4 divided doses)

In severe hyperthyroidism, Lugol's solution (0.05 mL/L drop 3 times a day) may be used to block release of thyroxine immediately. First dose should be given 1 hour after Methimazole. Additional therapy for severe cases may include prednisolone (1 to 2 mg/kg/day).

c. In mothers with Graves' disease or a past history of same, TRAb testing should be done at 18–20 weeks. A maternal TRAb value of at least 5 index units predicted neonatal thyrotoxicosis with a sensitivity of 100%, specificity of 76.0%, positive predictive value of 40.0%, and negative predictive value of 100%. Maternal FT4 levels should be maintained in the upper range of normal in the pregnancy.

d. Propylthiouracil (PTU) is used in the first trimester, followed by Methimazole (MMI). Antithyroid drugs should be given at low doses such that FHR is kept around 140/min. Beta blockers may be used in severe cases.

Adverse effects: PTU is hepatotoxic whereas MMI has teratogenic potential.

e. Methimazole is the drug of choice for treatment of hyperthyroidism in lactating women.

57. a. Neonatal hyperglycaemia is defined as whole blood glucose level higher than 125 mg/dL or plasma glucose values higher than 145 mg/dL.

Common causes of neonatal hyperglycemia: Iatrogenic, sepsis, ingestion of hyperosmolar formula, drugs (Steroids, caffeine, phenytoin) hypoxia, surgical procedures, neonatal diabetes mellitus (transient or permanent).

b. *Treatment:* We will decrease the GIR to 4 mg/kg/min. If high sugar values persist and reach the treatment threshold, we shall start insulin 0.05 to 0.1 unit/kg over 15 minutes, every 4 to 6 hours as needed. Monitor glucose every 30 minutes to 1 hour. If glucose remains >200 mg/dL even after 3 doses, initiate insulin infusion 0.05 to 0.2 unit/kg/h. Monitor strictly for hypoglycemia and hypokalemia.

Operational thresholds at which treatment should be initiated for neonatal hyperglycaemia:

- Any blood glucose measurement of ≥360 mg/dL
- Persistent blood glucose values ≥270 mg/dL
- Persistent blood glucose values >216 mg/dL with glycosuria ≥3+ on urinary dipstick testing. (Cloherty and Stark's Manual of Neonatal Care, South Asian Edition, Chapter 24, Page 333)

c. *Diagnosis of NDM (neonatal diabetes mellitus):* NDM is persisting hyperglycemia lasting more than 2 weeks presenting before 6 months of age, requiring insulin to maintain euglycemia.

Suspect NDM	• Growth restriction, polyuria, dehydration, failure to thrive • Glucose 200–250 mg/dL or more than few days (no alternative cause) • Glucose >300 mg/dL regardless of the time course • Need for insulin before 6–12 months of age
First-line tests	Urine ketones, serum glucose, C peptide, and insulin levels, pancreatic ultrasound, thyroid function tests, hepatic and renal functions, ophthalmological evaluation
Second-tier test	Glutamate decarboxylase, zinc transporter-8, insulin, and islet antigen-2 autoantibodies, IgE levels, X-rays spine, and limbs
Genetic analysis	For all NDM

d. Etiology of NDM:

Transient NDM: Genetic defect in *6q24, ABCC8, KCNJ11*

Permanent NDM: Genetic defect in *KCNJ11, ABCC8, GCK,* INS genes

Syndromic causes: IPE syndrome, Wolcott-Rallison syndrome, GLIS3

Treatment options for NDM: Sulfonylureas, insulin

e. IPEX syndrome (Immune dysregulation, polyendocrinopathy, enteropathy, X-linked syndrome.

Genetic defect in FOXP3-IPEX.

58. a. Congenital adrenal hyperplasia (CAH) and difference or disorders of sex development (DSD)

b. Investigations:

1. *Adrenocortical profile:* Serum 17-OHP, cortisol, 11-deoxycortisol, 17-OH pregnenolone, dihydroepiandrostenedione (DHEA) and androstenedione should be measured. Apart from 17-OH pregnenolone, the rest of the tests are available on the LC-MS/MS platform.
2. Karyotype/FISH
3. USG pelvis
4. Genetic confirmation of diagnosis by clinical exome sequencing can be offered

c. CAH due to 21-OH deficiency and 46,XX DSD.

Emergency management of adrenal crisis consists of management of shock with normal saline boluses followed by 1.5–2 times maintenance fluids in form of 5% dextrose with NS, correction of hypoglycemia and electrolyte disturbances and initiation of hydrocortisone replacement therapy (100 mg/m^2/day in four divided doses) after acquiring samples for confirmation of diagnosis.

Maintenance therapy consists of hydrocortisone 10–15 mg/m^2/day in three divided doses, Fludrocortisone 0.1–0.2 mg/day and salt supplementation in doses of 1–2.5 g per day, divided with feeds. This can be done by adding a pinch of common salt each time in expressed breast milk/feeds. Hydrocortisone and fludrocortisone are given lifelong. The normal family pot diet usually suffices for the sodium requirement after infancy and salt supplementation is usually required in the first year of life only.

d. Factors to be considered while taking decisions on the sex of rearing are underlying diagnosis, genital appearance, internal anatomy, likely gender identity, future fertility, the feasibility of surgical correction, and psychosocial factors. The sex of rearing in a 46,XX DSD neonate with CAH is best assigned as female due to likely female gender identity, preserved fertility, and the possibility of surgical correction.

e. All children with CAH should be monitored for steroid excess clinically. Physical examination should look for hyperpigmentation, cushingoid features, growth, body fat distribution, pigmented striae, and blood pressure for hypertension. Lab monitoring on follow-up should be done as below. Parents should be clearly instructed to increase the dose of hydrocortisone in stress such as febrile illness and gastroenteritis.

Monitoring of children with classical congenital adrenal hyperplasia	
Age, frequency	**Investigations**
First 3 months, monthly	Serum electrolytes, baseline 17-hydroxyprogesterone recorded
3–12 months, 3 monthly	• Serum electrolytes, serum 17-OHP, serum androstenedione, total testosterone, ACTH • Plasma renin activity
12–30 months, 4 monthly	• Skeletal age assessment annually after 24 months of age • Serum electrolytes, serum 17-OHP, serum androstenedione, total testosterone, ACTH • Plasma renin activity

   f. Prenatal dexamethasone administration to a pregnant woman with a prior CAH affected child for prevention of virilization of a female fetus should be considered only experimental and offered after a complete discussion with the family about possible maternal adverse effects, variable genital outcome and unknown long-term side effects of dexamethasone therapy. As of now, the use of prenatal steroids is not recommended and may be started only after a detailed discussion with the family

   g. Early genital surgery during infancy or early childhood is recommended for severely virilized (≥Prader stage 3) female babies. Corrective genital surgery includes vaginoplasty, clitoroplasty and labial surgery. Most children need a staged repair.

59. a. Hypopituitarism (Midline defects, hypoglycemia, persistent jaundice) Hypocortisolism due to ACTH deficiency, central hypothyroidism, central hypogonadism due to LH/FSH deficiency, growth hormone deficiency, prolactin and vasopressin deficiency.

   b. We shall start first with hydrocortisone supplementation and correction of cortisol levels, followed by levothyroxine supplementation. Cortisol deficiency should always be treated before thyroid hormone replacement (if there is an associated deficiency) to prevent adrenal crisis.

   c. Corpus callosum agenesis, septo optic dysplasia, holoprosencephaly.

   d. Random GH levels <7 ng/mL in the first week of life, in association with other pituitary hormone deficiency, can be used to diagnose neonatal growth hormone deficiency. There is no role of GH stimulation test in newborns.

   e. All neonates born at term gestation, have a higher level of gonadotropins, starting at around 4–6 weeks till 6 months in males and 2 years in females (mini puberty). The ideal time to evaluate is around 4 to 6 weeks. In males (14 days to 6 months), LH levels <0.8 IU/L and total testosterone <30 ng/dL can be taken as an indicator of central hypogonadism whereas in females (14 days to 2 years), a serum level of FSH <1.0 IU/L is diagnostic of hypogonadotropic hypogonadism (HH).

60. a. *In an apparent female baby*
- Clitoromegaly >1 cm
- Presence of inguinal hernia
- Posterior labial fusion

       In an apparent male baby
- Bilateral nonpalpable gonads
- Phallus length <2.5 cm (micropenis)
- Hypospadias associated with separation of scrotal sacs (bifid scrotum) or an undescended testis (not isolated hypospadias)
- Penoscrotal hypospadias (severe hypospadias)

   b. The external masculinizing score (EMS) is used to classify the degree of under masculinization 46,XY DSD infants. It is based on the size of the phallus, position of the urethral meatus, presence of gonads, and degree of scrotal fusion, each carrying scores from 0 to 3 to give a total score of 12. Lower scores indicate a more severe form of undervirilization and an EMS <9–10 indicates a need for further evaluation.

c. Detailed antenatal history including maternal drug use (antiandrogens, danazol, progesterone, and spironolactone). History of maternal virilization in the antenatal period (aromatase deficiency and luteoma of pregnancy). Detailed family chart and pedigree for any consanguinity, family history of DSD, sibling deaths, and infertility.

d. As this baby has a palpable gonad, this baby is likely to have 46,XY DSD. The presence of palpable gonad points to the presence of testis and Y chromosome material.

e. Causes of 46,XY DSD:
   - Androgen insensitivity
     - Partial
     - Complete
   - 5 alpha reductase deficiency
   - Testosterone biosynthetic defects
     - 17 beta-HSD deficiency
     - 3 beta-HSD
     - 17 alpha-hydroxylase/17,20 lyase deficiency
     - Congenital lipoid adrenal hyperplasia
   - Leydig cell hypoplasia
   - Drugs
   - Persistent Müllerian duct syndrome
   - Complete/partial gonadal dysgenesis.

f. Karyotype, USG pelvis, genitogram and cystourethrogram while planning surgery. Biochemical and hormonal evaluation is as follows:
   - *Adrenal hormones (after 48 hours):*
     - 17OHP
     - Cortisol
     - Adrenal steroid profile (in CAH)
   - *Electrolytes and blood sugar*
   - *Gonadotropins: LH and FSH (after 1 week)**
   - *Androgens (after 1 week)**
     - Androstenedione
     - Testosterone
     - DHT
   - *AMH*
   - *Inhibin B*

   *After beginning of minipuberty (preferably after 2 weeks)

61. a. *Differential diagnoses:* Sepsis with meningitis, dyselectrolytemia, intracranial bleed, neonatal stroke, cranial malformations, inborn errors of metabolism.

   Evaluation: RBS, Electrolytes (sodium, calcium, magnesium), CBC, CRP, Blood culture, CSF analysis for meningitis, USG cranium/MRI Brain, IEM workup.

   b. *Preliminary basic investigations when suspecting IEM:* Glucose, electrolytes, lactate, ammonia, arterial blood gas, urinary ketones ("GELAAK"), liver function tests, urine for reducing substances.

Second-line investigations for confirmation: Gas chromatography mass spectrometry (GSMS) of urine, plasma amino acid and acylcarnitine profile by Tandem Mass Spectrometry (TMS), CSF amino acid analysis, neuroimaging and MRS, EEG. Genetic testing for final confirmation.

c. Baby has respiratory alkalosis and hyperammonaemia. Probable diagnosis is urea cycle defect.

d. *Confirmation of diagnosis:* Gas chromatography mass spectrometry (GSMS) of urine, plasma amino acid and acylcarnitine profile by Tandem Mass Spectrometry (TMS).

Management:
- Stabilise baby, maintain airway/breathing/circulation, stop protein intake.
- Start IV glucose (GIR 8-10) or TPN with lipids but no protein initially
- Start first-line medications (sodium benzoate/sodium phenylbutyrate/L-arginine)

Sodium benzoate: Loading dose 250 mg/kg IV/oral. Maintenance dose: 250–400 mg/kg/day in 4 divided doses (IV/oral) (IV preparation is not available in India).

Sodium phenylbutyrate: Loading: 250 mg/kg. Maintenance: 250–500 mg/kg/day (Not available in India)

Arginine: 300 mg/kg/day oral/IV
- Peritoneal dialysis should be started as soon as possible with routine monitoring of ammonia levels. Hemodialysis is better.
- Energy intake—120% age adjusted requirements
- Use of special infant formula feeds (initially protein free) and later with reduced proteins.

e. *Probable diagnosis:* OTC (Ornithine transcarbamylase) deficiency. Further molecular genetic testing should be done to confirm the diagnosis.

f. *Long-term therapy:* Lifelong low protein diet and nitrogen scavenger therapy (sodium benzoate)

62. a. Vein of Galen Malformation (VOGM).

b. *Potential complications:* Hydrocephalus, cardiac failure, refractory PPHN

c. High output cardiac failure due to high-flow AV shunts of VOGM.

d. *Treatment:* Coil embolization. Both arterial and venous embolization is possible depending on number of feeders. Hydrocephalus is typically not shunted, as this may exacerbate cerebral ischemia by altering cerebral hemodynamics and increases risk of intraventricular hemorrhage.

e. Postembolization complications included cerebral hemorrhage/hematoma, cerebral ischemia, macrocephaly or hydrocephalus, leg ischemia, vessel perforation, pulmonary embolism, and nontarget embolization.

63. a. RBS, electrolytes (sodium, calcium, magnesium), CBC, CRP, blood culture, CSF analysis, USG cranium/MRI brain.

b. Benign neonatal seizures (nonfamilial).

c. Difference between familial and nonfamilial variants:

	Benign nonfamilial neonatal seizures	*Benign familial neonatal seizures*
Main seizures	Mostly clonic	Tonic-clonic
Onset	Fifth day of life	Second or third day of life
Duration of seizures	Status epilepticus (median 20 hours)	Repetitive isolated seizures
Main causes	Unknown, probably environmental	Autosomal dominant
Subsequent seizures	Practically nil (0.5%)	Relatively high (11%)
Psychomotor deficits	Minor	Practically nonexistent
Ictal EEG	Usually localized spikes	Usually generalized flattening
Interictal EEG	Usually theta pointu alternant	Normal or focal abnormalities

d. *Long-term prognosis:* The prognosis is usually excellent with normal development and no recurrence of seizures. Minor psychomotor deficits and occasional febrile or afebrile seizures (0.5%) have been reported.

64. a. Lissencephaly (smooth brain)
  b. Associations:
   - Type I lissencephaly with chromosomal defects of 17p (LIS1), Xq (XLIS)
   - Fetal CMV infection
   - IEMs like pyruvate dehydrogenase deficiency, Zellweger syndrome, glutaric aciduria
  c. The peak time period for neuronal migration disorders to occur is from 3rd to 5th month of gestation (12–24 weeks)
  d. Other disorders of neuronal migration:
   - Schizencephaly
   - Pachygyria
   - Polymicrogyria
   - Heterotopias
   - Focal cerebrocortical dysgenesis

65. a. *MRI findings:* Axial T1 (upper row) and T2 (lower row) images of the brain at the level of basal ganglia. It shows T2 hyperintense signals in right frontal and parietal lobes with effacement of sulci. Involvement of the right middle cerebral artery (MCA) in its cortical area, sparing deep gray matter.
  b. Diffusion restriction in DWI suggests right-sided acute infarct.
   Diagnosis: Neonatal stroke/perinatal arterial ischemic stroke
  c. *Maternal risk factors:* Infertility, oligohydramnios, prothrombotic disorder, preeclampsia, Diabetes, IUGR, chorioamnionitis, PROM, autoimmune disorders.
   Delivery risk factors: Fetal HR abnormalities, MSAF, placental infarcts
   Neonatal risk factors: Central venous/arterial catheters, congenital heart disease, sepsis, meningitis, birth asphyxia, RDS, dehydration, congenital nephritic/nephrotic syndrome, NEC, polycythemia, pulmonary hypertension, ECMO, medications like steroids

   d. Management: Mainly supportive.
- Neuroprotective management—maintain oxygenation, ventilation, and fluid status.
- Correct metabolic parameters—sugar and electrolytes.
- Treat specific causes like infection.
- Treat seizures—usually easily controlled and in most cases, medications can be stopped before discharge.
- Aspirin, unfractionated, or LMW heparin can be given if the risk of recurrence is high (thrombophilia, complex cyanotic heart disease)

   e. Current guidelines from American College of Chest Physicians recommend anticoagulation for neonates with perinatal arterial ischemic stroke (PAIS) only if there is ongoing cardioembolic source or if there is evidence of recurrent PAIS (thrombophilia, complex cyanotic heart disease).

   f. MR angiography, 2D ECHO

   g. Baseline CBC, PT, aPTT, Thromboplastin time and fibrinogen levels should be obtained shortly after the acute event. Additional tests for evaluation of thrombophilia (particularly in absence of any other cause or risk and strong family history) which may be considered:
- Antiphospholipid antibody panel, anticardiolipin and lupus anticoagulant
- *DNA-based assays:* Factor V Leiden mutation, prothrombin G
- *Protein based assays:* Protein C, protein S levels, antithrombin activity, lipoprotein (a), fasting homocysteine, plasminogen, Factor VIII activity, factor XII activity.

Timing: Baseline CBC, PT, aPTT, thromboplastin time and fibrinogen levels should be obtained shortly after the acute event.
- Antiphospholipid antibody panel, anticardiolipin and lupus anticoagulant may be performed from maternal serum during first few months of life
- DNA-based assays may be obtained at any time.
- Certain protein-based assays may aid in treatment (AT III and plasminogen) and may be performed during neonatal period. However, most other protein-based assays are affected by acute thrombosis and must be repeated at 3–6 months of life before definitive diagnosis is made. Therefore, it is recommended that complete evaluation (excluding DNA-based assays) be performed at *3–6 months* of life. If anticoagulation is being given, then these assays should be obtained 14–30 days after discontinuing the anticoagulant.
- Lipoprotein (a) concentrations increase during the first year of life and should be repeated at 8–12 months of life if values obtained at 3–6 months of life are low.

   h. *Findings:* Axial T1 and T2 images at the level of basal ganglia. There is atrophy with encephalomalacia changes in right fronto-parietal and insular lobes-likely sequelae of ischemic insult.

   i. *Long-term problems:* Motor deficits (Perinatal stroke is the most known cause for hemiplegic cerebral palsy (30%). About 50–60% of neonatal acute stroke and 80–90% of presumed strokes have unilateral weakness of some degree. Extent of disability is decided by location, size, and number of lesions), cognitive impairments, seizure disorder, behavioral abnormalities, visual impairment, delay in language development.

66. a. *Complications of meningitis:* Cerebral edema, ventriculitis, brain abscess, infarction, hemorrhage, hydrocephalus.

 b. USG brain can help in diagnosing IVH and in grading of type of IVH (Grade 1–4) which helps in prognosticating patients. USG brain also helps in monitoring Levene Index and thalamo-occipital distance in posthemorrhagic and postmeningitis hydrocephalus, which helps in determining need of serial lumbar puncture or neurosurgical intervention (shunt surgery).

 In ventriculitis in USG brain, we find ventricular dilatation with irregularity of ventricular margin and echogenic material.

 USG brain can also help in picking up brain abscess, which will be seen as cystic mass with internal debris and shaggy wall.

 c. *Diagnosis of ventriculitis:* Failure to respond to appropriate antibiotics clinically or bacteriologically (no clinical improvement/clinical worsening/worsening CSF counts/ persisting positive CSF culture or cytology) and signs of elevated ICP may suggest the diagnosis of ventriculitis. The definitive diagnosis is by ventricular tap and cytological, biochemical and microbiological analysis of ventricular cerebrospinal fluid (CSF). As this is invasive procedure, various noninvasive modalities in the form of neuroimaging have been used. In USG brain, there may be ventricular dilatation with irregularity of ventricular margin, ventricular septations, echogenic material. USG brain is usually the first imaging modality.

 Contrast enhanced MRI findings include intraventricular debris, pus, abnormal periventricular and subependymal signal intensity, and enhancement of the ventricular lining. MRI is usually not necessary for initial management.

 d. Recommended duration of treatment for ventriculitis: 4–6 weeks. Intraventricular antibiotics via EVD (external ventricular drain) or reservoir, may be needed in case baby is not responding to intravenous antibiotics alone and CSF counts/culture are worsening or persistent.

 e. T2-weighted image showing temporo-parieto-occipital mass lesion with a central hyperintense signal and a peripheral linear irregular hypointense wall signal. Perilesional edema and mass effect with midline shift towards the left. Diagnosis is brain abscess.

 f. *Management:* Neurosurgical consultation for need for surgical intervention (needle aspiration or excision). Duration of antibiotic therapy may need to be extended to 6–8 weeks, depending on clinical and radiographic response. Serial brain imaging at weekly or biweekly intervals should be performed to monitor the evolution of lesion.

67. a. Difference between central and peripheral hypotonia:
 - *Central hypotonia:* These hypotonic neonates show signs of abnormal consciousness, seizures, apnea, abnormal posturing, and feeding difficulties.

Muscle power is relatively preserved, and axial weakness is a significant clinical feature. The tendon reflexes are normal or hyperactive, and there is no evidence of muscle fasciculations. Postural reflexes are generally preserved in infants with cerebral hypotonia despite a paucity of spontaneous movements. In some acute encephalopathies, the Moro reflex may be exaggerated.

- *Peripheral hypotonia:* These infants appear more alert in comparison to those with CNS involvement. Babies with anterior horn cell disease usually have sparing of extra-ocular muscles while the disorders of neuromuscular junctions may have ptosis and extraocular muscle weakness. There is weakness in the antigravity limb muscles along with diminished or absent reflexes. They can have deformities of bones or joints (arthrogryposis). Fasciculations may be observed in the tongue. Postural reflexes are absent or diminished, and limbs that lack voluntary movement also cannot move reflexively.

b. Possible sites of involvement and D/D in peripheral hypotonia:

Antenor horn cell	Generalized weakness and absent deep tendon reflexes	Spinomuscular atrophy
Nerve	• Distal muscle weakness and wasting • Decreased tendon reflexes	Peripheral neuropathy
Neuromuscular junction	Involvement of facial muscles with or without generalized weakness	Myasthenia gravis botulism
Muscle	• Weakness • Decreased tendon reflexes • Fasciculations joint contractures	• Congenital muscular dystrophy • Congenital myotonic dystrophy • Congenital and metabolic myopathy

c. *D/D for central hypotonia:* Brain malformations, perinatal asphyxia, chromosomal disorders, stroke, inborn errors of metabolism.

d. *Probable diagnosis in this child:* Peripheral hypotonia with areflexia.

e. Approach to management:

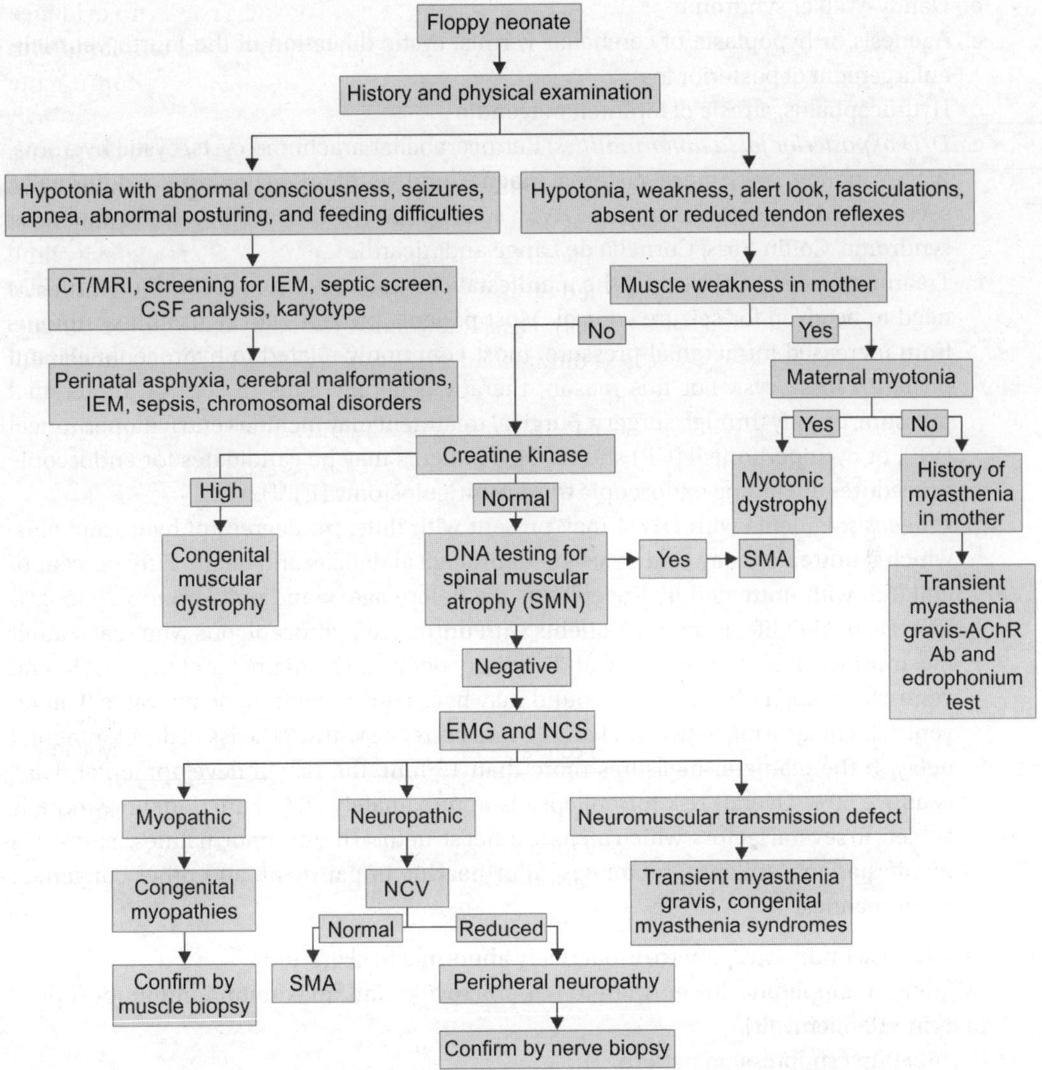

f. *FDA approved drugs for use in infants with SMA:* Nusinersen, Zolgensma

68. a. Ventriculomegaly and posterior fossa cyst
    b. Dandy-Walker syndrome
    c. Agenesis or hypoplasia of cerebellar vermis, cystic dilatation of the fourth ventricle, enlargement of posterior fossa.
    d. Hydrocephalus, atresia of foramen magendie
    e. *D/D of posterior fossa abnormalities:* Retrocerebellar arachnoid cysts, cystic hygroma, Blake's pouch cyst, mega cisterna magna, and vermian hypoplasia. Additionally, several syndromes correlate with DWM, such as Aase-Smith, cerebro-oculo-muscular syndrome, Coffin-Siris, Cornelia de Lange and Aicardi.
    f. Treatment consists of treating the manifestations and associated comorbidities. AEDs need to be given for seizure control. Most patients present with signs and symptoms from increased intracranial pressure, most commonly related to hydrocephalus and posterior fossa cyst. For this reason, therapy generally aims to control intracranial pressure, usually through surgery. Surgical treatment may include ventriculoperitoneal (VP), or cystoperitoneal (CP) shunts. Few patients may be candidates for endoscopic procedures, including endoscopic third ventriculostomy (ETV).
    g. *Prognosis:* Patients with DWM may present with different degrees of hydrocephalus, which if untreated may lead to severe neurological deficits and death. Fifty percent of children with untreated hydrocephalus die before age 3, and only around 20 to 23% will reach adult life. From the patients with untreated hydrocephalus who reach adult life, most will have motor, visual and auditory deficits. The diameter of the fetal lateral ventricle through obstetric ultrasound may have substantial prognostic value. Lateral ventricles measuring between 11 and 15 mm correlate with a 21% risk of developmental delay. If the diameter measures more than 15 mm, the risk of developmental delay is above 50%. Overall risk for epilepsy is approximately 30%. Functional outcome is subject to several factors, which include other structural brain abnormalities, extra-CNS manifestations, epilepsy, motor, visual or hearing impairment, and other congenital abnormalities.

69. **Fig. 41:** Discontinuous pattern/moderately abnormal background
    (Minimum amplitude/lower margin <5 microvolt and maximum amplitude/upper margin >10 microvolt)
    Fig. 42: Burst suppression pattern
    (Lower margin <5 and upper margin <10 and bursts with amplitude >25 microvolt)
    Fig. 43: Isoelectric trace/primarily inactive background
    (Minimum amplitude/lower margin <5 microvolt and maximum amplitude/upper margin <5 microvolt)
    Fig. 44: Seizures
    (Abrupt rise in the minimum amplitude and simultaneous rise in the maximum amplitude/sawtooth pattern; Raw EEG is a must to correlate findings)

70.
a. *Fetal ventriculomegaly:* Lateral ventricular width ≥10 mm on fetal ultrasonography.
b. Grading of severity:
  - *Mild:* 10-12 mm
  - *Moderate:* 13-15 mm
  - *Severe:* >15 mm

  This is a case of severe fetal ventriculomegaly.
c. *Prenatal evaluation:*
  - Comprehensive sonographic evaluation for complete search for associated CNS and non-CNS anomalies.
  - Fetal MRI, fetal echocardiography
  - Serological tests for TORCH infections
  - Amniocentesis—Karyotype or CMA/CMV and Toxoplasmosis PCR. For known syndromic forms of primary congenital hydrocephalus, targeted gene testing can be done. For unknown syndromic or nonsyndromic forms, SNP array and *L1CAM* gene mutation evaluation is suggested.
d. *Prognosis and counseling:* In mild isolated ventriculomegaly ≤12 mm size, the outcome is usually good. The risk for abnormal outcome increases when there are associated anomalies, the atrial width is >12 mm, or there is a progressive increase of the lateral ventricular width. The outcome of severe ventriculomegaly depends mainly on the presence of associated pathologies. When associated pathologies are diagnosed, the prognosis is usually poor unless the cause is intraventricular hemorrhage. Ventricular size does not seem to correlate with outcome and caution should be used in prognosticating outcome in isolated ventriculomegaly. Even when isolated, the risk of perinatal death or severe neurologic sequelae is in the range of 50% in survivors.
e. *Three most common causes of congenital hydrocephalus:* Aqueductal stenosis, myelomeningocele with Chiari type II malformation, Dandy-Walker malformation.
f. We would do postnatal MRI brain for detailed evaluation.
g. Ventriculoperitoneal shunt would be the mainstay of treatment in this baby.

Page numbers followed by *b* refer to box, *f* refer to figure, and *t* refer to table.